THE NutriBase

SODIUM
CALORIES & FAT
IN YOUR FOOD

DR. ART ULENE

Avery Publishing Group
Garden City Park, New York

.The information in this book is based upon the latest data made available by government agencies, food manufacturers, and trade associations. It is important to note that all nutrient breakdowns for processed foods are subject to change by manufacturers without notice and may therefore vary from printing to printing.

ISBN 0-89529-651-9

Copyright © 1995 by Cybersoft Corporation

Printed in the United States of America

10   9   8   7   6   5   4   3   2   1

Contents

INTRODUCTION

We have long known the important role that good nutrition plays in our attempts to achieve good health. But only in recent years have we really begun to appreciate the critical role played by individual nutrients such as sodium and fat. These two nutrients have come under special scrutiny, in part because—in proper amounts—they are essential for health, and in part because—when consumed in excess—they can cause disease.

Excessive sodium intake can cause hypertension (high blood pressure), and can aggravate many medical disorders, including congestive heart failure, certain forms of kidney disease, and premenstrual syndrome (PMS). Excessive fat intake contributes to the development of atherosclerosis (hardening of the arteries), coronary heart disease, stroke, obesity, and hypertension.

Some people are more susceptible than others to the problems that excessive fat and sodium can cause. Approximately 30 percent of Americans are "sodium-sensitive," which means that they are less able to eliminate excess dietary sodium from their body, and therefore more likely to develop problems like hypertension if they consume too much sodium. People who are not sodium-sensitive have a much lower risk of developing these problems. But because there are no simple, inexpensive tests for determining which you group fall into, the National Research Council recommends that we *all* limit our sodium intake to 2,400 milligrams per day—the equivalent of about one teaspoon of salt. This allows us to easily meet the minimum amount needed for good health (about 500 milligrams per day), but is far below what many Americans now consume (up to 7,000 milligrams per day).

A similar situation exists regarding fat. Some people inherit a tendency toward high blood cholesterol, so that excessive fat consumption can raise their blood cholesterol levels dramatically. Others are born with a different tendency: No matter how much fat they eat, their cholesterol levels stay in the healthy range—although they may gain excess weight because of the calories in the fat. People who are extremely active and those with a "rapid" metabolism can tolerate a higher intake of fat calories without gaining weight. That's because they burn more calories every day than do those who are sedentary or have a slower metabolism. It's a little easier to tell which group you fall into with respect to fat, but still not a simple or inexpensive task. That's why the American Heart Association has recommended that we *all* limit our fat consumption to the point where 30 percent or less of our total calories each day come from fat. Others—including myself—believe that it is even healthier to limit fat to 20 percent of total calories.

Even if you do not have hypertension, high cholesterol levels, heart disease, or any of the other conditions mentioned above, you can probably benefit from carefully watching your intake of sodium and fat. Talk to your family doctor about these issues to determine how much of each you should consume. Then use this book to help yourself stick to your budget.

This book is designed to provide you with the information you need to make wiser choices when you buy food and when you dine out. Use this book to learn more about the foods you should consume—or avoid—so that you can meet your particular nutritional requirements. Don't be intimidated by the huge number of foods listed, or by the impossible-to-memorize nutritional values that accompany the list. It is not necessary to memorize these numbers. Instead, just try to familiarize yourself with the foods and food categories that are best suited to your needs. Begin by looking up the foods that you eat most often or in the largest quantities. If these foods are not providing you with the amounts of salt and fat that are appropriate for you, use the book to find better alternatives that are just as tasty. Once you are familiar with the salt and fat contents of your most common food choices, gradually look up the remainder of the foods in your diet. You'll be surprised by how easy it is to learn about these foods and to make any necessary changes.

The following section will explain some of the basics about sodium and fat. After that, you will learn to use this book to locate the information you need to improve your diet.

UNDERSTANDING SODIUM

To most people, *sodium* is just another name for *salt*. Yet the two terms are not synonymous. Sodium is a mineral; its scientific abbreviation is *Na*. Salt is a combination of the two minerals sodium and chloride (*Cl*). This combination—commonly referred to as *NaCl*, or sodium chloride—is easily recognizable in its crystalline form. Almost any adult can guess its identity after seeing and tasting the characteristic white crystals. But much of the sodium we eat is not so easily identified. It exists not in the form of crystals, but naturally, as a part of the food itself. For example, a half cup of cooked lima beans contains about 19 milligrams of sodium, and one stalk of celery contains about 70 milligrams.

And because salt is both a preservative and a flavor enhancer, most processed foods, from canned soups to soft drinks, are high in sodium. This sodium is very well hidden in processed foods. It has not been hidden deliberately, though. It has simply dissolved and lost its crystalline form, so that it is no longer apparent to the eye.

Aside from buying and using processed foods, most of us create a sodium problem for ourselves by adding salt to our foods. Without even thinking, we add too much salt to our cooking. And, often without first tasting our food, we add salt at the table. As unimportant as these small additions may seem, they can add up to substantial amounts by the end of each day—amounts large enough to adversely affect our health.

While some sodium is essential for survival, inadequate sodium intake is a rare problem. We need less than 500 milligrams of sodium a day to stay healthy. This is enough to accomplish the vital functions that sodium performs in the body—helping maintain normal fluid levels, healthy muscle function, and proper acidity (pH) of the blood. A quick glance through some randomly selected pages of this book will show you how easy it is to reach the 500-milligram level. Better yet, read the nutrition labels on some of the foods in your refrigerator and pantry. You'll be surprised by the amount of salt found in the foods you are eating now, and by your typical daily intake.

When reducing your intake of sodium, it is important to be aware of two hidden sources of this mineral. One source includes a number of food ingredients and additives other than salt itself. For instance, both baking powder and baking soda contain sodium, as do the flavor enhancer monosodium glutamate (MSG) and the preservative sodium benzoate. In general, by looking for the word *sodium* among ingredients listings, you should be able to identify most sodium sources.

Medications—including over-the-counter cough, antacid, and pain relief preparations—constitute the second hidden source of sodium. Again, any ingredient that contains the word *sodium*—for example, sodium salicylate—should alert you to a possible problem.

This book will help you identify the high-sodium foods in your diet, and will guide you in selecting foods that will contribute to good health. The following guidelines should also help you lower your sodium intake:

■ Do not add salt while cooking. Instead, add it at the table, and do so only sparingly. This will decrease the amount that ends up in your food.

■ To prevent low-salt foods from tasting flat, add a little lemon juice or vinegar. These ingredients give the impression of saltiness.

■ When decreasing the amount of salt, increase the herbs and spices for added flavor. For instance, the pungency of pepper reduces the need for salt.

■ Avoid very salty foods, like salted nuts, potato chips, and corn chips; olives;

pickles; soy sauce; and canned foods. Because of the country's new health consciousness, low- and no-salt versions of many of these foods are now available. Keep your eye out for them when doing your food shopping.

UNDERSTANDING FATS

Recently, much attention has been focused on the need to reduce dietary fat. Nevertheless, the body does need fats—but only the right fats, and only in the appropriate quantities. Fats are essential for growth and development, and for the maintenance of healthy skin, hair, and nails. And, as one of the four nutrients, fat provides the body with the energy it needs to carry on all functions. Most of us know, though, that there are several kinds of dietary fat, and that some fats are more likely than others to contribute to hypertension and coronary heart disease. A basic understanding of the different types of fat is important for anyone who wants to maximize health through wise dietary choices.

Fats have been classified into three major categories—saturated fats, polyunsaturated fats, and monounsaturated fats. This classification is based on the number of hydrogen atoms each has in its chemical structure.

Saturated fats, which are usually solid at room temperature, are found primarily in animal products, including fatty meats like beef, veal, lamb, pork, and ham; and in dairy items, such as whole milk, cream, ice cream, and cheese. For example, the marbleized fat you can see in beef is saturated. Some types of vegetable products—including coconut oil, palm kernel oil, and vegetable shortening—are also high in saturates.

The liver uses saturated fats to manufacture cholesterol. Therefore, excessive dietary intake of saturated fats can significantly raise the blood cholesterol level, especially in people who have inherited a tendency toward high blood cholesterol. Guidelines issued by the National Cholesterol Education Program (NCEP), and widely supported by most experts, recommend that your intake of saturated fats should be kept below 10 percent of your total calorie intake. However, for people who have severe problems with high blood cholesterol, even that level may be too high.

Polyunsaturated fats are found in greatest abundance in corn, soybean, safflower, and sunflower oils. Certain fish oils, particularly the omega-3 fatty acids, are also high in polyunsaturates. Unlike the saturated fats, polyunsaturates may actually lower your total blood cholesterol level. In doing so, however, large amounts of polyunsaturates also have a tendency to reduce your HDLS—the "good" cholesterol that helps lower blood cholesterol levels. For this reason—and because, like all fats, polyunsaturates are high in calories for their weight and volume—the NCEP guidelines state that your intake of polyunsaturated fats should not exceed 10 percent of your total calorie intake.

Monounsaturated fats are found mostly in vegetable and nut oils such as olive, peanut, and canola. These fats appear to reduce blood levels of LDL cholesterol—the "bad" cholesterol that contributes to coronary heart disease—without affecting HDLs in any way. However, this positive impact upon LDL cholesterol is relatively modest. The NCEP guidelines recommend that your intake of monounsaturated fats be kept between 10 and 15 percent of your total calorie intake.

Although most foods—including some plant-derived foods—contain a combination of all three types of fats, one of the types usually predominates. Thus, a food is considered "saturated" or "high in saturates" when it is composed primarily of saturated fatty acids. Similarly, a food composed mostly of polyunsaturated fatty acids is called "polyunsaturated," while a food composed mostly of monounsaturated fatty acids is called "monounsaturated."

One other element, trans-fatty acids, might also play a role in blood cholesterol levels. Trans-fatty acids occur when polyunsaturated oils are altered through hydrogenation, a process used to harden liquid vegetable oils into solid foods like margarine and shortening. One recent study found that trans-monounsaturated fatty acids raise LDL cholesterol levels, behaving much like saturated fats. Simultaneously, these trans-fatty acids reduced HDL cholesterol readings. Much more research is necessary, since some studies have not produced clear-cut conclusions about these substances. But your dietary choices could become less matter-of-fact than they now appear. For now, however, it is clear that when your goal is to lower cholesterol, polyunsaturated and monounsaturated fats are much more desirable than saturated fats.

A final point about fat deserves mention. While most people should limit fat intake, children under the age of two should not have their fat intake restricted. At that age, the growing brain requires proportionately larger amounts of fat than is required in the adult years. Fat restriction before the age of two can result in abnormal brain development with serious consequences. You should consult with your child's pediatrician or with your family doctor before making any significant change in your child's diet—no matter how old your child is.

UNDERSTANDING CALORIES

When we talk about foods, we often mention the number of calories a certain food has. Yet calories are not nutrients, like carbohydrates and fat. What, then, are calories?

A calorie is an energy unit. As already mentioned, fats—as well as carbohydrates and protein—provide the body with the energy it needs to function. This energy is measured in calories. There are 4 calories in every gram of protein, 4 calories in every gram of carbohydrate, and 9 calories in every gram of fat. So on a gram-forgram basis, fat is more than twice as fattening as carbohydrates or protein. It is no wonder, then, that when people try to lose weight, it is important that they cut down on fatty foods.

In addition to fat's having more calories than protein or carbohydrates, fat is metabolized differently by the body. Therefore, the excess fat in your diet is more likely to be stored as fat in your body than is excess carbohydrate or protein. That's because dietary fat is similar in chemical composition to body fat, so it takes less energy to convert it to body fat. In fact, it takes only 3 percent of the calories in the fat you eat to turn that food into body fat, while it takes at least 25 percent of the carbohydrate and protein calories you eat to convert them into body fat.

THE FOOD GUIDE PYRAMID

Over the years, the United States Department of Agriculture (USDA) has tried to insure adequate nutrition by encouraging Americans to eat a "well-balanced diet"—a concept that has changed dramatically over the years. Most of us still remember the four food groups that the USDA once promoted. These food groups—fruits and vegetables; breads and cereals; meat, poultry, fish, and eggs; and dairy products—were developed to encourage a balanced diet that was rich in meat, poultry, and dairy products. Clearly, we now have a greater understanding of how such a diet affects our health, and the government now recommends a diet high in complex carbohydrates and low in fat. With this in mind, in May 1992, the government abandoned the four food groups in favor of the Food Guide Pyramid, which has dramatically changed the recommended amounts of foods in each group.

At the base of the Food Guide Pyramid is the bread, cereal, rice, and pasta group. Six to eleven servings from this group are recommended daily—more servings than from any other food group. The next level of the pyramid is occupied by the vegetable group, with three to five servings recommended daily, and the fruit group, with two to four servings recommended daily. Moving upward, the next pyramid level is shared by the milk, yogurt, and cheese group, and the meat, poultry, fish, dry beans, eggs, and nuts group, with two to three servings recommended daily from each group. Finally, at the peak of the pyramid—and occupying the smallest area—are fats, oils, and sweets, a group of foods that is to be eaten only sparingly.

Government health officials recommend that no more than 30 percent of your calories come from fat. Others, myself included, believe that levels of 20 percent would be even healthier. In contrast, it is recommended that about 60 percent of your calories come from complex carbodrates—those foods found in the two largest levels of the pyramid.

GUIDELINES FOR HEALTHY EATING

The remainder of this book will help you choose foods that are low in health-compromising sodium and fat. But, as the Food Guide Pyramid illustrates, to maximize your health, you must eat adequate servings from each of the pyramid's first three levels. The following guidelines should help:

■ When eating foods from the bread, cereal, rice, and pasta group, always choose whole-grain, high-fiber, low-fat breads and cereals—preferably without added sugar, coloring, or unnecessary preservatives. Choose brown rice over white rice, and whole-wheat or other whole-grain pastas over pastas made from white flour.

■ When eating fruits and vegetables, eat fresh raw produce as often as possible. Water-soluble vitamins, such as vitamin C, may leach out of foods during cooking, be damaged by overprocessing, or be destroyed when foods are overcooked. Even fat-soluble vitamins, which are fairly stable during low-temperature cooking, can be affected by frying. For this reason, it is best to steam or microwave vegetables rather than boiling or frying them. Unless the produce was grown organically, be sure to peel or thoroughly wash it to eliminate pesticide residues and waxes. Avoid canned produce, as large amounts of sodium may be added during processing.

■ When choosing foods from the milk, yogurt, and cheese group, select low-fat and nonfat brands, which provide the most nutrients and the least amount of fat. When possible, choose low-salt cheeses, and avoid processed cheeses like American cheese, as these are higher in sodium than are natural cheeses. When eating meat, poultry, and fish, choose the leanest cuts available, trim off any excess fat, and bake or broil the foods instead of frying them. Keep in mind that cured meats, such as sausages and luncheon meats, are far higher in sodium than are fresh meats.

■ Select as few foods as possible from the fats, oils, and sweets group. When you do use fats and oils, though, choose monounsaturated and polyunsaturated fats instead of saturated fats. Limit your intake of sweets, choosing fresh fruits instead of cakes, cookies, and other high-fat desserts.

THE NEW FOOD LABELING

For many years, consumers complained about the confusing nature of food labels. For instance, the word "light" might mean light in calories when used by one manufacturer, and light in taste or color when used by another. Serving sizes, too, varied greatly, making it nearly impossible to compare the nutrient values of one product with those of another.

Because of this confusion, as of 1994, new food labels were required on all processed foods regulated by the Food and Drug Administration (FDA) and on all processed meat products regulated by the U.S. Department of Agriculture (USDA). Let's take a look at the most significant features of the new food label.

Nutrition Facts

One of the new label's features is a revamped nutrition panel, identified by its "Nutrition Facts" heading. The new nutrition panel features more consistent serving sizes, in both household and metric measures, and states how many servings are found in each container. In addition, the panel lists the following dietary components:

- Total calories
- Calories from fat
- Total fat
- Saturated fat
- Cholesterol

- Sodium
- Total carbohydrates
- Dietary fiber
- Sugars
- Protein

- Vitamin A
- Vitamin C
- Calcium
- Iron

For the last four nutrients listed above—vitamin A, vitamin C, calcium, and iron—the amount is expressed only as a percentage of its Daily Value, a recommended daily amount based on a 2,000-calorie diet. For most of the other nutrients listed, the amount is expressed both in grams or milligrams and as a percentage of its Daily Value. To educate the consumer, reference values are provided at the bottom of the label to show how much total fat, saturated fat, cholesterol, sodium, total carbohydrates, and dietary fiber should be included in both a 2,000-calorie and a 2,500-calorie diet.

Nutrient Content Descriptions

On the new food label, terms once used inconsistently, and often misleadingly, now must be applied uniformly to insure that such terms mean the same on each product on which they appear. Following are definitions of some of the most frequently used terms.

■ **Free.** The product contains no amount of, or only "physiologically inconsequential" amounts of one or more of these components: fat, saturated fat, cholesterol, sodium, sugars, and calories. For instance, "calorie free" means that there are fewer than 5 calories per serving, and "sugar free" and "fat free" indicate that there is less than 0.5 gram per serving.

■ **Low.** This food could be eaten frequently without exceeding dietary guidelines for one or more of the following components: fat, saturated fat, cholesterol, sodium, and calories. Thus, the following terms are used:

Low fat. 3 grams or less per serving.

Low saturated fat. 1 gram or less per serving.

Low sodium. Less than 140 milligrams per serving.

Very low sodium. Less than 35 milligrams per serving.

Low cholesterol. Less than 20 milligrams per serving.

Low calorie. 40 calories or less per serving.

■ **Lean and extra lean.** The following terms can be used to describe the fat content of meat, poultry, seafood, and game meats:

Lean. Less than 10 grams of fat, less than 4 grams of saturated fat, and less than 95 milligrams of cholesterol per serving and per 100 grams.

Extra lean. Less than 5 grams of fat, less than 2 grams of saturated fat, and less than 95 milligrams of cholesterol per serving and per 100 grams.

■ **High.** One serving of the food contains 20 percent or more of the Daily Value for a particular nutrient.

■ **Good source.** One serving of the food contains 10 to 19 percent of the Daily Value for a particular nutrient.

■ **Reduced.** A nutritionally altered product contains 25 percent less of a nutrient or of calories than the regular, or reference, product.

■ **Less.** A food, whether altered or not, contains 25 percent less of a nutrient or of calories than the reference food.

■ **Light.** A nutritionally altered product contains one-third fewer calories or half of the fat of the reference food, or the sodium content of a low-calorie, low-fat food has been reduced by 50 percent.

■ **More.** One serving of the food, altered or not, contains a nutrient in a quantity that is at least 10 percent of the Daily Value more than the reference food.

The following section should provide you with the details you need to better access and understand the data contained in this volume. I hope this book inspires you to learn more about your unique nutritional needs and the foods you are using to meet those needs. You will enjoy the sense of control this knowledge gives you. More important, you will make better food choices and take a major step toward better health. I wish you good health always.

Arthur Ulene, MD

HOW TO USE THIS BOOK

This book was designed to provide nutritional information on a wide range of foods, both generic and brand name, raw and prepared. The information provided here was gleaned from a number of government agencies, from hundreds of manufacturers, and from food trade associations. This information was compiled and later supplemented through countless hours of follow-up that involved hundreds of additional sources. Because scientific techniques are constantly being improved and nutritional theory continues to advance, this book will be continuously updated to reflect the most current nutritional data available.

FINDING THE LISTING YOU WANT

This easy-to-use guide is divided into two parts. Part One is an A-to-Z reference to the calorie, sodium, and fat contents of a wide variety of foods. Part Two is an A-to-Z reference to the calorie, sodium, and fat contents of restaurant-chain foods. In this section, foods are listed alphabetically under the name of the appropirate restaurant.

All of the foods in this reference have been listed alphabetically. For instance, if you were looking for the nutrient values of ground beef, you would turn to the *B's* and look under *Beef.* For convenience, similar foods have been grouped together in categories such as *Baby Foods, Breads, Candies, Cereals, Cheese, Cookies, Pasta,* and *Sauces.* Therefore, if the food you are looking for is not listed individually by its own name, you should try looking it up under a logical category.

Some foods are known by two or more names. In most cases, the food is listed under just one name, and cross-references have been provided to guide you to the proper listing. For instance, garbanzo beans are also called chick peas and ceci beans. In this book, you will find the nutrient information under *Garbanzo beans,* with cross-references under *Ceci beans* and *Chick peas.*

If you are unable to find a particular food, look for the listing of a similar food. The nutritional data should be close, if not exact, for any product not listed. When doing this, make sure you are comparing weight measure against weight measure and volume measure against volume measure.

After you locate the listing of the food you are interested in, you may find that abbreviations have been used to provide you with the information you need. Refer to page xvi for a complete key to the abbreviations used throughout this book.

UNDERSTANDING FISH, MEAT, AND VEGETABLE LISTINGS

When examining the nutrient values of *cooked* fish, meat, poultry, and vegetables, keep in mind that unless otherwise noted, no additional ingredients have been added. Also be aware that unless otherwise noted, the food values for fish, meats, and poultry are for meat only, and do not include skin or bones.

We hope that you will find *The Nutribase Guide to Sodium, Calories, & Fat in Your Food* a valuable companion that provides the information you need to take control of your eating habits. Should you have any comments about this book, feel free to write to the following address: Nutribase Comments, c/o Avery Publishing Group, 120 Old Broadway, Garden City Park, NY 11040.

Codes and Abbreviations

>	greater than		na	not available
<	less than		oz	ounce
%	percentage		pkg	package
approx	approximately		prep	prepared according to directions
cal	calories			
diam	diameter		sod	sodium
fl	fluid		tbsp	tablespoon
gm	gram		tr	trace
lb	pound		(tr)	may contain a trace amount
mcg	microgram(s)		tsp	teaspoon
med	medium-sized		w/	with
mgs	milligrams		w/o	without
(mq)	may contain a measurable quantity		wt	weight

A

Food Name	Serv. Size	Total Cal.	Sod. MGS	Fat GMS
ABALONE, MIXED SPECIES, raw	3 oz	89	256	0.7
ABALONE MUSHROOM. See MUSHROOM, OYSTER.				
ACEROLA CHERRY/Barbados cherry				
trimmed	1 cup	31	7	0.3
trimmed	1 oz	9	2	0.1
trimmed	1 fruit	2	0	0.0
untrimmed	1 lb	114	26	1.1
ACEROLA CHERRY JUICE/Barbados cherry juice				
	1 cup	51	7	0.7
	1 oz	6	1	0.1
ACORN FLOUR, full fat	1 oz	142	0	8.6
ACORN SQUASH. See SQUASH, ACORN.				
ADZUKI BEAN				
boiled, mature seeds	1/2 cup	147	9	0.1
raw	1 oz	93	1	0.2
raw (Arrowhead Mills)	2 oz	190	3	1.0
raw, mature seeds	1/2 cup	322	5	0.5
yokan, mature seeds, 1/4-inch slice	1 slice	36	12	0.0
ADZUKI BEAN, CANNED				
mature seeds, sweetened	1/2 cup	351	323	0.0
organic, no salt added (Eden Foods)	1/2 cup	80	10	<1.0
organic, w/liquid (Eden Foods)	1/2 cup	100	20	<1.0
AGAR				
dried	100 gm	306	102	0.3
raw	1 lb	116	40	0.1
raw	100 gm	26	9	0.0
raw	1 oz	7	3	tr
AHI. See TUNA, YELLOWFIN.				
AKU. See TUNA, SKIPJACK.				
ALBACORE. See TUNA, CANNED; TUNA, FROZEN.				
ALCOHOL-FREE BEVERAGES				
BEER				
(Cutter)	12 oz	76	<1	0.0
(Kaliber)	12 oz	71	3	0.0
(Sharp's)	12 oz	86	5	0.0
MIXED-DRINK MIXERS				
Banana Daiquiri, frozen, diluted w/water (Bacardi)	7 oz	150	0	1.0
Bloody Mary				
bottled (Mr. & Mrs. T)	4.5 oz	20	670	0.0
bottled, rich & spicy (Mr. & Mrs. T)	4.5 oz	30	500	0.0
bottled 'Smooth N' Spicy' (Holland House)	1 oz	3	329	0.0

Food Name	Serv. Size	Total Cal.	Sod. MGS	Fat GMS
Daiquiri				
bottled *(Holland House)*	1 oz	36	111	0.0
instant, dry *(Holland House)*	.56 oz	65	21	0.0
Grenadine				
syrup *(Roses)*	1 oz	65	27	0.0
syrup *(Roses)*	.5 oz	32	14	<1.0
Lime Daiquiri, shelf stable, w/water *(Bacardi)*	7 oz	130	10	0.0
Mai Tai				
bottled *(Holland House)*	1 oz	32	60	0.0
instant, dry *(Holland House)*	.56 oz	64	4	0.0
Manhattan, bottled *(Holland House)*	1 oz	28	5	0.0
Margarita				
bottled *(Holland House)*	1 oz	27	92	0.0
bottled *(Mr. & Mrs. T)*	3 oz	80	35	<1.0
frozen, diluted w/water *(Bacardi)*	7 oz	90	0	0.0
instant, dry *(Holland House)*	.5 oz	57	4	0.0
shelf stable, w/water *(Bacardi)*	7 oz	130	10	0.0
Old Fashioned, bottled *(Holland House)*	1 oz	33	6	0.0
Peach Daiquiri, frozen, diluted w/water *(Bacardi)*	7 oz	130	5	0.0
Piña Colada				
bottled *(Holland House)*	1 oz	33	4	0.0
bottled *(Mr. & Mrs. T)*	4 oz	150	120	<1.0
frozen, diluted w/water *(Bacardi)*	7 oz	200	25	6.0
instant, dry *(Holland House)*	.56 oz	82	<1	3.0
shelf stable, w/water *(Bacardi)*	7 oz	170	20	2.0
Raspberry Daiquiri, bottled *(Holland House)*	1 oz	30	4	0.0
Rum Runner, shelf stable, w/water *(Bacardi)*	7 oz	140	15	0.0
Strawberry Colada, shelf stable, w/water *(Bacardi)*	7 oz	150	15	1.0
Strawberry Daiquiri				
bottled *(Holland House)*	1 oz	31	3	0.0
frozen, diluted w/water *(Bacardi)*	7 oz	140	0	0.0
shelf stable, w/water *(Bacardi)*	7 oz	130	15	0.0
Strawberry Margarita				
bottled *(Holland House)*	1 oz	31	3	0.0
bottled *(Mr. & Mrs. T)*	3.5 oz	100	10	<1.0
instant, dry *(Holland House)*	.56 oz	66	<1	0.0
Sweet and Sour				
bottled *(Mr. & Mrs. T)*	3 oz	70	45	<1.0
liquid *(Holland House)*	1 oz	34	107	0.0
Tom Collins				
bottled *(Holland House)*	1 oz	47	96	0.0

Food Name	Serv. Size	Total Cal.	Sod. MGS	Fat GMS
instant, dry *(Holland House)*	.56 oz	65	14	0.0
Whiskey Sour				
bottled *(Holland House)*	1 oz	37	105	0.0
instant, dry *(Holland House)*	.56 oz	64	16	0.0

ALCOHOLIC BEVERAGES. See also ALCOHOL-FREE BEVERAGES.

BEER, ALE, and MALT LIQUOR

Food Name	Serv. Size	Total Cal.	Sod. MGS	Fat GMS
(Anheuser Marzen)	12 oz	168	12	0.0
(Beck's)	12 oz	148	14	0.0
(Budweiser)	12 oz	144	12	0.0
(Budweiser) 'Bud Light'	12 oz	110	12	0.0
(Busch)	12 oz	144	12	0.0
(Carlsberg)	12 oz	149	12	0.0
(Carlsberg) 'Light'	12 oz	110	12	0.0
(Coors)	12 oz	137	<1	0.0
(Coors) 'Dry'	12 oz	119	<1	0.0
(Coors) 'Dry' 3.2%	12 oz	101	<1	0.0
(Coors) 'Extra Gold'	12 oz	151	<1	0.0
(Coors) 'Extra Gold' 3.2%	12 oz	121	<1	0.0
(Coors) 'Light'	12 oz	103	<1	0.0
(Coors) 'Light' 3.2%	12 oz	98	<1	0.0
(Coors) 3.2%	12 oz	119	<1	0.0
(Coqui)	12 oz	208	13	0.0
(Dribeck's)	12 oz	94	14	0.0
(Elephant)	12 oz	208	12	0.0
(Keystone)	12 oz	121	<1	0.0
(Keystone) 'Dry'	12 oz	121	<1	0.0
(Keystone) 'Light'	12 oz	100	<1	0.0
(Keystone) 'Light' 3.2%	12 oz	99	<1	0.0
(Keystone) 3.2%	12 oz	104	<1	0.0
(Killian's)	12 oz	161	<1	0.0
(Killian's) 3.2%	12 oz	128	<1	0.0
(King Cobra)	12 oz	182	12	0.0
(Knickerbocker)	12 oz	140	9	0.0
(LA) light alcohol	12 oz	114	12	0.0
(Lite) 'Genuine Draft'	12 oz	98	6	0.0
(Lite) 'Lite'	12 oz	96	6	0.0
(Lowenbräu) 'Dark Special'	12 oz	158	7	0.0
(Lowenbräu) 'Special'	12 oz	158	7	0.0
(McSorley's)	12 oz	166	6	0.0
(Meister Brau)	12 oz	141	6	0.0
(Meister Brau) 'Light'	12 oz	98	6	0.0

Food Name	Serv. Size	Total Cal.	Sod. MGS	Fat GMS
(Michelob)	12 oz	156	12	0.0
(Michelob) 'Classic Dark'	12 oz	158	12	0.0
(Michelob) 'Dry'	12 oz	133	12	0.0
(Michelob) 'Light'	12 oz	134	12	0.0
(Miller) 'Genuine Draft'	12 oz	147	7	0.0
(Miller) 'High Life'	12 oz	147	7	0.0
(Miller) 'Magnum'	12 oz	162	8	0.0
(Milwaukee) 'Milwaukee's Best'	12 oz	133	6	0.0
(Milwaukee) 'Milwaukee's Best Light'	12 oz	98	6	0.0
(Natural Light)	12 oz	110	12	0.0
(Ortlieb's)	12 oz	140	9	0.0
(Prior) 'Double Dark'	12 oz	171	10	0.0
(Rheingold)	12 oz	148	9	0.0
(Rheingold) 'Light'	12 oz	96	7	0.0
(Rolling Rock) 'Light'	12 oz	104	<1	0.0
(Rolling Rock) 'Premium'	12 oz	145	<1	0.0
(Schmidt's)	12 oz	148	9	0.0
(Schmidt's) 'Classic'	12 oz	144	10	0.0
(Schmidt's) 'Light'	12 oz	96	7	0.0
(Tiger Head)	12 oz	166	6	0.0
(Zima)	12 oz	148	2	na
CHAMPAGNE				
brut *(Jacques Bonet)*	4 oz	92	4	0.0
brut *(Lejon)*	4 oz	92	4	0.0
extra dry *(Jacques Bonet)*	4 oz	97	4	0.0
extra dry *(Lejon)*	4 oz	97	4	0.0
pink *(Jacques Bonet)*	4 oz	98	4	0.0
pink *(Lejon)*	4 oz	98	4	0.0
LIQUOR AND LIQUEUR				
Bourbon				
80 proof, distilled	1 oz	65	tr	0.0
86 proof, distilled	1 oz	70	tr	0.0
90 proof, distilled	1 oz	74	tr	0.0
94 proof, distilled	1 oz	77	tr	0.0
100 proof, distilled	1 oz	83	tr	0.0
Brandy				
80 proof, distilled	1 oz	65	tr	0.0
86 proof, distilled	1 oz	70	tr	0.0
90 proof, distilled	1 oz	74	tr	0.0
94 proof, distilled	1 oz	77	tr	0.0
100 proof, distilled	1 oz	83	tr	0.0

Food Name	Serv. Size	Total Cal.	Sod. MGS	Fat GMS
Coffee Liqueur				
53 proof	1 oz	117	3	0.1
63 proof	1 oz	107	3	0.1
Creme de Menthe, 72 proof	1 oz	125	2	0.1
Gin				
80 proof, distilled	1 oz	64	0	0.0
86 proof, distilled	1 oz	69	0	0.0
90 proof, distilled	1 oz	73	0	0.0
94 proof, distilled	1 oz	76	0	0.0
100 proof, distilled	1 oz	82	0	0.0
Rum				
80 proof, distilled	1 oz	64	0	0.0
86 proof, distilled	1 oz	69	0	0.0
90 proof, distilled	1 oz	73	0	0.0
94 proof, distilled	1 oz	76	0	0.0
100 proof, distilled	1 oz	82	0	0.0
Rye Whiskey				•
80 proof, distilled	1 oz	65	tr	0.0
86 proof, distilled	1 oz	70	tr	0.0
90 proof, distilled	1 oz	74	tr	0.0
94 proof, distilled	1 oz	77	tr	0.0
100 proof, distilled	1 oz	83	tr	0.0
Scotch				
80 proof, distilled	1 oz	65	tr	0.0
86 proof, distilled	1 oz	70	tr	0.0
90 proof, distilled	1 oz	74	tr	0.0
94 proof, distilled	1 oz	77	tr	0.0
100 proof, distilled	1 oz	83	tr	0.0
Tequila				
80 proof, distilled	1 oz	65	tr	0.0
86 proof, distilled	1 oz	70	tr	0.0
90 proof, distilled	1 oz	74	tr	0.0
94 proof, distilled	1 oz	77	tr	0.0
100 proof, distilled	1 oz	83	tr	0.0
Vodka				
80 proof, distilled	1 oz	64	0	0.0
86 proof, distilled	1 oz	69	0	0.0
90 proof, distilled	1 oz	73	0	0.0
94 proof, distilled	1 oz	76	0	0.0
100 proof, distilled	1 oz	82	0	0.0

Food Name	Serv. Size	Total Cal.	Sod. MGS	Fat GMS
Whiskey				
80 proof, distilled	1 oz	64	0	0.0
86 proof, distilled	1 oz	69	0	0.0
90 proof, distilled	1 oz	73	0	0.0
94 proof, distilled	1 oz	76	0	0.0
100 proof, distilled	1 oz	82	0	0.0
MIXED DRINKS. See also ALCOHOL-FREE BEVERAGES, MIXED-DRINK MIXERS.				
Banana Daiquiri				
frozen, prepared w/1/2-can rum, diluted as directed				
(Bacardi)	7 oz	210	0	1.0
Bloody Mary, prepared from recipe	5 oz	115	332	0.2
Bourbon and Soda, prepared from recipe	4 oz	104	16	0.0
Daiquiri				
instant, prepared as directed (Bar-Tender's)	3.5 oz	177	50	0.0
prepared from recipe	1 oz	56	2	0.0
Gin and Tonic, prepared from recipe	1 oz	23	1	0.0
Lime Daiquiri, mix, shelf stable, prepared w/1/2-can rum				
(Bacardi)	7 oz	210	10	0.0
Manhattan, prepared from recipe	1 oz	64	1	0.0
Margarita				
frozen, prepared w/1/2-can rum, diluted as directed				
(Bacardi)	7 oz	160	5	0.0
shelf stable, prepared w/1/2-can rum (Bacardi)	7 oz	210	10	0.0
Martini, prepared from recipe	1 oz	63	1	0.0
Peach Daiquiri				
frozen, prepared w/1/2-can rum, diluted as directed				
(Bacardi)	7 oz	200	5	0.0
Piña Colada				
frozen, prepared w/1/2-can rum, diluted as directed				
(Bacardi)	7 oz	260	25	6.0
mix, shelf stable, prepared w/1/2-can rum (Bacardi)	7 oz	240	20	2.0
prepared from recipe	1 oz	58	2	0.6
Rum Runner, shelf stable, prepared w/1/2-can rum				
(Bacardi)	7 oz	210	15	0.0
Screwdriver, prepared from recipe	1 oz	25	0	0.0
Strawberry Colada				
mix, shelf stable, prepared w/1/2-can rum (Bacardi)	7 oz	230	15	1.0
Strawberry Daiquiri				
frozen, prepared w/1/2-can rum, diluted as directed				
(Bacardi)	7 oz	200	0	0.0
mix, shelf stable, prepared w/1/2-can rum (Bacardi)	7 oz	200	15	0.0

Food Name	Serv. Size	Total Cal.	Sod. MGS	Fat GMS
Tequila Sunrise, prepared from recipe	1 oz	34	1	0.0
Tom Collins, prepared from recipe	1 oz	16	5	0.0
Whiskey Sour				
mix, powder, instant, prepared w/whiskey (Bar-Tender's)	3.5 oz	177	50	0.0
prepared from recipe	1 oz	41	3	0.0
WINE. See also WINE, COOKING.				
'Arriba' (Mission Bell)	2 oz	95	4	0.0
'Diamond Red' (Mission Bell)	2 oz	95	4	0.0
'Silver Satin' (Mission Bell)	2 oz	83	4	0.0
'Silver Satin Bitter Lemon' (Mission Bell)	2 oz	83	4	0.0
'Swiss Up' (Mission Bell)	2 oz	84	4	0.0
Barbera, white (Colony)	4 oz	91	4	0.0
Burgundy				
(Bravo)	4 oz	91	4	0.0
(Carlo Rossi)	4 oz	92	na	0.0
(Colony) 'Classic'	4 oz	90	4	0.0
(Gallo)	4 oz	88	na	0.0
(Gallo) 'Hearty'	4 oz	92	na	0.0
(Gambarelli & Davitto) 'Parma'	4 oz	91	4	0.0
(Petri)	4 oz	91	4	0.0
Cabernet Sauvignon				
(Colony)	4 oz	88	4	0.0
(Gallo)	4 oz	88	na	0.0
Carbonated				
(Carlo Rossi) 'Paisano'	4 oz	92	na	0.0
(Jacques Bonet) almond	4 oz	104	4	0.0
(Jacques Bonet) apricot	4 oz	111	4	0.0
(Jacques Bonet) cherry	4 oz	106	4	0.0
(Jacques Bonet) peach	4 oz	111	4	0.0
(Jacques Bonet) raspberry	4 oz	106	4	0.0
Chablis				
(Bravo)	4 oz	86	4	0.0
(Carlo Rossi)	4 oz	84	na	0.0
(Carlo Rossi) pink	4 oz	92	na	0.0
(Colony)	4 oz	98	4	0.0
(Colony) 'Classic'	4 oz	84	4	0.0
(Colony) emerald	4 oz	102	4	0.0
(Colony) gold	4 oz	97	4	0.0
(Colony) ruby	4 oz	104	4	0.0
(Gallo)	4 oz	80	na	0.0
(Gallo) 'Blanc'	4 oz	80	na	0.0

Food Name	Serv. Size	Total Cal.	Sod. MGS	Fat GMS
(Gambarelli & Davitto) 'Parma'	4 oz	86	4	0.0
(Petri)	4 oz	98	4	0.0
(Petri) 'Blanc'	4 oz	86	4	0.0
Chardonnay (Gallo)	4 oz	88	na	0.0
Chenin Blanc				
(Colony)	4 oz	86	4	0.0
(Gallo)	4 oz	88	na	0.0
Chianti				
(Carlo Rossi) 'Light'	4 oz	92	na	0.0
(Petri)	4 oz	91	4	0.0
Cold duck				
(Jacques Bonet)	4 oz	108	4	0.0
(Lejon)	4 oz	108	4	0.0
French colombard				
(Colony)	4 oz	84	4	0.0
(Gallo)	4 oz	88	na	0.0
Gewurztraminer (Gallo)	4 oz	88	na	0.0
Marsala (Gambarelli & Davitto)	4 oz	77	4	0.0
Moselle (Colony) 'Rhineskeller'	4 oz	97	4	0.0
Muscatel (Italian Swiss Colony)	2 oz	122	4	0.0
Pastoso (Petri)	4 oz	92	4	0.0
Port				
(Gallo)	2 oz	64	na	0.0
(Gallo) white	2 oz	86	na	0.0
(Italian Swiss Colony)	2 oz	85	4	0.0
(Italian Swiss Colony) white	2 oz	86	4	0.0
(Livingston Cellars) tawny	2 oz	86	na	0.0
Rhine				
(Bravo)	4 oz	97	4	0.0
(Carlo Rossi)	4 oz	84	na	0.0
(Colony) 'Classic'	4 oz	89	4	0.0
(Gallo)	4 oz	80	na	0.0
(Gambarelli & Davitto) 'Parma'	4 oz	92	4	0.0
(Petri)	4 oz	97	4	0.0
Reisling (Gallo) 'Johannisberg'	4 oz	84	na	0.0
Rosé				
(Bravo)	4 oz	92	4	0.0
(Carlo Rossi) 'Vin Rosé'	4 oz	88	na	0.0
(Colony) 'Classic'	4 oz	89	4	0.0
(Gallo) 'Grenache'	4 oz	88	na	0.0
(Gallo) 'Red Rosé'	4 oz	112	na	0.0

Food Name	Serv. Size	Total Cal.	Sod. MGS	Fat GMS
(Gallo) 'Vin Rosé'	4 oz	88	na	0.0
(Gambarelli & Davitto) 'Parma'	4 oz	92	4	0.0
(Petri)	4 oz	92	4	0.0
Sauvignon Blanc, *(Gallo)*	4 oz	80	na	0.0
Sherry				
(Gallo)	2 oz	64	na	0.0
(Italian Swiss Colony) cream	2 oz	85	4	0.0
(Italian Swiss Colony) dry	2 oz	63	4	0.0
(Livingston Cellars) cream	2 oz	78	na	0.0
(Livingston Cellars) 'Very Dry'	2 oz	60	na	0.0
Tokay *(Italian Swiss Colony)*	2 oz	82	4	0.0
Vermouth				
(Gallo) dry	2 oz	56	na	0.0
(Gallo) sweet	2 oz	90	na	0.0
(Gambarelli & Davitto) dry	2 oz	64	4	0.0
(Gambarelli & Davitto) sweet	2 oz	77	4	0.0
(Lejon) dry	2 oz	64	4	0.0
(Lejon) sweet	2 oz	77	4	0.0
Zinfandel				
(Colony)	4 oz	91	4	0.0
(Colony) white	4 oz	82	4	0.0
(Gallo)	4 oz	92	na	0.0
WINE COOLERS				
(Bartles & Jaymes) Berry Cooler 'Light'	12 oz	150	na	0.0
(Bartles & Jaymes) Black Cherry Cooler 'Light'	12 oz	139	na	0.0
(Bartles & Jaymes) Citrus Cooler 'Light'	6 oz	67	na	<1.0
(Bartles & Jaymes) Tropical Cooler 'Light'	12 oz	151	na	0.0
ALE. See ALCOHOLIC BEVERAGES.				
ALFALFA SEEDS				
(Arrowhead Mills)	1 cup	40	na	1.0
sprouted, raw	1 lb	132	29	3.1
sprouted, raw	1/2 cup	5	1	0.1
sprouted, raw	1 tbsp	1	0	0.0
sprouted, raw	1 oz	8	2	0.2
ALLSPICE				
ground	1 oz	75	22	2.5
ground	1 tbsp	16	5	0.5
ground	1 tsp	5	1	0.2
ground *(Durkee)*	1 tsp	7	0	tr
ground *(Laurel Leaf)*	1 tsp	7	0	tr
ground *(Spice Islands)*	1 tsp	6	1	0.1

Food Name	Serv. Size	Total Cal.	Sod. MGS	Fat GMS
ALMOND				
(Beer Nuts)	1 oz	180	51	14.4
(Dole)	1 oz	170	4	14.0
(Fisher)	1 oz	170	0	15.0
chopped	1 cup	766	14	67.9
in shell	1 lb	1069	19	94.7
sliced	1 cup	554	10	49.1
slivered, tightly packed	1 cup	795	15	70.5
whole kernels	1 cup	836	16	74.1
whole kernels, approx 24	1 oz	167	3	14.8
Blanched				
sliced	1 cup	615	11	55.2
whole kernels	1 cup	850	15	76.2
whole kernels	1 oz	166	3	14.9
Dry roasted				
(Planters)	1 oz	170	200	15.0
whole kernels	1 cup	810	15	71.2
whole kernels	1 oz	167	3	14.7
Honey roasted				
(Planters)	1 oz	170	180	13.0
whole kernels	1 cup	855	187	71.9
whole kernels	1 oz	168	37	14.1
Oil roasted				
whole kernels	1 cup	970	16	90.5
whole kernels, approx 22	1 oz	176	3	16.4
Oil roasted and blanched				
toasted	1 cup	870	17	80.3
toasted	1 oz	167	3	14.4
whole kernels, approx 24	1 oz	174	3	16.1
Raw				
blanched (Planters)	1 oz	170	0	15.0
sliced (Planters)	1 oz	170	0	15.0
slivered (Planters)	1 oz	170	0	15.0
whole (Planters)	1 oz	170	0	15.0
Toasted				
(Dole)	1 oz	170	4	14.0
unblanched	1 oz	167	3	14.4
ALMOND BUTTER				
Plain				
	1/2 cup	791	14	73.9
	1 oz	179	3	16.8

Food Name	Serv. Size	Total Cal.	Sod. MGS	Fat GMS
blanched, toasted *(Hain)*	2 tbsp	220	10	19.0
gourmet *(Roaster Fresh)*	1 oz	184	4	16.0
no salt, crunchy 'Natural' *(Westbrae)*	2 tbsp	190	0	17.0
no salt, smooth 'Natural' *(Westbrae)*	2 tbsp	190	0	17.0
raw 'Natural' *(Hain)*	2 tbsp	190	5	18.0
raw, organic *(Maranatha Natural)*	2 tbsp	190	5	15.0
roasted *(Maranatha Natural)*	2 tbsp	190	5	15.0
salted	1 cup	791	563	73.9
salted	1 oz	179	128	16.8
salted	1 tbsp	101	72	9.5
Honey and cinnamon				
	1/2 cup	753	14	65.3
	1 oz	171	3	14.8
salted	1/2 cup	753	213	65.3
salted	1 oz	171	48	14.8
ALMOND MEAL				
partially defatted	4 oz	463	8	20.8
partially defatted, salted	4 oz	463	846	20.8
ALMOND OIL				
	1/2 cup	964	0	109.0
	1 oz	251	0	28.4
	1 tbsp	120	0	13.6
(Hain)	1 tbsp	120	0	14.0
(Spectrum Naturals)	1 tbsp	120	0	14.0
ALMOND PASTE				
	4 oz	506	10	30.8
	1 oz	127	3	7.7
firmly packed	1 cup	1012	20	61.7
ALMOND POWDER				
full-fat	1 oz	168	2	14.7
full-fat, not packed	1 cup	385	4	33.6
partially defatted	1 oz	112	3	4.5
partially defatted, not packed	1 cup	255	7	10.4
ALOE VERA JUICE				
sodium free, certified 100% juice *(Sunburst)*	2 oz	5	<3	0.0
ALPINE SPICED CIDER *(Krusteaz)*	8 oz	80	20	0.0
AMARANTH				
boiled, drained	1/2 cup	14	14	0.1
raw	1 cup	7	6	0.1
AMARANTH DINNER, CANNED				
w/garden vegetables 'Fast Menu' fat-free *(Health Valley)*	7.5 oz	120	138	3.0

Food Name	Serv. Size	Total Cal.	Sod. MGS	Fat GMS
w/garden vegetables 'Fast Menu' fat-free *(Health Valley)* ..... 5 oz		70	90	0.0
AMARANTH FLOUR *(Arrowhead Mills)* .... 2 oz		200	<1	3.0
AMARANTH SEED *(Arrowhead Mills)* .... 2 oz		200	1	3.0
AMBERJACK				
raw .... 1 lb		386	(mq)	4.1
raw .... 1 oz		24	(mq)	0.3
AMBROSIA SALAD *(Sunfresh)* in light syrup .... 2/3 cup		70	30	0.0
AMBROSIA JUICE *(Knudsen & Sons)* .... 8 oz		110	na	0.0
ANASAZI BEAN raw *(Arrowhead Mills)* .... 2 oz		200	3	1.0
ANCHOVY, European, meat only, raw .... 1 oz		37	29	1.4
ANCHOVY, CANNED				
in olive oil; drained .... 1 oz		60	1040	2.8
in olive oil, drained, 5 medium .... .7 oz		42	734	1.9
in olive oil, drained, yield from 2-oz can .... 1.6 oz		94	1651	4.4
ANGLER FISH. See MONKFISH.				
ANISE SEED				
whole .... 1 oz		95	5	4.5
whole .... 1 tbsp		23	1	1.1
whole .... 1 tsp		7	0	0.3
APPLE				
boiled, peeled slices .... 1/2 cup		60	1	0.4
boiled, unpeeled slices .... 1/2 cup		46	1	0.3
microwaved, peeled slices .... 1/2 cup		64	1	0.5
microwaved, unpeeled slices .... 1/2 cup		48	1	0.4
raw, peeled .... 1 oz		16	tr	0.1
raw, peeled slices .... 1 cup		63	0	0.3
raw, peeled whole fruit, approx 3 per lb .... 1 med		73	0	0.4
raw, unpeeled .... 1 oz		17	tr	0.1
raw, unpeeled slices .... 1 cup		65	0	0.4
raw, unpeeled whole fruit, approx 3 per lb .... 1 med		81	0	0.5
raw, unpeeled whole fruit .... 1 lb		244	2	1.5
APPLE, CANNED				
Chipped				
(Lucky Leaf) .... 4 oz		50	10	0.0
(Musselman's) .... 4 oz		50	10	0.0
(White House) in water .... 4 oz		50	5	0.0
Diced				
(Lucky Leaf) .... 4 oz		50	10	0.0
(Musselman's) .... 4 oz		50	10	0.0
Rings, spiced				
(Lucky Leaf) green .... 4 oz		100	20	0.0

od Name	Serv. Size	Total Cal.	Sod. MGS	Fat GMS
(Lucky Leaf) red	4 oz	100	20	0.0
(Musselman's) green	4 oz	100	20	0.0
(Musselman's) red	4 oz	100	20	0.0
(White House)	3.5 oz	180	25	0.0
Sliced				
(Lucky Leaf) dessert	4 oz	70	25	0.0
(Lucky Leaf) sweetened, in syrup	4 oz	50	35	0.0
(Lucky Leaf) sweetened, in water	4 oz	50	10	0.0
(Lucky Leaf) sweetened, unpeeled	4 oz	90	15	0.0
(Musselman's) dessert	4 oz	70	25	0.0
(Musselman's) sweetened, in syrup	4 oz	50	35	0.0
(Musselman's) sweetened, in water	4 oz	50	10	0.0
(Musselman's) sweetened, unpeeled	4 oz	90	15	0.0
(White House) sweetened	4 oz	54	10	0.0
(White House) sweetened, in water	4 oz	40	5	0.0
Whole				
(Lucky Leaf) baked	1 apple	110	35	0.0
(Lucky Leaf) sweetened, peeled, cored	1 apple	90	10	0.0
(Musselman's) baked	1 apple	110	35	0.0
(Musselman's) sweetened, peeled, cored	1 apple	90	10	0.0
(White House) baked	3.5 oz	118	11	0.0
PPLE, DEHYDRATED/SULFURED				
chips *(Weight Watchers)*	.75 oz	70	200	0.0
cooked	4 oz	84	29	0.1
stewed, low moisture	1/2 cup	72	25	0.1
uncooked	4 oz	392	141	0.7
uncooked, low moisture	1/2 cup	104	37	0.2
PPLE, DRIED				
chunks *(Sun•Maid)*	2 oz	150	40	0.0
chunks *(SunSweet)*	2 oz	150	40	0.0
sliced, uncooked *(Del Monte)*	2 oz	140	50	0.0
sulfured, stewed	1/2 cup	73	26	0.1
sulfured, uncooked	4 oz	276	99	0.4
sulfured, uncooked	1 cup	209	75	0.3
sulfured, uncooked, approx 2.3 oz	10 rings	155	56	0.2
PPLE, FROZEN				
escalloped *(Stouffer's)*	4 oz	130	15	2.0
glazed, in raspberry sauce 'Side Dish' *(Budget Gourmet)*	5 oz	110	210	3.0
unsweetened	4 oz	54	3	0.4
unsweetened, heated	4 oz	53	3	0.4
unsweetened, heated, sliced	1/2 cup	48	3	0.3

Food Name	Serv. Size	Total Cal.	Sod. MGS	Fa GM
unsweetened, sliced	1/2 cup	41	3	0.5
APPLE APRICOT JUICE (Knudsen & Sons)	8 oz	120	na	0.0
APPLE BANANA JUICE (Knudsen & Sons)	8 oz	85	na	0.0
APPLE BLACKBERRY JUICE				
(Knudsen & Sons)	8 oz	100	na	0.0
(Santa Cruz Natural) organic	8 oz	120	na	1.0
APPLE BOYSENBERRY JUICE				
(Knudsen & Sons)	8 oz	110	na	0.0
(Santa Cruz Natural) organic	8 oz	120	na	1.0
APPLE BUTTER				
	1 cup	519	0	0.5
	1 tbsp	33	0	0.
APPLE CHERRY BERRY DRINK (Veryfine)	8 oz	130	25	0.0
APPLE CHERRY CIDER				
(Indian Summer)	6 oz	100	10	<1.0
(McCain) 100% juice 'Junior'	4.2 oz	50	5	0.0
(Musselman's) 'Breakfast Cocktail'	6 oz	100	5	0.0
(Red Cheek) 'Naturally 100%'	6 oz	113	11	0.0
APPLE CIDER				
(Indian Summer) can or bottle	6 oz	80	10	<1.0
(Indian Summer) can or bottle, cinnamon	6 oz	90	10	<1.
(Lucky Leaf) can or bottle	6 oz	90	0	0.
(Lucky Leaf) can or bottle, sparkling	6 oz	80	45	0.0
(Musselman's) can or bottle	6 oz	90	0	0.0
(S. Martinelli) 'Sparkling'	6 oz	100	5	0.0
(Tree Top) canned or frozen, diluted as directed	6 oz	90	10	0.0
APPLE CIDER MIX (Swiss Miss)	.776 oz	84	58	0.
APPLE CITRUS JUICE (Tree Top) canned or frozen	6 oz	90	10	0.
APPLE CRANBERRY CIDER (Indian Summer)	6 oz	100	10	<1.0
APPLE CRANBERRY DRINK				
(Mott's)	10 oz	176	3	0.0
(Mott's)	9.5 oz	167	3	0.
(Tropicana)	6 oz	110	15	<1.0
(Tropicana) 'Single Serve'	10 oz	175	3	0.0
APPLE CRANBERRY JUICE				
(Apple & Eve)	6 oz	80	5	0.
(Knudsen & Sons)	8 oz	110	na	0.
(Lucky Leaf)	6 oz	130	10	0.
(Mott's)	9.5 oz	147	27	0.
(Mott's)	6 oz	83	17	0.
(Mott's) aseptic box	8.45 oz	136	24	0.

Food Name	Serv. Size	Total Cal.	Sod. MGS	Fat GMS
(Santa Cruz Natural) organic	8 oz	115	na	<1.0
(Smucker's) 'Naturally 100%'	8 oz	120	10	0.0
(Tree Top) canned	6 oz	100	10	0.0
(Tree Top) frozen	6 oz	100	10	0.0
(Veryfine) cocktail	8 oz	130	10	0.0
APPLE DRINK				
(Hi-C) 'Candy Apple Cooler'	8.45 oz	132	25	<.1
(Hi-C) 'Candy Apple Cooler'	6 oz	94	17	<.1
(Hi-C) 'Jamin' Apple Drink,' aseptic box	6 oz	90	20	<.1
(10-K)	8 oz	60	55	0.0
APPLE DUMPLING, frozen *(Pepperidge Farm)*	3 oz	260	230	13.0
APPLE GRAPE CHERRY JUICE				
(Welch's) 'Orchard Cocktail'	6 oz	110	20	0.0
(Welch's) 'Orchard Cocktail-in-a-Box'	8.45 oz	150	20	0.0
(Welch's) 'Orchard Cocktail' frozen	6 oz	90	10	0.0
APPLE GRAPE JUICE				
(Juicy Juice)	6 oz	90	10	0.0
(Juicy Juice) box	8.45 oz	120	10	0.0
(Mott's)	9.5 oz	139	27	0.0
(Mott's)	6 oz	86	17	0.0
(Mott's) aseptic box	8.45 oz	128	24	0.0
(Musselman's) 'Breakfast Cocktail'	6 oz	110	5	0.0
(Red Cheek)	6 oz	109	9	0.0
(Tree Top) canned	6 oz	100	10	0.0
(Tree Top) frozen	6 oz	100	10	0.0
(Welch's) 'Orchard Cocktail'	6 oz	110	20	0.0
(Welch's) 'Orchard Cocktail,' frozen	6 oz	110	10	0.0
(Welch's) 'Orchard Cocktail,' frozen, w/raspberry	6 oz	90	10	0.0
(Welch's) 'Orchard Cocktail-in-a Box' w/raspberry	8.45 oz	140	20	0.0
APPLE JUICE				
Can, bottle, or box				
(Heinz) strained, 'Saver Size'	4.2 oz	70	15	0.0
(IGA) 'Unsweetened'	6 oz	74	10	0.0
(Indian Summer)	6 oz	90	10	<1.0
(J. Hungerford)	9.03 oz	128	6	0.0
(J. Hungerford) 50% juice	9.03 oz	119	8	0.0
(J. Hungerford) 100% juice	9.03 oz	112	17	0.0
(Juicy Juice)	6 oz	90	5	0.0
(Knudsen & Sons) Gravenstein	8 oz	110	na	0.0
(Knudsen & Sons) 'Natural'	8 oz	85	na	0.0
(Kraft) 'Pure 100%'	6 oz	80	5	0.0

Food Name	Serv. Size	Total Cal.	Sod. MGS	Fa GM
(Lucky Leaf) 'Individual Portion Control'	3.8 oz	60	0	0.
(Lucky Leaf) 100% vitamin C enriched	6 oz	90	0	0.
(Lucky Leaf) regular	6 oz	90	0	0.
(McCain) 100% juice 'Junior'	4.2 oz	50	5	0.
(Minute Maid) aseptic box	6 oz	80	30	0.
(Minute Maid) 'Juices to Go'	6 oz	80	30	0.
(Mott's)	10 oz	148	22	0.
(Mott's)	9.5 oz	141	20	0.
(Mott's)	8.45 oz	124	18	0.
(Mott's)	6 oz	88	13	0.
(Mott's) natural style	6 oz	76	28	0.
(Musselman's) 'Individual Portion Control'	3.8 oz	60	0	0.
(Musselman's) 100% vitamin C enriched	6 oz	90	0	0.
(Musselman's) regular	6 oz	90	0	0.
(Ocean Spray)	6 oz	90	15	0.
(Red Cheek) 'Natural'	6 oz	97	16	0.
(Red Cheek) '100% Pure'	6 oz	97	7	0.
(S&W) '100% Pure Unsweetened'	6 oz	85	5	0.
(S. Martinelli)	6 oz	100	5	0.
(S. Martinelli) 'Sparkling'	6 oz	100	5	0.
(Sippin' Pak) 100% pure, from concentrate	8.45 oz	110	25	0.
(Snapple) 'Apple Crisp'	8 oz	140	30	0.
(Tree Top)	6 oz	90	10	0.
(TreeSweet)	6 oz	90	15	0.
(Tropicana) '100% Pure'	8 oz	116	17	0.
(Tropicana) 100% pure	6 oz	80	15	<1.
(Veryfine) '100%'	8 oz	107	10	0.
(Welch's) sparkling	6 oz	100	5	0.
(White House)	6 oz	87	5	0.
Chilled or frozen				
(A&P) diluted as directed	6 oz	90	0	<1.
(Knudsen & Sons) clear	8 oz	90	na	0.
(Minute Maid) diluted as directed	6 oz	80	15	0.0
(Sunkist) diluted as directed	8 oz	79	12	0.
(Tree Top) diluted as directed	6 oz	90	10	0.
(Welch's) 'Orchard Cocktail'	10 oz	170	95	0.
APPLE KIT				
Candy *(Concord)* microwaveable	1 apple	50	0	0.
Caramel *(Concord)* microwaveable	1 apple	150	105	3.
APPLE ORANGE PINEAPPLE COCKTAIL				
(Welch's) 'Orchard Tropical Cocktails'	8.45 oz	140	20	0.0

Food Name	Serv. Size	Total Cal.	Sod. MGS	Fat GMS
(Welch's) 'Orchard Tropical Cocktails'	6 oz	100	20	0.0
APPLE PASTRY				
Fresh				
(Entenmann's) 'Apple Puffs'	1 puff	280	320	13.0
(Tastykake) pocket	3 oz	323	222	17.6
Frozen				
(Hormel) 'Apple Dulcita'	4 oz	290	350	10.0
(Mrs. Paul's) 'Apple Fritter'	2 pieces	240	500	9.0
(Pepperidge Farm) 'Apple Dumpling'	3 oz	260	230	13.0
(Pepperidge Farm) apple fruit square	1 piece	220	170	12.0
(Pepperidge Farm) 'Berkshire' apple crisps	1 ramekin	250	130	8.0
(Weight Watchers) 'Sweet Celebrations' apple crisps	3.5 oz	190	190	5.0
APPLE PEACH JUICE *(Knudsen & Sons)*	8 oz	140	na	0.0
APPLE PEAR JUICE *(Tree Top)* frozen	6 oz	90	10	0.0
APPLE PIE SPICE *(Tone's)*	1 tsp	9	1	0.2
APPLE PUNCH				
(Minute Maid) chilled	6 oz	90	20	0.0
(Minute Maid) frozen concentrate	6 oz	90	0	0.0
APPLE PUNCH DRINK *(Red Cheek)*	6 oz	113	7	0.0
APPLE RASPBERRY DRINK				
(Mott's)	10 oz	158	17	0.0
(Mott's)	9.5 oz	150	16	0.0
APPLE RASPBERRY JUICE				
(Knudsen & Sons)	8 oz	110	na	0.0
(Mott's)	9.5 oz	134	76	0.0
(Mott's)	6 oz	83	48	0.0
(Mott's) aseptic box	8.45 oz	124	67	0.0
(Red Cheek)	6 oz	113	8	0.0
(Santa Cruz Natural) organic	8 oz	120	na	1.0
(Tree Top) canned or frozen	6 oz	80	10	0.0
(Veryfine) cocktail	8 oz	110	15	0.0
APPLE STRAWBERRY JUICE				
(Knudsen & Sons)	8 oz	110	na	0.0
(Santa Cruz Natural) organic	8 oz	120	na	<1.0
APPLE STRAWBERRY NECTAR *(Kern's)* can or bottle	6 oz	110	0	0.0
APPLE STRUDEL				
(Aunt Fanny's) individual	3 oz	330	210	18.0
(Entenmann's) old fashioned	1.5 oz	120	110	5.0
APPLE-WHITE GRAPE JUICE				
(Welch's) 'No Sugar Added' frozen cocktail	6 oz	40	5	0.0

Food Name	Serv. Size	Total Cal.	Sod. MGS	Fat GMS
APPLESAUCE				
(A&P)				
regular	1/2 cup	110	15	<1.0
unsweetened	1/2 cup	50	0	<1.0
(Del Monte)				
'Lite'	1/2 cup	50	10	0.0
regular	1/2 cup	90	5	0.0
(Featherweight)	1/2 cup	50	3	0.0
(Finast)				
regular	1/2 cup	105	10	0.0
unsweetened	1/2 cup	56	na	0.2
(Lucky Leaf)				
chunky	4 oz	80	20	0.0
'Juice Pack'	4 oz	50	0	0.0
'Natural' individual portion control	4 oz	50	0	0.0
regular	4 oz	80	20	0.0
'Regular' individual portion control	4 oz	80	0	0.0
unsweetened	4 oz	50	0	0.0
(Mott's)				
chunky	6 oz	86	11	0.0
cinnamon	6 oz	152	<1	0.0
'Natural'	6 oz	80	3	0.0
'Natural Single Serve'	4 oz	53	2	0.0
regular	6 oz	150	<1	0.0
'Single Serve'	4 oz	100	<1	0.0
'Single Serve' cinnamon	4 oz	101	<1	0.0
(Musselman's)				
chunky	4 oz	80	20	0.0
'Juice Pack'	4 oz	50	0	0.0
'Natural' individual portion control	4 oz	50	0	0.0
regular	4 oz	80	20	0.0
'Regular' individual portion control	4 oz	80	0	0.0
unsweetened	4 oz	50	0	0.0
(S&W)				
regular	1/2 cup	90	10	0.0
unsweetened	1/2 cup	55	5	0.0
(S&W Nutradiet)	1/2 cup	55	10	0.0
(Stokely)				
regular	1/2 cup	90	30	0.0
unsweetened	1/2 cup	45	5	0.0
(Tree Top) 'Original'	1/2 cup	80	0	0.0

Food Name	Serv. Size	Total Cal.	Sod. MGS	Fat GMS
(White House)				
chunky	4 oz	80	5	0.0
in apple juice	4 oz	50	5	0.0
'Regular'	4 oz	80	5	0.0
unsweetened	4 oz	50	5	0.0
APRICOT				
candied	100 gm	338	1	0.2
pitted	1 oz	14	<1	0.1
raw, halves	1 cup	74	2	0.6
untrimmed	1 lb	202	2	1.7
APRICOT, CANNED				
In extra heavy syrup				
peeled	4 oz	109	15	<.1
peeled, whole	1/2 cup	118	16	0.1
In extra light syrup				
unpeeled	4 oz	56	2	0.1
unpeeled, halves	1/2 cup	61	3	0.1
In heavy syrup				
peeled	4 oz	94	12	0.1
peeled, halves	1 cup	214	10	0.2
peeled, whole	1/2 cup	107	14	0.1
peeled, whole *(S&W)*	1/2 cup	100	15	0.0
unpeeled	4 oz	94	5	0.1
unpeeled *(A&P)*	1/2 cup	110	15	1.0
unpeeled, halves	1/2 cup	107	5	0.1
unpeeled, halves *(IGA)*	1 cup	220	15	0.0
unpeeled, halves *(S&W)*	1/2 cup	110	15	0.0
In juice				
peeled *(Featherweight)*	1/2 cup	50	10	0.0
unpeeled	4 oz	54	5	<.1
unpeeled, halves	1/2 cup	60	5	<.1
unpeeled, 'Lite' *(Libby's)*	1/2 cup	60	5	0.0
In light syrup				
unpeeled	4 oz	71	5	0.1
unpeeled, halves	1/2 cup	80	5	0.1
unpeeled, halves 'No Frills' *(Pathmark)*	1/2 cup	80	5	0.0
In water				
peeled	1/2 cup	25	12	<.1
peeled, whole *(S&W Nutradiet)*	1/2 cup	28	5	0.0
unpeeled	4 oz	31	3	0.2
unpeeled, halves	1/2 cup	33	4	0.2

Food Name	Serv. Size	Total Cal.	Sod. MGS	Fat GMS
unpeeled, halves (S&W)	1/2 cup	35	5	0.0
unpeeled, halves (S&W Nutradiet)	1/2 cup	35	5	0.0
APRICOT, DEHYDRATED/SULFURED				
cooked	4 oz	143	6	0.3
stewed, low-moisture	1/2 cup	156	6	0.3
uncooked	4 oz	363	15	0.7
uncooked, low-moisture	1/2 cup	192	8	0.4
APRICOT, DRIED				
sulfured, cooked	4 oz	96	3	0.2
sulfured, stewed, halves	1/2 cup	106	4	0.2
sulfured, uncooked	4 oz	270	11	0.5
sulfured, uncooked, approx 1.2 oz	10 halves	83	3	0.2
sulfured, uncooked, halves	1 cup	309	13	0.6
(Del Monte)	2 oz	140	10	0.0
(Mariani) California, sun dried, premium	1/4 cup	140	10	0.0
(Mariani) Mediterranean, sun dried, premium	1/4 cup	140	10	0.0
(Sun•Maid)	2 oz	140	10	0.0
(SunSweet)	2 oz	140	10	0.0
APRICOT, FROZEN				
sweetened	4 oz	111	5	0.1
sweetened, unthawed	1 cup	237	10	0.2
APRICOT KERNEL OIL				
	1/2 cup	964	0	109.0
	1 oz	251	0	28.4
	1 tbsp	120	0	13.6
(Hain)	1 tbsp	120	0	14.0
(Spectrum Naturals)	1 tbsp	120	0	14.0
APRICOT NECTAR				
(Del Monte)	6 oz	100	10	0.0
(Kern's)	6 oz	110	0	0.0
(Knudsen & Sons)	8 oz	105	na	0.0
(Libby's)	6 oz	110	0	0.0
(S&W)	6 oz	100	10	0.0
APRICOT PINEAPPLE NECTAR				
(Kern's)	6 oz	110	5	0.0
(S&W Nutradiet)	4 oz	35	20	0.0
ARCTIC BONITO. See TUNA, SKIPJACK.				
ARROWHEAD				
boiled, drained	4 oz	88	20	0.1
boiled, drained	1 med	9	2	0.0
raw	1 large	25	6	0.1

Food Name	Serv. Size	Total Cal.	Sod. MGS	Fat GMS
raw	1 med	12	3	0.0
raw, trimmed	1 oz	28	6	0.1
raw, untrimmed	1 lb	337	75	1.0
ARROWROOT, powdered *(Tone's)*	1 tsp	10	1	0.0
ARROWROOT FLOUR				
	1/3 cup	154	1	(mq)
	1 oz	101	1	(mq)
ARTICHOKE HEARTS				
boiled, drained	4 oz	57	108	0.2
boiled, drained	1/2 cup	42	80	0.1
canned, marinated *(S&W)*	3.5 oz	225	15	26.0
frozen, boiled, drained	4 oz	51	60	0.6
frozen, 'Deluxe' *(Birds Eye)*	3 oz	30	140	0.4
frozen *(Seabrook)*	3 oz	25	6	0.0
ARTICHOKES, FRENCH				
boiled, drained	1 med	60	114	0.2
boiled, drained, hearts	1/2 cup	42	80	0.1
frozen, boiled, drained	3 oz	36	42	0.4
raw	1 large	76	152	0.2
raw	1 med	60	120	0.2
ARTICHOKES, GLOBE				
boiled, drained	1 med	60	114	0.2
boiled, drained, hearts	1/2 cup	42	80	0.1
boiled, drained, trimmed	4 oz	57	108	0.2
boiled, drained, untrimmed	4 oz	23	43	0.1
fresh *(Dole)*	1 large	23	65	0.1
frozen, boiled, drained	3 oz	36	42	0.4
frozen, unprepared	9 oz	97	120	1.1
raw	1 large	76	152	0.2
raw	1 med	60	120	0.2
raw, untrimmed	1 lb	85	171	0.3
ARTICHOKES, JERUSALEM				
raw, slices	1/2 cup	57	3	0.0
trimmed	1 oz	22	na	tr
untrimmed	1 lb	238	na	<.1
ARUGULA/rocket/roquette/ruculo/rugula				
raw	1 leaf	1	1	0.0
raw	1/2 cup	3	3	0.1
(Frieda's)	1 lb	104	68	1.4
(Frieda's)	1 oz	7	4	<.1

Food Name	Serv. Size	Total Cal.	Sod. MGS	Fat GMS
ASPARAGUS				
boiled, drained	1/2 cup	22	10	0.3
boiled, drained, cuts and spears	4 oz	28	5	0.4
fresh (Dole)	5 spears	18	0	0.0
raw, cuts and spears	1/2 cup	15	1	0.2
raw, trimmed	1 oz	6	1	0.1
raw, untrimmed	1 lb	54	5	0.5
ASPARAGUS, CANNED				
Cuts and tips (Finast)	1 cup	35	720	0.0
Points, all green (S&W Nutradiet)	1/2 cup	17	10	0.0
Spears				
and tips, all green (Del Monte)	1/2 cup	20	355	0.0
colossal, all green 'Fancy' (S&W)	1/2 cup	20	320	0.0
cut (Green Giant)	1/2 cup	18	420	0.0
cut, 50% less salt (Green Giant)	1/2 cup	18	210	0.0
cut, green (Pathmark)	1/2 cup	20	450	0.0
cut, green 'No Salt Added' (Pathmark)	1/2 cup	20	5	0.0
green (Stokely)	1/2 cup	20	380	0.0
green 'Fancy' (S&W)	1/2 cup	18	320	0.0
green, w/liquid (Green Giant)	1/2 cup	20	420	0.0
'No Salt or Sugar Added' (Stokely)	1/2 cup	20	5	0.0
white (Green Giant)	1/2 cup	16	410	0.0
white, w/liquid (Green Giant)	1/2 cup	16	410	0.0
w/liquid, 50% less salt (Green Giant)	1/2 cup	20	210	0.0
w/liquid, green, tipped (Del Monte)	1/2 cup	20	355	0.0
ASPARAGUS, FROZEN				
boiled, drained	10-oz pkg	82	12	1.2
boiled, drained, cuts and spears	4 oz	32	5	0.5
cuts (Birds Eye)	3.3 oz	25	5	0.0
cuts (Seabrook)	3.3 oz	25	6	0.0
cuts 'Harvest Fresh' (Green Giant)	1/2 cup	25	95	0.0
cuts and spears (Frosty Acres)	3.3 oz	25	6	0.0
spears (Birds Eye)	3.3 oz	25	0	0.0
spears (Finast)	3.3 oz	25	5	0.0
spears (Frosty Acres)	3.3 oz	25	4	0.0
spears (Seabrook)	3.3 oz	25	4	0.0
spears (Southern)	3.5 oz	27	20	0.2
unprepared	10-oz pkg	68	23	0.7

ASPARAGUS BEAN. See YARDLONG BEAN.

Food Name	Serv. Size	Total Cal.	Sod. MGS	Fat GMS
AVOCADO				
All commercial varieties				
puréed	1/2 cup	185	12	17.6
trimmed	1 oz	46	3	4.3
untrimmed	1 lb	540	35	51.4
California				
puréed	1/2 cup	204	14	19.9
trimmed	1 oz	50	3	4.9
untrimmed	1 lb	610	42	59.8
Florida				
puréed	1/2 cup	129	6	10.2
trimmed	1 oz	32	1	2.5
untrimmed	1 lb	339	14	26.9
AVOCADO OIL				
	1/2 cup	964	0	109.0
	1 oz	251	0	28.4
	1 tbsp	124	0	14.0
(Hain)	1 tbsp	120	0	14.0
(Spectrum Naturals)	1 tbsp	120	0	14.0
AWA/milkfish				
dry-heat cooked	3 oz	161	78	7.3
raw	1 lb	673	(mq)	30.5
raw	1 oz	42	(mq)	1.9

B

Food Name	Serv. Size	Total Cal.	Sod. MGS	Fat GMS
BABASSU OIL. See PALM KERNEL OIL.				
BABY FOOD				
CEREAL				
Barley				
dry	1 tbsp	9	42	2.3
dry	.5 oz	52	7	0.5
instant, dry, '1st Foods' *(Gerber)*	.5 oz	60	na	1.0
instant, dry, 'Stage 1' *(Beech-Nut)*	.5 oz	60	10	0.0
instant, .5 oz cereal prepared w/2.4 oz formula, 'Stage 1' *(Beech-Nut)*	1 serving	120	25	4.0
instant, .5 oz cereal prepared w/2.4 oz whole milk *(Gerber)*	1 serving	100	na	4.0
instant, .5 oz cereal prepared w/2.4 oz formula	1 serving	110	na	4.0

Food Name	Serv. Size	Total Cal.	Sod. MGS	Fat GMS
instant *(Heinz)*	3.5 oz	370	15	3.7
prepared w/whole milk	3.5 oz	111	49	3.3
Cereal w/applesauce and bananas, '3rd Foods' *(Gerber)*	7 tbsp	82	3	0.6
Cereal w/egg yolks				
junior	7.5 oz	111	70	3.8
junior	1 oz	15	9	0.5
strained	1 oz	14	9	0.5
w/bacon, junior	4.5 oz	101	61	6.4
w/bacon, junior	1 oz	22	14	1.4
w/bacon, strained	7.5 oz	179	98	11.1
w/bacon, strained	1 oz	24	13	1.5
Cereal w/eggs				
strained	4.5 oz	74	49	1.9
strained	1 oz	16	11	0.4
Corn				
instant, dry, 'Tropical Foods' *(Gerber)*	.5 oz	60	na	1.0
instant, dry, 'Tropical Foods' *(Gerber)*	3.5 oz	390	55	4.6
instant, prepared w/milk, 'Tropical Foods' *(Gerber)*	2.4 oz	110	na	4.0
Grits and egg yolks				
strained	4.5 oz	73	45	2.9
strained	1 oz	16	10	0.7
High-protein				
instant, dry	1 tbsp	9	1	0.1
instant, dry	.5 oz	51	7	0.8
instant, 1 oz cereal prepared w/whole milk	1 serving	31	14	1.1
instant, w/apple and orange, dry	1 tbsp	9	3	0.2
instant, w/apple and orange, dry	.5 oz	53	15	0.9
instant, w/apple and orange, 1 oz cereal prepared w/whole milk	1 serving	32	16	1.1
Mixed				
dry	1 tbsp	9	1	0.1
dry	.5 oz	54	6	0.6
instant, dry *(Earth's Best)*	.5 oz	60	0	0.0
instant, dry, '2nd Foods' *(Gerber)*	.5 oz	60	na	1.0
instant, dry, 'Stages 2' *(Beech-Nut)*	.5 oz	60	10	0.0
instant, .5 oz cereal prepared w/2.4 oz formula, 'Stages 2' *(Beech-Nut)*	1 serving	120	25	4.0
instant, .5 oz cereal prepared w/2.5 oz formula (Earth's Best)	1 serving	110	15	3.0
instant, .5 oz cereal prepared w/2.4 oz whole milk, 'Stages 2' *(Beech-Nut)*	1 serving	100	50	3.0

Food Name	Serv. Size	Total Cal.	Sod. MGS	Fat GMS
instant *(Heinz)*	3.5 oz	373	12	4.9
instant, prepared w/apple juice, '2nd Foods' *(Gerber)*	2.4 oz	90	na	1.0
1 oz cereal prepared w/whole milk	1 serving	32	13	1.0
w/apples and bananas, 'Stages 2' *(Beech-Nut)*	4.5 oz	90	0	1.0
w/apples and bananas, strained *(Heinz)*	3.5 oz	70	3	0.3
w/applesauce and bananas, junior	7.75 oz	183	79	0.9
w/applesauce and bananas, junior	1 oz	24	10	0.1
w/applesauce and bananas, '2nd Foods' *(Gerber)*	4 oz	90	na	1.0
w/applesauce and bananas, '2nd Foods' *(Gerber)*	7 tbsp	81	2	0.6
w/applesauce and bananas, strained	4.75 oz	111	3	0.7
w/applesauce and bananas, strained	1 oz	23	1	0.1
w/applesauce and bananas, '3rd Foods' *(Gerber)*	7 tbsp	82	3	0.6
w/bananas, dry	1 tbsp	9	3	0.1
w/bananas, dry	.5 oz	56	17	0.7
w/bananas, instant, dry, '2nd Foods' *(Gerber)*	.5 oz	60	na	1.0
w/bananas, 1 oz cereal prepared w/whole milk	1 serving	33	17	1.0
w/fruit and nuts, no sugar added, 1-4 yr., dry *(Familia)*	1.5 oz	170	4	3.0
w/fruit and nuts, no sugar added, 1-4 yr., 1.5 oz cereal prepared w/whole milk *(Familia)*	1 serving	270	77	8.0
w/fruit and nuts, 1-4 yr., 1.5 oz cereal prepared w/2/3 cup milk *(Familia)*	1 serving	270	74	8.0
w/fruit and nuts, 100% natural, 1-4 yr., dry *(Familia)*	1.5 oz	170	1	3.0
w/honey, dry	1 tbsp	9	1	0.1
w/honey, dry	.5 oz	56	6	0.7
w/honey, 1 oz cereal prepared w/whole milk	1 serving	33	14	1.0
Oatmeal				
instant, dry	1 tbsp	10	1	0.2
instant, dry	.5 oz	57	5	1.1
prepared w/whole milk	1 oz	33	13	1.2
w/apples and bananas, 'Stages 2' *(Beech-Nut)*	4.5 oz	90	5	1.0
w/apples and bananas, strained *(Heinz)*	3.5 oz	76	3	0.6
w/apples and cinnamon, instant, '3rd Foods' *(Gerber)*	1 pkt	90	50	2.0
w/applesauce and bananas, '2nd Foods' *(Gerber)*	4 oz	90	na	1.0
w/applesauce and bananas, '2nd Foods' *(Gerber)*	7 tbsp	83	2	0.8
w/applesauce and bananas, '3rd Foods' *(Gerber)*	7 tbsp	80	3	0.8
w/applesauce and bananas, junior	7.75 oz	165	68	1.5
w/applesauce and bananas, junior	1 oz	21	9	0.2
w/applesauce and bananas, strained	4.75 oz	99	3	0.9
w/applesauce and bananas, strained	1 oz	21	1	0.2
w/bananas, dry	1 tbsp	9	3	0.1
w/bananas, dry	.5 oz	56	17	0.9

Food Name	Serv. Size	Total Cal.	Sod. MGS	Fat GMS
w/bananas, instant, '3rd Foods' (Gerber)	1 pkt	90	50	2.0
w/bananas, prepared w/whole milk	1 oz	33	17	1.1
w/bananas, prepared w/whole milk	3.5 oz	116	61	3.8
w/bananas, 100% natural, organic, dry (Healthy Times)	.5 oz	60	0	0.0
w/bananas, organic, .5 oz cereal prepared w/2.4 oz formula (Healthy Times)	.5 oz	100	15	3.0
w/honey, dry	1 tbsp	9	1	0.2
w/honey, dry	.5 oz	56	7	1.0
w/honey, prepared w/whole milk	1 oz	33	14	1.1
Rice				
dry	1 tbsp	9	1	0.1
dry	.5 oz	56	5	0.7
dry (Earth's Best)	.5 oz	60	0	0.0
dry (Health Valley)	1 tbsp	60	5	1.0
dry, .5 oz cereal prepared w/2.5 oz formula (Earth's Best)	3 oz	110	15	3.0
dry, prepared w/whole milk	1 oz	33	13	1.0
instant, dry, '1st Foods' (Gerber)	.5 oz	60	na	1.0
instant, dry, '1st Foods' (Gerber)	3.5 oz	380	7	3.3
instant, dry, 'Stages 1' (Beech-Nut)	.5 oz	60	15	0.0
instant, .5 oz cereal prepared w/2.4 oz formula (Beech-Nut)	.5 oz	120	20	4.0
instant, .5 oz cereal prepared w/2.4 oz whole milk (Beech-Nut)	2.9 oz	110	30	3.0
instant (Heinz)	3.5 oz	376	12	4.1
sprouted (Health Valley)	1 tbsp	60	5	1.0
w/apples, instant, dry, 'Stages 2' (Beech-Nut)	.5 oz	60	15	0.0
w/apples, instant, .5 oz cereal prepared w/2.4 oz formula (Beech-Nut)	.5 oz	120	20	4.0
w/apples, instant, .5 oz cereal prepared w/2.4 oz whole milk (Beech-Nut)	2.9 oz	110	50	3.0
w/apples and bananas, 'Stages 2' (Beech-Nut)	4.5 oz	100	25	0.0
w/apples and bananas, strained (Heinz)	3.5 oz	70	5	0.2
w/applesauce and bananas, '2nd Foods' (Gerber)	4 oz	90	na	0.0
w/applesauce and bananas, '2nd Foods' (Gerber)	7 tbsp	79	9	0.2
w/applesauce and bananas, strained	4.75 oz	107	38	0.5
w/applesauce and bananas, strained	1 oz	22	8	0.1
w/bananas, dry	1 tbsp	10	2	0.1
w/bananas, dry	.5 oz	57	14	0.6
w/bananas, instant, dry, '2nd Foods' (Gerber)	.5 oz	60	na	1.0
w/bananas, instant, dry, 'Stages 2' (Beech-Nut)	.5 oz	60	15	0.0

Food Name	Serv. Size	Total Cal.	Sod. MGS	Fat GMS
w/bananas, instant, .5 oz cereal prepared w/2.4 oz formula *(Beech-Nut)*	.5 oz	120	20	4.0
w/bananas, instant, .5 oz cereal prepared w/2.4 oz whole milk *(Beech-Nut)*	2.9 oz	100	50	3.0
w/bananas, prepared w/whole milk	1 oz	33	16	1.0
w/formula, instant, '1st Foods' *(Gerber)*	2.4 oz	110	na	4.0
w/honey, dry	1 tbsp	9	1	0.1
w/honey, dry	.5 oz	56	7	0.4
w/honey, prepared w/whole milk	1 oz	33	14	0.9
w/mango, instant, dry, 'Tropical Foods' *(Gerber)*	3.5 oz	386	20	2.6
w/mango, instant, prepared w/milk, 'Tropical Foods' *(Gerber)*	2.4 oz	100	na	3.0
w/mixed fruit, junior	7.75 oz	185	24	0.4
w/mixed fruit, junior	1 oz	24	3	0.1
w/mixed fruit, junior *(Gerber)*	6 oz	140	17	1.0
w/mixed fruit, '3rd Foods' *(Gerber)*	7 tbsp	79	10	0.2
DESSERTS AND SNACKS				
Apple betty				
junior	7.75 oz	154	20	0.0
junior	1 oz	20	3	0.0
strained	4.75 oz	97	14	0.0
strained	1 oz	20	3	0.0
Apple Juice Dessert, w/yogurt, '2nd Foods' *(Gerber)*	4 oz	100	na	2.0
Apple yogurt				
apple yogurt dessert, 'Stages 2' *(Beech-Nut)*	4.5 oz	120	25	2.0
'Breakfast' *(Earth's Best)*	4.5 oz	100	20	2.0
Banana yogurt				
'2nd Foods' *(Gerber)*	7 tbsp	74	22	0.4
'Stages 2' *(Beech-Nut)*	4.5 oz	120	30	2.0
strained *(Heinz)*	3.5 oz	83	20	0.5
Banana-apple dessert, '2nd Foods' *(Gerber)*	7 tbsp	68	7	0.1
Banana-pineapple dessert, 'Stages 2' *(Beech-Nut)*	4.5 oz	110	15	0.0
Banana-vanilla dessert, 'Tropical Foods' *(Gerber)*	7 tbsp	85	11	0.9
Blueberry yogurt, 'Breakfast' *(Earth's Best)*	4.5 oz	100	20	2.0
Cereal snack				
apple-banana finger snacks, 'Graduates' *(Gerber)*	3.2 oz	405	86	4.8
apple-cinnamon finger snacks, 'Graduates' *(Gerber)*	3.2 oz	407	84	5.0
Cherry vanilla dessert				
junior	7.75 oz	152	33	0.4
junior	1 oz	20	4	0.1
strained	4.75 oz	92	22	0.4

Food Name	Serv. Size	Total Cal.	Sod. MGS	Fat GMS
strained	1 oz	19	5	0.1
Cookies and crackers				
animal-shaped, baked, chunky *(Gerber)*	3.5 oz	443	187	13.1
apple, organic, 'Hugga Bears' *(Healthy Times)*	1 oz	120	38	3.0
arrowroot	1 oz	125	105	4.1
arrowroot, baked finger snacks, 'Graduates' *(Gerber)*	3.5 oz	452	324	15.3
arrowroot, w/maple, wheat-free *(Healthy Times)*	1 cookie	120	38	3.0
baked, chunky, 'Biter Biscuit' *(Gerber)*	1 biscuit	50	na	1.0
cinnamon animal crackers, baked, 'Graduates' *(Gerber)*	3.5 oz	449	369	12.3
pretzel	1 oz	113	76	0.6
pretzel, baked, finger snacks, 'Graduates' *(Gerber)*	3.5 oz	403	597	3.3
strawberry, organic, 'Hugga Bears' *(Healthy Times)*	1 oz	120	38	3.0
teething biscuit	1 biscuit	43	40	0.5
teething biscuit	1 oz	111	103	1.2
zwieback, baked, chunky *(Gerber)*	3.5 oz	432	210	11.5
Cottage cheese w/pineapple				
junior	7.75 oz	172	112	1.5
junior	1 oz	22	14	0.2
strained	4.75 oz	93	70	1.1
strained	1 oz	20	15	0.2
'Stages 2' *(Beech-Nut)*	4.5 oz	130	15	1.0
'Stages 3' *(Beech-Nut)*	6 oz	170	20	2.0
Custard/pudding				
banana pudding, 'Stages 2' *(Beech-Nut)*	4.5 oz	100	10	0.0
banana pudding, strained *(Heinz)*	3.5 oz	74	9	0.5
caramel pudding, junior	7.75 oz	168	60	1.9
caramel pudding, junior	1 oz	22	8	0.3
caramel pudding, strained	4.75 oz	104	36	0.9
caramel pudding, strained	1 oz	22	8	0.2
cherry vanilla pudding, '2nd Foods' *(Gerber)*	7 tbsp	69	9	0.2
cherry vanilla pudding, strained *(Gerber)*	4.5 oz	90	12	1.0
chocolate custard, junior	7.75 oz	196	55	3.5
chocolate custard, junior	1 oz	25	7	0.5
chocolate custard, junior *(Heinz)*	3.5 oz	75	27	1.2
chocolate custard, strained	4.75 oz	108	29	2.2
chocolate custard, strained	1 oz	24	7	0.5
orange pudding, strained	4.75 oz	108	27	1.2
orange pudding, strained	1 oz	23	6	0.3
pineapple pudding, junior	7.75 oz	191	48	0.9
pineapple pudding, junior	1 oz	25	6	0.1
pineapple pudding, strained	4.75 oz	104	24	0.4

Food Name	Serv. Size	Total Cal.	Sod. MGS	Fat GMS
pineapple pudding, strained	1 oz	23	5	0.1
vanilla custard, junior	7.75 oz	196	64	5.1
vanilla custard, junior	1 oz	25	8	0.7
vanilla custard, junior *(Gerber)*	6 oz	150	41	2.0
vanilla custard, '2nd Foods' *(Gerber)*	7 tbsp	88	25	0.9
vanilla custard, 'Stages 2' *(Beech-Nut)*	4.5 oz	140	60	4.0
vanilla custard, 'Stages 3' *(Beech-Nut)*	6 oz	180	80	5.0
vanilla custard, strained	4.75 oz	109	36	2.6
vanilla custard, strained	1 oz	24	8	0.6
vanilla custard, strained *(Gerber)*	4.5 oz	100	32	1.0
vanilla custard, '3rd Foods' *(Gerber)*	7 tbsp	89	24	0.9
vanilla custard, strained *(Heinz)*	3.5 oz	75	27	1.2
Dutch apple dessert				
junior	7.75 oz	152	35	2.2
junior	1 oz	20	5	0.3
junior *(Heinz)*	3.5 oz	69	5	0.4
'2nd Foods' *(Gerber)*	7 tbsp	79	14	1.0
'Stages 2' *(Beech-Nut)*	4.5 oz	100	15	0.0
strained	4.75 oz	92	22	1.2
strained	1 oz	19	5	0.3
strained *(Heinz)*	3.5 oz	69	5	0.4
'3rd Foods' *(Gerber)*	7 tbsp	77	14	0.9
Fruit dessert				
junior *(Gerber)*	6 oz	130	12	1.0
junior *(Heinz)*	3.5 oz	65	14	0.2
'2nd Foods' *(Gerber)*	7 tbsp	82	9	0.2
'Stages 2' *(Beech-Nut)*	4.5 oz	80	0	0.0
'Stages 3' *(Beech-Nut)*	6 oz	120	5	0.0
strained *(Gerber)*	4.5 oz	100	13	1.0
strained *(Heinz)*	3.5 oz	66	11	0.2
'3rd Foods' *(Gerber)*	7 tbsp	73	7	0.2
w/o ascorbic acid, junior	7.75 oz	139	29	0.0
w/o ascorbic acid, junior	1 oz	18	4	0.0
w/o ascorbic acid, strained	4.75 oz	80	19	0.0
w/o ascorbic acid, strained	1 oz	17	4	0.0
Guava dessert, w/tapioca, 'Tropical Foods' *(Gerber)*	7 tbsp	69	3	0.1
Hawaiian dessert				
junior *(Gerber)*	6 oz	150	32	1.0
'2nd Foods' *(Gerber)*	7 tbsp	86	17	0.2
'3rd Foods' *(Gerber)*	7 tbsp	87	15	0.1
strained *(Gerber)*	4.5 oz	120	23	1.0

Food Name	Serv. Size	Total Cal.	Sod. MGS	Fat GMS
Mango dessert, w/tapioca 'Tropical Foods' (Gerber)	7 tbsp	75	2	0.2
Mango-banana dessert, w/passion fruit,				
'Tropical Foods' (Gerber)	7 tbsp	73	9	0.1
Mixed fruit yogurt, '2nd Foods' (Gerber)	7 tbsp	79	15	0.3
Papaya dessert, w/tapioca, 'Tropical Foods' (Gerber)	7 tbsp	62	7	0.2
Papaya-pineapple dessert, 'Tropical Foods' (Gerber)	7 tbsp	76	8	0.0
Peach cobbler				
junior	7.75 oz	147	20	0.0
junior	1 oz	19	3	0.0
'2nd Foods' (Gerber)	7 tbsp	77	8	0.2
strained	4.75 oz	88	9	0.0
strained	1 oz	18	2	0.0
strained (Heinz)	3.5 oz	72	6	0.3
'3rd Foods' (Gerber)	7 tbsp	77	9	0.1
Peach melba				
junior	7.75 oz	132	20	0.0
junior	1 oz	17	3	0.0
strained	4.75 oz	81	12	0.0
strained	1 oz	17	3	0.0
Peach yogurt				
'2nd Foods' (Gerber)	7 tbsp	76	14	0.4
'Stages 2' (Beech-Nut)	4.5 oz	120	30	2.0
Peach-mango dessert, 'Tropical Foods' (Gerber)	7 tbsp	60	7	0.2
Pear yogurt				
'Stages 2' (Beech-Nut)	4.5 oz	130	35	2.0
strained (Heinz)	3.5 oz	80	19	0.4
Pineapple-banana dessert, 'Tropical Foods' (Gerber)	7 tbsp	79	9	0.1
Pineapple-orange dessert				
strained	4.75 oz	90	13	0.0
strained	1 oz	20	3	0.0
Tropical fruit dessert				
junior	7.75 oz	132	15	0.0
junior	1 oz	17	2	0.0
medley, 'Tropical Foods' (Gerber)	7 tbsp	64	6	0.1
w/tapioca, strained	4.5 oz	80	6	0.0
Tropical yogurt, 'Breakfast' (Earth's Best)	4.5 oz	110	20	2.0
Tutti frutti dessert, junior (Heinz)	3.5 oz	67	12	0.4
DINNERS AND MAIN DISHES				
Apples and chicken dinner, 'Simple Recipe'				
'2nd Foods' (Gerber)	7 tbsp	66	13	1.4

Food Name	Serv. Size	Total Cal.	Sod. MGS	Fat GMS
Apples and ham dinner, 'Simple Recipe'				
'2nd Foods' (Gerber)	7 tbsp	67	9	0.8
Apples and turkey dinner				
'Simple Recipe,' '2nd Foods' (Gerber)	4 oz	80	20	2.0
'Simple Recipe,' '2nd Foods' (Gerber)	7 tbsp	67	13	1.2
Beans and rice dinner				
'Tropical Foods' (Gerber)	7 tbsp	52	8	1.5
w/green beans (Earth's Best)	4.5 oz	70	0	0.0
Beef and egg noodle dinner				
'2nd Foods' (Gerber)	7 tbsp	62	10	2.0
'3rd Foods' (Gerber)	7 tbsp	64	14	1.9
strained (Heinz)	3.5 oz	49	15	1.8
Beef and rice dinner				
toddler	6.25 oz	145	632	5.1
toddler	1 oz	23	101	0.8
Beef dinner				
junior (Gerber)	2.5 oz	80	38	4.0
'Stages 1' (Beech-Nut)	2.8 oz	90	40	5.0
'Stages 3' (Beech-Nut)	6 oz	150	45	8.0
supreme, 'Stages 2' (Beech-Nut)	4.5 oz	120	40	6.0
'3rd Foods' (Gerber)	7 tbsp	103	52	4.6
w/vegetables, lean meat, junior (Gerber)	4.5 oz	100	29	3.0
w/vegetables, lean meat, strained (Gerber)	4.5 oz	90	32	3.0
Beef lasagna dinner				
toddler	6.25 oz	136	804	3.7
toddler	1 oz	22	129	0.6
Beef noodle dinner				
junior	7.5 oz	121	36	4.1
junior	1 oz	16	5	0.5
strained	4.5 oz	68	37	2.2
strained	1 oz	15	8	0.5
Beef stew				
'Stages Table Time' (Beech-Nut)	6 oz	150	380	6.0
toddler	6.25 oz	90	611	2.1
toddler	1 oz	14	98	0.3
Beef vegetable dinner				
high-meat, junior	4.5 oz	109	42	5.9
high-meat, junior	1 oz	24	9	1.3
high-meat, strained	4.5 oz	96	46	5.4
high-meat, strained	1 oz	21	10	1.2

Food Name	Serv. Size	Total Cal.	Sod. MGS	Fat GMS
Beef vegetable entrée				
'Stages 2' *(Beech-Nut)*	4.5 oz	90	35	4.0
'Stages 3' *(Beech-Nut)*	6 oz	160	70	7.0
Broccoli-chicken dinner, 'Simple Recipe'				
'2nd Foods' *(Gerber)*	7 tbsp	42	20	1.5
Carrots and beef dinner, 'Simple Recipe'				
'2nd Foods' *(Gerber)*	7 tbsp	59	40	2.5
Chicken dinner				
junior *(Gerber)*	2.5 oz	110	28	7.0
'3rd Foods' *(Gerber)*	7 tbsp	132	39	7.9
vegetable entrée, 'Stages 2' *(Beech-Nut)*	4.5 oz	90	65	3.0
vegetable entrée, 'Stages 3' *(Beech-Nut)*	6 oz	90	70	2.0
w/vegetables, lean meat, junior *(Gerber)*	4.5 oz	90	32	3.0
w/vegetables, lean meat, strained *(Gerber)*	4.5 oz	90	31	3.0
Chicken noodle dinner				
junior	7.5 oz	109	36	3.0
junior	1 oz	14	5	0.4
'2nd Foods' *(Gerber)*	7 tbsp	55	14	1.2
strained	4.5 oz	67	20	1.9
strained	1 oz	15	5	0.4
'3rd Foods' *(Gerber)*	7 tbsp	56	14	1.3
Chicken rice dinner				
'Stages 2' *(Beech-Nut)*	4.5 oz	80	40	3.0
'Tropical Foods' *(Gerber)*	7 tbsp	48	14	1.3
Chicken stew dinner				
toddler	6 oz	133	683	6.3
toddler	1 oz	22	114	1.0
w/noodles, 'Graduates'	3.2 oz	69	308	2.0
Chicken vegetable dinner				
high-meat, junior	4.5 oz	118	33	7.0
high-meat, junior	1 oz	26	7	1.6
high-meat, strained	4.5 oz	100	35	4.6
high-meat, strained	1 oz	22	8	1.0
Green bean dinner, w/turkey, 'Simple Recipe'				
'2nd Foods' *(Gerber)*	7 tbsp	55	11	1.5
Ham dinner				
ham and vegetable entrée, 'Stages 2' *(Beech-Nut)*	4.5 oz	80	30	3.0
w/vegetables, lean meat, junior *(Gerber)*	4.5 oz	110	27	4.0
w/vegetables, lean meat, strained *(Gerber)*	4.5 oz	100	26	4.0
Ham vegetable dinner				
high-meat, junior	4.5 oz	99	28	4.2

Food Name	Serv. Size	Total Cal.	Sod. MGS	Fat GMS
high-meat, junior	1 oz	22	6	0.9
high-meat, strained	4.5 oz	97	28	4.5
high-meat, strained	1 oz	22	6	1.0
Lamb and vegetable entrée, 'Stages 2' (Beech-Nut)	4.5 oz	90	40	4.0
Lamb noodle dinner				
junior	7.5 oz	138	38	4.7
junior	1 oz	18	5	0.6
Macaroni dinner				
tomato beef, '2nd Foods' (Gerber)	7 tbsp	57	32	1.1
tomato beef, '3rd Foods' (Gerber)	7 tbsp	60	12	0.9
tomatoes and beef, junior (Heinz)	3.5 oz	52	14	1.2
w/bacon, junior	7.5 oz	160	166	7.0
w/bacon, junior	1 oz	21	22	0.9
w/beef, 'Stages 2' (Beech-Nut)	4.5 oz	90	40	4.0
w/beef, 'Stages 3' (Beech-Nut)	6 oz	160	85	8.0
w/cheese (Earth's Best)	4.5 oz	100	10	4.0
w/cheese, junior	7.5 oz	130	162	4.3
w/cheese, junior	1 oz	17	22	0.6
w/cheese, strained	4.5 oz	76	93	2.7
w/cheese, strained	1 oz	17	21	0.6
w/cheese, '2nd Foods' (Gerber)	7 tbsp	63	88	2.0
Macaroni main dish				
alphabets w/beef and tomato sauce, chunky (Gerber)	7 tbsp	80	199	2.0
w/beef, in sauce, 'Graduates' (Gerber)	3.2 oz	78	302	1.7
w/ham, junior	7.5 oz	128	100	3.0
w/ham, junior	1 oz	17	13	0.4
w/tomato and beef, junior	7.5 oz	126	36	2.3
w/tomato and beef, junior	1 oz	17	5	0.3
w/tomato and beef, strained	4.5 oz	70	22	1.4
w/tomato and beef, strained	1 oz	16	5	0.3
Mixed vegetable dinner				
junior	7.5 oz	70	19	0.0
junior	1 oz	9	3	0.0
strained	4.5 oz	52	10	0.1
strained	1 oz	12	2	0.0
Noodle main dish				
w/beef, chunky, 'Homestyle' (Gerber)	7 tbsp	88	216	3.5
w/chicken, carrots, and peas, chunky (Gerber)	7 tbsp	65	207	1.5
Pasta dinner (Earth's Best)	4.5 oz	90	20	3.0
Potato dinner, w/green beans (Earth's Best)	4.5 oz	100	25	3.0

Food Name	Serv. Size	Total Cal.	Sod. MGS	Fat GMS
Ravioli				
beef, w/tomato sauce, 'Graduates' *(Gerber)*	3.2 oz	97	322	2.0
beef, w/tomato sauce, 'Graduates' micro cup *(Gerber)*	6 oz	170	590	4.0
cheese, w/tomato sauce, 'Graduates' *(Gerber)*	3.2 oz	99	297	2.2
cheese, w/tomato sauce, 'Graduates' micro cup *(Gerber)*	6 oz	170	510	4.0
Rice and lentil dinner, *(Earth's Best)*	4.5 oz	80	25	2.0
Rice main dish				
saucy, w/chicken, chunky *(Gerber)*	7 tbsp	67	222	1.5
w/beef and tomato sauce, chunky *(Gerber)*	7 tbsp	79	202	1.9
Spaghetti				
rings, in meat sauce, 'Stages Table Time' *(Beech-Nut)*	6 oz	160	390	4.0
w/beef, 'Stages 3' *(Beech-Nut)*	6 oz	170	75	8.0
w/mini meatballs and sauce,'Graduates' *(Gerber)*	6 oz	160	590	5.0
w/mini meatballs and sauce, 'Graduates' *(Gerber)*	3.2 oz	91	300	2.8
w/tomato and meat, junior	7.5 oz	134	43	2.8
w/tomato and meat, junior	1 oz	18	6	0.4
w/tomato and meat, toddler	6.25 oz	133	634	1.8
w/tomato and meat, toddler	1 oz	21	101	0.3
w/tomato sauce and beef, chunky *(Gerber)*	7 tbsp	85	223	1.9
w/tomato sauce and beef, junior *(Gerber)*	6 oz	120	41	3.0
w/tomato sauce and beef, '3rd Foods' *(Gerber)*	7 tbsp	64	20	1.2
w/tomato sauce and meat, junior *(Heinz)*	3.5 oz	58	19	1.3
Split pea and ham dinner				
junior	7.5 oz	151	30	2.8
junior	1 oz	20	4	0.4
Sweet potato dinner, w/chicken *(Earth's Best)*	4.5 oz	90	30	2.0
Turkey dinner				
junior *(Gerber)*	2.5 oz	100	37	6.0
supreme, 'Stages 2' *(Beech-Nut)*	4.5 oz	120	35	6.0
Turkey rice dinner				
junior	7.5 oz	104	32	3.0
junior	1 oz	14	4	0.4
junior *(Gerber)*	6 oz	110	34	4.0
'2nd Foods' *(Gerber)*	7 tbsp	55	15	1.5
'Stages 2' *(Beech-Nut)*	4.5 oz	70	35	2.0
'Stages 3' *(Beech-Nut)*	6 oz	110	65	4.0
strained	4.5 oz	63	22	1.7
strained	1 oz	14	5	0.4
strained *(Gerber)*	4.5 oz	80	20	3.0
'3rd Foods' *(Gerber)*	7 tbsp	55	17	1.4
w/vegetables, junior *(Heinz)*	3.5 oz	42	20	0.6

Food Name	Serv. Size	Total Cal.	Sod. MGS	Fat GMS
w/vegetables, strained *(Heinz)*	3.5 oz	47	21	1.1
Turkey stew main dish, w/rice, 'Graduates' *(Gerber)*	3.2 oz	59	298	1.0
Turkey vegetable dinner				
high-meat, junior	4.5 oz	115	55	6.4
high-meat, junior	1 oz	26	12	1.4
high-meat, strained	4.5 oz	111	38	6.1
high-meat, strained	1 oz	25	9	1.4
lean meat, junior *(Gerber)*	4.5 oz	100	31	4.0
lean meat, strained *(Gerber)*	4.5 oz	100	31	4.0
Veal-vegetable dinner				
high-meat, junior	4.5 oz	93	32	4.0
high-meat, junior	1 oz	21	7	0.9
high-meat, strained	4.5 oz	88	31	3.5
high-meat, strained	1 oz	20	7	0.8
Vegetable bacon dinner				
junior	7.5 oz	151	96	8.3
junior	1 oz	20	13	1.1
'2nd Foods' *(Gerber)*	7 tbsp	73	49	3.3
strained	4.5 oz	88	55	4.2
'3rd Foods' *(Gerber)*	7 tbsp	77	52	3.4
Vegetable beef dinner				
(Earth's Best)	4.5 oz	90	15	3.0
junior	7.5 oz	113	51	3.6
junior	1 oz	15	7	0.5
'2nd Foods' *(Gerber)*	7 tbsp	65	11	2.4
strained	4.5 oz	68	27	2.6
strained	1 oz	15	6	0.6
'3rd Foods' *(Gerber)*	7 tbsp	62	16	1.6
Vegetable chicken dinner				
junior	7.5 oz	107	19	2.3
junior	1 oz	14	3	0.3
'2nd Foods' *(Gerber)*	7 tbsp	58	10	1.3
strained	4.5 oz	55	14	1.4
strained	1 oz	12	3	0.3
'3rd Foods' *(Gerber)*	7 tbsp	51	17	1.1
vegetable dinner, 'Summer' *(Earth's Best)*	4.5 oz	90	15	3.0
Vegetable dumpling dinner				
w/beef, junior	7.5 oz	102	111	1.7
w/beef, junior	1 oz	14	15	0.2
w/beef, junior *(Heinz)*	3.5 oz	47	16	1.2
w/beef, strained	4.5 oz	61	63	1.1

Food Name	Serv. Size	Total Cal.	Sod. MGS	Fat GMS
w/beef, strained	1 oz	14	14	0.3
w/beef, strained *(Heinz)*	3.5 oz	49	15	1.3
Vegetable ham dinner				
junior	7.5 oz	111	38	3.6
junior	1 oz	15	5	0.5
'2nd Foods' *(Gerber)*	7 tbsp	59	9	1.9
strained	4.5 oz	61	15	2.2
strained	1 oz	14	3	0.5
'3rd Foods' *(Gerber)*	7 tbsp	61	12	1.8
toddler	6.25 oz	127	531	5.3
toddler	1 oz	20	85	0.9
Vegetable lamb dinner				
junior	7.5 oz	109	28	3.6
junior	1 oz	14	4	0.5
strained	4.5 oz	67	26	2.6
strained	1 oz	15	6	0.6
Vegetable liver dinner				
junior	7.5 oz	94	28	1.3
junior	1 oz	12	4	0.2
strained	4.5 oz	50	23	0.5
strained	1 oz	11	5	0.1
Vegetable main dish				
w/beef, chunky *(Gerber)*	7 tbsp	70	201	2.0
w/chicken, chunky *(Gerber)*	7 tbsp	66	202	1.4
w/ham, chunky *(Gerber)*	7 tbsp	70	200	2.3
w/turkey, chunky *(Gerber)*	7 tbsp	61	190	4.4
Vegetable noodle dinner				
w/chicken, junior	7.5 oz	136	55	4.7
w/chicken, junior	1 oz	18	7	0.6
w/chicken, junior *(Heinz)*	3.5 oz	57	21	1.8
w/chicken, strained	4.5 oz	81	26	3.2
w/chicken, strained	1 oz	18	6	0.7
w/chicken, strained *(Heinz)*	3.5 oz	54	24	1.7
w/turkey, junior	7.5 oz	111	36	3.2
w/turkey, junior	1 oz	15	5	0.4
w/turkey, junior *(Heinz)*	3.5 oz	48	21	2.0
w/turkey, strained	4.5 oz	56	27	1.5
w/turkey, strained	1 oz	12	6	0.3
w/turkey, strained *(Heinz)*	3.5 oz	47	22	1.6
Vegetable stew				
w/beef, 'Graduates' *(Gerber)*	3.2 oz	71	290	1.4

Food Name	Serv. Size	Total Cal.	Sod. MGS	Fat GMS
w/beef, 'Graduates' micro cup *(Gerber)*	6 oz	130	500	3.0
w/chicken, 'Stages Table Time' *(Beech-Nut)*	6 oz	190	340	8.0
Vegetable turkey dinner				
(Earth's Best)	4.5 oz	60	15	1.0
junior	7.5 oz	100	36	2.6
junior	1 oz	13	5	0.3
'2nd Foods' *(Gerber)*	7 tbsp	49	12	1.2
'3rd Foods' *(Gerber)*	7 tbsp	53	13	1.0
strained	4.5 oz	54	17	1.5
strained	1 oz	12	4	0.3
toddler	6.25 oz	142	591	6.0
toddler	1 oz	23	95	1.0
EGG YOLK				
'2nd Foods' *(Gerber)*	7 tbsp	193	42	16.8
strained	3.3 oz	191	37	16.3
strained	1 oz	58	11	4.9
FRUIT				
Apple *(Earth's Best)*	4.5 oz	60	5	1.0
Apple, peach, and strawberry, 'Stages 2' *(Beech-Nut)*	4.5 oz	100	0	0.0
Apple, pear, and banana, 'Stages 2' *(Beech-Nut)*	4.5 oz	100	0	0.0
Apple and apricot				
(Earth's Best)	4.5 oz	70	5	1.0
strained *(Heinz)*	3.5 oz	55	3	0.3
Apple and banana				
(Earth's Best)	4.5 oz	80	15	1.0
'2nd Foods' *(Gerber)*	4 oz	60	na	0.0
Apple and blueberry				
(Earth's Best)	4.5 oz	60	na	1.0
junior	7.75 oz	136	29	0.4
junior	1 oz	18	4	0.1
junior *(Gerber)*	6 oz	80	2	1.0
'2nd Foods' *(Gerber)*	7 tbsp	51	0	0.2
strained	4.75 oz	82	3	0.3
strained	1 oz	17	1	0.1
strained *(Gerber)*	4.5 oz	60	1	1.0
'3rd Foods' *(Gerber)*	7 tbsp	50	1	0.2
Apple and cranberry, w/tapioca, strained *(Heinz)*	3.5 oz	66	6	0.3
Apple and pear				
(Heinz)	3.5 oz	56	2	0.2
junior	3.5 oz	57	1	0.2
Apple and plum *(Earth's Best)*	4.5 oz	70	10	1.0

Food Name	Serv. Size	Total Cal.	Sod. MGS	Fat GMS
Apple and raspberry				
w/sugar, junior	7.75 oz	128	4	0.4
w/sugar, junior	1 oz	16	1	0.1
w/sugar, strained	4.75 oz	78	3	0.3
w/sugar, strained	1 oz	16	1	0.1
Applesauce				
'Beginner Foods' (Heinz)	3.5 oz	73	1	0.1
'1st Foods' (Gerber)	2.5 oz	35	0	0.0
'1st Foods' (Gerber)	7 tbsp	56	0	0.2
golden delicious, 'Baby's First' (Beech-Nut)	2.5 oz	50	0	0.0
golden delicious, 'Stages 1' (Beech-Nut)	4.5 oz	70	0	0.0
golden delicious, 'Stages 1' (Beech-Nut)	2.8 oz	50	0	0.0
junior	7.5 oz	79	4	0.0
junior	1 oz	10	1	0.0
junior (Gerber)	6 oz	90	3	1.0
junior (Heinz)	3.5 oz	53	2	0.2
'2nd Foods' (Gerber)	7 tbsp	52	22	0.2
'Stages 3' (Beech-Nut)	6 oz	90	0	0.0
strained	4.5 oz	52	3	0.3
strained	1 oz	12	1	0.1
strained (Gerber)	4.5 oz	60	3	1.0
strained (Heinz)	3.5 oz	53	2	0.2
'3rd Foods' (Gerber)	7 tbsp	51	1	0.2
w/apricot, junior	7.75 oz	103	7	0.4
w/apricot, junior	1 oz	13	1	0.1
w/apricot, '2nd Foods' (Gerber)	7 tbsp	53	1	0.2
w/apricot, 'Stages 2' (Beech-Nut)	4.5 oz	80	0	0.0
w/apricot, strained	4.75 oz	61	4	0.3
w/apricot, strained	1 oz	13	1	0.1
w/apricot, strained (Gerber)	4.5 oz	70	3	1.0
w/banana, 'Stages 2' (Beech-Nut)	4.5 oz	80	0	0.0
w/banana, 'Stages 3' (Beech-Nut)	6 oz	100	0	0.0
w/cherry, junior	7.75 oz	106	7	0.0
w/cherry, junior	1 oz	14	1	0.0
w/cherry, 'Stages 2' (Beech-Nut)	4.5 oz	70	5	0.0
w/cherry, 'Stages 3' (Beech-Nut)	6 oz	100	0	0.0
w/cherry, strained	4.75 oz	65	3	0.0
w/cherry, strained	1 oz	14	1	0.0
w/pineapple, junior	7.5 oz	83	4	0.2
w/pineapple, junior	1 oz	11	1	0.0
w/pineapple, strained	4.5 oz	47	3	0.1

Food Name	Serv. Size	Total Cal.	Sod. MGS	Fat GMS
w/pineapple, strained	1 oz	10	1	0.0
Apricot				
w/pear, 'Stages 3' (Beech-Nut)	6 oz	120	0	0.0
w/pear and applesauce, 'Stages 2' (Beech-Nut)	4.5 oz	90	0	0.0
w/tapioca, junior	7.75 oz	139	13	0.0
w/tapioca, junior	1 oz	18	2	0.0
w/tapioca, junior (Gerber)	6 oz	130	9	1.0
w/tapioca, junior (Heinz)	3.5 oz	66	10	0.2
w/tapioca, '2nd Foods' (Gerber)	7 tbsp	67	6	0.2
w/tapioca, strained	4.75 oz	81	11	0.0
w/tapioca, strained	1 oz	17	2	0.0
w/tapioca, strained (Gerber)	4.5 oz	90	8	1.0
w/tapioca, strained (Heinz)	3.5 oz	64	7	0.2
w/tapioca, '3rd Foods' (Gerber)	7 tbsp	71	5	0.2
Banana				
'Beginner Foods' (Heinz)	3.5 oz	107	3	0.2
Chiquita, 'Baby's First' (Beech-Nut)	2.5 oz	70	0	0.0
Chiquita, 'Stages 1' (Beech-Nut)	4.5 oz	110	0	0.0
Chiquita, 'Stages 1' (Beech-Nut)	2.8 oz	70	0	0.0
(Earth's Best)	4.5 oz	100	60	0.0
'1st Foods' (Gerber)	2.5 oz	70	na	0.0
'1st Foods' (Gerber)	7 tbsp	100	3	0.3
w/pineapple and tapioca, '2nd Foods' (Gerber)	7 tbsp	52	na	0.1
w/pineapple and tapioca, '3rd Foods' (Gerber)	7 tbsp	52	4	0.1
w/tapioca, junior	7.75 oz	147	20	0.4
w/tapioca, junior	1 oz	19	3	0.1
w/tapioca, junior (Gerber)	6 oz	140	15	1.0
w/tapioca, junior (Heinz)	3.5 oz	73	8	0.2
w/tapioca, '2nd Foods' (Gerber)	7 tbsp	78	5	0.2
w/tapioca, '3rd Foods' (Gerber)	7 tbsp	77	5	0.2
w/tapioca, strained	4.75 oz	77	12	0.1
w/tapioca, strained	1 oz	16	3	0.0
w/tapioca, strained (Gerber)	4.5 oz	110	12	1.0
w/tapioca, strained (Heinz)	3.5 oz	73	8	0.2
Banana and apple, strained (Gerber)	4.5 oz	90	9	1.0
Banana and pear, w/applesauce, 'Stages 2' (Beech-Nut)	4.5 oz	100	0	0.0
Banana and pineapple				
'Stages 2' (Beech-Nut)	4.5 oz	110	15	0.0
w/tapioca, junior	4.75 oz	92	11	0.1
w/tapioca, junior	1 oz	19	2	0.0
w/tapioca, junior (Gerber)	6 oz	90	7	1.0

Food Name	Serv. Size	Total Cal.	Sod. MGS	Fat GMS
w/tapioca, strained	7.75 oz	143	13	0.0
w/tapioca, strained	1 oz	18	2	0.0
w/tapioca, strained *(Gerber)*	4.5 oz	60	5	0.0
w/tapioca, strained *(Heinz)*	3.5 oz	64	8	0.2
Guava				
w/tapioca, strained	4.5 oz	86	3	0.0
w/tapioca, strained	1 oz	19	1	0.0
w/tapioca, strained *(Gerber)*	4.5 oz	90	3	1.0
w/tapioca, strained, 'Stages 2' *(Beech-Nut)*	4.5 oz	100	10	0.0
Guava and papaya				
w/tapioca, strained	4.5 oz	81	5	0.1
w/tapioca, strained	1 oz	18	1	0.0
Mango				
tropical fruit dessert, 'Stages 2' *(Beech-Nut)*	4.5 oz	100	15	0.0
w/tapioca, strained	4.75 oz	108	5	0.3
w/tapioca, strained	1 oz	23	1	0.1
w/tapioca, strained *(Gerber)*	4.5 oz	90	4	1.0
Mango and banana, w/passion fruit and tapioca,				
strained *(Gerber)*	4.5 oz	100	12	0.0
Papaya				
'Stages 2' *(Beech-Nut)*	4.5 oz	100	15	0.0
w/tapioca, strained *(Gerber)*	4.5 oz	80	9	1.0
Papaya and applesauce				
w/tapioca, strained	4.5 oz	90	6	0.1
w/tapioca, strained	1 oz	20	1	0.0
Peach				
'Beginner Foods' *(Heinz)*	3.5 oz	80	2	0.2
'1st Foods' *(Gerber)*	2.5 oz	30	na	0.0
'1st Foods' *(Gerber)*	7 tbsp	43	1	0.2
junior *(Gerber)*	6 oz	110	5	1.0
junior *(Heinz)*	3.5 oz	68	7	0.3
'2nd Foods' *(Gerber)*	7 tbsp	66	3	0.2
'Stages 3' *(Beech-Nut)*	6 oz	90	0	0.0
strained *(Gerber)*	4.5 oz	90	4	1.0
strained *(Heinz)*	3.5 oz	68	7	0.3
'3rd Foods' *(Gerber)*	7 tbsp	65	2	0.2
w/mango and tapioca, strained *(Gerber)*	4.5 oz	100	9	1.0
w/oatmeal and banana *(Earth's Best)*	4.5 oz	70	5	1.0
w/sugar, junior	7.75 oz	156	11	0.4
w/sugar, junior	1 oz	20	1	0.1
w/sugar, strained	4.75 oz	96	8	0.3

Food Name	Serv. Size	Total Cal.	Sod. MGS	Fat GMS
w/sugar, strained	1 oz	20	2	0.1
w/yogurt, 'Stages 2' (Beech-Nut)	4.5 oz	120	30	2.0
yellow cling, 'Baby's First' (Beech-Nut)	2.5 oz	45	0	0.0
yellow cling, 'Stages 1' (Beech-Nut)	4.5 oz	70	0	0.0
yellow cling, 'Stages 1' (Beech-Nut)	2.8 oz	50	0	0.0
Pear				
Bartlett, 'Baby's First' (Beech-Nut)	2.5 oz	50	0	0.0
Bartlett, 'Stages 1' (Beech-Nut)	4.5 oz	70	0	0.0
Bartlett, 'Stages 1' (Beech-Nut)	2.8 oz	50	0	0.0
Bartlett, 'Stages 3' (Beech-Nut)	6 oz	100	5	0.0
Bartlett, w/applesauce, 'Stages 2' (Beech-Nut)	4.5 oz	80	0	0.0
Bartlett, w/pineapple, 'Stages 2' (Beech-Nut)	4.5 oz	90	0	0.0
'Beginner Foods' (Heinz)	3.5 oz	76	3	0.2
(Earth's Best)	4.5 oz	60	11	0.0
'1st Foods' (Gerber)	2.5 oz	40	2	0.0
'1st Foods' (Gerber)	7 tbsp	57	1	0.3
junior	7.5 oz	92	4	0.2
junior	1 oz	12	1	0.0
junior (Gerber)	6 oz	100	2	1.0
junior (Heinz)	3.5 oz	60	3	0.2
'2nd Foods' (Gerber)	7 tbsp	55	0	0.2
strained	4.5 oz	52	3	0.3
strained	1 oz	12	1	0.1
strained (Gerber)	4.5 oz	80	3	1.0
strained (Heinz)	3.5 oz	60	3	0.2
'3rd Foods' (Gerber)	7 tbsp	55	2	0.2
Pear and pineapple				
junior	7.5 oz	94	2	0.4
junior	1 oz	12	0	0.1
junior (Gerber)	6 oz	100	3	1.0
'2nd Foods' (Gerber)	7 tbsp	55	1	0.2
strained	4.5 oz	52	5	0.1
strained	1 oz	12	1	0.0
strained (Gerber)	4.5 oz	80	3	1.0
'3rd Foods' (Gerber)	7 tbsp	54	2	0.2
Pears and raspberries (Earth's Best)	4.5 oz	60	0	0.0
Plum				
w/banana and rice (Earth's Best)	4.5 oz	90	15	0.0
w/rice, 'Stages 2' (Beech-Nut)	4.5 oz	150	0	0.0
w/tapioca, junior (Gerber)	6 oz	130	3	1.0
w/tapioca, '2nd Foods' (Gerber)	7 tbsp	74	3	0.2

Food Name	Serv. Size	Total Cal.	Sod. MGS	Fat GMS
w/tapioca, strained *(Gerber)*	4.5 oz	90	5	0.0
w/tapioca, strained *(Heinz)*	3.5 oz	67	9	0.2
w/tapioca, '3rd Foods' *(Gerber)*	7 tbsp	75	2	0.2
w/tapioca, w/o ascorbic acid, junior	7.75 oz	163	18	0.0
w/tapioca, w/o ascorbic acid, junior	1 oz	21	2	0.0
w/tapioca, w/o ascorbic acid, strained	4.75 oz	96	8	0.0
w/tapioca, w/o ascorbic acid, strained	1 oz	20	2	0.0
Prune				
'1st Foods' *(Gerber)*	2.5 oz	70	na	0.0
'1st Foods' *(Gerber)*	7 tbsp	101	6	0.2
w/oatmeal *(Earth's Best)*	4.5 oz	100	20	0.0
w/pear, 'Stages 2' *(Beech-Nut)*	4.5 oz	90	0	0.0
w/tapioca, '2nd Foods' *(Gerber)*	7 tbsp	77	4	0.2
w/tapioca, strained *(Gerber)*	4.5 oz	100	5	1.0
w/tapioca, strained *(Heinz)*	3.5 oz	90	8	0.2
w/tapioca, w/o ascorbic acid, junior	7.75 oz	154	4	0.2
w/tapioca, w/o ascorbic acid, junior	1 oz	20	1	0.0
w/tapioca, w/o ascorbic acid, strained	4.75 oz	94	7	0.1
w/tapioca, w/o ascorbic acid, strained	1 oz	20	1	0.0
INFANT FORMULA				
Mix				
liquid, iron-fortified, prepared, 'Follow-Up' *(Carnation)*	5 oz	100	39	4.1
liquid, iron-fortified, prepared, 'Good Start' *(Carnation)*	5 oz	100	24	5.1
liquid, low-iron, prepared *(Enfamil)*	5 oz	100	27	5.6
liquid, low-iron, prepared *(Gerber)*	5 oz	100	47	5.3
liquid, low-iron, prepared *(Similac)*	5 oz	100	27	5.4
liquid, soy, iron-fortified, milk-free *(Nursoy)*	5 oz	100	30	5.3
liquid, soy, iron-fortified, milk-free, prepared *(Gerber)*	5 oz	100	47	5.3
liquid, soy, iron-fortified, milk-free, prepared *(ProSobee)*	5 oz	100	36	5.3
liquid, soy, w/iron, milk-free, prepared *(Isomil)*	5 oz	100	44	5.4
liquid, w/iron, prepared *(Enfamil)*	5 oz	100	27	5.6
liquid, w/iron, prepared *(Gerber)*	5 oz	100	33	5.4
liquid, w/iron, prepared *(Similac)*	5 oz	100	27	5.4
powder, iron-fortified, prepared, 'Follow-Up' *(Carnation)*	5 oz	100	39	4.1
powder, iron-fortified, prepared, 'Good Start' *(Carnation)*	5 oz	100	24	5.1
powder, low-iron, prepared *(Enfamil)*	5 oz	100	27	5.6
powder, low-iron, prepared *(Gerber)*	5 oz	100	47	5.3
powder, low-iron, prepared *(Similac)*	5 oz	100	27	5.4
powder, soy, iron-fortified, milk-free, prepared *(Gerber)*	5 oz	100	47	5.3
powder, soy, iron-fortified, milk-free, prepared *(ProSobee)*	5 oz	100	36	5.3
powder, soy, w/iron, milk-free, prepared *(Isomil)*	5 oz	100	44	5.5

Food Name	Serv. Size	Total Cal.	Sod. MGS	Fat GMS
powder, w/iron, prepared *(Enfamil)*	5 oz	100	27	5.6
powder, w/iron, prepared *(Gerber)*	5 oz	100	33	5.4
powder, w/iron, prepared *(Similac)*	5 oz	100	27	5.4
Ready to use				
iron-fortified, 'Follow-Up' *(Carnation)*	5 oz	100	39	4.1
iron-fortified, 'Good Start' *(Carnation)*	5 oz	100	24	5.1
low-iron *(Enfamil)*	5 oz	100	27	5.6
low-iron *(Gerber)*	5 oz	100	47	5.3
low-iron *(Similac)*	5 oz	100	27	5.4
soy, iron-fortified, milk-free *(Gerber)*	5 oz	100	47	5.3
soy, iron-fortified, milk-free *(ProSobee)*	5 oz	100	36	5.3
soy, w/iron, milk-free *(Isomil)*	5 oz	100	44	5.4
w/iron *(Enfamil)*	5 oz	100	27	5.6
w/iron *(Gerber)*	5 oz	100	33	5.4
w/iron *(Similac)*	5 oz	100	27	5.4
JUICE				
Apple				
	4.2 oz	61	4	0.1
	1 oz	15	1	0.0
(Earth's Best)	4.2 oz	60	20	0.0
'Graduates' *(Gerber)*	6 oz	80	0	0.0
'Graduates' *(Gerber)*	3.2 oz	48	2	0.1
100% juice, 'Junior' *(McCain)*	4.2 oz	50	5	0.0
'Stages 1' *(Beech-Nut)*	4.2 oz	60	5	0.0
strained, '1st Foods' *(Gerber)*	4 oz	60	2	0.0
strained, '1st Foods' *(Gerber)*	3.2 oz	46	1	0.1
strained *(Heinz)*	3.5 oz	48	5	0.2
strained, 'Saver Size' *(Heinz)*	4.2 oz	70	15	0.0
w/yogurt, 2nd Foods' *(Gerber)*	3.2 oz	73	32	0.9
Apple-apricot, strained *(Heinz)*	3.5 oz	47	8	0.2
Apple-banana				
(Earth's Best)	4.2 oz	60	2	0.0
'Graduates' *(Gerber)*	6 oz	90	10	0.0
'Graduates' *(Gerber)*	3.2 oz	51	2	0.1
'2nd Foods' *(Gerber)*	3.2 oz	51	2	0.1
strained *(Heinz)*	3.5 oz	52	6	0.2
Apple-carrot				
'3rd Foods' *(Gerber)*	4 oz	50	15	0.0
'3rd Foods' *(Gerber)*	3.2 oz	42	10	0.1
Apple-cherry				
	4.2 oz	53	4	0.3

Food Name	Serv. Size	Total Cal.	Sod. MGS	Fat GMS
.... 1 oz	13	1	0.1
'Graduates' *(Gerber)* .... 6 oz	80	25	0.0
'Graduates' *(Gerber)* .... 3.2 oz	51	3	0.1
100% juice, 'Junior' *(McCain)* .... 4.2 oz	50	5	0.0
'2nd Foods' *(Gerber)* .... 4 oz	60	na	0.0
'2nd Foods' *(Gerber)* .... 3.2 oz	48	5	0.1
'Stages 2' *(Beech-Nut)* .... 4 oz	60	5	0.0
strained *(Heinz)* .... 3.5 oz	45	7	0.2
Apple-cranberry			
'Stages 2' *(Beech-Nut)* .... 4 oz	60	5	0.0
strained *(Heinz)* .... 3.5 oz	48	7	0.2
Apple-grape			
.... 4.2 oz	60	4	0.3
.... 1 oz	14	1	0.1
(Earth's Best) .... 4.2 oz	60	15	0.0
'Graduates' *(Gerber)* .... 6 oz	90	40	0.0
'Graduates' *(Gerber)* .... 3.2 oz	51	3	0.1
'2nd Foods' *(Gerber)* .... 4 oz	60	na	0.0
'2nd Foods' *(Gerber)* .... 3.2 oz	48	7	0.1
'Stages 2' *(Beech-Nut)* .... 4 oz	70	15	0.0
strained *(Heinz)* .... 3.5 oz	47	7	0.2
Apple-peach			
.... 4.2 oz	55	1	0.1
.... 1 oz	13	0	0.0
'2nd Foods' *(Gerber)* .... 3.2 oz	47	5	0.1
'2nd Foods' *(Gerber)* .... 4 oz	60	na	0.0
strained *(Heinz)* .... 3.5 oz	44	7	0.2
Apple-pineapple, strained *(Heinz)* .... 3.5 oz	47	6	0.2
Apple-plum			
.... 4.2 oz	64	1	0.0
.... 1 oz	15	0	0.0
'2nd Foods' *(Gerber)* .... 4 oz	60	na	0.0
'2nd Foods' *(Gerber)* .... 3.2 oz	48	8	0.1
Apple-prune			
.... 4.2 oz	95	7	0.1
.... 1 oz	23	2	0.0
'2nd Foods' *(Gerber)* .... 4 oz	60	na	0.0
'2nd Foods' *(Gerber)* .... 3.2 oz	53	4	0.1
strained *(Heinz)* .... 3.5 oz	50	7	0.2
Apple-sweet potato, '3rd Foods' *(Gerber)* ...... 3.2 oz	48	5	0.1

ood Name	Serv. Size	Total Cal.	Sod. MGS	Fat GMS
Banana				
w/yogurt, '2nd Foods' *(Gerber)*	4 oz	110	na	2.0
w/yogurt, '2nd Foods' *(Gerber)*	3.2 oz	84	37	1.0
Grape				
'Juice Plus,' 'Stages 2' *(Beech-Nut)*	4 oz	90	10	0.0
red, '1st Foods' *(Gerber)*	4 oz	80	na	0.0
red, '1st Foods' *(Gerber)*	3.2 oz	65	5	0.1
white, '1st Foods' *(Gerber)*	4 oz	80	na	0.0
white, '1st Foods' *(Gerber)*	3.2 oz	65	6	0.1
white, 'Stages 1' *(Beech-Nut)*	4.2 oz	80	10	0.0
white, strained *(Heinz)*	3.5 oz	58	6	0.2
Guava, w/mixed fruit 'Tropical Foods' *(Gerber)*	3.2 oz	58	6	0.1
Mango, w/mixed fruit 'Tropical Foods' *(Gerber)*	3.2 oz	59	5	0.1
Mango nectar, w/grape and pear juice				
'Stages 2' *(Beech-Nut)*	4 oz	80	5	0.0
Mixed fruit				
	4.2 oz	61	5	0.1
	1 oz	15	1	0.0
100% juice, 'Junior' *(McCain)*	4.2 oz	60	5	0.0
'2nd Foods' *(Gerber)*	4 oz	60	na	0.0
'2nd Foods' *(Gerber)*	3.2 oz	49	4	0.1
'Stages 2' *(Beech-Nut)*	4 oz	70	10	0.0
strained *(Heinz)*	3.5 oz	50	6	0.2
w/yogurt, '2nd Foods' *(Gerber)*	4 oz	100	na	2.0
w/yogurt, '2nd Foods' *(Gerber)*	3.2 oz	75	36	0.9
Orange				
	4.2 oz	57	1	0.4
	1 oz	14	0	0.1
'2nd Foods' *(Gerber)*	4 oz	60	na	0.0
'2nd Foods' *(Gerber)*	3.2 oz	46	2	0.3
'Stages 3' *(Beech-Nut)*	4 oz	60	0	0.0
strained *(Heinz)*	3.5 oz	48	5	0.3
Orange-apple				
	4.2 oz	56	4	0.3
	1 oz	13	1	0.1
strained *(Heinz)*	3.5 oz	50	8	0.3
w/banana	4.2 oz	61	5	0.1
w/banana	1 oz	15	1	0.0
Orange-apricot				
	4.2 oz	60	8	0.1
	1 oz	14	2	0.0

Food Name	Serv. Size	Total Cal.	Sod. MGS	Fat GMS
Orange-banana				
....	4.2 oz	65	4	0.1
....	1 oz	15	1	0.0
Orange-carrot, '3rd Foods' (Gerber)	3.2 oz	43	10	0.1
Orange-pineapple				
....	4.2 oz	62	3	0.1
....	1 oz	15	1	0.0
Papaya, w/mixed fruit, 'Tropical Foods' (Gerber)	3.2 oz	57	5	0.2
Papaya nectar, w/pear and grape juice, 'Stages 2' (Beech-Nut)	4 oz	70	10	0.0
Peach nectar, w/pear and grape juice, 'Stages 2' (Beech-Nut)	4 oz	70	10	0.0
Pear				
(Earth's Best)	4.2 oz	60	0	0.0
'Stages 1' (Beech-Nut)	4 oz	60	5	0.0
strained (Heinz)	3.5 oz	49	9	0.2
strained, '1st Foods' (Gerber)	4 oz	60	6	0.0
strained, '1st Foods' (Gerber)	3.2 oz	46	1	0.1
strained, 'Saver Size' (Heinz)	4.2 oz	70	25	1.0
Pear-grape, strained (Heinz)	3.5 oz	43	4	0.1
Pear-peach				
w/yogurt, '2nd Foods' (Gerber)	4 oz	90	na	1.0
w/yogurt, '2nd Foods' (Gerber)	3.2 oz	72	34	0.9
Pineapple-carrot				
'3rd Foods' (Gerber)	4 oz	60	15	0.0
'3rd Foods' (Gerber)	3.2 oz	47	10	0.1
Prune-orange				
....	4.2 oz	91	3	0.4
....	1 oz	22	1	0.1
Tropical blend, 'Stages 2' (Beech-Nut)	4 oz	70	5	0.0
Tropical blend nectar, 'Stages 2' (Beech-Nut)	4 oz	90	10	0.0
MEAT				
Beef				
junior	3.5 oz	105	65	4.8
junior	1 oz	30	19	1.4
'2nd Foods' (Gerber)	7 tbsp	100	52	4.7
strained	3.5 oz	106	80	5.3
strained	1 oz	30	23	1.5
'3rd Foods' (Gerber)	7 tbsp	103	52	4.6
w/beef heart, strained	3.5 oz	93	62	4.4
w/beef heart, strained	1 oz	27	18	1.3

Food Name	Serv. Size	Total Cal.	Sod. MGS	Fat GMS
w/broth, junior *(Heinz)*	3.5 oz	123	53	7.2
w/broth, 'Stages 1' *(Beech-Nut)*	2.5 oz	80	40	5.0
w/broth, strained *(Heinz)*	3.5 oz	123	53	7.2
w/egg yolks, strained *(Gerber)*	2.5 oz	80	38	4.0
Chicken				
junior	3.5 oz	148	50	9.5
junior	1 oz	42	14	2.7
'2nd Foods' *(Gerber)*	7 tbsp	128	40	7.9
'Stages 1' *(Beech-Nut)*	2.8 oz	80	55	4.0
strained	3.5 oz	129	47	7.8
strained	1 oz	37	13	2.2
'3rd Foods' *(Gerber)*	7 tbsp	132	39	7.9
w/broth, junior *(Heinz)*	3.5 oz	143	59	9.7
w/broth, 'Stages 1' *(Beech-Nut)*	2.5 oz	70	55	4.0
w/broth, strained *(Heinz)*	3.5 oz	143	59	9.7
Chicken sticks				
finger snacks, 'Graduates' *(Gerber)*	10 sticks	143	445	8.3
junior	1 stick	19	48	1.4
Ham				
junior	3.5 oz	124	66	6.6
junior	1 oz	35	19	1.9
junior *(Gerber)*	2.5 oz	90	30	5.0
'2nd Foods' *(Gerber)*	7 tbsp	120	42	7.1
strained	3.5 oz	110	41	5.7
strained	1 oz	31	12	1.6
'3rd Foods' *(Gerber)*	7 tbsp	123	42	7.2
w/egg yolks, strained *(Gerber)*	2.5 oz	90	30	5.0
Lamb				
junior	3.5 oz	111	72	5.2
junior	1 oz	32	21	1.5
'2nd Foods' *(Gerber)*	7 tbsp	104	51	4.8
'Stages 1' *(Beech-Nut)*	2.8 oz	70	50	3.0
strained	3.5 oz	102	61	4.7
strained	1 oz	29	18	1.3
w/broth, 'Stages 1' *(Beech-Nut)*	2.5 oz	60	50	3.0
w/broth, strained *(Heinz)*	3.5 oz	129	59	7.6
w/egg yolks, strained *(Gerber)*	2.5 oz	70	36	3.0
Liver				
strained	3.5 oz	100	73	3.8
strained	1 oz	29	21	1.1
w/liver broth, strained *(Heinz)*	3.5 oz	100	49	3.2

Food Name	Serv. Size	Total Cal.	Sod. MGS	Fat GMS
Meat sticks				
finger snacks, 'Graduates' *(Gerber)*	10 sticks	150	451	9.6
junior	1 stick	18	55	1.5
Pork				
strained	3.5 oz	123	42	7.0
strained	1 oz	35	12	2.0
Turkey				
junior	3.5 oz	128	71	7.0
junior	1 oz	37	20	2.0
'2nd Foods' *(Gerber)*	7 tbsp	109	54	5.9
'Stages 1' *(Beech-Nut)*	2.8 oz	100	50	6.0
strained	3.5 oz	113	54	5.7
strained	1 oz	32	16	1.6
'3rd Foods' *(Gerber)*	7 tbsp	115	52	6.1
w/broth, 'Stages 1' *(Beech-Nut)*	2.5 oz	90	40	6.0
w/broth, strained *(Heinz)*	3.5 oz	137	49	8.6
w/egg yolks, strained *(Gerber)*	2.5 oz	100	38	6.0
Turkey sticks				
finger snacks, 'Graduates' *(Gerber)*	10 sticks	141	425	8.5
junior	1 stick	18	48	1.4
Veal				
junior	3.5 oz	109	68	4.9
junior	1 oz	31	20	1.4
junior *(Gerber)*	2.5 oz	80	39	4.0
'2nd Foods' *(Gerber)*	7 tbsp	102	55	5.1
'Stages 1' *(Beech-Nut)*	2.8 oz	60	50	2.0
strained	3.5 oz	100	63	4.8
strained	1 oz	29	18	1.4
'3rd Foods' *(Gerber)*	7 tbsp	108	56	5.0
w/broth, 'Stages 1' *(Beech-Nut)*	2.5 oz	70	50	3.0
w/broth, strained *(Heinz)*	3.5 oz	130	57	7.9
w/egg yolks, strained *(Gerber)*	2.5 oz	80	38	4.0
Veal and beef				
junior *(Gerber)*	6 oz	110	31	3.0
strained *(Gerber)*	4.5 oz	90	17	4.0
Veal and ham				
junior *(Gerber)*	6 oz	120	24	4.0
strained *(Gerber)*	4.5 oz	80	14	3.0
Veal and turkey				
junior *(Gerber)*	6 oz	100	24	3.0
strained *(Gerber)*	4.5 oz	70	17	2.0

Food Name	Serv. Size	Total Cal.	Sod. MGS	Fat GMS
SOUP				
Chicken				
hearty, w/stars, 'Stages Table Time' (Beech-Nut)	6 oz	180	350	9.0
strained	4.5 oz	64	20	2.2
strained	1 oz	14	5	0.5
strained (Heinz)	3.5 oz	49	20	1.7
Cream of broccoli, '3rd Foods' (Gerber)	3.2 oz	26	83	1.1
Cream of chicken				
strained	4.5 oz	74	24	2.0
strained	1 oz	16	5	0.5
Cream of potato, '3rd Foods' (Gerber)	3.2 oz	33	69	0.8
Cream of tomato, '3rd Foods' (Gerber)	3.2 oz	41	73	0.7
Cream of vegetable, '3rd Foods' (Gerber)	3.2 oz	29	48	0.8
VEGETABLES				
Beet				
'2nd Foods' (Gerber)	7 tbsp	39	91	0.2
strained	4.5 oz	44	106	0.1
strained	1 oz	10	24	0.0
strained (Gerber)	4.5 oz	60	115	1.0
strained (Heinz)	3.5 oz	40	34	0.2
Broccoli, carrot, and cheese, '3rd Foods' (Gerber)	7 tbsp	44	46	1.0
Carrot				
(Earth's Best)	4.5 oz	40	70	1.0
'Beginner Foods' (Heinz)	3.5 oz	30	32	0.3
buttered, junior	7.5 oz	70	34	1.3
buttered, junior	1 oz	9	5	0.2
buttered, strained	4.5 oz	46	23	0.8
buttered, strained	1 oz	10	5	0.2
diced, 'Graduates' (Gerber)	3.2 oz	22	26	0.1
'1st Foods' (Gerber)	2.5 oz	25	na	0.0
'1st Foods' (Gerber)	7 tbsp	34	78	0.3
junior	7.5 oz	68	104	0.4
junior	1 oz	9	14	0.1
junior (Gerber)	6 oz	80	83	1.0
junior (Heinz)	3.5 oz	23	44	0.2
'Regal Imperial,' 'Baby's First' (Beech-Nut)	2.5 oz	25	80	0.0
'Regal Imperial,' 'Stages 1' (Beech-Nut)	4.5 oz	40	130	0.0
'Regal Imperial,' 'Stages 1' (Beech-Nut)	2.8 oz	30	80	0.0
'2nd Foods' (Gerber)	7 tbsp	30	40	0.2
'Stages 3' (Beech-Nut)	6 oz	60	170	0.0
strained	4.5 oz	35	47	0.1

Food Name	Serv. Size	Total Cal.	Sod. MGS	Fat GMS
strained	1 oz	8	10	0.0
strained (Gerber)	4.5 oz	35	46	0.0
strained (Heinz)	3.5 oz	23	44	0.2
'3rd Foods' (Gerber)	7 tbsp	29	49	0.2
Carrot and parsnip (Earth's Best)	4.5 oz	60	30	0.0
Corn, creamed				
junior	7.5 oz	138	111	0.9
junior	1 oz	18	15	0.1
junior (Heinz)	3.5 oz	65	14	0.5
'2nd Foods' (Gerber)	7 tbsp	62	8	0.5
'Stages 2' (Beech-Nut)	4.5 oz	100	25	1.0
strained	4.5 oz	73	55	0.5
strained	1 oz	16	12	0.1
strained (Gerber)	4.5 oz	80	12	1.0
strained (Heinz)	3.5 oz	63	16	0.4
Garden vegetable				
(Earth's Best)	4.5 oz	70	15	0.0
'2nd Foods' (Gerber)	7 tbsp	39	20	0.4
'Stages 2' (Beech-Nut)	4.5 oz	60	35	0.0
strained	4.5 oz	47	45	0.3
strained	1 oz	10	10	0.1
strained (Gerber)	4.5 oz	50	26	1.0
Green bean				
'Beginner Foods' (Heinz)	3.5 oz	30	3	0.3
buttered, junior	7.25 oz	66	4	1.9
buttered, junior	1 oz	9	1	0.3
buttered, strained	4.5 oz	42	4	1.0
buttered, strained	1 oz	9	1	0.2
creamed, junior	7.5 oz	68	26	0.9
creamed, junior	1 oz	9	3	0.1
creamed, junior (Gerber)	6 oz	80	14	1.0
creamed, junior (Heinz)	3.5 oz	41	13	1.0
creamed, '3rd Foods' (Gerber)	7 tbsp	45	8	0.2
diced, 'Graduates' (Gerber)	3.2 oz	21	23	0.1
'1st Foods' (Gerber)	2.5 oz	25	na	0.0
'1st Foods' (Gerber)	7 tbsp	32	1	0.2
junior	7.25 oz	52	4	0.2
junior	1 oz	7	1	0.0
'2nd Foods' (Gerber)	7 tbsp	30	1	0.2
'Stages 3' (Beech-Nut)	6 oz	45	80	0.0
'Stages 1' (Beech-Nut)	4.5 oz	35	0	0.0

Food Name	Serv. Size	Total Cal.	Sod. MGS	Fat GMS
strained	4.5 oz	32	3	0.1
strained	1 oz	7	1	0.0
strained *(Heinz)*	3.5 oz	25	2	0.2
Mixed				
junior	7.5 oz	87	77	0.9
junior	1 oz	12	10	0.1
junior *(Gerber)*	6 oz	70	32	1.0
'2nd Foods' *(Gerber)*	7 tbsp	42	17	0.4
'Stages 2' *(Beech-Nut)*	4.5 oz	50	30	0.0
strained	4.5 oz	52	17	0.6
strained	1 oz	12	4	0.1
strained *(Gerber)*	4.5 oz	60	15	1.0
strained *(Heinz)*	3.5 oz	44	21	0.4
'3rd Foods' *(Gerber)*	7 tbsp	39	14	0.2
Peas				
'Beginner Foods' *(Heinz)*	3.5 oz	55	13	0.5
buttered, junior	7.25 oz	124	10	2.7
buttered, junior	1 oz	17	1	0.4
buttered, strained	4.5 oz	72	10	1.4
buttered, strained	1 oz	16	2	0.3
buttered, tender, sweet, 'Stages 1' *(Beech-Nut)*	4.5 oz	60	0	0.0
buttered, tender, sweet, 'Stages 1' *(Beech-Nut)*	2.8 oz	40	0	0.0
creamed, strained	4.5 oz	68	18	2.4
creamed, strained	1 oz	15	4	0.5
creamed, strained *(Heinz)*	3.5 oz	52	11	1.5
diced, 'Graduates' *(Gerber)*	3.2 oz	44	9	0.1
'1st Foods' *(Gerber)*	2.5 oz	30	na	0.0
'1st Foods' *(Gerber)*	7 tbsp	47	6	0.4
junior *(Gerber)*	6 oz	90	5	1.0
'2nd Foods' *(Gerber)*	7 tbsp	47	5	0.5
strained	4.5 oz	51	5	0.4
strained	1 oz	11	1	0.1
strained *(Gerber)*	4.5 oz	60	6	1.0
tender, sweet, 'Baby's First' *(Beech-Nut)*	2.5 oz	40	0	0.0
'3rd Foods' *(Gerber)*	7 tbsp	47	6	0.4
Peas and brown rice *(Earth's Best)*	4.5 oz	80	10	0.0
Peas and carrots, 'Stages 2' *(Beech-Nut)*	4.5 oz	60	35	0.0
Potato, diced, 'Graduates' *(Gerber)*	3.2 oz	38	6	0.1
Spinach, creamed				
junior	7.5 oz	89	117	3.0
junior	1 oz	12	16	0.4

Food Name	Serv. Size	Total Cal.	Sod. MGS	Fat GMS
'2nd Foods' (Gerber)	7 tbsp	47	57	0.6
strained	4.5 oz	47	63	1.7
strained	1 oz	10	14	0.4
strained (Gerber)	4.5 oz	60	73	1.0
Spinach and potato (Earth's Best)	4.5 oz	60	25	2.0
Squash				
'Beginner Foods' (Heinz)	3.5 oz	36	5	0.2
buttered, junior	7.5 oz	64	4	1.3
buttered, junior	1 oz	9	1	0.2
buttered, strained	4.5 oz	37	3	0.4
buttered, strained	1 oz	8	1	0.1
butternut, and corn (Earth's Best)	4.5oz	90	0	2.0
butternut, 'Baby's First' (Beech-Nut)	2.5 oz	30	0	0.0
butternut, 'Stages 1' (Beech-Nut)	4.5 oz	50	0	0.0
butternut, 'Stages 1' (Beech-Nut)	2.8 oz	30	0	0.0
'1st Foods' (Gerber)	2.5 oz	25	na	0.0
'1st Foods' (Gerber)	7 tbsp	33	1	0.3
junior	7.5 oz	51	2	0.4
junior	1 oz	7	0	0.1
junior (Gerber)	6 oz	60	3	1.0
'2nd Foods' (Gerber)	7 tbsp	32	1	0.2
strained	4.5 oz	31	3	0.3
strained	1 oz	7	1	0.1
strained (Gerber)	4.5 oz	35	3	0.0
strained (Heinz)	3.5 oz	32	2	0.3
'3rd Foods' (Gerber)	7 tbsp	33	1	0.2
winter (Earth's Best)	4.5 oz	50	10	0.0
Sweet potato				
(Earth's Best)	4.5 oz	60	15	1.0
'Baby's First' (Beech-Nut)	2.5 oz	50	10	0.0
'Beginner Foods' (Heinz)	3.5 oz	69	14	0.2
buttered, junior	7.75 oz	125	18	1.5
buttered, junior	1 oz	16	2	0.2
buttered, strained	4.75 oz	76	11	0.9
buttered, strained	1 oz	16	2	0.2
'1st Foods' (Gerber)	2.5 oz	45	na	0.0
'1st Foods' (Gerber)	7 tbsp	67	15	0.2
junior	7.75 oz	132	48	0.2
junior	1 oz	17	6	0.0
junior (Gerber)	6 oz	110	39	1.0
junior (Heinz)	3.5 oz	69	11	0.3

Food Name	Serv. Size	Total Cal.	Sod. MGS	Fat GMS
'2nd Foods' (Gerber)	7 tbsp	62	17	0.2
'Stages 1' (Beech-Nut)	2.8 oz	60	10	0.0
'Stages 1' (Beech-Nut)	4.5 oz	90	80	0.0
'Stages 3' (Beech-Nut)	6 oz	110	80	0.0
strained	4.75 oz	77	27	0.1
strained	1 oz	16	6	0.0
strained (Gerber)	4.5 oz	80	22	1.0
strained (Heinz)	3.5 oz	69	11	0.3
'3rd Foods' (Gerber)	7 tbsp	63	23	0.2
WATER, w/fluoride, sodium-free (Beech-Nut)	4 oz	0	0	0.0
BACON				
cooked, yield from 1 lb raw	4.5 oz	732	2026	62.5
cured, approx 20 slices per lb, cooked	3 slices	109	303	9.4
cured, breakfast strips, cooked	3 slices	156	714	12.5
cured, broiled	4.5 oz	732	2027	62.5
cured, broiled	3 med slices	109	303	9.4
cured, canned	100 gm	685	680	71.5
cured, pan-fried	4.5 oz	732	2027	62.5
cured, pan-fried	3 med slices	109	303	9.4
cured, roasted	4.5 oz	732	2027	62.5
cured, roasted	3 med slices	109	303	9.4
cured, strips, cooked	6 oz	780	3568	62.4
cured, 12 slices per lb, raw	1 slice	211	277	21.9
cured, strips, 15 slices per 12 oz, raw	3 slices	264	671	25.3
raw	1 oz	158	194	16.3
(Hormel)				
'Black Label' cooked	1 oz	142	192	14.0
'Black Label' low salt, cooked	1.76 oz	250	260	25.0
'Black Label' sliced, cooked	2 slices	60	298	5.0
'Range' thick sliced, cooked	1 oz	152	199	16.0
(JM)				
cooked	2 slices	100	370	9.0
'Lower Sodium' cooked	2 slices	100	260	9.0
'Lower Sodium' raw	2 slices	290	250	30.0
raw	2 slices	280	530	29.0
(Jones Dairy Farm), raw	1 slice	165	187	17.0
(Kahn's), 'American Beauty,' cooked	2 slices	100	(mq)	9.0
(Oscar Mayer)				
'Center Cut' cooked, approx .2-oz slices	1 slice	25	113	1.8
'Center Cut' cooked, yield from 1 lb raw	6 oz	852	3813	62.5
cooked, approx .2-oz slices	1 slice	33	138	2.8

Food Name	Serv. Size	Total Cal.	Sod. MGS	Fat GMS
cooked, yield from 16-oz pkg raw	5 oz	784	3236	64.9
'Lower Salt' cooked, approx .2-oz slices	1 slice	33	104	2.6
'Lower Salt' cooked, yield from 1 lb raw	5.6 oz	870	2768	70.3
thick sliced, cooked, approx .4-oz slices	1 slice	58	259	4.8
thick sliced, cooked, yield from 1 lb raw	5 oz	811	3656	67.1
(Range Brand) 'Sliced' cooked	2 slices	110	392	9.0
(Red Label) cooked	3 slices	110	(mq)	10.0
BACON, ALTERNATIVE				
BEEF				
heated (JM)	2 slices	100	320	7.0
heated (Sizzlean)	2 strips	70	480	5.0
heated, yield from 12-oz pkg	6 oz	764	700	58.5
raw	1 oz	115	271	11.0
raw (JM)	2 slices	200	430	18.0
unheated	1 oz	115	271	11.0
PORK				
80% fat-free (Louis Rich)	1 slice	35	185	2.0
heated (Sizzlean)	2 strips	90	530	8.0
heated, brown sugar cured (Sizzlean)	2 strips	110	490	9.0
heated, yield from 12-oz pkg	6 oz	780	3568	62.4
raw	1 oz	110	280	10.5
TURKEY, heated (Louis Rich)	1 slice	32	186	2.4
VEGETARIAN				
	1 cup	446	2110	42.5
	1 oz	88	415	8.4
(Morningstar Farms) 'Breakfast Strips' frozen	3 strips	80	350	6.0
(White Wave SoyFood) 'Healthy'	1 oz	27	310	1.0
(Worthington) 'Stripples' frozen	4 strips	120	460	9.0
Canadian style				
(Heartline)	2 oz	176	260	7.0
(Heartline) 'Canadian Bacon Style' lite	.5 oz	22	135	0.0
BACON, CANADIAN-STYLE				
cured, grilled	2 slices	86	719	3.9
cured, grilled, yield from 6 oz raw	4.9 oz	257	2149	11.7
cured, packed 6 slices per 6 oz, unheated	2 slices	89	799	4.0
cured, unheated	6 oz	267	2395	11.9
unheated	1 oz	45	399	2.0
(Hormel) 'Sliced'	1 oz	45	315	2.0
(Jones Dairy Farm) unheated	1 slice	25	144	1.0
(Light & Lean)	2 slices	35	(mq)	1.0
(Oscar Mayer)	.8 oz	28	305	1.0

Food Name	Serv. Size	Total Cal.	Sod. MGS	Fat GMS
BACON BITS				
(Hormel)	1 oz	117	1008	7.0
(Hormel)	1 tbsp	30	313	2.0
(Libby's) 'Bacon Crumbles'	1 tbsp	25	(mq)	1.0
(Oscar Mayer)	3 oz	248	2224	12.4
(Oscar Mayer)	1 tbsp	20	183	1.0
BACON BITS, ALTERNATIVE				
(Bac•Os)	2 tsp	25	90	1.0
(McCormick) 'Bac'N Pieces' no cholesterol	1 1/2 tbsp	30	240	1.0
(Schilling) 'Bac'N Pieces'	1 tsp	26	51	0.4
BACON PIECES (Hormel)	1 oz	94	654	5.0
BAGEL				
BLUEBERRY				
(Earth Grains) 3 oz	1 bagel	245	210	0.0
(Western Bagel)	1 bagel	240	410	4.0
CINNAMON-RAISIN				
(Dunkin' Donuts)	1 bagel	250	370	2.0
(Earth Grains) 3 oz	1 bagel	245	210	0.0
(Thomas') 'Deli Style'	1 bagel	170	230	2.0
(Western Bagel)	1 bagel	230	410	4.0
EGG				
	1 oz	79	143	0.6
(Dunkin' Donuts)	1 bagel	250	380	2.0
(Lender's) 'Bagel Shop'	1 bagel	230	460	2.5
(Lender's) 'Bakery Style'	1 bagel	210	450	2.0
HONEY WHEAT (Earth Grains) 3 oz	1 bagel	240	210	0.0
ONION				
enriched, 3.5 inch diam	1 bagel	195	379	1.1
enriched, w/calcium proprianate, 3.5 inch diam	1 bagel	195	379	1.1
enriched, w/calcium proprianate, toasted	1 oz	84	163	0.5
unenriched, 3.5 inch diam	1 bagel	195	379	1.1
unenriched, w/calcium proprianate, 3.5 inch diam	1 bagel	195	379	1.1
(Dunkin' Donuts)	1 bagel	230	480	1.0
(Earth Grains) 3 oz	1 bagel	240	210	0.0
(Lender's) 'Bagel Shop'	1 bagel	220	460	2.0
(Western Bagel)	1 bagel	220	430	4.0
PLAIN				
enriched, 3.5 inch diam	1 bagel	195	379	1.1
enriched, w/calcium proprianate, 3.5 inch diam	1 bagel	195	379	1.1
unenriched, 3.5 inch diam	1 bagel	195	379	1.1
unenriched, w/calcium proprianate, 3.5 inch diam	1 bagel	195	379	1.1

Food Name	Serv. Size	Total Cal.	Sod. MGS	Fat GMS
(Dunkin' Donuts)	1 bagel	240	450	1.0
(Earth Grains) 3 oz	1 bagel	240	210	0.0
(Lender's) 'Bagel Shop'	1 bagel	210	350	1.5
(Lender's) 'Bakery Style'	1 bagel	210	450	2.0
POPPY SEED				
enriched, 3.5 inch diam	1 bagel	195	379	1.1
enriched, w/calcium proprianate, 3.5 inch diam	1 bagel	195	379	1.1
enriched, w/calcium proprianate, toasted	1 oz	84	163	0.5
unenriched, 3.5 inch diam	1 bagel	195	379	1.1
unenriched, w/calcium proprianate, 3.5 inch diam	1 bagel	195	379	1.1
RAISIN				
(Lender's) 'Bagel Shop'	1 bagel	240	350	3.0
(Lender's) 'Bakery Style'	1 bagel	220	380	2.0
RAISIN-HONEY CINNAMON (Finast) 2.5 oz	1 bagel	200	305	1.0
SESAME				
enriched, 3.5 inch diam	1 bagel	195	379	1.1
enriched, w/calcium proprianate, 3.5 inch diam	1 bagel	195	379	1.1
enriched, w/calcium proprianate, toasted	1 oz	84	163	0.5
unenriched, 3.5 inch diam	1 bagel	195	379	1.1
unenriched, w/calcium proprianate, 3.5 inch diam	1 bagel	195	379	1.1
WATER (Western Bagel)	1 bagel	230	420	4.0
BAGEL, FROZEN				
BLUEBERRY (Lender's) 2.5 oz	1 bagel	190	250	1.0
CINNAMON-RAISIN				
(Lender's) 'Big'n Crusty' 3 1/8 oz	1 bagel	250	370	2.0
(Sara Lee) 3.1 oz	1 bagel	240	280	2.0
(Sara Lee) 2.5 oz	1 bagel	200	230	2.0
EGG				
(Lender's) 2 oz	1 bagel	150	360	1.0
(Lender's) 'Big'n Crusty' 3 1/8 oz	1 bagel	250	380	2.0
(Sara Lee) 3.1 oz	1 bagel	250	450	2.0
(Sara Lee) 2.5 oz	1 bagel	200	360	2.0
GARLIC				
(Lender's) 2 oz	1 bagel	160	340	1.0
(Lender's) 'Big'n Crusty' 3 1/8 oz	1 bagel	250	530	1.0
OAT BRAN				
(Lender's) 2.5 oz	1 bagel	170	290	2.0
(Sara Lee) 3 oz	1 bagel	220	450	1.0
(Sara Lee) 2.5 oz	1 bagel	180	360	1.0
ONION				
(Lender's) 2 oz	1 bagel	160	290	1.0

Food Name	Serv. Size	Total Cal.	Sod. MGS	Fat GMS
(Lender's) 'Bagelettes' .9 oz	1 bagel	70	135	<1.0
(Lender's) 'Big'n Crusty' 3 1/8 oz	1 bagel	230	480	1.0
(Sara Lee) 3.1 oz	1 bagel	230	560	1.0
(Sara Lee) 2.5 oz	1 bagel	190	450	1.0
PLAIN				
(Lender's) 2 oz	1 bagel	150	320	1.0
(Lender's) 'Bagelettes' .9 oz	1 bagel	70	170	<1.0
(Lender's) 'Big'n Crusty'	1 bagel	240	450	1.0
(Lender's) soft, 2.5 oz	1 bagel	210	350	3.0
(Sara Lee) 3.1 oz	1 bagel	230	580	1.0
(Sara Lee) 2.5 oz	1 bagel	190	460	1.0
POPPY SEED				
(Lender's) 2 oz	1 bagel	160	370	1.0
(Sara Lee) 3.1 oz	1 bagel	230	560	1.0
(Sara Lee) 2.5 oz	1 bagel	190	450	1.0
PUMPERNICKEL *(Lender's)* 2 oz	1 bagel	160	330	1.0
RAISIN *(Lender's)* 'Bagelettes' .9 oz	1 bagel	70	110	<1.0
RAISIN-HONEY *(Lender's)* 2.5 oz	1 bagel	200	310	1.0
RYE *(Lender's)* 2 oz	1 bagel	150	310	1.0
SESAME				
(Lender's) 2 oz	1 bagel	160	320	1.0
(Sara Lee) 3.1 oz	1 bagel	240	550	2.0
(Sara Lee) 2.5 oz	1 bagel	190	440	1.0
WHEAT-RAISIN *(Lender's)* 2.5 oz	1 bagel	190	310	1.0
BAGEL CHIP				
(Burns & Ricker) cinnamon raisin 'Original Bagel Crisps'	1 oz	130	170	4.0
(Burns & Ricker) garlic 'Original Bagel Crisps'	1 oz	130	190	4.0
BAKED BEANS, CANNED. See also BEANS, CANNED.				
(Allens)	1/2 cup	170	330	6.0
(Grandma Brown's)	1 cup	301	655	3.0
(Green Giant)	1/2 cup	150	670	2.0
(Open Range)	4.656 oz	152	425	2.3
(Van Camp's)	1 cup	260	1020	2.0
bacon and brown sugar, 'Premium' *(Van Camp's)*	6 oz	170	790	2.0
barbecue *(B&M)*	8 oz	260	1000	6.0
barbecue *(Campbell's)*	7 7/8 oz	210	900	4.0
Boston *(Health Valley)*	4 oz	213	74	1.0
Boston, 'No Salt Added' *(Health Valley)*	4 oz	213	25	1.0
Boston, w/ham 'Homestyle' *(Hunt's)*	9.03 oz	248	740	1.9
'Brick Oven' *(S&W)*	1/2 cup	160	560	2.0
brown sugar *(Van Camp's)*	1 cup	290	640	5.1

Food Name	Serv. Size	Total Cal.	Sod. MGS	Fat GMS
'Deluxe' *(Van Camp's)*	1 cup	320	970	4.0
'Dry Beans in Sauce' *(Green Giant)*	1/2 cup	130	570	1.0
'Dry Beans in Sauce' *(Joan of Arc)*	1/2 cup	130	570	1.0
'Home Style' *(Campbell's)*	8 oz	220	820	4.0
honey *(B&M)*	8 oz	240	940	2.0
hot 'n spicy *(B&M)*	8 oz	240	990	3.0
in homestyle sauce *(Bush's Best)*	4 oz	110	350	1.0
in molasses, brown sugar, 'Old Fashioned' *(Campbell's)*	8 oz	230	730	3.0
in tomato sauce *(B&M)*	8 oz	230	1010	3.0
in tomato sauce *(Campbell's)*	8 oz	200	770	3.0
in tomato sauce *(Pathmark)*	1/2 cup	150	440	2.0
in tomato sauce, 40-oz can *(Finast)*	1/2 cup	120	930	1.0
in tomato sauce, 'No Frills' *(Pathmark)*	1/2 cup	160	390	2.0
in tomato sauce, 16-oz can *(Finast)*	1 cup	270	1180	3.0
maple *(B&M)*	8 oz	240	890	2.0
maple *(Friends)*	8 oz	240	890	2.0
no salt added, fat-free *(Health Valley)*	7.5 oz	190	20	0.0
pea beans *(B&M)*	8 oz	270	750	6.0
pea, small *(Friends)*	8 oz	360	1040	4.0
pea, small, w/pork *(Friends)*	8 oz	260	890	5.0
pork and beans, 'Deluxe' *(Bush's Best)*	4 oz	110	350	1.0
pork and beans, 'Showboat' *(Bush's Best)*	4 oz	80	470	<1.0
regular, fat-free *(Health Valley)*	7.5 oz	190	290	0.0
'Saucepan' *(Grandma Brown's)*	1 cup	307	592	4.8
vegetarian	1/2 cup	118	504	0.6
vegetarian *(A&P)*	1/2 cup	130	420	<1.0
vegetarian *(Allens)*	1/2 cup	110	380	1.0
vegetarian *(B&M)*	8 oz	230	370	3.0
vegetarian *(Campbell's)*	7.75 oz	170	780	1.0
vegetarian, 'Vegetarian Style' *(Van Camp's)*	1 cup	206	950	0.6
vegetarian, w/miso 'Vegetarian' *(Health Valley)*	4 oz	90	134	1.0
w/beef	1/2 cup	161	632	4.6
w/franks	1/2 cup	182	550	8.4
w/franks, 'Beanee Weenee' *(Van Camp's)*	1 cup	326	990	15.4
w/onions, approx 1/2 cup *(Bush's Best)*	4 oz	110	550	1.0
w/pork	1/2 cup	134	522	2.0
w/pork *(A&P)*	1/2 cup	150	440	2.0
w/pork *(Hunt's)*	4 oz	140	400	1.0
w/pork *(S&W)*	1/2 cup	130	135	2.0
w/pork *(Van Camp's)*	1 cup	216	1000	1.9
w/pork 'Extra Fancy' *(Allens)*	1/2 cup	125	540	1.0

Food Name	Serv. Size	Total Cal.	Sod. MGS	Fat GMS
w/pork, 'Extra Standard' *(Allens)*	1/2 cup	90	350	1.0
w/pork, 'Fancy' *(Allens)*	1/2 cup	110	430	1.0
w/pork, 'Micro-Cup' *(Hormel)*	7.5 oz	254	650	5.0
w/pork and sweet sauce	1/2 cup	140	423	1.8
w/pork and tomato sauce	1/2 cup	123	554	1.3
w/pork and tomato sauce *(Green Giant)*	1/2 cup	90	420	1.0
w/pork and tomato sauce *(Joan of Arc)*	1/2 cup	90	420	1.0
BAKING POWDER				
	1 tbsp	11	1050	0.0
	1 tsp	3	290	0.0
commercial	3 1/2 oz	109	16804	0.0
commercial *(Calumet)*	1/4 tsp	0	100	0.0
cream of tartar, w/tartaric acid	1 tbsp	7	694	0.0
double-acting, sodium aluminum sulfate	1 tsp	2	488	0.0
double-acting, straight phosphate	1 tsp	2	363	0.0
'Low Salt' *(Featherweight)*	1 tsp	8	2	0.0
low-sodium	1 tsp	5	5	0.0
low-sodium, commercial	1 tbsp	23	1	0.0
low-sodium, commercial	1 tsp	7	0	0.0
low-sodium, non-commercial	1 tsp	2	0	0.0
w/monohydrate	1 tbsp	14	1205	0.0
w/monohydrate	1 tsp	4	329	0.0
w/straight phosphate	1 tbsp	15	1028	0.0
w/straight phosphate	1 tsp	5	312	0.0
BAKING SODA				
	1 tsp	0	1259	0.0
(Arm & Hammer)	1/2 tsp	0	476	0.0
BALSAM PEAR/bitter melon				
Leafy tips				
boiled, drained	4 oz	40	15	0.2
boiled, drained	1/2 cup	10	4	0.1
raw	1/2 cup	7	3	0.2
raw, trimmed	1 oz	9	3	0.2
raw, untrimmed	1 lb	52	18	1.2
Pods				
boiled, drained	4 oz	22	7	0.2
boiled, drained, 1/2-inch pieces	1/2 cup	12	4	0.1
raw	1 pear	21	6	0.2
raw, approx 9 3/8 inch x 1 1/2 inch, 5.3 oz each	1 pod	21	6	0.2
raw, 1/2-inch pieces	1 cup	16	5	0.2
raw, trimmed	1 oz	5	1	0.1

Food Name	Serv. Size	Total Cal.	Sod. MGS	Fat GMS
raw, untrimmed	1 lb	64	20	0.6
BAMBOO SHOOTS				
boiled, drained	4 oz	14	5	0.2
boiled, drained, 1/2-inch slices	1 cup	14	5	0.3
canned (LaChoy)	1.5 oz	8	3	0.2
canned (LaChoy)	2 tbsp	3	0	0.1
canned, drained solids, 1/8-inch slices	1 cup	25	9	0.5
raw, 1/2-inch slices	1 cup	41	6	0.5
raw, trimmed	1 oz	8	1	0.1
raw, w/sheath	1 lb	36	6	0.4
BANANA				
fresh (Dole)	1 fruit	120	na	1.0
mashed	1/2 cup	104	1	0.5
peeled	1 oz	26	<1	0.1
powdered	1 oz	98	1	0.5
powdered	1/4 cup	87	1	0.5
powdered	1 tbsp	21	tr	0.1
raw, w/o skin and seeds	1 fruit	105	1	0.6
unpeeled	1 lb	271	3	1.4
BANANA, COOKING. See PLANTAIN.				
BANANA, DEHYDRATED				
	1 oz	98	1	0.5
	1/4 cup	87	1	0.5
BANANA, RED				
raw	100 gm	90	1	0.2
raw, approx 7.25 inch x 1.5 inch	1 med	118	1	0.3
raw, sliced	1/2 cup	68	1	0.2
BANANA BERRY DRINK				
'Stompin' Banana Berry Drink' (Hi-C)	6 oz	90	25	0.0
BANANA BREAD. See BREAD, QUICK.				
BANANA CHIPS				
	1 oz	147	2	9.5
freeze-dried (Mountain House)	1/2 cup	248	na	8.0
premium (Mariani)	1 oz	150	<10	9.0
BANANA NECTAR (Libby's)	6 oz	110	15	0.0
BANANA PEPPER. See PEPPER, BANANA.				
BANANA PINEAPPLE NECTAR (Kern's)	6 oz	110	0	0.0
BANANA SQUASH. See SQUASH, BANANA.				
BARBADOS CHERRY. See ACEROLA CHERRY.				
BARBADOS CHERRY JUICE. See ACEROLA CHERRY JUICE.				

Food Name	Serv. Size	Total Cal.	Sod. MGS	Fat GMS
BARBECUE SAUCE				
(Bull's Eye)	.5 oz	22	47	0.0
(Cattleman's) mild	1 tbsp	25	260	0.0
(Enrico's) 'Original'	1 tbsp	18	4	1.0
(Healthy Choice) original	1.1 oz	25	229	0.2
(Heinz) 'Old Fashioned'	1 tbsp	18	180	0.1
(Heinz) 'Select'	1 oz	40	275	0.0
(Heinz) 'Thick and Rich' old fashioned	1 oz	35	350	0.0
(Heinz) 'Thick and Rich' original	1 oz	35	390	0.0
(Hunt's) 'Bold' original	1.2 oz	46	315	0.3
(Hunt's) 'Light' original	1.1 oz	26	223	0.1
(Hunt's) original	1.2 oz	40	410	0.3
(Kraft)	2 tbsp	45	460	1.0
(Kraft) 'Thick 'n Spicy' original	2 tbsp	50	430	1.0
(Open Range) original	1.2 oz	38	333	0.2
(Ott's)	1 tbsp	14	147	0.1
(Skipper's)	1 tbsp	25	226	1.0
CAJUN STYLE				
(Golden Dipt)	1 oz	90	360	8.0
(Heinz)	1 tbsp	15	108	0.1
(Heinz) 'Thick and Rich'	1 oz	35	360	0.0
CHUNKY				
(Heinz) 'Thick and Rich'	1 oz	30	380	0.0
(Kraft) 'Thick 'n Spicy'	2 tbsp	60	420	1.0
COUNTRY STYLE				
(Hunt's)	1.2 oz	39	399	0.3
(Hunt's)	1 tbsp	20	140	<1.0
DIJON AND HONEY				
(Estee)	1 tbsp	18	5	<1.0
(Lawry's)	1/2 cup	203	1768	1.2
GARLIC (Kraft)	2 tbsp	40	420	0.0
HAWAIIAN STYLE				
(Heinz)	1 tbsp	19	108	0.1
(Heinz) 'Thick and Rich'	1 oz	40	210	0.0
HICKORY				
(Healthy Choice)	1.1 oz	26	229	0.2
(Heinz) 'Select'	1 oz	35	260	0.0
(Hunt's)	1 tbsp	20	160	<1.0
(Hunt's) bold	1.2 oz	46	283	0.4
(Hunt's) 'Light'	1.1 oz	27	245	0.2
(Open Range)	1.2 oz	37	423	0.2

Food Name	Serv. Size	Total Cal.	Sod. MGS	Fat GMS
HICKORY SMOKE				
(Heinz)	1 tbsp	19	56	0.1
(Heinz) 'Thick and Rich'	1 oz	35	380	0.0
(Heinz) 'Thick and Rich'	1 tbsp	20	220	0.0
(Kraft)	2 tbsp	45	440	1.0
(Kraft) 'Thick 'n Spicy'	2 tbsp	50	430	1.0
(Kraft) w/onion bits	2 tbsp	50	340	1.0
HOMESTYLE (Hunt's)	1.2 oz	41	381	0.1
HONEY				
(Hain)	1 tbsp	14	120	1.0
(Kraft) 'Thick 'n Spicy'	2 tbsp	60	340	1.0
HONEY MUSTARD (Hunt's)	1.2 oz	48	450	0.2
HOT				
(Healthy Choice) and spicy	1.1 oz	25	229	0.2
(Heinz) 'Thick and Rich'	1 tbsp	20	220	0.0
(Hunt's) and spicy	1.2 oz	48	450	0.2
(Kraft)	2 tbsp	45	520	1.0
(Kraft) hickory smoke	2 tbsp	45	360	1.0
ITALIAN SEASONING (Kraft)	2 tbsp	50	280	1.0
KANSAS CITY STYLE				
(Hunt's)	1.2 oz	43	220	0.2
(Kraft)	2 tbsp	50	270	1.0
(Kraft) 'Thick 'n Spicy'	2 tbsp	60	270	1.0
MESQUITE SMOKE				
(Enrico's)	1 tbsp	18	4	1.0
(Heinz) 'Thick and Rich'	1 oz	30	380	0.0
(Hunt's)	2 tbsp	40	360	0.0
(Kraft)	2 tbsp	45	410	1.0
(Kraft) 'Thick 'n Spicy'	2 tbsp	50	430	1.0
MUSHROOM				
(Heinz)	1 tbsp	14	219	0.1
(Heinz) 'Thick and Rich'	1 oz	30	460	0.0
NEW ORLEANS STYLE (Hunt's)	1.2 oz	41	383	0.2
ONION				
(Heinz)	1 tbsp	15	255	0.1
(Heinz) 'Thick and Rich'	1 oz	30	420	0.0
(Kraft) w/onion bits	2 tbsp	50	340	1.0
ORANGE JUICE, 'California Grill' (Lawry's)	1/4 cup	34	3846	0.7
ORIENTAL (LaChoy)	1 tbsp	16	304	<.1
SALSA STYLE (Kraft)	2 tbsp	45	420	0.0
SLOPPY JOE, w/beef (Libby's)	1/3 cup	110	190	7.0

Food Name	Serv. Size	Total Cal.	Sod. MGS	Fat GMS
SMOKY				
(Cattleman's)	1 tbsp	25	300	0.0
(Maull's)	1 tbsp	20	139	<1.0
(Ott's)	1 tbsp	14	149	0.1
SOUTHERN STYLE (Hunt's)	1 tbsp	20	170	<1.0
TEXAS STYLE				
(Heinz) hot 'Thick and Rich'	1 oz	30	390	0.0
(Hunt's)	1 tbsp	25	150	<1.0
WESTERN STYLE (Hunt's)	1 tbsp	20	170	<1.0
BARBECUE SPICE (Tone's)	1 tsp	9	713	0.4
BARLEY				
	1 cup	651	22	4.2
flakes (Arrowhead Mills)	2 oz	200	1	1.0
pearled, cooked	1 cup	193	5	0.7
pearled, cooked	4 oz	139	1	0.5
pearled, raw	1 cup	704	18	2.3
pearled, raw	1 oz	100	3	0.3
pearled, raw (Arrowhead Mills)	2 oz	200	1	1.0
pearled, raw, medium 'Scotch Brand' 1.7 oz (Quaker)	1/4 cup	172	0	0.5
pearled, raw, quick 'Scotch Brand' (Quaker)	1/3 cup	172	0	0.5
raw	1 oz	100	3	0.7
BARLEY FLOUR (Arrowhead Mills)	2 oz	200	1	1.0
BASELLA. See VINE SPINACH.				
BASIL				
dried (Golden Dipt)	2 grams	8	36	0.0
dried, crumbled	1 oz	71	10	1.1
dried, crumbled	1 tbsp	11	2	0.2
dried, crumbled (Spice Islands)	1 tsp	3	<1	<.1
dried, ground (Durkee)	1 tsp	5	0	tr
dried, ground (Laurel Leaf)	1 tsp	5	0	tr
fresh	2 tbsp	1	0	0.0
fresh	5 leaves	1	0	0.0
BASS, FRESHWATER, MIXED SPECIES				
dry-heat cooked	3 oz	124	77	4.0
raw	1 lb	516	317	16.7
raw	3 oz	97	59	3.1
raw	1 oz	32	20	1.0
BASS, SEA, MIXED SPECIES				
baked	4 oz	141	99	2.9
broiled	4 oz	141	99	2.9
dry-heat cooked	3 oz	105	74	2.2

Food Name	Serv. Size	Total Cal.	Sod. MGS	Fat GMS
microwaved	4 oz	141	99	2.9
raw	1 lb	439	308	9.1
raw	3 oz	82	58	1.7
raw	1 oz	27	19	0.6
BASS, STRIPED				
dry-heat cooked	3 oz	105	75	2.5
raw	1 lb	439	313	10.6
raw	3 oz	82	59	2.0
raw	1 oz	27	23	0.7
BATTER MIX				
beer, dry mix (Golden Dipt)	1 oz	100	650	0.0
corn dog, dry mix (Golden Dipt)	1 oz	100	490	0.0
fish and chips, dry mix (Golden Dipt)	1.25 oz	120	910	0.0
onion ring, dry mix (Golden Dipt)	1 oz	100	570	0.0
original, dry mix (Golden Dipt)	1 oz	100	740	0.0
tempura, dry mix (Golden Dipt)	1 oz	100	130	0.0
BAY LEAF				
dried, crumbled	1 oz	89	7	2.4
dried, crumbled	1 tbsp	6	0	0.2
dried, crumbled	1 tsp	2	0	0.1
dried, crumbled (Durkee)	1 tsp	2	0	tr
dried, crumbled (Laurel Leaf)	1 tsp	2	0	tr
dried, crumbled (Spice Islands)	1 tsp	5	<1	0.1
BEAN. See individual listings.				
BEAN DINNER, W/FRANKFURTERS, FROZEN				
(Banquet)	10 oz	520	1230	25.0
(Morton)	10 oz	350	1490	13.0
(Swanson)	10.5 oz	440	900	19.0
BEAN ENTRÉE, MICROWAVE				
w/frankfurters, in sauce, 'Diner' micro cup (Libby's)	7.75 oz	330	930	15.0
w/wieners, microwave cup (Kid's Kitchen)	7.5 oz	310	750	13.0
BEAN MIX				
Cajun, w/sauce, dry (Lipton)	1/4 pkg	130	400	<1.0
Cajun, w/sauce, prepared (Lipton)	1/2 cup	160	440	3.0
chicken and sauce, dry (Lipton)	1/4 pkg	120	470	1.0
chicken and sauce, prepared (Lipton)	1/2 cup	150	500	4.0
'Kettle Creations' bean medley with pasta, dry (Lipton)	1/4 cup	130	690	1.5
BEAN SALAD, CANNED				
four-bean (Joan of Arc)	1/2 cup	100	660	1.0
four-bean (Read)	1/2 cup	100	660	1.0
green bean, German-style (Joan of Arc)	1 cup	180	920	7.0

Food Name	Serv. Size	Total Cal.	Sod. MGS	Fat GMS
green bean, German-style *(Read)*	1 cup	180	920	7.0
three-bean *(Joan of Arc)*	1/2 cup	90	710	0.0
three-bean *(Read)*	1/2 cup	90	710	0.0
'Three Bean Salad' *(Green Giant)*	1/2 cup	70	470	<1.0
BEAN SPROUTS, CANNED				
(LaChoy)	2 oz	6	17	0.1
(LaChoy)	2.928 oz	12	20	0.1
BEANS, BAKED. See BAKED BEANS, CANNED.				
BEANS, CANNED. See also BAKED BEANS, CANNED; BEAN SPROUTS, CANNED; BEAN SALAD, CANNED; and individual listings.				
barbecue *(Open Range)*	4.75 oz	185	687	3.3
'Beans 'N Fixins' *(Big John's)*	4.7 oz	127	590	3.5
'Big John's Beans 'n Fixin's' *(Hunt's)*	4 oz	170	490	6.0
'Mexe-Beans' *(Old El Paso)*	1/2 cup	163	627	1.0
'Mix and Serve' *(Hunt's)*	4.75 oz	125	575	2.8
mixed *(Bush's Best)*	1/2 cup	70	410	0.0
'Pork and Beans' *(Hunt's)*	4.5 oz	130	516	1.2
'Pork and Beans' *(Open Range)*	4.6 oz	157	621	4.8
ranch *(Open Ranch)*	4.7 oz	124	628	3.2
spiced *(Gebhardt)*	4.5 oz	100	654	1.6
vegetarian, 'Deluxe' *(Bush's Best)*	4 oz	110	350	0.0
'Vegetarian Style' *(Van Camp's)*	1 cup	206	950	0.6
w/beef, 'Homestyle' *(Hunt's)*	9 oz	246	944	6.5
w/franks, 'Homestyle' *(Hunt's)*	9 oz	319	735	9.9
w/sausage, 'Homestyle' *(Hunt's)*	9 oz	306	567	9.8
BEARNAISE. See SAUCE.				
BEECHNUT, DRIED				
in shell	1 lb	1595	(mq)	138.4
shelled	1 oz	164	11	14.2
BEEF				
(NOTE: TRIMMED = Lean; separable fat removed after cooking. UNTRIMMED = Separable fat not removed.)				
BRAIN				
pan-fried	3 oz	167	134	13.5
raw	4 oz	142	116	10.5
simmered	4 oz	181	136	14.2
BRISKET, FLAT HALF				
Trimmed				
all grades, 0-inch fat, braised	4 oz	217	71	7.0
all grades, 0-inch fat, braised	3 oz	162	54	5.3
all grades, 1/4-inch fat, braised	3 oz	189	54	8.2

Food Name	Serv. Size	Total Cal.	Sod. MGS	Fat GMS
all grades, 1/2-inch fat, braised	3 oz	180	54	7.3
Untrimmed				
all grades, 0-inch fat, braised	4 oz	244	70	10.7
all grades, 1/4-inch fat, braised	11.5 oz	1189	183	93.1
all grades, 1/4-inch fat, braised	3 oz	309	48	24.2
all grades, 1/4-inch fat, raw	4 oz	328	70	26.7
all grades, 1/2-inch fat, braised	3 oz	311	48	24.6
all grades, 1/2-inch fat, raw	1 lb	1338	277	110.7
all grades, 1/2-inch fat, raw	1 oz	84	17	6.9
BRISKET, POINT HALF				
Trimmed				
all grades, 0-inch fat, braised	4 oz	277	87	15.6
all grades, 0-inch fat, braised	3 oz	207	65	11.7
all grades, 1/4-inch fat, braised	3 oz	222	65	13.3
all grades, 1/2-inch fat, braised	3 oz	224	65	13.5
all grades, 1-inch fat, braised	4 oz	296	87	17.8
Untrimmed				
all grades, 0-inch fat, braised	3 oz	304	58	24.2
all grades, 1/4-inch fat, braised	3 oz	343	55	29.1
all grades, 1/4-inch fat, raw	1 lb	1501	295	131.9
all grades, 1/4-inch fat, raw	1 oz	94	18	8.3
all grades, 1/2-inch fat, braised	3 oz	347	55	29.6
all grades, 1/2-inch fat, raw	1 lb	1601	290	143.5
all grades, 1/2-inch fat, raw	1 oz	100	18	9.0
BRISKET, WHOLE				
Trimmed				
all grades, 0-inch fat, braised	4 oz	247	79	11.4
all grades, 0-inch fat, braised	3 oz	185	59	8.6
all grades, 1/4-inch fat, braised	4 oz	274	79	14.5
all grades, 1/4-inch fat, braised	3 oz	206	59	10.9
all grades, 1/2-inch fat, braised	3 oz	205	61	10.9
Untrimmed				
all grades, 0-inch fat, braised	3 oz	247	55	16.6
all grades, 1/4-inch fat, braised	3 oz	327	52	26.8
all grades, 1/4-inch fat, raw	1 lb	1415	290	120.4
all grades, 1/4-inch fat, raw	1 oz	88	18	7.5
all grades, 1/2-inch fat, braised	3 oz	332	52	27.6
all grades, 1/2-inch fat, raw	1 lb	1474	281	127.7
all grades, 1/2-inch fat, raw	1 oz	92	18	8.0

Food Name	Serv. Size	Total Cal.	Sod. MGS	Fat GMS
CHUCK, ARM POT ROAST				
Trimmed				
all grades, 0-inch fat, braised	3 oz	178	56	6.5
all grades, 1/4-inch fat, braised	3 oz	184	56	7.1
all grades, 1/2-inch fat, braised	3 oz	196	56	8.5
choice, 0-inch fat, braised	3 oz	186	56	7.4
choice, 1/4-inch fat, braised	3 oz	191	56	7.9
choice, 1/2-inch fat, braised	3 oz	199	56	8.8
prime, 1/2-inch fat, braised	3 oz	222	56	11.4
prime, 1/2-inch fat, raw	1 lb	699	304	31.6
prime, 1/2-inch fat, raw	1 oz	44	19	2.0
select, 0-inch fat, braised	3 oz	168	56	5.3
select, 1/4-inch fat, braised	3 oz	175	56	6.1
select, 1/2-inch fat, braised	3 oz	189	56	7.6
Untrimmed				
all grades, 0-inch fat, braised	3 oz	238	53	14.5
all grades, 1/4-inch fat, braised	3 oz	282	51	20.2
all grades, 1/4-inch fat, raw	1 lb	1111	268	83.3
all grades, 1/4-inch fat, raw	1 oz	69	17	5.2
all grades, 1/2-inch fat, braised	3 oz	297	51	22.1
all grades, 1/2-inch fat, raw	1 lb	1166	268	89.8
all grades, 1/2-inch fat, raw	1 oz	73	17	5.6
choice, 0-inch fat, braised	3 oz	249	53	15.8
choice, 1/4-inch fat, braised	3 oz	296	50	21.9
choice, 1/4-inch fat, raw	1 lb	1157	268	88.8
choice, 1/4-inch fat, raw	1 oz	72	17	5.6
choice, 1/2-inch fat, braised	3 oz	301	50	22.5
choice, 1/2-inch fat, raw	1 lb	1188	263	92.9
choice, 1/2-inch fat, raw	1 oz	74	16	5.8
prime, 1/2-inch fat, braised	3 oz	332	49	26.3
prime, 1/2-inch fat, raw	1 lb	1334	259	109.6
prime, 1/2-inch fat, raw	1 oz	83	16	6.8
select, 0-inch fat, braised	3 oz	221	54	12.4
select, 1/4-inch fat, braised	3 oz	268	51	18.5
select, 1/4-inch fat, raw	1 lb	1061	268	77.4
select, 1/4-inch fat, raw	1 oz	66	17	4.8
select, 1/2-inch fat, braised	3 oz	286	51	20.8
select, 1/2-inch fat, raw	1 lb	1075	272	79.2
select, 1/2-inch fat, raw	1 oz	67	17	4.9

Food Name	Serv. Size	Total Cal.	Sod. MGS	Fat GMS
CHUCK, BLADE ROAST				
Trimmed				
all grades, 0-inch fat, braised	3 oz	215	60	11.3
all grades, 1/4-inch fat, braised	3 oz	213	60	11.1
all grades, 1/2-inch fat, braised	3 oz	229	60	13.0
choice, 0-inch fat, braised	3 oz	225	60	12.5
choice, 1/4-inch fat, braised	3 oz	224	60	12.2
choice, 1/2-inch fat, braised	3 oz	234	60	13.4
prime, 1/2-inch fat, braised	3 oz	270	60	17.5
prime, 1/2-inch fat, raw	1 lb	921	349	60.8
prime, 1/2-inch fat, raw	1 oz	58	22	3.8
select, 0-inch fat, braised	3 oz	202	60	9.9
select, 1/4-inch fat, braised	3 oz	201	60	9.9
select, 1/2-inch fat, braised	3 oz	218	60	11.6
Untrimmed				
all grades, 0-inch fat, braised	3 oz	284	55	20.5
all grades, 1/4-inch fat, braised	3 oz	293	54	21.8
all grades, 1/4-inch fat, raw	1 lb	1152	304	91.2
all grades, 1/4-inch fat, raw	1 oz	72	19	5.7
all grades, 1/2-inch fat, braised	3 oz	326	54	25.8
all grades, 1/2-inch fat, raw	1 lb	1288	299	107.0
all grades, 1/2-inch fat, raw	1 oz	81	19	6.7
choice, 0-inch fat, braised	3 oz	296	55	22.0
choice, 1/4-inch fat, braised	3 oz	309	54	23.6
choice, 1/4-inch fat, raw	1 lb	1234	299	100.8
choice, 1/4-inch fat, raw	1 oz	77	19	6.3
choice, 1/2-inch fat, braised	3 oz	330	54	26.4
choice, 1/2-inch fat, raw	1 lb	1320	295	110.7
choice, 1/2-inch fat, raw	1 oz	83	18	6.9
prime, 1/2-inch fat, braised	3 oz	354	54	29.0
prime, 1/2-inch fat, raw	1 lb	1488	290	129.6
prime, 1/2-inch fat, raw	1 oz	93	18	8.1
select, 0-inch fat, braised	3 oz	266	56	18.4
select, 1/4-inch fat, braised	3 oz	277	55	19.9
select, 1/4-inch fat, raw	1 lb	1066	308	81.3
select, 1/4-inch fat, raw	1 oz	67	19	5.1
select, 1/2-inch fat, braised	3 oz	311	54	24.1
select, 1/2-inch fat, raw	1 lb	1179	304	94.4
select, 1/2-inch fat, raw	1 oz	74	19	5.9

Food Name	Serv. Size	Total Cal.	Sod. MGS	Fat GMS
FLANK				
Trimmed				
choice, 0-inch fat, braised	3 oz	201	61	11.0
choice, 0-inch fat, broiled	3 oz	176	71	8.6
Untrimmed				
choice, 0-inch fat, braised	3 oz	224	59	14.0
choice, 0-inch fat, broiled	3 oz	192	69	10.6
choice, 0-inch fat, raw	1 oz	51	20	3.0
choice, 0-inch fat, raw	4 oz	203	80	12.0
HEART				
raw	4 oz	132	71	4.3
simmered	3 oz	149	54	4.8
KIDNEY				
raw	4 oz	121	202	3.5
simmered	3 oz	122	114	2.9
LEAN CUTS				
bottom round steak, 'Lite' (Heritage Lifestyle) uncooked	3 oz	108	40	4.0
(Brae Beef) raw	4 oz	120	60	2.0
brisket 'Lite' (Heritage Lifestyle) uncooked	3 oz	98	40	3.0
burger (Lean and Free) raw	4 oz	174	64	9.3
chuck, arm pot roast, 'Lite' (Heritage Lifestyle) uncooked	3 oz	101	40	3.0
chuck blade roast, 'Lite' (Heritage Lifestyle) uncooked	3 oz	128	45	7.0
cube steak (Lean and Free) raw	4 oz	109	(mq)	1.0
eye round steak, 'Lite' (Heritage Lifestyle) uncooked	3 oz	111	38	4.0
ground, lean, 'Lite' (Heritage Lifestyle) uncooked	3 oz	118	45	5.0
lean cuts, raw (Lean and Free)	4 oz	161	(mq)	7.5
rib eye (Lean and Free) raw	4 oz	121	59	2.6
rib roast, large end, 'Lite' (Heritage Lifestyle) uncooked	3 oz	142	40	8.0
rib steak, small end, 'Lite' (Heritage Lifestyle) uncooked	3 oz	118	35	5.0
rolled (Lean and Free) raw	4 oz	125	60	2.8
round steak (Lean and Free) raw	4 oz	111	60	1.1
round tip roast, 'Lite' (Heritage Lifestyle) uncooked	3 oz	91	43	1.5
sirloin steak (Lean and Free) raw	4 oz	111	67	1.8
sirloin steak, 'Lite' (Heritage Lifestyle) uncooked	3 oz	103	45	3.0
sirloin tip (Lean and Free) raw	4 oz	110	62	1.2
strip loin steak (Lean and Free) raw	4 oz	113	61	1.8
T-bone (Lean and Free) raw	4 oz	125	54	2.7
tenderloin fillet steak (Lean and Free) raw	4 oz	116	68	2.4
tenderloin steak, 'Lite' (Heritage Lifestyle) uncooked	3 oz	109	40	4.0
top loin steak, 'Lite' (Heritage Lifestyle) uncooked	3 oz	114	40	4.0
top round (Lean and Free) raw	4 oz	134	49	4.5

Food Name	Serv. Size	Total Cal.	Sod. MGS	Fat GMS
top round steak, 'Lite' *(Heritage Lifestyle)* uncooked	3 oz	100	40	3.0
LIVER				
braised	3 oz	137	59	4.2
pan-fried	3 oz	184	90	6.8
pan-fried in vegetable oil	4 oz	246	120	9.1
raw	4 oz	162	82	4.3
LUNG				
braised	3 oz	102	86	3.2
raw	4 oz	104	224	2.8
PANCREAS				
braised	3 oz	230	51	14.6
raw	4 oz	266	76	21.0
PORTERHOUSE				
Trimmed				
choice, 1/4-inch fat, broiled	3 oz	185	56	9.2
choice, 1/2-inch fat, broiled	3 oz	185	56	9.2
Untrimmed				
choice, 1/4-inch fat, broiled	3 oz	259	52	18.8
choice, 1/4-inch fat, raw	1 lb	1229	222	98.4
choice, 1/4-inch fat, raw	1 oz	77	14	6.2
choice, 1/2-inch fat, broiled	3 oz	254	52	18.0
choice, 1/2-inch fat, raw	1 lb	1288	222	105.6
choice, 1/2-inch fat, raw	1 oz	81	14	6.6
RIB, LARGE END				
Trimmed				
all grades, ribs 6-9, 0-inch fat, roasted	3 oz	202	62	11.4
all grades, ribs 6-9, 1/4-inch fat, broiled	3 oz	190	61	11.0
all grades, ribs 6-9, 1/4-inch fat, roasted	3 oz	201	62	11.2
all grades, ribs 6-9, 1/2-inch fat, broiled	3 oz	198	59	12.1
all grades, ribs 6-9, 1/2-inch fat, roasted	3 oz	207	62	11.9
choice, ribs 6-9, 0-inch fat, roasted	3 oz	215	62	12.7
choice, ribs 6-9, 1/4-inch fat, broiled	3 oz	204	61	12.4
choice, ribs 6-9, 1/4-inch fat, roasted	3 oz	213	62	12.5
choice, ribs 6-9, 1/2-inch fat, broiled	3 oz	203	59	12.6
choice, ribs 6-9, 1/2-inch fat, roasted	3 oz	211	62	12.3
prime, ribs 6-9, 1/4-inch fat, broiled	3 oz	250	59	17.7
prime, ribs 6-9, 1/4-inch fat, roasted	3 oz	241	62	15.6
prime, ribs 6-9, 1/2-inch fat, broiled	3 oz	250	59	17.7
prime, ribs 6-9, 1/2-inch fat, roasted	3 oz	241	62	15.6
select, ribs 6-9, 0-inch fat, roasted	3 oz	187	62	9.7
select, ribs 6-9, 1/4-inch fat, broiled	3 oz	175	61	9.3

Food Name	Serv. Size	Total Cal.	Sod. MGS	Fat GMS
select, ribs 6-9, 1/4-inch fat, roasted	3 oz	187	62	9.7
select, ribs 6-9, 1/2-inch fat, broiled	3 oz	183	59	10.4
select, ribs 6-9, 1/2-inch fat, roasted	3 oz	197	62	10.8
Untrimmed				
all grades, ribs 6-9, 0-inch fat, roasted	3 oz	300	55	24.0
all grades, ribs 6-9, 1/4-inch fat, broiled	3 oz	295	54	24.2
all grades, ribs 6-9, 1/4-inch fat, raw	1 lb	1465	249	127.9
all grades, ribs 6-9, 1/4-inch fat, raw	1 oz	92	16	8.0
all grades, ribs 6-9, 1/4-inch fat, roasted	3 oz	310	54	25.3
all grades, ribs 6-9, 1/2-inch fat, broiled	3 oz	321	51	27.5
all grades, ribs 6-9, 1/2-inch fat, raw	1 lb	1588	240	142.3
all grades, ribs 6-9, 1/2-inch fat, raw	1 oz	99	15	8.9
all grades, ribs 6-9, 1/2-inch fat, roasted	3 oz	313	54	25.5
choice, ribs 6-9, 0-inch fat, roasted	10.2 oz	1080	186	88.4
choice, ribs 6-9, 0-inch fat, roasted	3 oz	316	54	25.9
choice, ribs 6-9, 1/4-inch fat, broiled	3 oz	312	54	26.2
choice, ribs 6-9, 1/4-inch fat, raw	1 lb	1565	240	139.8
choice, ribs 6-9, 1/4-inch fat, raw	1 oz	98	15	8.7
choice, ribs 6-9, 1/4-inch fat, roasted	3 oz	326	54	27.2
choice, ribs 6-9, 1/2-inch fat, broiled	3 oz	326	51	28.1
choice, ribs 6-9, 1/2-inch fat, raw	1 lb	1615	240	145.6
choice, ribs 6-9, 1/2-inch fat, raw	1 oz	101	15	9.1
choice, ribs 6-9, 1/2-inch fat, roasted	3 oz	316	54	25.9
prime, ribs 6-9, 1/4-inch fat, broiled	3 oz	351	52	30.8
prime, ribs 6-9, 1/4-inch fat, raw	1 lb	1710	240	156.5
prime, ribs 6-9, 1/4-inch fat, raw	1 oz	107	15	9.8
prime, ribs 6-9, 1/4-inch fat, roasted	3 oz	342	54	28.9
prime, ribs 6-9, 1/2-inch fat, broiled	3 oz	361	51	32.1
prime, ribs 6-9, 1/2-inch fat, raw	1 lb	1737	236	159.6
prime, ribs 6-9, 1/2-inch fat, raw	1 oz	109	15	10.0
prime, ribs 6-9, 1/2-inch fat, roasted	3 oz	346	54	29.4
select, ribs 6-9, 0-inch fat, roasted	3 oz	281	55	21.7
select, ribs 6-9, 1/4-inch fat, broiled	3 oz	275	54	21.9
select, ribs 6-9, 1/4-inch fat, raw	1 lb	1379	249	117.7
select, ribs 6-9, 1/4-inch fat, raw	1 oz	86	16	7.4
select, ribs 6-9, 1/4-inch fat, roasted	3 oz	289	55	22.7
select, ribs 6-9, 1/2-inch fat, broiled	3 oz	301	52	25.1
select, ribs 6-9, 1/2-inch fat, raw	1 lb	1488	245	130.7
select, ribs 6-9, 1/2-inch fat, raw	1 oz	93	15	8.2
select, ribs 6-9, 1/2-inch fat, roasted	3 oz	303	54	24.5

Food Name	Serv. Size	Total Cal.	Sod. MGS	Fat GMS
RIB, SHORTRIB				
Trimmed, choice, braised	3 oz	251	49	15.4
Untrimmed				
choice, braised	3 oz	400	43	35.7
choice, raw	1 lb	1760	222	164.3
choice, raw	1 oz	110	14	10.3
RIB, SMALL END				
Trimmed				
all grades, ribs 10-12, 0-inch fat, broiled	3 oz	181	59	8.8
all grades, ribs 10-12, 1/4-inch fat, roasted	3 oz	185	60	9.8
all grades, ribs 10-12, 1/2-inch fat, broiled	3 oz	188	59	9.5
all grades, ribs 10-12, 1/2-inch fat, roasted	3 oz	201	64	11.5
all grades, ribs 10-12, 1/4-inch fat, broiled	3 oz	188	59	9.5
choice, ribs 10-12, 0-inch fat, broiled	3 oz	191	59	9.9
choice, ribs 10-12, 1/4-inch fat, broiled	3 oz	198	59	10.7
choice, ribs 10-12, 1/4-inch fat, roasted	3 oz	197	60	11.1
choice, ribs 10-12, 1/2-inch fat, broiled	3 oz	191	59	9.9
choice, ribs 10-12, 1/2-inch fat, roasted	3 oz	207	64	12.1
prime, ribs 10-12, 1/4-inch fat, broiled	3 oz	221	59	13.2
prime, ribs 10-12, 1/4-inch fat, roasted	3 oz	258	64	17.9
prime, ribs 10-12, 1/2-inch fat, broiled	3 oz	221	59	13.2
prime, ribs 10-12, 1/2-inch fat, roasted	3 oz	258	64	17.9
select, ribs 10-12, 0-inch fat, broiled	3 oz	168	59	7.4
select, ribs 10-12, 1/4-inch fat, broiled	3 oz	176	59	8.2
select, ribs 10-12, 1/4-inch fat, roasted	3 oz	173	60	8.3
select, ribs 10-12, 1/2-inch fat, broiled	3 oz	178	59	8.4
select, ribs 10-12, 1/2-inch fat, roasted	3 oz	184	64	9.6
Untrimmed				
all grades, ribs 10-12, 0-inch fat, broiled	3 oz	252	54	17.9
all grades, ribs 10-12, 1/4-inch fat, broiled	3 oz	286	53	22.1
all grades, ribs 10-12, 1/4-inch fat, raw	1 lb	1352	240	113.9
all grades, ribs 10-12, 1/4-inch fat, raw	1 oz	84	15	7.1
all grades, ribs 10-12, 1/4-inch fat, roasted	3 oz	295	54	23.8
all grades, ribs 10-12, 1/2-inch fat, broiled	3 oz	277	53	21.1
all grades, ribs 10-12, 1/2-inch fat, raw	1 lb	1388	245	117.8
all grades, ribs 10-12, 1/2-inch fat, raw	1 oz	87	15	7.4
all grades, ribs 10-12, 1/2-inch fat, roasted	3 oz	305	55	24.9
choice, ribs 10-12, 0-inch fat, broiled	3 oz	265	54	19.4
choice, ribs 10-12, 1/4-inch fat, broiled	3 oz	297	53	23.5
choice, ribs 10-12, 1/4-inch fat, raw	1 lb	1429	240	122.8
choice, ribs 10-12, 1/4-inch fat, raw	1 oz	89	15	7.7

Food Name	Serv. Size	Total Cal.	Sod. MGS	Fat GMS
choice, ribs 10-12, 1/4-inch fat, roasted	3 oz	312	53	25.7
choice, ribs 10-12, 1/2-inch fat, broiled	3 oz	282	53	21.6
choice, ribs 10-12, 1/2-inch fat, raw	1 lb	1415	240	121.2
choice, ribs 10-12, 1/2-inch fat, raw	1 oz	88	15	7.6
choice, ribs 10-12, 1/2-inch fat, roasted	3 oz	312	55	25.7
prime, ribs 10-12, 1/4-inch fat, broiled	3 oz	307	53	24.4
prime, ribs 10-12, 1/4-inch fat, raw	1 lb	1551	240	136.4
prime, ribs 10-12, 1/4-inch fat, raw	1 oz	97	15	8.5
prime, ribs 10-12, 1/4-inch fat, roasted	3 oz	354	55	30.5
prime, ribs 10-12, 1/2-inch fat, broiled	3 oz	309	53	24.7
prime, ribs 10-12, 1/2-inch fat, raw	1 lb	1583	240	140.2
prime, ribs 10-12, 1/2-inch fat, raw	1 oz	99	15	8.8
prime, ribs 10-12, 1/2-inch fat, roasted	3 oz	357	54	30.8
select, ribs 10-12, 0-inch fat, broiled	3 oz	242	54	16.8
select, ribs 10-12, 1/4-inch fat, broiled	3 oz	273	53	20.6
select, ribs 10-12, 1/4-inch fat, raw	1 lb	1297	245	107.4
select, ribs 10-12, 1/4-inch fat, raw	1 oz	81	15	6.7
select, ribs 10-12, 1/4-inch fat, roasted	3 oz	281	54	22.2
select, ribs 10-12, 1/2-inch fat, broiled	3 oz	263	54	19.4
select, ribs 10-12, 1/2-inch fat, raw	1 lb	1288	245	106.4
select, ribs 10-12, 1/2-inch fat, raw	1 oz	81	15	6.7
select, ribs 10-12, 1/2-inch fat, roasted	3 oz	283	56	22.3

RIB, WHOLE
Trimmed

Food Name	Serv. Size	Total Cal.	Sod. MGS	Fat GMS
all grades, ribs 6-12, 1/4-inch fat, broiled	3 oz	190	60	10.4
all grades, ribs 6-12, 1/4-inch fat, roasted	3 oz	195	61	10.6
all grades, ribs 6-12, 1/2-inch fat, broiled	3 oz	194	59	11.0
all grades, ribs 6-12, 1/2-inch fat, roasted	3 oz	204	63	11.7
choice, ribs 6-12, 1/4-inch fat, broiled	3 oz	201	60	11.7
choice, ribs 6-12, 1/4-inch fat, roasted	3 oz	207	61	11.9
choice, ribs 6-12, 1/2-inch fat, broiled	3 oz	198	59	11.5
choice, ribs 6-12, 1/2-inch fat, roasted	3 oz	209	63	12.2
prime, ribs 6-12, 1/4-inch fat, broiled	3 oz	238	59	15.9
prime, ribs 6-12, 1/4-inch fat, roasted	3 oz	248	63	16.5
prime, ribs 6-12, 1/2-inch fat, broiled	3 oz	238	59	15.9
prime, ribs 6-12, 1/2-inch fat, roasted	3 oz	248	63	16.5
select, ribs 6-12, 1/4-inch fat, broiled	3 oz	175	60	8.9
select, ribs 6-12, 1/4-inch fat, roasted	3 oz	181	61	9.1
select, ribs 6-12, 1/2-inch fat, broiled	3 oz	181	59	9.6
select, ribs 6-12, 1/2-inch fat, roasted	3 oz	191	63	10.3

Food Name	Serv. Size	Total Cal.	Sod. MGS	Fat GMS
Untrimmed				
all grades, ribs 6-12, 1/4-inch fat, broiled	3 oz	291	54	23.3
all grades, ribs 6-12, 1/4-inch fat, raw	1 lb	1420	245	122.4
all grades, ribs 6-12, 1/4-inch fat, raw	1 oz	89	15	7.7
all grades, ribs 6-12, 1/4-inch fat, roasted	3 oz	304	54	24.7
all grades, ribs 6-12, 1/2-inch fat, broiled	3 oz	308	52	25.5
all grades, ribs 6-12, 1/2-inch fat, raw	1 lb	1501	240	132.2
all grades, ribs 6-12, 1/2-inch fat, raw	1 oz	94	15	8.3
all grades, ribs 6-12, 1/2-inch fat, roasted	3 oz	324	54	27.0
choice, ribs 6-12, 1/4-inch fat, broiled	3 oz	306	53	25.1
choice, ribs 6-12, 1/4-inch fat, raw	1 lb	1510	240	133.2
choice, ribs 6-12, 1/4-inch fat, raw	1 oz	94	15	8.3
choice, ribs 6-12, 1/4-inch fat, roasted	3 oz	320	54	26.5
choice, ribs 6-12, 1/2-inch fat, broiled	3 oz	313	52	26.1
choice, ribs 6-12, 1/2-inch fat, raw	1 lb	1533	240	135.5
choice, ribs 6-12, 1/2-inch fat, raw	1 oz	96	15	8.5
choice, ribs 6-12, 1/2-inch fat, roasted	3 oz	328	54	27.6
prime, ribs 6-12, 1/4-inch fat, broiled	3 oz	333	53	28.2
prime, ribs 6-12, 1/4-inch fat, raw	1 lb	1651	240	149.0
prime, ribs 6-12, 1/4-inch fat, raw	1 oz	103	15	9.3
prime, ribs 6-12, 1/4-inch fat, roasted	3 oz	348	54	29.6
prime, ribs 6-12, 1/2-inch fat, broiled	3 oz	347	51	29.9
prime, ribs 6-12, 1/2-inch fat, raw	1 lb	1678	236	152.4
prime, ribs 6-12, 1/2-inch fat, raw	1 oz	105	15	9.5
prime, ribs 6-12, 1/2-inch fat, roasted	3 oz	361	54	31.4
select, ribs 6-12, 1/4-inch fat, broiled	3 oz	275	54	21.4
select, ribs 6-12, 1/4-inch fat, raw	1 lb	1347	249	113.7
select, ribs 6-12, 1/4-inch fat, raw	1 oz	84	16	7.1
select, ribs 6-12, 1/4-inch fat, roasted	3 oz	286	54	22.5
select, ribs 6-12, 1/2-inch fat, broiled	3 oz	289	52	23.3
select, ribs 6-12, 1/2-inch fat, raw	1 lb	1411	245	121.2
select, ribs 6-12, 1/2-inch fat, raw	1 oz	88	15	7.6
select, ribs 6-12, 1/2-inch fat, roasted	3 oz	306	54	24.9
RIB EYE, SMALL END				
Trimmed				
choice, ribs 10-12, 0-inch fat, broiled	3 oz	191	59	9.9
choice, ribs 10-12, 1/4-inch fat, broiled	4 oz	255	78	13.3
Untrimmed				
choice, ribs 10-12, 0-inch fat, broiled	3 oz	261	54	18.9
choice, ribs 10-12, 0-inch fat, raw	1 lb	1243	254	100.1
choice, ribs 10-12, 0-inch fat, raw	1 oz	78	16	6.3

Food Name	Serv. Size	Total Cal.	Sod. MGS	Fat GMS
ROUND, BOTTOM				
Trimmed				
all grades, 0-inch fat, braised	3 oz	173	43	6.5
all grades, 0-inch fat, roasted	3 oz	156	56	5.7
all grades, 1/4-inch fat, braised	3 oz	178	43	7.0
all grades, 1/4-inch fat, roasted	3 oz	161	56	6.3
all grades, 1/2-inch fat, braised	3 oz	189	43	8.2
choice, 0-inch fat, braised	3 oz	181	43	7.4
choice, 0-inch fat, roasted	3 oz	164	56	6.6
choice, 1/4-inch fat, braised	3 oz	187	43	8.0
choice, 1/4-inch fat, roasted	3 oz	168	56	7.1
choice, 1/2-inch fat, braised	3 oz	191	43	8.5
prime, 1/2-inch fat, braised	3 oz	212	43	10.8
prime, 1/2-inch fat, raw	1 lb	721	268	33.1
prime, 1/2-inch fat, raw	1 oz	45	17	2.1
select, 0-inch fat, braised	3 oz	163	43	5.3
select, 0-inch fat, roasted	3 oz	145	56	4.6
select, 1/4-inch fat, braised	3 oz	167	43	5.8
select, 1/4-inch fat, roasted	10.5 oz	534	197	18.5
select, 1/4-inch fat, roasted	3 oz	152	56	5.3
select, 1/2-inch fat, braised	3 oz	182	43	7.4
Untrimmed				
all grades, 0-inch fat, braised	3 oz	181	43	7.5
all grades, 0-inch fat, roasted	3 oz	160	56	6.3
all grades, 1/4-inch fat, braised	3 oz	234	43	14.4
all grades, 1/4-inch fat, raw	1 lb	943	249	60.9
all grades, 1/4-inch fat, raw	1 oz	59	16	3.8
all grades, 1/4-inch fat, roasted	3 oz	211	54	12.7
all grades, 1/2-inch fat, braised	3 oz	222	43	12.6
all grades, 1/2-inch fat, raw	1 lb	1021	249	70.5
all grades, 1/2-inch fat, raw	1 oz	64	16	4.4
choice, 0-inch fat, braised	3 oz	193	43	9.0
choice, 0-inch fat, roasted	3 oz	173	55	7.7
choice, 1/4-inch fat, braised	3 oz	241	43	15.2
choice, 1/4-inch fat, raw	1 lb	989	249	66.7
choice, 1/4-inch fat, raw	1 oz	62	16	4.2
choice, 1/4-inch fat, roasted	3 oz	221	54	13.9
choice, 1/2-inch fat, braised	3 oz	224	43	12.9
choice, 1/2-inch fat, raw	1 lb	1030	249	71.5
choice, 1/2-inch fat, raw	1 oz	64	16	4.5
prime, 1/2-inch fat, braised	3 oz	252	43	16.2

Food Name	Serv. Size	Total Cal.	Sod. MGS	Fat GMS
prime, 1/2-inch fat, raw	1 lb	1021	249	69.8
prime, 1/2-inch fat, raw	1 oz	64	16	4.4
select, 0-inch fat, braised	3 oz	171	43	6.4
select, 0-inch fat, roasted	3 oz	150	56	5.1
select, 1/4-inch fat, braised	3 oz	220	43	12.8
select, 1/4-inch fat, raw	1 lb	885	254	54.3
select, 1/4-inch fat, raw	1 oz	55	16	3.4
select, 1/4-inch fat, roasted	3 oz	199	54	11.3
select, 1/2-inch fat, braised	3 oz	215	43	11.8
select, 1/2-inch fat, raw	1 lb	984	249	66.0
select, 1/2-inch fat, raw	1 oz	62	16	4.1

ROUND, EYE OF
Trimmed

Food Name	Serv. Size	Total Cal.	Sod. MGS	Fat GMS
all grades, 0-inch fat, roasted	3 oz	141	53	4.0
all grades, 1/4-inch fat, roasted	3 oz	143	53	4.2
all grades, 1/2-inch fat, roasted	3 oz	156	53	5.5
choice, 0-inch fat, roasted	3 oz	149	53	4.8
choice, 1/4-inch fat, roasted	3 oz	149	53	4.8
choice, 1/2-inch fat, roasted	3 oz	156	53	5.7
prime, 1/2-inch fat, roasted	3 oz	213	50	12.7
prime, 1/2-inch fat, raw	1 lb	676	240	28.4
prime, 1/2-inch fat, raw	1 oz	42	15	1.8
prime, 1/2-inch fat, roasted	3 oz	168	53	7.0
select, 0-inch fat, roasted	3 oz	132	53	3.0
select, 0-inch fat, roasted	10.4 oz	460	184	10.4
select, 1/4-inch fat, roasted	3 oz	136	53	3.4
select, 1/2-inch fat, roasted	3 oz	151	53	5.1

Untrimmed

Food Name	Serv. Size	Total Cal.	Sod. MGS	Fat GMS
all grades, 0-inch fat, roasted	3 oz	145	53	4.6
all grades, 1/4-inch fat, raw	1 lb	966	222	64.8
all grades, 1/4-inch fat, raw	1 oz	60	14	4.1
all grades, 1/4-inch fat, roasted	3 oz	195	50	10.8
all grades, 1/2-inch fat, raw	1 lb	903	227	57.1
all grades, 1/2-inch fat, raw	1 oz	56	14	3.6
all grades, 1/2-inch fat, roasted	3 oz	207	50	12.1
choice, 0-inch fat, braised	3 oz	176	38	4.9
choice, 0-inch fat, roasted	3 oz	153	53	5.4
choice, 1/4-inch fat, raw	1 lb	989	222	67.1
choice, 1/4-inch fat, raw	1 oz	62	14	4.2
choice, 1/4-inch fat, roasted	3 oz	205	50	12.0
choice, 1/2-inch fat, raw	1 lb	916	227	58.8

Food Name	Serv. Size	Total Cal.	Sod. MGS	Fat GMS
choice, 1/2-inch fat, raw	1 oz	57	14	3.7
choice, 1/2-inch fat, roasted	3 oz	207	50	12.2
prime, 1/2-inch fat, raw	1 lb	1002	227	68.3
prime, 1/2-inch fat, raw	1 oz	63	14	4.3
select, 0-inch fat, roasted	3 oz	137	53	3.5
select, 1/4-inch fat, raw	1 lb	916	227	59.1
select, 1/4-inch fat, raw	1 oz	57	14	3.7
select, 1/4-inch fat, roasted	1 oz	184	51	9.6
select, 1/4-inch fat, roasted	4 oz	246	68	12.8
select, 1/2-inch fat, raw	1 lb	853	227	51.4
select, 1/2-inch fat, raw	1 oz	53	14	3.2
select, 1/2-inch fat, roasted	3 oz	201	50	11.5
ROUND, FULL CUT				
Trimmed				
choice, 1/4-inch fat, broiled	3 oz	162	54	6.2
select, 1/4-inch fat, broiled	3 oz	146	54	4.4
select, 1/2-inch fat, broiled	3 oz	156	54	5.9
Untrimmed				
choice, 1/4-inch fat, broiled	3 oz	204	52	11.6
choice, 1/4-inch fat, raw	1 lb	921	240	58.1
choice, 1/4-inch fat, raw	1 oz	58	15	3.6
choice, 1/2-inch fat, broiled	3 oz	233	51	15.5
choice, 1/2-inch fat, raw	1 lb	1093	231	79.6
choice, 1/2-inch fat, raw	1 oz	68	14	5.0
select, 1/4-inch fat, broiled	3 oz	190	53	10.0
select, 1/4-inch fat, raw	1 lb	866	240	52.6
select, 1/4-inch fat, raw	1 oz	54	15	3.3
select, 1/2-inch fat, broiled	3 oz	223	51	14.3
select, 1/2-inch fat, raw	1 lb	1048	231	74.1
select, 1/2-inch fat, raw	1 oz	65	14	4.6
ROUND, TIP				
Trimmed				
all grades, 0-inch fat, roasted	3 oz	150	55	5.0
all grades, 1/4-inch fat, roasted	3 oz	157	55	5.9
all grades, 1/2-inch fat, roasted	3 oz	161	55	6.4
choice, 0-inch fat, roasted	3 oz	153	55	5.4
choice, 1/4-inch fat, roasted	3 oz	160	55	6.2
choice, 1/2-inch fat, roasted	3 oz	164	55	6.6
prime, 1/4-inch fat, roasted	3 oz	181	55	8.6
prime, 1/2-inch fat, roasted	3 oz	181	55	8.6
select, 0-inch fat, roasted	3 oz	144	55	4.5

Food Name	Serv. Size	Total Cal.	Sod. MGS	Fat GMS
select, 1/4-inch fat, roasted	3 oz	153	55	5.4
select, 1/2-inch fat, roasted	3 oz	156	55	5.7
Untrimmed				
all grades, 0-inch fat, roasted	3 oz	162	54	6.7
all grades, 1/4-inch fat, raw	1 lb	912	259	59.8
all grades, 1/4-inch fat, raw	1 oz	57	16	3.7
all grades, 1/4-inch fat, roasted	3 oz	199	54	11.3
all grades, 1/2-inch fat, raw	1 lb	934	259	62.4
all grades, 1/2-inch fat, raw	1 oz	58	16	3.9
all grades, 1/2-inch fat, roasted	3 oz	213	53	13.0
choice, 0-inch fat, roasted	3 oz	170	54	7.6
choice, 1/4-inch fat, raw	1 lb	962	259	65.2
choice, 1/4-inch fat, raw	1 oz	60	16	4.1
choice, 1/4-inch fat, roasted	3 oz	210	53	12.6
choice, 1/2-inch fat, raw	1 lb	948	259	64.0
choice, 1/2-inch fat, raw	1 oz	59	16	4.0
choice, 1/2-inch fat, roasted	3 oz	216	53	13.3
prime, 1/4-inch fat, raw	1 lb	971	263	66.1
prime, 1/4-inch fat, raw	1 oz	61	16	4.1
prime, 1/4-inch fat, roasted	3 oz	233	53	15.2
prime, 1/2-inch fat, raw	1 lb	1012	259	72.9
prime, 1/2-inch fat, raw	1 oz	63	16	4.6
prime, 1/2-inch fat, roasted	3 oz	241	52	16.3
select, 0-inch fat, roasted	3 oz	158	54	6.2
select, 1/4-inch fat, raw	1 lb	848	256	51.2
select, 1/4-inch fat, raw	1 oz	53	16	3.2
select, 1/4-inch fat, roasted	3 oz	191	54	10.3
select, 1/2-inch fat, raw	1 lb	875	263	55.7
select, 1/2-inch fat, raw	1 oz	55	16	3.5
select, 1/2-inch fat, roasted	3 oz	205	53	12.0
ROUND, TOP				
Trimmed				
all grades, 0-inch fat, braised	3 oz	169	38	4.3
all grades, 1/4-inch fat, braised	3 oz	174	38	4.8
all grades, 1/4-inch fat, broiled	3 oz	153	52	4.2
all grades, 1/2-inch fat, broiled	3 oz	162	52	5.3
choice, 1/4-inch fat, braised	3 oz	181	38	5.5
choice, 1/4-inch fat, broiled	3 oz	161	52	5.0
choice, 1/4-inch fat, pan-fried	3 oz	193	60	7.3
choice, 1/4-inch fat, pan-fried in vegetable oil	4 oz	257	81	9.7
choice, 1/2-inch fat, broiled	3 oz	165	52	5.5

Food Name	Serv. Size	Total Cal.	Sod. MGS	Fat GMS
choice, 1/2-inch fat, pan-fried	3 oz	193	60	7.3
prime, 1/4-inch fat, broiled	3 oz	183	52	7.5
prime, 1/2-inch fat, broiled	3 oz	183	52	7.5
select, 0-inch fat, braised	3 oz	161	38	3.4
select, 1/4-inch fat, braised	3 oz	167	38	3.9
select, 1/4-inch fat, broiled	3 oz	144	52	3.2
select, 1/2-inch fat, broiled	3 oz	156	52	4.6
Untrimmed				
all grades, 0-inch fat, braised	3 oz	178	38	5.4
all grades, 1/4-inch fat, braised	3 oz	211	38	9.7
all grades, 1/4-inch fat, broiled	3 oz	184	51	8.2
all grades, 1/4-inch fat, raw	1 lb	798	227	42.5
all grades, 1/4-inch fat, raw	1 oz	50	14	2.7
all grades, 1/2-inch fat, broiled	3 oz	179	51	7.5
all grades, 1/2-inch fat, raw	1 lb	780	227	39.7
all grades, 1/2-inch fat, raw	1 oz	49	14	2.5
choice, 0-inch fat, braised	3 oz	184	38	6.0
choice, 1/4-inch fat, broiled	3 oz	190	51	9.0
choice, 1/4-inch fat, pan-fried	3 oz	235	58	13.1
choice, 1/4-inch fat, pan-fried in vegetable oil	4 oz	314	77	17.4
choice, 1/4-inch fat, raw	1 lb	821	227	45.0
choice, 1/4-inch fat, raw	1 oz	51	14	2.8
choice, 1/2-inch fat, braised	3 oz	221	38	10.9
choice, 1/2-inch fat, broiled	3 oz	181	51	7.7
choice, 1/2-inch fat, pan-fried	3 oz	247	57	14.5
choice, 1/2-inch fat, raw	1 lb	789	227	40.7
choice, 1/2-inch fat, raw	1 oz	49	14	2.5
prime, 1/4-inch fat, broiled	3 oz	195	51	9.1
prime, 1/4-inch fat, raw	1 lb	816	231	42.9
prime, 1/4-inch fat, raw	1 oz	51	14	2.7
prime, 1/2-inch fat, broiled	3 oz	201	51	9.9
prime, 1/2-inch fat, raw	1 lb	853	227	47.9
prime, 1/2-inch fat, raw	1 oz	53	14	3.0
select, 0-inch fat, braised	3 oz	170	38	4.5
select, 1/4-inch fat, braised	3 oz	199	38	8.4
select, 1/4-inch fat, broiled	3 oz	175	51	7.2
select, 1/4-inch fat, raw	1 lb	744	227	36.2
select, 1/4-inch fat, raw	1 oz	46	14	2.3
select, 1/2-inch fat, broiled	3 oz	176	51	7.1
select, 1/2-inch fat, raw	1 lb	748	227	36.3
select, 1/2-inch fat, raw	1 oz	47	14	2.3

Food Name	Serv. Size	Total Cal.	Sod. MGS	Fat GM
SIRLOIN, TOP				
Trimmed				
all grades, 0-inch fat, broiled	3 oz	162	56	5.
all grades, 1/4-inch fat, broiled	3 oz	166	56	6.
all grades, 1/2-inch fat, broiled	3 oz	177	56	7.
choice, 0-inch fat, broiled	4 oz	227	75	8.
choice, 0-inch fat, broiled	3 oz	170	56	6.
choice, 1/4-inch fat, broiled	4 oz	229	75	9.
choice, 1/4-inch fat, broiled	3 oz	172	56	6.
choice, 1/4-inch fat, pan-fried	3 oz	202	65	9.
choice, 1/4-inch fat, pan-fried in vegetable oil	4 oz	270	87	12.
choice, 1/2-inch fat, broiled	3 oz	179	56	7.
choice, 1/2-inch fat, pan-fried	3 oz	202	65	9.
prime, 1/2-inch fat, broiled	3 oz	201	56	10.
prime, 1/2-inch fat, raw	1 lb	703	263	32.
prime, 1/2-inch fat, raw	1 oz	44	16	2.
select, 0-inch fat, broiled	3 oz	153	56	4.
select, 1/4-inch fat, broiled	3 oz	158	56	5.
select, 1/2-inch fat, broiled	3 oz	170	56	6.
Untrimmed				
all grades, 0-inch fat, broiled	3 oz	183	55	8.
all grades, 1/4-inch fat, broiled	3 oz	219	54	13.
all grades, 1/4-inch fat, raw	1 lb	984	240	68.
all grades, 1/4-inch fat, raw	1 oz	62	15	4.
all grades, 1/2-inch fat, broiled	3 oz	238	54	15.
all grades, 1/2-inch fat, raw	1 lb	1179	236	91.
all grades, 1/2-inch fat, raw	1 oz	74	15	5.
choice, 0-inch fat, broiled	3 oz	195	54	9.
choice, 1/4-inch fat, broiled	3 oz	229	53	14.
choice, 1/4-inch fat, pan-fried	3 oz	277	59	19.
choice, 1/4-inch fat, pan-fried in vegetable oil	4 oz	370	79	25.
choice, 1/4-inch fat, raw	1 lb	1030	240	73.
choice, 1/4-inch fat, raw	1 oz	64	15	4.
choice, 1/2-inch fat, broiled	3 oz	241	53	15.
choice, 1/2-inch fat, pan-fried	3 oz	288	58	20.
choice, 1/2-inch fat, raw	1 lb	1198	231	93.
choice, 1/2-inch fat, raw	1 oz	75	14	5.
prime, 1/2-inch fat, broiled	3 oz	271	53	19.
prime, 1/2-inch fat, raw	1 lb	1320	231	108.
prime, 1/2-inch fat, raw	1 oz	83	14	6.
select, 0-inch fat, broiled	3 oz	166	55	6.

Food Name	Serv. Size	Total Cal.	Sod. MGS	Fat GMS
select, 1/4-inch fat, broiled	3 oz	208	54	11.8
select, 1/4-inch fat, raw	1 lb	939	245	62.5
select, 1/4-inch fat, raw	1 oz	59	15	3.9
select, 1/2-inch fat, broiled	3 oz	232	53	14.8
select, 1/2-inch fat, raw	1 lb	1116	236	84.0
select, 1/2-inch fat, raw	1 oz	70	15	5.3
SHANK CROSSCUTS				
Trimmed				
choice, 1/4-inch fat, simmered	4 oz	228	73	7.2
choice, 1/4-inch fat, simmered	3 oz	171	54	5.4
choice, 1/2-inch fat, simmered	3 oz	171	54	5.4
Untrimmed				
choice, 1/4-inch fat, raw	1 oz	50	17	2.8
choice, 1/4-inch fat, raw	3 oz	150	51	8.4
choice, 1/4-inch fat, simmered	3 oz	224	52	12.5
choice, 1/2-inch fat, raw	1 lb	721	277	35.1
choice, 1/2-inch fat, raw	1 oz	45	17	2.2
choice, 1/2-inch fat, simmered	3 oz	207	53	10.3
T-BONE				
Trimmed				
choice, 1/4-inch fat, broiled	3 oz	182	56	8.8
choice, 1/2-inch fat, broiled	3 oz	182	56	8.8
Untrimmed				
choice, 1/4-inch fat, broiled	3 oz	253	52	18.0
choice, 1/4-inch fat, raw	1 lb	1234	222	99.2
choice, 1/4-inch fat, raw	1 oz	77	14	6.2
choice, 1/2-inch fat, broiled	3 oz	275	51	20.9
choice, 1/2-inch fat, raw	1 lb	1393	218	118.5
choice, 1/2-inch fat, raw	1 oz	87	14	7.4
TENDERLOIN				
Trimmed				
all grades, 0-inch fat, broiled	3 oz	175	54	8.1
all grades, 1/4-inch fat, broiled	3 oz	179	54	8.5
all grades, 1/4-inch fat, roasted	3 oz	189	52	9.8
all grades, 1/2-inch fat, broiled	3 oz	173	54	7.9
all grades, 1/2-inch fat, roasted	3 oz	186	50	9.6
choice, 0-inch fat, broiled	3 oz	180	54	8.6
choice, 1/4-inch fat, broiled	3 oz	189	54	9.5
choice, 1/4-inch fat, roasted	4 oz	262	82	14.2
choice, 1/4-inch fat, roasted	3 oz	196	61	10.6
choice, 1/2-inch fat, broiled	3 oz	176	54	8.1

Food Name	Serv. Size	Total Cal.	Sod. MGS	Fat GMS
choice, 1/2-inch fat, roasted	3 oz	190	50	9.9
prime, 1/4-inch fat, broiled	3 oz	197	54	10.5
prime, 1/4-inch fat, roasted	3 oz	217	50	13.0
prime, 1/2-inch fat, broiled	3 oz	197	54	10.5
prime, 1/2-inch fat, roasted	3 oz	217	50	13.0
select, 0-inch fat, broiled	3 oz	170	54	7.5
select, 1/4-inch fat, broiled	3 oz	169	54	7.4
select, 1/4-inch fat, roasted	3 oz	179	52	8.8
select, 1/2-inch fat, broiled	3 oz	167	54	7.1
select, 1/2-inch fat, roasted	3 oz	177	50	8.6
Untrimmed				
all grades, 0-inch fat, broiled	3 oz	200	53	11.2
all grades, 1/4-inch fat, broiled	3 oz	247	50	17.2
all grades, 1/4-inch fat, raw	1 lb	1284	218	104.4
all grades, 1/4-inch fat, raw	1 oz	80	14	6.5
all grades, 1/4-inch fat, roasted	3 oz	282	48	21.8
all grades, 1/2-inch fat, broiled	3 oz	226	52	14.6
all grades, 1/2-inch fat, raw	1 lb	1093	222	81.6
all grades, 1/2-inch fat, roasted	3 oz	258	48	18.7
choice, 0-inch fat, broiled	3 oz	207	52	12.2
choice, 1/4-inch fat, broiled	4 oz	356	69	25.6
choice, 1/4-inch fat, broiled	3 oz	258	50	18.6
choice, 1/4-inch fat, raw	1 lb	1306	218	106.8
choice, 1/4-inch fat, raw	1 oz	82	14	6.7
choice, 1/4-inch fat, roasted	3 oz	288	55	22.4
choice, 1/2-inch fat, broiled	3 oz	230	51	15.1
choice, 1/2-inch fat, raw	1 lb	1116	222	83.9
choice, 1/2-inch fat, roasted	3 oz	262	48	19.2
prime, 1/4-inch fat, broiled	3 oz	269	50	19.9
prime, 1/4-inch fat, raw	1 lb	1288	218	104.6
prime, 1/4-inch fat, raw	1 oz	81	14	6.5
prime, 1/4-inch fat, roasted	3 oz	300	47	23.7
prime, 1/2-inch fat, broiled	3 oz	270	50	19.9
prime, 1/2-inch fat, raw	1 lb	1306	218	106.8
prime, 1/2-inch fat, roasted	3 oz	304	47	24.4
select, 0-inch fat, broiled	3 oz	195	53	10.6
select, 1/4-inch fat, broiled	3 oz	230	51	15.2
select, 1/4-inch fat, raw	1 lb	1261	218	101.6
select, 1/4-inch fat, raw	1 oz	79	14	6.3
select, 1/4-inch fat, roasted	3 oz	275	48	21.0
select, 1/2-inch fat, broiled	3 oz	216	52	13.4

Food Name	Serv. Size	Total Cal.	Sod. MGS	Fat GMS
select, 1/2-inch fat, raw	1 lb	1043	222	75.7
select, 1/2-inch fat, roasted	3 oz	245	48	17.3
THYMUS				
braised	3 oz	271	99	21.2
raw	4 oz	267	108	23.0
TONGUE				
potted or deviled	100 gm	290	1430	23.0
raw	4 oz	253	78	18.2
simmered	3 oz	241	51	17.6
smoked	100 gm	328	73	28.8
whole, canned or pickled	100 gm	267	1021	20.3
TOP LOIN				
Trimmed				
all grades, 0-inch fat, broiled	3 oz	168	58	7.1
all grades, 1/4-inch fat, broiled	3 oz	176	58	8.0
all grades, 1/2-inch fat, broiled	3 oz	173	58	7.6
choice, 0-inch fat, broiled	4 oz	237	77	10.9
choice, 0-inch fat, broiled	3 oz	178	58	8.2
choice, 1/4-inch fat, broiled	4 oz	243	77	11.5
choice, 1/4-inch fat, broiled	3 oz	182	58	8.6
choice, 1/2-inch fat, broiled	3 oz	176	58	8.0
prime, 1/4-inch fat, broiled	3 oz	208	58	11.6
prime, 1/2-inch fat, broiled	3 oz	208	58	11.6
select, 0-inch fat, broiled	3 oz	156	58	5.9
select, 1/4-inch fat, broiled	3 oz	164	58	6.6
select, 1/2-inch fat, broiled	3 oz	161	58	6.4
Untrimmed				
all grades, 0-inch fat, broiled	3 oz	180	57	8.7
all grades, 1/4-inch fat, broiled	3 oz	244	54	16.8
all grades, 1/4-inch fat, raw	1 lb	1102	240	81.3
all grades, 1/2-inch fat, broiled	3 oz	238	54	16.0
all grades, 1/2-inch fat, raw	1 lb	1284	236	103.6
choice, 0-inch fat, broiled	3 oz	194	57	10.2
choice, 1/4-inch fat, broiled	3 oz	253	54	17.8
choice, 1/4-inch fat, raw	1 lb	1179	240	90.4
choice, 1/2-inch fat, broiled	3 oz	243	54	16.6
choice, 1/2-inch fat, raw	1 lb	1311	231	106.7
prime, 1/4-inch fat, broiled	3 oz	275	54	20.3
prime, 1/4-inch fat, raw	1 lb	1383	236	114.2
prime, 1/2-inch fat, broiled	3 oz	288	53	22.0
prime, 1/2-inch fat, raw	1 lb	1461	231	123.7

Food Name	Serv. Size	Total Cal.	Sod. MGS	Fat GMS
select, 0-inch fat, broiled	3 oz	169	57	7.5
select, 1/4-inch fat, broiled	3 oz	226	54	14.6
select, 1/4-inch fat, raw	1 lb	1043	245	74.6
select, 1/2-inch fat, broiled	3 oz	223	54	14.2
select, 1/2-inch fat, raw	1 lb	1198	236	93.0
TRIPE				
canned *(Armour)*	6 oz	180	230	4.0
pickled	100 gm	62	46	1.3
raw	4 oz	111	52	4.5
BEEF, ALTERNATIVE				
(Heartline) 'Beef Fillet Style'	2 oz	176	480	7.0
(Heartline) 'Beef Fillet Style' lite	.5 oz	22	135	0.0
(Heartline) 'Ground Beef Style'	2 oz	176	480	7.0
(Heartline) 'Ground Beef Style' lite	.5 oz	22	135	0.0
(Heartline) 'Teriyaki Beef Style'	2 oz	176	450	7.0
Canned				
(Worthington) 'Prime Stakes'	3.25-oz piece	160	410	10.0
(Worthington) 'Savory Slices' 2-oz slices	2 slices	100	340	6.0
(Worthington) 'Vegetable Steaks' approx 1.28-oz pieces	3.2 oz	110	400	2.0
Frozen				
(Worthington) roll, approx 1.25-oz slices	2 slices	130	750	6.0
(Worthington) roll, smoked, frozen, approx 2/3-oz slices	3 slices	120	790	6.0
(Worthington) 'Stakelets'	2.5 oz	150	460	8.0
BEEF, CANNED, chopped *(Armour)*	3 oz	280	1290	24.0
BEEF, CORNED				
(Healthy Deli)	1 oz	35	210	1.0
(Hillshire Farm)	1 oz	31	230	0.4
(Oscar Mayer)	.6 oz	17	204	0.3
brisket, cured, cooked	3 oz	213	964	16.1
brisket, cured, raw	1 lb	898	553	67.6
brisket, cured, raw	1 oz	56	35	4.2
canned *(Dinty Moore)*	2 oz	130	(mq)	8.0
canned, cured	1 oz	71	285	4.2
canned, '7 oz can' *(Libby's)*	2.3 oz	160	720	9.0
canned, '12 oz can' *(Libby's)*	2.4 oz	160	750	9.0
'St. Paddy's' *(Healthy Deli)*	1 oz	24	290	0.4
'Slender Sliced' *(Eckrich)*	1 oz	40	270	1.0
BEEF, CORNED, ALTERNATIVE				
roll, frozen *(Worthington)*	2.5 oz	150	660	7.0
roll, frozen *(Worthington)* approx .5-oz slices	4 slices	120	740	6.0

Food Name	Serv. Size	Total Cal.	Sod. MGS	Fat GMS
BEEF, CORNED, HASH				
canned *(Armour)*	7.5 oz	390	900	27.0
canned, '15 oz can' *(Libby's)*	7 1/2 oz	400	1260	27.0
canned, '15 oz can' *(Mary Kitchen)*	7 1/2 oz	360	1386	24.0
canned *(Mary Kitchen)*	1 oz	47	111	3.0
canned *(Nalley's)*	8 oz	420	940	27.0
canned, 'No Frills' *(Pathmark)*	7 1/2 oz	410	1250	26.0
canned, '25 oz can' *(Mary Kitchen)*	8 1/3 oz	400	1429	27.0
canned, '24 oz can' *(Libby's)*	8 oz	420	1330	28.0
canned, w/potato	1 cup	398	1188	24.9
microwave cup *(Dinty Moore)*	7.5 oz	350	850	22.0
25% less salt, 'Premium' *(Armour)*	7.5 oz	350	790	21.0
BEEF, CORNED, SPREAD, canned *(Hormel)*	.5 oz	35	(mq)	3.0
BEEF, DRIED				
chipped, cooked, creamed	1 cup	377	1754	25.2
cured	1 oz	47	984	1.1
sliced *(Armour)*	1.1 oz	60	na	2.0
BEEF, GROUND				
Extra lean				
baked, medium-cooked	3 oz	213	42	13.7
baked, well-done	3 oz	233	54	13.6
broiled, medium-cooked	3 oz	218	59	13.9
broiled, well-done	3 oz	225	70	13.4
pan-fried, medium-cooked	3 oz	217	59	14.0
pan-fried, well-done	3 oz	224	69	13.6
raw	1 oz	66	19	4.8
raw	4 oz	264	75	19.3
Lean				
baked, medium-cooked	3 oz	228	48	15.6
baked, well-done	3 oz	248	60	15.6
broiled, medium-cooked	3 oz	231	65	15.7
broiled, well-done	3 oz	238	76	15.0
pan-fried, medium-cooked	3 oz	234	65	16.2
pan-fried, well-done	3 oz	235	74	15.0
raw	1 oz	75	20	5.9
raw	4 oz	298	78	23.4
Regular				
baked, medium-cooked	3 oz	244	51	17.8
baked, well-done	3 oz	269	64	18.3
broiled, frozen patty, medium-cooked	3 oz	240	65	16.7
broiled, medium-cooked	3 oz	246	71	17.6

Food Name	Serv. Size	Total Cal.	Sod. MGS	Fat GMS
broiled, well-done	3 oz	248	79	16.5
pan-fried, medium-cooked	3 oz	260	71	19.2
pan-fried, well-done	3 oz	243	79	16.1
raw	1 oz	88	19	7.5
raw	4 oz	350	77	30.0
raw, frozen patty	3 oz	240	58	19.7
BEEF DINNER, FROZEN. See also BEEF ENTRÉE, FROZEN.				
and gravy (Swanson)	11.25 oz	310	770	6.0
chopped (Banquet)	11 oz	420	600	32.0
chopped steak, 'Hungry Man' (Swanson)	16.75 oz	640	1600	37.0
'Extra Helping' (Banquet)	16 oz	870	810	61.0
in barbecue sauce (Swanson)	11 oz	460	860	17.0
Mexicana (Budget Gourmet)	12.8 oz	560	1290	23.0
patty, charbroiled (Freezer Queen)	10 oz	300	1260	17.0
Salisbury steak (Banquet)	11 oz	500	600	34.0
Salisbury steak (Freezer Queen)	10 oz	380	1260	22.0
Salisbury steak (Healthy Choice)	11.5 oz	300	480	7.0
Salisbury steak (Le Menu)	10.5 oz	370	880	20.0
Salisbury steak (Morton)	10 oz	300	1420	17.0
Salisbury steak (Swanson)	10.75 oz	400	880	17.0
Salisbury steak, charbroiled flavor 'Healthy Balance' (Banquet)	10.5 oz	270	800	8.0
Salisbury steak 'Classics' (Armour)	11.25 oz	350	1430	17.0
Salisbury steak 'Classics Lite' (Armour)	11.5 oz	300	1020	2.0
Salisbury steak 'Extra Helping' (Banquet)	18 oz	910	740	60.0
Salisbury steak 'Hungry Man' (Swanson)	16.5 oz	680	1730	41.0
Salisbury steak 'Lightstyle' (Le Menu)	10 oz	280	400	9.0
Salisbury steak, parmigiana 'Classics' (Armour)	11.5 oz	410	1120	21.0
Salisbury steak, sirloin (Budget Gourmet)	11.5 oz	410	890	22.0
Salisbury steak, w/mushroom gravy 'Extra Helping' (Banquet)	18 oz	890	685	58.0
sirloin, chopped (Le Menu)	12.25 oz	430	1010	24.0
sirloin, chopped (Swanson)	10.75 oz	340	790	16.0
sirloin, roast, 'Classics' (Armour)	10.45 oz	190	970	4.0
sirloin, w/barbecue sauce (Healthy Choice)	11 oz	280	240	4.0
sirloin tips (Healthy Choice)	11.25 oz	270	360	7.0
sliced (Morton)	10 oz	220	950	5.0
sliced, 'Hungry Man' (Swanson)	15.25 oz	450	1060	12.0
sliced, w/gravy (Freezer Queen)	10 oz	210	1010	7.0
steak Diane, 'Classics Lite' (Armour)	10 oz	290	440	9.0
tips (Le Menu)	11.5 oz	400	760	18.0

Food Name	Serv. Size	Total Cal.	Sod. MGS	Fat GMS
tips 'Classics' (Armour)	10.25 oz	230	820	7.0
tips, in Burgundy sauce (Budget Gourmet)	11 oz	310	720	11.0
BEEF ENTRÉE, ALTERNATIVE				
'Country Stew' (Worthington)	9.5 oz	220	760	10.0
pie, frozen (Worthington)	8 oz	360	1940	16.0
BEEF ENTRÉE, CANNED				
chow mein (LaChoy)	3/4 cup	40	960	2.0
chow mein, 'Bi-Pack' (LaChoy)	8.748 oz	83	998	0.9
chow mein, 'Bi-Pack' (LaChoy)	3/4 cup	70	840	1.0
Oriental, w/noodles, 'Bi-Pack' (LaChoy)	9 oz	148	1101	1.2
pepper, 'Bi-Pack' (LaChoy)	3/4 cup	80	950	2.0
pepper Oriental, 'Bi-Pack' (LaChoy)	8.783 oz	101	1219	2.0
pepper Oriental, 'Bi-Pack' (LaChoy)	3/4 cup	80	950	2.0
stew (Armour)	8 oz	210	1200	11.0
stew (Dinty Moore)	8 oz	220	870	13.0
stew (Estee)	7.5 oz	210	65	11.0
stew (Featherweight)	7.5 oz	160	400	3.0
stew (Wolf Brand)	1 cup	179	1043	7.5
stew, 'Big Chunk' (Nalley's)	7.5 oz	200	790	7.0
stew, '15-oz can' (Dinty Moore)	7.5 oz	200	810	12.0
stew, '15-oz pkg' (Libby's)	7.5 oz	160	870	5.0
stew, 'Homestyle' (Nalley's)	8 oz	180	810	5.0
stew, '40-oz can' (Dinty Moore)	8 oz	210	971	11.0
stew, 'No Frills' (Pathmark)	8 oz	190	625	4.0
stew, '24-oz can' (Dinty Moore)	8 oz	220	980	12.0
stew, '24-oz pkg' (Libby's)	8 oz	170	930	5.0
pepper Oriental (LaChoy)	3/4 cup	100	1340	4.0
BEEF ENTRÉE, FREEZE-DRIED				
beef and rice w/onions, prepared (Mountain House)	1 cup	330	265	12.0
stew, prepared (Mountain House)	1 cup	260	75	9.0
BEEF ENTRÉE, FROZEN. See also BEEF DINNER, FROZEN.				
and broccoli, w/rice, 'Fresh & Lite' (LaChoy)	11 oz	260	1299	5.0
Cantonese, w/rice, 'Stir Fry' (Weight Watchers)	9 oz	200	530	4.0
casserole, 'Microwave Classic' (Pillsbury)	1 pkg	430	1100	25.0
champignon, 'Gourmet Selection' (Tyson)	10.5 oz	370	830	15.0
creamed, chipped (Myers)	3.5 oz	136	863	8.0
creamed, chipped (Stouffer's)	5.5 oz	230	850	17.0
creamed, chipped, 'Cookin' Bag' (Banquet)	4 oz	100	(mq)	4.0
creamed, chipped, 'Cook-In-Pouch' (Freezer Queen)	5 oz	80	500	2.0
Dijon, w/pasta and vegetables (Right Course)	9.5 oz	290	580	9.0
fiesta, w/corn pasta (Right Course)	8 7/8 oz	270	590	7.0

Food Name	Serv. Size	Total Cal.	Sod. MGS	Fat GMS
homestyle, w/noodles, gravy, and vegetable *(Stouffer's)*	8 3/8 oz	230	720	7.0
Jade garden, 'Stir Fry' *(Weight Watchers)*	9 oz	150	490	3.0
London broil *(Ultimate 200)*	7.5 oz	110	320	3.0
London broil, in mushroom sauce *(Weight Watchers)*	7.37 oz	140	510	3.0
Oriental, w/vegetables and rice *(Lean Cuisine)*	8 5/8 oz	290	590	9.0
patty, charbroiled, w/mushroom and onion gravy *(Banquet)*	8 oz	300	(mq)	21.0
patty, charbroiled, w/ mushroom and onion gravy *(Freezer Queen)*	7 oz	200	960	12.0
patty, charbroiled, w/mushroom gravy *(Banquet)*	8 oz	290	(mq)	21.0
patty, charbroiled, w/mushroom gravy *(Banquet)*	5 oz	210	(mq)	15.0
patty, charbroiled, w/ mushroom gravy *(Freezer Queen)*	7 oz	180	1050	11.0
patty, charbroiled, w/ mushroom gravy *(Freezer Queen)*	5 oz	90	900	3.0
pepper, Oriental *(Chun King)*	13 oz	310	1300	3.0
pie *(Banquet)*	7 oz	510	870	33.0
pie *(Myers)*	3.5 oz	123	343	6.0
pie *(Stouffer's)*	10 oz	460	1130	27.0
pie, 'Supreme Microwave' *(Banquet)*	7 oz	440	730	29.0
'Platters' *(Banquet)*	10 oz	460	630	34.0
pot pie *(Swanson)*	7 oz	370	730	19.0
pot pie, 'Hungry Man' *(Swanson)*	16 oz	610	1360	31.0
ragoût, w/rice pilaf *(Right Course)*	10 oz	300	550	8.0
rib, boneless, seasoned, w/barbecue sauce *(Healthy Choice)*	11 oz	330	530	6.0
Romanoff supreme, w/pasta and vegetables *(Weight Watchers)*	9 oz	230	540	7.0
Salisbury steak *(Dining Lite)*	9 oz	200	1000	8.0
Salisbury steak, charbroiled, w/vegetable medley 'Single Serve' *(Freezer Queen)*	9 oz	330	990	22.0
Salisbury steak, homestyle, w/gravy, macaroni and cheese *(Stouffer's)*	9 5/8 oz	350	1130	17.0
Salisbury steak, 'Homestyle Recipe' *(Swanson)*	10 oz	320	980	16.0
Salisbury steak, supreme 'Gourmet Selection' *(Tyson)*	10 oz	430	810	26.0
Salisbury steak, w/gravy 'Cook-In-Pouch' *(Freezer Queen)*	5 oz	160	850	11.0
Salisbury steak, w/gravy 'Cookin' Bags' *(Banquet)*	5 oz	190	(mq)	14.0
Salisbury steak, w/gravy 'Family Entrées' *(Banquet)*	8 oz	300	(mq)	22.0
Salisbury steak, w/gravy 'Family Suppers' *(Freezer Queen)*	7 oz	200	1110	13.0
Salisbury steak, w/gravy and scalloped potatoes *(Lean Cuisine)*	9.5 oz	240	580	7.0
Salisbury steak, w/mushroom gravy 'Classics' *(Healthy Choice)*	11 oz	280	500	6.0
sirloin roast *(Budget Gourmet)*	9.5 oz	330	700	14.0

Food Name	Serv. Size	Total Cal.	Sod. MGS	Fat GMS
sirloin tips (Ultimate 200)	7.5 oz	200	560	6.0
sirloin tips, w/Burgundy sauce, Homestyle Recipe (Swanson)	7 oz	160	550	5.0
sirloin tips, w/country-style vegetables (Budget Gourmet)	10 oz	310	570	18.0
sliced beef, w/barbecue sauce, 'Cookin' Bag' (Banquet)	4 oz	100	(mq)	2.0
sliced beef, w/gravy, 'Cookin' Bag' (Banquet)	4 oz	100	(mq)	5.0
sliced beef, w/gravy, 'Cook-In-Pouch' (Freezer Queen)	4 oz	60	500	1.0
sliced beef, w/gravy, 'Deluxe Family Suppers' (Freezer Queen)	7 oz	130	870	3.0
sliced beef, w/gravy, 'Family Entrées' (Banquet)	8 oz	160	(mq)	5.0
steak, breaded (Hormel)	4 oz	370	(mq)	30.0
steak and mushroom hand-held pie, 'Aussie Pie' (Mrs. Paterson's)	5.5 oz	410	820	20.0
Szechuan (Chun King)	13 oz	340	1810	3.0
teriyaki (Chun King)	13 oz	380	2200	2.0
teriyaki (Dining Lite)	9 oz	270	850	5.0
teriyaki, w/rice and vegetables, 'Fresh & Lite' (LaChoy)	10 oz	240	1198	5.0
stew, 'Family Entrées' (Banquet)	7 oz	140	(mq)	5.0
stew, 'Family Suppers' (Freezer Queen)	7 oz	150	820	6.0
BEEF ENTRÉE, MICROWAVE				
beef and mushrooms, 'Health Selections' micro cup (Hormel)	7 oz	210	390	3.0
ribs, boneless, microwave bowl (Top Shelf)	1 serving	440	550	24.0
roast, tender, microwave bowl (Top Shelf)	1 serving	240	980	7.0
roast beef, w/gravy and potatoes, 'American Classics' (Dinty Moore)	10 oz	260	910	6.0
Salisbury steak, w/potatoes, microwave bowl (Top Shelf)	1 serving	254	1211	6.0
stew (Armour)	7.5 oz	150	870	5.0
stew, chunky, microwave cup (Weight Watchers)	7.5 oz	120	450	2.0
stew, 'Diner' microwave cup (Libby's)	7.75 oz	240	790	12.0
stew, hearty, 'Microeasy,' 1/4 pkg prepared w/1.5 lbs beef (Lipton)	1 serving	370	800	20.0
stew, hearty, microwave cup (Lunch Bucket)	7.5 oz	180	870	11.0
stew, micro cup (Hormel)	7.5 oz	230	1140	15.0
stew, microwave bowl (Dinty Moore)	10 oz	260	1180	14.0
stew, microwave cup (Dinty Moore)	7.5 oz	180	830	9.0
sukiyaki, microwave bowl (Top Shelf)	1 serving	330	1700	10.0
w/macaroni, 'Diner' microwave cup (Libby's)	7.75 oz	230	670	6.0
BEEF ENTRÉE, PACKAGED				
Salisbury steak (Top Shelf)	10 oz	320	910	15.0

Food Name	Serv. Size	Total Cal.	Sod. MGS	Fat GMS
Salisbury steak, w/mushroom gravy *(Ultra Slim Fast)* ..... 10.5 oz		290	830	5.0
BEEF JERKY				
'Arrowhead' *(Pemmican)* .... .7-oz piece		70	580	3.0
'Big Jerk' *(Slim Jim)* .... .25-oz piece		25	220	1.0
'Giant Jerk' *(Slim Jim)* .... .63-oz piece		60	510	2.0
jalapeño *(Pemmican)* .... 1.3-oz piece		110	1150	3.0
jalapeño *(Pemmican)* .... 1.1 oz		90	960	2.0
jalapeño flavored steak *(Pemmican)* .... .25 oz		25	220	1.0
'Lumberjack' *(Hormel)* .... 1 oz		101	304	9.0
natural *(Pemmican)* .... 1.3-oz piece		110	1150	3.0
natural *(Pemmican)* .... 1.1 oz		90	960	2.0
natural *(Pemmican)* .... 1 oz		80	880	2.0
natural flavored steak *(Pemmican)* .... .25 oz		25	220	1.0
peppered *(Pemmican)* .... 1.3-oz piece		110	1150	3.0
peppered *(Pemmican)* .... 1.1 oz		90	960	2.0
peppered steak *(Pemmican)* .... .25 oz		25	220	1.0
regular *(Frito-Lay's)* .... .21 oz		25	200	1.0
regular *(Hickory Farms)* .... 1 oz		100	1360	3.0
regular *(Slim Jim)* .... .14-oz piece		20	120	1.0
regular 'Super Jerk' approx .31 oz *(Slim Jim)* .... 1 piece		30	250	1.0
'Steakers' *(Pemmican)* .... 1.1-oz pouch		80	470	1.0
'Steakers' *(Pemmican)* .... 1 strip		40	160	1.0
Tabasco *(Pemmican)* .... 1.3-oz piece		110	1150	3.0
Tabasco *(Pemmican)* .... 1.1 oz		90	960	2.0
Tabasco flavored steak *(Pemmican)* .... .25 oz		25	220	1.0
Tabasco 'Super Jerk' *(Slim Jim)* .... .31-oz piece		30	250	1.0
'Tender' *(Frito-Lay's)* .... .7 oz		120	370	10.0
'Tender Brave' *(Pemmican)* .... 1 oz		80	830	2.0
'Tender Chief' *(Pemmican)* .... 1 oz		80	830	2.0
'Tender Tomahawk' *(Pemmican)* .... .25-oz piece		20	210	1.0
'Tender Trail' *(Pemmican)* .... 1 oz		80	830	2.0
'Tender Tribe' *(Pemmican)* .... 1 oz		80	830	2.0
teriyaki, natural style *(Pemmican)* .... 1 oz		80	800	2.0
teriyaki, natural style *(Pemmican)* .... .25-oz piece		20	200	1.0
teriyaki, natural style, slab *(Pemmican)* .... 1.3 oz		100	1030	2.0
BEEF JERKY, ALTERNATIVE				
'Jerquee' vegetable protein product *(Stonewall's)* .... .5 oz		50	125	2.0
'Spicy Italian Style' *(Cajun Jerky)* .... .5 oz		50	125	2.0
BEEF POT PIE. See BEEF ENTRÉE, FROZEN.				
BEEF SEASONING MIX				
(French's) dry ground, w/onions .... 1/4 pkg		25	440	0.0

Food Name	Serv. Size	Total Cal.	Sod. MGS	Fat GMS
(Lawry's) marinade	1 pkg	49	7284	0.2
(Schilling) Stroganoff	1/4 pkg	32	1078	0.3
BEEF STEW. See BEEF ENTRÉE, CANNED; BEEF ENTRÉE, DRIED; BEEF ENTRÉE, FROZEN; BEEF ENTRÉE, MICROWAVE.				
BEEF STEW MIX, hearty, 'Microeasy' *(Lipton)* dry	1/4 pkg	70	730	<1.0
BEEF STEW SEASONING MIX				
(French's) dry mix	1/6 pkg	25	770	0.0
(Lawry's) 'Seasoning Blends'	1 pkg	131	3181	0.7
(Schilling)	1/2 pkg	33	806	0.3
(Schilling) 'Bag'n Season'	1 pkg	87	4320	1.0
BEER. See ALCOHOLIC BEVERAGES.				
BEER, NONALCOHOLIC. See ALCOHOL-FREE BEVERAGES.				
BEER SALAMI. See LUNCHEON MEAT.				
BEERWURST				
beef	1 oz	92	264	8.3
beef, 4-inch diam	1/8-inch slice	76	236	6.9
beef, 2.75-inch diam	1/16-inch slice	20	62	1.8
pork	1 oz	67	352	5.3
pork, 4-inch diam	1/8-inch slice	55	285	4.3
pork, 2.75-inch diam	1/16-inch slice	14	74	1.1
pork, cured, 4-inch diam	1/8-inch slice	55	285	4.3
pork, cured, 2.75-inch diam	1/16-inch slice	14	74	1.1
BEET				
boiled, drained	4 oz	35	56	0.1
boiled, drained, sliced	1/2 cup	37*	65	0.2
raw, sliced	1/2 cup	29	53	0.1
raw, trimmed	1 oz	12	20	<1
raw, untrimmed	1 lb	133	220	0.4
BEET, CANNED				
cut *(Stokely)*	1/2 cup	40	300	0.0
diced *(S&W)*	1/2 cup	40	270	0.0
diced *(Stokely)*	1/2 cup	35	300	0.0
Harvard *(Stokely)*	1/2 cup	70	135	0.0
Harvard, sliced, w/liquid	1/2 cup	90	199	0.1
julienne *(S&W)*	1/2 cup	40	270	0.0
'No Salt or Sugar Added' *(Stokely)*	1/2 cup	40	40	0.0
pickled *(Freshlike)*	1/2 cup	40	650	0.0
pickled *(Stokely)*	1/2 cup	100	400	0.0
pickled *(Veg•All)*	1/2 cup	100	650	0.0
pickled, crinkle sliced, w/liquid *(Del Monte)*	1/2 cup	80	375	0.0
pickled 'Jars' *(Stokely)*	1/2 cup	90	280	0.0

Food Name	Serv. Size	Total Cal.	Sod. MGS	Fat GMS
pickled, sliced, w/liquid	1/2 cup	74	301	0.1
pickled, sliced, w/red wine vinegar 'Party' (S&W)	1/2 cup	70	215	0.0
pickled, sliced, w/red wine vinegar 'Regular' (S&W)	1/2 cup	70	215	0.0
pickled, whole, extra small (S&W)	1/2 cup	70	215	0.0
regular pack, w/liquid	1/2 cup	36	323	0.1
sliced (A&P)	1/2 cup	40	300	<1.0
sliced (Featherweight)	1/2 cup	45	55	0.0
sliced (Finast)	1/2 cup	40	390	0.0
sliced (Pathmark)	1/2 cup	45	330	0.0
sliced (S&W Nutradiet)	1/2 cup	35	40	0.0
sliced (Stokely)	1/2 cup	40	300	0.0
sliced, drained	1/2 cup	26	233	0.1
sliced, 'No Salt Added' (A&P)	1/2 cup	35	50	<1.0
sliced, 'No Salt Added' (Finast)	1/2 cup	40	40	0.0
sliced, 'No Salt Added' (Pathmark)	1/2 cup	35	35	0.0
sliced, water packed, w/o salt (Freshlike)	1/2 cup	40	50	0.0
sliced, water packed, w/o sugar or salt (Freshlike)	1/2 cup	40	50	0.0
sliced, w/liquid, 'No Salt Added' (Del Monte)	1/2 cup	35	100	0.0
small, sliced (Freshlike)	1/2 cup	40	260	0.0
small, sliced, 'Premium' (S&W)	1/2 cup	40	270	0.0
small, whole (Freshlike)	1/2 cup	40	260	0.0
small, whole (S&W)	1/2 cup	40	270	0.0
special dietary pack, w/liquid	1/2 cup	36	57	0.1
tiny, whole, w/liquid (Del Monte)	1/2 cup	35	290	0.0
whole (A&P)	1/2 cup	40	300	<1.0
whole (IGA)	1/2 cup	40	275	0.0
whole (Stokely)	1/2 cup	40	300	0.0
whole, sliced, w/liquid (Del Monte)	1/2 cup	35	290	0.0
BEET GREENS				
boiled, drained	4 oz	31	273	0.2
boiled, drained, 1-inch pieces	1/2 cup	19	174	0.1
raw, approx 2 oz	1 leaf	6	64	<.1
raw, 1-inch pieces	1/2 cup	4	38	0.0
raw, untrimmed	1 lb	49	510	0.2
raw, untrimmed	1 oz	5	57	<.1
BEET ROOT JUICE, bottled (Biotta)	6 oz	75	128	0.1
BELLYFISH. See MONKFISH.				
BERRY DRINK				
'Berries & Berries' (Tropicana)	6 oz	90	20	<1.0
'Berries & Berries' juice (Tropicana)	10 oz	156	3	0.0
'Berry B. Wild' (Squeezit)	6.75 oz	120	5	0.0

Food Name	Serv. Size	Total Cal.	Sod. MGS	Fat GMS
berry blend juice, 'Fruit Box' *(Tang)*	8.45 oz	140	10	0.0
berry citrus drink, frozen, prepared *(Five Alive)*	6 oz	90	5	0.0
berry juice, bottled *(Juicy Juice)*	6 oz	90	10	0.0
berry juice, boxed *(Juicy Juice)*	8.45 oz	130	15	0.0
berry juice, canned *(Juicy Juice)*	6 oz	90	10	0.0
berry nectar, organic *(Santa Cruz Natural)*	8 oz	90	na	<1.0
berry punch, aseptic box or chilled *(Minute Maid)*	6 oz	90	20	0.0
berry punch, frozen concentrate *(Minute Maid)*	6 oz	90	0	0.0
'Bopin' Berry' *(Hi-C)*	6 oz	90	25	0.0
'Great Bluedini' *(Kool-Aid)* 'Kool Bursts'	6.75 oz	110	10	0.0
'Great Bluedini' *(Kool-Aid)* 'Koolers'	8.45 oz	110	10	0.0
Mountain Berry Punch *(Kool-Aid)* 'Koolers'	8.45 oz	140	10	0.0
'Very Berry' *(Hawaiian Punch)*	6 oz	90	30	0.0

BERRY DRINK MIX

Food Name	Serv. Size	Total Cal.	Sod. MGS	Fat GMS
berry blend, sugar-free w/NutraSweet, prepared *(Crystal Light)*	8 oz	4	0	0.0
'Berry Blue' sugar-free w/NutraSweet, prepared *(Kool-Aid)*	8 oz	4	5	0.0
'Berry Blue' sugar-sweetened, prepared *(Kool-Aid)*	8 oz	80	5	0.0
'Berry Blue' unsweetened, prepared w/sugar *(Kool-Aid)*	8 oz	100	0	0.0
'Berry Blue' unsweetened, prepared w/o sugar *(Kool-Aid)*	8 oz	2	0	0.0
'Great Bluedini' sugar-free w/NutraSweet, prepared *(Kool-Aid)*	8 oz	4	0	0.0
'Great Bluedini' sugar-sweetened, prepared *(Kool-Aid)*	8 oz	70	0	0.0
'Great Bluedini' unsweetened, prepared w/sugar *(Kool-Aid)*	8 oz	100	0	0.0
'Great Bluedini' unsweetened, prepared w/o sugar *(Kool-Aid)*	8 oz	2	0	0.0
Mountain Berry Punch, sugar-free w/NutraSweet, prepared *(Kool-Aid)*	8 oz	4	35	0.0
Mountain Berry Punch, sugar-sweetened, prepared *(Kool-Aid)*	8 oz	80	15	0.0
Mountain Berry Punch, unsweetened, prepared w/sugar *(Kool-Aid)*	8 oz	100	15	0.0
Mountain Berry Punch, unsweetened, prepared w/o sugar *(Kool-Aid)*	8 oz	2	15	0.0
'Surfin' Berry' sugar-free w/NutraSweet, prepared *(Kool-Aid)*	8 oz	4	10	0.0
'Surfin' Berry' unsweetened, prepared w/sugar *(Kool-Aid)*	8 oz	100	25	0.0
'Surfin' Berry' unsweetened, prepared w/o sugar *(Kool-Aid)*	8 oz	2	25	0.0

Food Name	Serv. Size	Total Cal.	Sod. MGS	Fat GMS
BEVERAGES. See ALCOHOL-FREE BEVERAGES; ALCOHOLIC BEVERAGES; COFFEE; DIET DRINK; MILK; SOFT DRINKS AND MIXERS; SPORTS DRINK; TEA; WATER; and individual listings.				
BISCUIT				
buttermilk, commercially baked	1 oz	103	298	4.7
mixed grain, dough, baked	1 oz	86	221	1.8
plain, commercially baked	1 oz	103	298	4.7
(Awrey's) country	3-inch biscuit	160	530	5.0
(Awrey's) round	1 oz	80	260	3.0
(Awrey's) sliced	2 oz	160	520	5.0
(Awrey's) square	1 oz	80	260	3.0
(Awrey's) unsliced	2 oz	160	520	5.0
(Mrs. Winner's)	1 biscuit	245	503	5.0
(Weight Watchers) buttermilk	1.8 oz	100	410	1.0
(Wonder)	1 biscuit	80	140	1.0
BISCUIT, FROZEN (Bridgford)	2 oz	180	632	6.0
BISCUIT, REFRIGERATED				
(Ballard) buttermilk, extra lights, 'Ovenready'	1 biscuit	50	180	0.0
(Ballard) buttermilk, 'Ovenready'	1 biscuit	50	180	1.0
(Ballard) extra lights, 'Ovenready'	1 biscuit	50	180	0.0
(Ballard) 'Ovenready'	1 biscuit	50	180	1.0
(Big Country) 'Butter Tastin'	1 biscuit	100	320	4.0
(Big Country) buttermilk	1 biscuit	100	320	4.0
(Big Country) Southern style	1 biscuit	100	320	4.0
(1869 Brand) baking powder	1 biscuit	100	310	5.0
(1869 Brand) 'Butter Tastin'	1 biscuit	100	300	5.0
(1869 Brand) buttermilk	1 biscuit	100	310	5.0
(Good 'N Buttery) fluffy	1 biscuit	90	270	5.0
(Grands Inch) 'Butter Tastin'	1 biscuit	190	560	9.0
(Grands Inch) cinnamon raisin	1 biscuit	190	540	7.0
(Grands Inch) flaky	1 biscuit	190	530	8.0
(Hungry Jack) buttermilk, 'Extra Rich'	1 biscuit	50	180	1.0
(Hungry Jack) buttermilk, flaky	1 biscuit	90	300	4.0
(Hungry Jack) buttermilk, fluffy	1 biscuit	90	280	4.0
(Hungry Jack) flaky, 'Butter Tastin'	1 biscuit	90	280	4.0
(Hungry Jack) flaky	1 biscuit	80	300	4.0
(Hungry Jack) honey, flaky, 'Honey Tastin'	1 biscuit	90	290	4.0
(Hungry Jack) Southern style, flaky	1 biscuit	80	300	4.0
(Pillsbury) 'Big Premium Heat 'n Eat'	2 biscuits	280	610	15.0
(Pillsbury) butter	1 biscuit	50	180	1.0
(Pillsbury) buttermilk, 'Heat 'n Eat'	2 biscuits	170	530	5.0

Food Name	Serv. Size	Total Cal.	Sod. MGS	Fat GMS
(Pillsbury) buttermilk	1 biscuit	50	180	1.0
(Pillsbury) buttermilk, 'Tender Layer'	1 biscuit	50	170	1.0
(Pillsbury) 'Country'	1 biscuit	50	180	1.0
(Roman Meal) oat bran, honey nut	1 biscuit	131	278	4.7
(Roman Meal) white	2 biscuits	180	456	3.8
(Roman Meal) white, 'Premium'	1 biscuit	127	308	4.7
BISCUIT, TOASTER				
(Oroweat) 'Australian'	1 biscuit	180	440	5.0
(Oroweat) cinnamon raisin	1 biscuit	200	410	5.0
(Oroweat) cornbread	1 biscuit	200	230	3.0
BISCUIT MIX				
(Arrowhead Mills)	2 oz	100	96	1.0
(Bisquick)	1/2 cup	240	700	8.0
(Gold Medal) 'Pouch Mix,' prepared w/skim milk	1/8 recipe	90	270	3.0
(Health Valley) buttermilk, 'Biscuit & Pancake'	1 oz	100	170	1.0
(Krusteaz) cinnamon raisin, w/glaze, prepared from mix	3-inch biscuit	200	150	4.0
(Krusteaz) prepared from mix	2-inch biscuit	90	260	3.0
(Martha White) prepared from mix, 'BixMix,' made w/2% milk, rolled	2-inch biscuit	90	240	2.0
(Robin Hood) 'Pouch Mix,' prepared w/skim milk	1/8 recipe	90	270	3.0
BLACK BEAN				
boiled	4 oz	150	1	0.6
boiled	1/2 cup	114	1	0.5
raw	1/2 cup	331	5	1.4
raw	1 oz	97	1	0.4
raw (Arrowhead Mills)	2 oz	190	9	1.0
BLACK BEAN, CANNED				
(Eden Foods) organic, very low sodium, no salt added	1/2 cup	70	15	<1.0
(Green Giant)	1/2 cup	90	580	0.0
(Joan of Arc)	1/2 cup	90	580	0.0
(Progresso)	1/2 cup	90	350	1.0
BLACK BEAN DINNER, CANNED				
Western, w/garden vegetables, 'Fast Menu' (Health Valley)	7.5 oz	120	170	1.0
BLACK BEAN MIX, INSTANT				
prepared w/o added ingredients (Fantastic Foods)	1/2 cup	157	400	2.0
prepared w/2 tbsp salted butter (Fantastic Foods)	1/2 cup	207	469	8.0
BLACK CHERRY DRINK MIX				
unsweetened, prepared w/sugar (Kool-Aid)	8 oz	100	0	0.0
unsweetened, prepared w/o sugar (Kool-Aid)	8 oz	2	0	0.0

Food Name	Serv. Size	Total Cal.	Sod. MGS	Fat GMS
BLACK CHERRY JUICE				
(Knudsen & Sons)	8 oz	150	na	0.0
(Smucker's) 'Naturally 100%'	8 oz	130	10	0.0
BLACK PUDDING. See BLOOD SAUSAGE.				
BLACK TURTLE BEAN				
boiled	1/2 cup	120	3	0.3
canned	1/2 cup	109	461	0.4
raw	1/2 cup	312	8	0.8
BLACK WALNUT FLAVOR DRINK				
canned, liquid nutrition (Ensure)	8 oz	250	na	8.8
BLACKBERRY				
raw	1/2 cup	37	0	0.3
trimmed	1 oz	15	tr	0.1
untrimmed	1 lb	225	1	1.7
BLACKBERRY, CANNED				
in heavy syrup	4 oz	104	3	0.2
in heavy syrup, w/liquid	1/2 cup	118	4	0.2
in water (Allens)	1/2 cup	25	15	<1.0
BLACKBERRY, FROZEN				
unsweetened	18-oz pkg	326	5	2.2
unsweetened	1 cup	97	2	0.7
unsweetened	1/2 cup	49	1	0.3
BLACKBERRY SYRUP (Knott's Berry Farm)	1 oz	120	0	0.0
BLACK-EYED PEAS/cowpeas/yellow-eyed peas				
boiled, drained	1/2 cup	79	3	0.3
boiled, drained	4 oz	110	5	0.4
leafy tips, boiled, drained	4 oz	25	7	0.1
leafy tips, raw, chopped	1/2 cup	5	1	<.1
leafy tips, raw, trimmed	1 oz	8	2	0.1
leafy tips, raw, untrimmed	1 lb	68	16	0.6
raw, in pods	1 lb	208	9	0.8
raw, trimmed	1 oz	26	1	0.1
raw, trimmed	1/2 cup	65	3	0.3
young pods w/seeds, raw, approx 11 7/8 inches x 5/16 inch	1 pod	5	tr	<.1
young pods, w/seeds, raw, trimmed	1 oz	12	1	0.1
young pods, w/seeds, raw, trimmed	1/2 cup	21	2	0.1
young pods, w/seeds, raw, untrimmed	1 lb	182	17	1.2
BLACK-EYED PEAS, CANNED				
(A&P) mature	7.5 oz	120	410	1.0
(Allens)	1/2 cup	100	370	<1.0

Food Name	Serv. Size	Total Cal.	Sod. MGS	Fat GMS
(Allens) mature	1/2 cup	105	300	1.0
(Allens) w/snaps	1/2 cup	100	370	<1.0
(Bush's Best) packed from fresh shelled	1/2 cup	70	350	0.0
(Bush's Best) packed from soaked dry	1/2 cup	70	350	0.0
(Bush's Best) seasoned w/bacon	1/2 cup	90	420	1.0
(Green Giant) mature	1/2 cup	90	300	1.0
(Joan of Arc) mature	1/2 cup	90	300	1.0
(Luck's) mature, w/pork	1/2 cup	200	760	6.0
BLACK-EYED PEAS, DRIED				
mature, boiled	1/2 cup	100	3	0.5
mature, boiled	4 oz	132	5	0.6
mature, boiled *(A&P)*	1 cup	230	15	1.0
mature, raw	1 oz	95	5	0.4
mature, raw	1/2 cup	283	14	1.1
BLACK-EYED PEAS, FROZEN				
	10-oz pkg	396	17	2.0
boiled, drained	1/2 cup	112	5	0.6
boiled, drained	4 oz	150	6	0.7
(Freshlike)	3.3 oz	130	5	1.0
(Frosty Acres)	3.3 oz	130	6	1.0
(Seabrook)	3.3 oz	130	6	1.0
(Southern)	3.5 oz	136	20	0.7
(Veg•All)	3.3 oz	130	5	1.0
BLINTZ				
(Golden) blueberry	1 blintz	90	150	1.0
(Golden) cheese, low fat	1 blintz	80	135	2.0
(Golden) cherry	1 blintz	95	145	1.0
(King Kold) frozen	2.5 oz	113	272	1.6
(King Kold) frozen 'No Salt Added'	1.5 oz	96	78	0.5
BLOOD PUDDING. See BLOOD SAUSAGE.				
BLOOD SAUSAGE/black pudding/blood pudding				
	1 oz	107	193	9.8
approx 5 inches x 4 5/8 inches	1/16-inch slice	94	170	8.6
BLOODY MARY. See ALCOHOLIC BEVERAGES.				
BLUEBERRY				
trimmed	1 pint	225	24	1.5
trimmed	1 cup	81	9	0.6
trimmed	1/2 cup	41	5	0.3
trimmed	1 oz	16	2	0.1
untrimmed	1 lb	250	27	1.7
untrimmed	1 pint	226	24	1.5

Food Name	Serv. Size	Total Cal.	Sod. MGS	Fat GMS
BLUEBERRY, CANNED				
in heavy syrup	4 oz	100	3	0.4
in heavy syrup (A&P)	1/2 cup	110	25	<1.0
in heavy syrup (S&W)	1/2 cup	111	10	0.0
in heavy syrup, w/liquid	1/2 cup	113	4	0.4
in water (Lucky Leaf)	4 oz	40	0	0.0
in water (Musselman's)	4 oz	40	0	0.0
BLUEBERRY, FROZEN				
sweetened	10-oz pkg	230	3	0.4
sweetened	1/2 cup	94	2	0.2
unsweetened	20-oz pkg	289	6	3.6
unsweetened	1 cup	79	2	1.0
unsweetened	1/2 cup	39	1	0.5
BLUEBERRY NECTAR (Knudsen & Sons)	8 oz	135	na	0.0
BLUEBERRY SYRUP				
(Estee) 'Breakfast'	1 tbsp	12	10	0.0
(Featherweight)	1 tbsp	16	35	0.0
(Knott's Berry Farm)	1 oz	120	0	0.0
(Knott's Berry Farm) 'Light'	1 oz	50	0	0.0
(Knudsen & Sons)	1 oz	75	na	<1.0
BLUEFISH				
dry-heat cooked	3 oz	135	65	4.6
raw	1 lb	562	272	19.2
raw	3 oz	105	51	3.6
raw	1 oz	35	17	1.2
BLUEGILL				
raw	1 lb	404	368	3.2
raw	1.7-oz fillet	43	38	0.3
raw	1 oz	25	23	0.3
BOBWHITE. See QUAIL.				
BOCKWURST				
	1 oz	87	313	7.8
7 links per lb	1 link	200	718	17.9
BOK CHOY				
boiled, drained	4 oz	14	39	0.2
boiled, drained, shredded	1/2 cup	10	29	0.1
raw, shredded	1 cup	9	46	0.1
raw, shredded	1/2 cup	5	23	0.1
raw, shredded (Dole)	1/2 cup	5	23	0.1
raw, trimmed	1 oz	4	19	0.1
raw, untrimmed	1 lb	52	257	0.8

Food Name	Serv. Size	Total Cal.	Sod. MGS	Fat GMS
BOLOGNA. See LUNCHEON MEAT.				
BONITO. See also TUNA, SKIPJACK.				
Caribbean, raw	1 lb	626	(mq)	19.1
Caribbean, raw	1 oz	39	(mq)	1.2
Japanese, raw	1 lb	585	200	9.1
Japanese, raw	1 oz	37	12	0.6
BORAGE				
boiled, drained	4 oz	28	98	0.9
boiled, drained	3.5 oz	25	88	0.8
raw, 1-inch pieces	1/2 cup	9	35	0.3
raw, trimmed	1 oz	6	23	0.2
raw, untrimmed	1 lb	76	290	2.5
BORECOLE. See KALE.				
BORLOTTI BEAN. See CRANBERRY BEAN.				
BOSTON CREAM PIE. See CAKE.				
BOTTLE GOURD. See GOURD, BOTTLE.				
BOUILLON. See SOUP.				
BOURBON. See ALCOHOLIC BEVERAGES.				
BOYSENBERRY, CANNED, in heavy syrup	1/2 cup	113	4	0.2
BOYSENBERRY, FROZEN				
unsweetened, unthawed	10-oz pkg	142	3	0.7
unsweetened, unthawed	1 cup	66	1	0.3
BOYSENBERRY DRINK				
boysenberry juice, 'Naturally 100%' (Smucker's)	8 oz	120	10	0.0
boysenberry nectar (Knudsen & Sons)	8 oz	110	na	0.0
BOYSENBERRY SYRUP				
(Knott's Berry Farm)	1 oz	120	0	0.0
(Knott's Berry Farm) 'Light'	1 oz	50	0	0.0
BRAMBLE. See RASPBERRY.				
BRANDY. See ALCOHOLIC BEVERAGES.				
BRATWURST				
(Eckrich)	1 link	310	820	30.0
(Hickory Farms) 'Brotwurst'	1 oz	90	277	8.0
(Hickory Farms) cheddar, 'Cheddy Brots'	1 oz	98	259	9.0
(Hillshire Farm) fresh	2 oz	190	410	17.0
(Hillshire Farm) 'Fully Cooked'	2 oz	170	380	16.0
(Hickory Farms) hot, 'Hot Brots'	1 oz	96	269	9.0
(Hillshire Farm) smoked	2 oz	190	540	17.0
(Hillshire Farm) spicy	2 oz	180	(mq)	17.0
(Kahn's)	1 link	190	490	17.0

Food Name	Serv. Size	Total Cal.	Sod. MGS	Fat GMS
BRAUNSCHWEIGER				
(Hormel)	1 oz	80	322	7.0
(JM)	1 oz	80	260	6.0
(Oscar Mayer) 'German Brand'	1 oz	96	329	8.7
(Oscar Mayer) liver sausage	1 oz	100	230	9.0
(Oscar Mayer) 'Slices'	1 oz	96	327	8.7
(Oscar Mayer) 'Tube'	1 oz	97	301	8.7
BRAZIL NUT/butternut/cream nut/paranut				
in shell, unblanched	1 lb	1428	3	144.2
shelled, unblanched, approx 6–8 kernels	1 oz	186	tr	18.8
shelled, unblanched, approx 32 kernels	1 cup	919	2	92.7
BREAD. See also BAGEL; BISCUIT; BUN; CROISSANT; ENGLISH MUFFIN; ROLL; MUFFIN/PASTRY, TOASTER.				
APPLE-WALNUT (Arnold)	1 slice	64	103	1.3
BARBECUE, 'BBQ Loaf' (Colombo Brand)	2 oz	139	318	1.6
BRAN				
and oat, 'Light' (Oatmeal Goodness)	1 slice	40	90	<1.0
'Bran'nola' (Brownberry)	1 slice	85	137	1.4
'Bran'nola Original' (Arnold)	1 slice	85	137	1.4
'Gold'N Bran' (Earth Grains)	1 oz	70	150	1.0
honey bran, '1.5-lb loaf' (Pepperidge Farm)	1 slice	90	160	1.0
original, natural 'Bran'nola' (Oroweat)	1 slice	100	160	1.0
raisin (Brownberry)	1 slice	61	108	1.3
BROWN				
Boston, w/white corn meal, 3.25 inch diam	1/2-inch slice	95	113	0.6
Boston, w/yellow corn meal, 3.25 inch diam	1/2-inch slice	95	113	0.6
canned (B&M)	1.6 oz	94	320	0.0
canned (Friends)	1.6 oz	94	320	0.0
canned, Boston	1 oz	55	179	0.4
canned, 'New England' (S&W)	2 slices	76	172	0.4
canned, raisin (B&M)	1.6 oz	92	345	0.0
canned, raisin (Friends)	1.6 oz	92	345	0.0
plain (B&M)	1/2-inch slice	92	345	0.0
plain (Friends)	1/2-inch slice	92	345	0.0
raisin (B&M)	1/2-inch slice	94	320	0.0
raisin (Friends)	1/2-inch slice	94	320	0.0
BUTTERMILK				
(Grant's Farm)	1-oz slice	70	190	1.0
(Oroweat)	1 slice	100	210	1.0
CRESCENT (Pillsbury)	1 serving	100	230	6.0
CRISP, hard crispbread or toast	4 oz	473	278	9.8

Food Name	Serv. Size	Total Cal.	Sod. MGS	Fat GMS
EGG	1 oz	81	139	1.7
FRENCH				
enriched	1 oz	78	173	0.9
enriched, 5 inches x 2.5 inches	1 slice	101	203	1.0
extra sour *(Colombo Brand)*	2 oz	150	311	1.3
extra sour, sliced *(Colombo Brand)*	2 oz	153	310	1.6
'Hearth' *(Pepperidge Farm)*	1 oz	75	160	1.0
'Parisian' *(DiCarlo)*	1 slice	70	180	1.0
sweet, 'French Stick' *(Colombo Brand)*	2 oz	154	331	1.9
twin *(Farm Hearth)*	1 oz	80	160	1.0
unenriched, 5 inches x 2.5 inches	1 slice	101	203	1.0
GARLIC *(Colombo Brand)*	2 oz	185	331	10.1
GRAIN				
'Bran'nola' *(Arnold)*	1 slice	85	144	1.6
'Bran'nola Nutty Grains' *(Brownberry)*	1 slice	85	144	1.6
honey grain *(Grant's Farm)*	1-oz slice	70	170	1.0
honey grain, 'Family Recipe' *(Colonial)*	1-oz slice	70	180	1.0
honey grain, 'Family Recipe' *(Kilpatrick's)*	1-oz slice	70	180	1.0
honey grain, 'Family Recipe' *(Rainbo)*	1-oz slice	70	180	1.0
5-grain, organic *(BreadMill Bakery)*	1 slice	122	298	1.0
mixed grain, 'Round Top' *(Roman Meal)*	1 slice	67	140	0.8
mixed grain, 'Thin Sliced Sandwich' *(Roman Meal)*	1 slice	55	114	0.7
mixed grain, toasted	1 oz	77	150	1.2
mixed grain, whole grain	1 oz	71	138	1.1
multi-grain *(Hearty Grains)*	1 slice	80	230	2.0
multi-grain *(Weight Watchers)*	1 slice	40	100	<1.0
9-grain, 'Light' *(Oroweat)*	1 slice	40	135	0.0
7-grain *(Aunt Hattie's)*	1 slice	100	200	2.0
7-grain *(Grant's Farm)*	1-oz slice	60	140	1.0
7-grain, 'Hearty Slice' *(Pepperidge Farm)*	2 slices	180	340	2.0
7-grain, 'Light' *(Grant's Farm)*	.75-oz slice	40	115	<1.0
'Sun Grain' *(Roman Meal)*	1 slice	68	140	1.4
12-grain *(Earth Grains)*	1 oz	70	140	1.0
12-grain *(Oroweat)*	1 slice	110	210	2.0
GRANOLA, oat and honey *(Pepperidge Farm)*	1 slice	60	105	2.0
HAWAIIAN *(King's Hawaiian Bread)*	2 oz	180	160	4.0
HEALTH NUT				
(Brownberry)	1 slice	71	158	2.6
(Oroweat)	1 slice	110	200	2.0
HIGH-CALCIUM				
dark	1 oz	69	161	0.7

Food Name	Serv. Size	Total Cal.	Sod. MGS	Fat GMS
light	1 oz	64	196	0.6
HOLLYWOOD				
'Dark' (Hollywood)	1 slice	70	160	1.0
'Light' (Hollywood)	1 slice	70	150	1.0
HONEY NUT, and oat bran (Aunt Hattie's)	1 slice	100	180	na
HONEY OAT NUT (Earth Grains)	1 oz	80	85	2.0
HONEY WHEAT BRAN (Grant's Farm)	1-oz slice	70	120	1.0
HONEY WHEATBERRY				
(Earth Grains)	1 oz	70	160	1.0
(Oroweat)	1 slice	90	180	1.0
INDIAN FRY, Navajo, 5 inch diam	1 slice	296	626	8.6
ITALIAN				
'Family' (Wonder)	1 slice	70	160	1.0
'Francisco International' (Arnold)	1-oz slice	72	190	1.1
'Hearth' (Pepperidge Farm)	1 oz	80	150	1.0
'Hi-Fibre' (Monk's)	1 slice	70	80	1.0
light, 'Bakery' (Arnold)	1 slice	45	90	0.5
'Light' (Brownberry)	1 slice	44	89	0.5
thick sliced, 'Francisco International' (Arnold)	1 slice	66	111	0.8
OAT				
'Bran'nola Country' (Arnold)	1 slice	90	166	2.0
'Bran'nola Country' (Brownberry)	1 slice	90	166	2.0
country oat, 'Light' (Oroweat)	1 slice	40	135	0.0
crunchy (Pepperidge Farm)	2 slices	190	290	4.0
split top, 'Family Recipe' (Colonial)	1-oz slice	70	140	1.0
split top, 'Family Recipe' (Kilpatrick's)	1-oz slice	70	140	1.0
split top, 'Family Recipe' (Rainbo)	1-oz slice	70	140	1.0
OAT BRAN				
country oat, natural, 'Bran'nola' (Oroweat)	2 slices	230	390	4.0
honey (Roman Meal)	1 slice	71	130	1.2
honey (Earth Grains)	1 oz	80	105	1.0
honey, w/whole wheat, organic (BreadMill Bakery)	1 slice	121	315	1.0
honey nut (Roman Meal)	1 slice	72	130	1.6
organic, 'Light' (BreadMill Bakery)	1 slice	113	229	1.0
plain (Awrey's)	1 slice	50	130	0.0
plain (Grant's Farm)	1-oz slice	70	140	1.0
plain (Weight Watchers)	1 slice	40	100	<1.0
'Split-Top' (Roman Meal)	1 slice	68	140	0.9
OATMEAL				
cinnamon (Oatmeal Goodness)	1 slice	90	140	2.0
country twists (Hearty Grains)	1 slice	80	120	2.0

Food Name	Serv. Size	Total Cal.	Sod. MGS	Fat GMS
light, 'Bakery' (Arnold)	1 slice	44	98	0.6
light, 'Light Style' (Pepperidge Farm)	1 slice	45	95	0.0
'1.5 lb loaf' (Pepperidge Farm)	1 slice	90	200	1.0
plain (Pepperidge Farm)	1 slice	70	160	1.0
raisin, 'Hearty Grain' (Pillsbury)	1 slice	90	210	2.0
toasted almond (Grant's Farm)	1-oz slice	80	135	1.0
'Very Thin' (Pepperidge Farm)	1 slice	40	80	1.0
w/bran (Oatmeal Goodness)	1 slice	90	140	2.0
w/sunflower seed (Oatmeal Goodness)	1 slice	90	140	2.0
OATNUT (Orowheat)	1 slice	100	200	2.0
PITA				
oat bran (Sahara)	1/2 pita	66	163	0.3
onion, no fats, no oils, pre-sliced, 1.2 oz (Kangaroo)	1 pocket	75	160	0.0
white (Sahara)	1/2 pita	79	147	0.5
white, enriched	1 oz	78	152	0.3
white, enriched	1 pita	165	322	0.7
white, mini (Sahara)	1 pita	79	147	0.5
white, unenriched	1 oz	78	152	0.3
white, unenriched	1 pita	165	322	0.7
whole-wheat	1 oz	75	151	0.7
whole-wheat	1 pita	170	340	1.7
whole-wheat, approx 2 oz (Sahara)	1 pita	150	320	2.0
PROTEIN, includes gluten	1 oz	69	155	0.6
PUMPERNICKEL				
	1 oz	71	190	0.9
'Family' (Pepperidge Farm)	1 slice	80	230	1.0
plain (Arnold)	1 slice	70	198	0.9
small, 'Party' (Pepperidge Farm)	4 slices	60	160	1.0
RAISIN				
cinnamon (Arnold)	1 slice	67	86	1.4
cinnamon (Brownberry)	1 slice	66	107	1.3
cinnamon (Monk's)	1 slice	70	85	2.0
cinnamon (Pepperidge Farm)	1 slice	90	100	2.0
cinnamon swirl (Pepperidge Farm)	1 slice	90	100	2.0
orange (Brownberry)	1 slice	67	83	1.2
unenriched	1 oz	84	120	1.4
walnut (Brownberry)	1 slice	68	96	2.7
walnut, royal (Northridge)	1 slice	90	90	2.0
whole wheat, organic (BreadMill Bakery)	1 slice	120	327	1.0
RICE BRAN				
golden (Monk's)	1 slice	70	80	1.0

Food Name	Serv. Size	Total Cal.	Sod. MGS	Fat GMS
honey nut *(Roman Meal)*	1 slice	71	127	1.6
plain *(Roman Meal)*	1 slice	70	132	1.5
RYE				
caraway, 'Natural' *(Brownberry)*	1 slice	73	185	0.8
Dijon *(Pepperidge Farm)*	1 slice	50	170	1.0
Dijon, 'Hearty' *(Pepperidge Farm)*	1 slice	70	260	1.0
dill *(Arnold)*	1 slice	71	187	1.0
'Hearty' *(Beefsteak)*	1 slice	70	180	1.0
hearty rye, 'Light' *(Oroweat)*	1 slice	40	135	0.0
honey cracked *(Grant's Farm)*	1-oz slice	70	190	1.0
Jewish, seeded *(Levy's)*	1 slice	76	181	0.9
Jewish, seedless *(Levy's)*	1 slice	75	178	0.8
'Mild' *(Beefsteak)*	1 slice	70	180	1.0
'Old Allegheny' *(Braun's)*	1 slice	70	160	1.0
onion *(Beefsteak)*	1 slice	70	170	1.0
plain *(Weight Watchers)*	1 slice	40	100	<1.0
seeded, 'Family' *(Pepperidge Farm)*	1 slice	80	220	1.0
seedless, 'Family' *(Pepperidge Farm)*	1 slice	80	210	1.0
seedless, 'Natural Thin Sliced' *(Brownberry)*	1 slice	45	118	0.6
small, 'Party' *(Pepperidge Farm)*	4 slices	60	250	1.0
'Soft' *(Beefsteak)*	1 slice	70	170	1.0
very thin, light *(Earth Grains)*	1 oz	70	230	1.0
wheatberry *(Beefsteak)*	1 slice	70	160	1.0
SOURDOUGH				
French *(Boudin)*, approx 2-oz slices	2 slices	130	297	1.0
'Light' *(Earth Grains)*	.75 oz	40	115	1.0
'Light' *(Rainbo)*	.75-oz slice	40	110	<1.0
plain *(DiCarlo)*	1 slice	70	140	1.0
SUNFLOWER				
and bran *(Monk's)*	1 slice	70	80	1.0
'Texas Toast' *(Golden Corral)*	1 serving	170	230	6.0
whole wheat, organic *(BreadMill Bakery)*	1 slice	129	287	2.0
VIENNA				
light, 'Light Style' *(Pepperidge Farm)*	1 slice	45	100	0.0
thick sliced, 'Hearth' *(Pepperidge Farm)*	1 slice	70	125	1.0
WHEAT				
	1 oz	74	150	1.2
apple honey *(Brownberry)*	1 slice	69	148	1.9
'Brick Oven' *(Arnold)*	1 slice	57	104	1.5
'Butter Top' *(Home Pride)*	1 slice	70	140	1.0
buttertop *(Aunt Hattie's)*	1 slice	70	140	1.0

Food Name	Serv. Size	Total Cal.	Sod. MGS	Fat GMS
cracked	1 oz	74	153	1.1
cracked (Earth Grains)	1 oz	70	180	1.0
cracked (Pepperidge Farm)	1 slice	70	140	1.0
cracked (Wonder)	1 slice	70	180	1.0
cracked wheat and honey twists (Hearty Grains)	1 serving	80	120	2.0
dark, 'Bran'nola' (Arnold)	1 slice	83	166	1.0
'Family Recipe' (Colonial)	1-oz slice	70	150	1.0
'Family Recipe' (Kilpatrick's)	1-oz slice	70	150	1.0
'Family Recipe' (Rainbo)	1-oz slice	70	150	1.0
'Family,' 2-lb loaf (Pepperidge Farm)	1 slice	70	130	1.0
fat-free, 'Light' (Wonder)	1 slice	40	120	<1.0
'Hearth' (Brownberry)	1 oz	70	150	1.4
'Hearty' (Beefsteak)	1 slice	70	160	1.0
hearty, 'Bran'nola' (Arnold)	1 slice	88	197	1.9
hearty, 'Bran'nola' (Brownberry)	1 slice	88	197	1.9
honey buttered, split top, 'Family Recipe' (Colonial)	1-oz slice	70	140	1.0
honey buttered, split top, 'Family Recipe' (Kilpatrick's)	1-oz slice	70	140	1.0
honey buttered, split top, 'Family Recipe' (Rainbo)	1-oz slice	70	140	1.0
honey wheatberry (Arnold)	1 slice	77	143	1.2
'Light' (Grant's Farm)	.75-oz slice	40	115	<1.0
'Light' (Rainbo)	.75-oz slice	40	100	<1.0
light, golden, 'Bakery' (Arnold)	1 slice	44	86	0.5
'Light Style' (Pepperidge Farm)	1 slice	45	90	0.0
'Light 35' (Earth Grains)	1 oz	35	100	<1.0
loaf (Pipin' Hot)	1-inch slice	70	170	2.0
multi-grain (Beefsteak)	1 slice	70	130	1.0
'Natural' (Brownberry)	1 slice	80	183	1.3
oatmeal (Oatmeal Goodness)	1 slice	90	140	2.0
oatmeal, 'Light' (Oatmeal Goodness)	1 slice	40	90	<1.0
1.5-lb loaf (Pepperidge Farm)	1 slice	90	190	2.0
plain (Country Grain)	1 slice	70	160	1.0
plain (Fresh & Natural)	1 slice	70	140	1.0
plain (Weight Watchers)	1 slice	40	100	<1.0
sesame, 'Hearty' (Pepperidge Farm)	2 slices	190	340	3.0
'7-Grain' (Home Pride)	1 slice	70	140	1.0
'Soft' (Beefsteak)	1 slice	70	160	1.0
soft (Brownberry)	1 slice	74	127	1.8
soft, made w/buttermilk (Aunt Hattie's)	1 slice	70	130	1.0
sprouted (Pepperidge Farm)	1 slice	70	100	2.0
stone ground (Grant's Farm)	1-oz slice	60	150	1.0
stone ground, 'Family Recipe' (Colonial)	1-oz slice	70	150	1.0

Food Name	Serv. Size	Total Cal.	Sod. MGS	Fat GMS
stone ground, 'Family Recipe' (Kilpatrick's)	1-oz slice	70	150	1.0
stone ground, 'Family Recipe' (Rainbo)	1-oz slice	70	150	1.0
'Stoneground' (Home Pride)	1 slice	70	140	1.0
very thin (Earth Grains)	1 oz	70	150	1.0
WHEAT GERM	1 oz	74	157	0.8
WHEATBERRY (Grant's Farm)	1-oz slice	70	150	1.0
WHITE				
	1 oz	76	153	1.0
'Brick Oven' (Arnold)	1 slice	61	134	1.2
'Butter Top' (Home Pride)	1 slice	70	140	1.0
buttermilk (Wonder)	1 slice	70	160	1.0
buttertop, 'Homestyle' (Aunt Hattie's)	1 slice	70	140	1.0
'Country White' (Arnold)	1 slice	98	204	1.8
enriched, 'Country Style' (Holsum)	1 slice	70	135	1.0
extra fiber, 'Brick Oven' (Arnold)	1 slice	55	93	0.8
'Hearty Country' (Pepperidge Farm)	2 slices	190	340	2.0
'High Fiber' (Wonder)	1 slice	40	80	0.0
honey buttered, split-top, 'Family Recipe' (Colonial)	1-oz slice	80	140	1.0
honey buttered, split-top, 'Family Recipe' (Kilpatrick's)	1-oz slice	80	140	1.0
honey buttered, split-top, 'Family Recipe' (Rainbo)	1-oz slice	80	140	1.0
'Large Family,' 2-lb loaf (Pepperidge Farm)	1 slice	70	150	1.0
'Light' (Grant's Farm)	.75-oz slice	40	115	<1.0
'Light' (Rainbo)	.75-oz slice	40	100	<1.0
'Light' (Wonder)	1 slice	40	110	0.0
'Light Premium' (Arnold)	1 slice	42	89	0.5
'Light Premium' (Brownberry)	1 slice	42	89	0.5
'Light 35' (Earth Grains)	1 oz	35	105	<1.0
'Natural' (Brownberry)	1 slice	59	136	1.1
old fashioned (Northridge)	1 slice	70	125	1.0
plain (Monk's)	1 slice	60	95	1.0
plain (Weight Watchers)	1 slice	40	100	<1.0
plain (Wonder)	1 slice	70	140	1.0
'Robust' (Beefsteak)	1 slice	70	140	1.0
sandwich (Pepperidge Farm)	2 slices	130	260	2.0
special recipe, 'Iron Kids' (Rainbo)	1 slice	60	140	1.0
thin (Holsum)	1 slice	70	160	1.0
'Thin Sliced' (Wonder)	1 slice	50	120	1.0
'Thin Sliced,' 1-lb size (Pepperidge Farm)	1 slice	80	130	2.0
toasting (Pepperidge Farm)	1 slice	90	200	1.0
very thin (Earth Grains)	1 oz	80	160	1.0
'Very Thin' (Pepperidge Farm)	1 slice	40	80	0.0

Food Name	Serv. Size	Total Cal.	Sod. MGS	Fat GMS
white loaf *(Pipin' Hot)*	1-inch slice	70	170	2.0
w/buttermilk, 'Homestyle' *(Aunt Hattie's)*	1 slice	80	140	1.0
WHOLE BRAN, 'Natural' *(Brownberry)*	1 slice	58	167	1.4
WHOLE WHEAT				
	1 oz	70	149	1.2
'Family' *(Wonder)*	1 slice	70	140	1.0
'High Fiber' *(Wonder)*	1 slice	40	80	0.0
'Light' *(Wonder)*	1 slice	40	120	0.0
100% *(Northridge)*	1 slice	60	120	1.0
'100% Stone Ground' *(Monk's)*	1 slice	70	110	1.0
100% whole wheat *(Earth Grains)*	1 oz	70	150	1.0
'100%' *(Wonder)*	1 slice	70	160	1.0
plain *(Aunt Hattie's)*	1 slice	90	170	2.0
plain *(Daily)*	2-oz slice	140	0	0.0
'Soft 100%' *(Wonder)*	1 slice	70	140	1.0
'Stoneground 100%' *(Arnold)*	1 slice	48	97	0.7
stoneground, 100% *(Oroweat)*	1 slice	60	125	1.0
'Thin Sliced,' 1-lb loaf *(Pepperidge Farm)*	1 slice	60	110	1.0
'Very Thin' *(Pepperidge Farm)*	1 slice	35	75	0.0
BREAD, BROWN AND SERVE				
'Austrian' *(Du Jour)*	1 oz	70	140	1.0
'French' *(Du Jour)*	1 oz	70	140	1.0
'Italian' *(Pepperidge Farm)*	1 oz	80	150	1.0
BREAD, QUICK, MIX				
APPLE CINNAMON				
(Pillsbury) mix only, dry	1/12 pkg	140	160	1.0
(Pillsbury) prepared as directed	1/12 loaf	170	200	6.0
(Pillsbury) prepared w/1/4 cup oil, 1/4 cup egg substitute	1/12 loaf	190	170	6.0
(Pillsbury) prepared w/water, 1/4 cup oil, 1 egg	1/12 loaf	180	170	6.0
(Pillsbury) prepared w/water, 1/4 cup oil, 1/4 cup egg substitute	1/12 loaf	190	170	6.0
BANANA				
(Pillsbury) mix only, dry	1/12 pkg	120	190	1.0
(Pillsbury) prepared w/water, 3 tbsp oil, 1/2 cup egg substitute	1/12 loaf	170	210	6.0
(Pillsbury) prepared w/water, 3 tbsp oil, and 2 eggs	1/12 loaf	170	200	5.0
BANANA NUT *(Krusteaz)* prepared as directed	3/4-inch slice	190	300	6.0
BLUEBERRY NUT				
(Pillsbury) mix only, dry	1/12 pkg	130	160	1.0
(Pillsbury) prepared as directed	1/12 loaf	150	150	4.0
(Pillsbury) prepared w/1/4 cup oil, 1/4 cup egg substitute	1/12 loaf	180	170	6.0

Food Name	Serv. Size	Total Cal.	Sod. MGS	Fat GMS
(Pillsbury) prepared w/water, 1/4 cup oil, 1 egg .... 1/12 loaf		180	160	6.0
(Pillsbury) prepared w/water, 1/4 cup oil, 1/4 cup egg substitute .... 1/12 loaf		180	170	6.0
CHERRY NUT *(Pillsbury)* prepared as directed .... 1/12 loaf		180	150	5.0
CORNBREAD				
(Aunt Jemima) 'Easy,' prepared as directed .... 1 piece		196	679	6.3
(Ballard) mix only, dry .... 1/16 pkg		120	560	2.0
(Ballard) prepared as directed .... 1/8 pan		140	570	3.0
(Ballard) prepared w/1 cup milk, 1 egg .... 1/16 pan		150	580	3.0
(Dromedary) mix only, dry .... 3 tbsp		100	280	2.0
(Dromedary) prepared as directed .... 2-inch square		130	480	3.0
(Gold Medal) white, 'Pouch Mix, prepared w/egg and whole milk .... 1/6 pan		150	490	5.0
(Gold Medal) yellow, 'Pouch Mix,' prepared w/egg and whole milk .... 1/6 pan		150	500	5.0
(Krusteaz) honey, prepared as directed .... 1/16 pan		120	230	3.0
(Krusteaz) Southern, prepared as directed .... 2-inch square		140	450	3.0
(Martha White) buttermilk, prepared w/water .... 1/6 pan		110	360	2.0
(Martha White) 'Cotton Pickin' prepared as directed ...... 1/4 pan		170	540	3.0
(Martha White) 'Cotton Pickin' prepared w/water .... 1/6 pan		110	360	2.0
(Martha White) Mexican, prepared w/2% milk .... 1/6 pan		140	410	4.0
(Martha White) yellow, 'Light Crust,' prepared as directed .... 2 oz		140	400	4.0
(Robin Hood) white, 'Pouch Mix,' prepared w/egg and whole milk .... 1/6 pan		150	490	5.0
CRANBERRY				
(Pillsbury) mix only, dry .... 1/12 pkg		140	150	1.0
(Pillsbury) prepared as directed .... 1/12 loaf		160	160	4.0
(Pillsbury) prepared w/water, 2 tbsp oil, 1 egg .... 1/12 loaf		160	150	4.0
(Pillsbury) prepared w/water, 2 tbsp oil, 1/4 cup egg substitute .... 1/12 loaf		170	160	4.0
DATE				
(Pillsbury) prepared w/water, 1 tbsp oil, 1 egg .... 1/12 pkg		160	150	3.0
(Pillsbury) prepared w/water, 1 tbsp oil, 1/4 cup egg substitute .... 1/12 loaf		160	150	3.0
DATE NUT				
(Dromedary) mix only, dry .... 1/12 pkg		166	242	7.0
(Dromedary) prepared as directed .... 1/12 loaf		183	248	8.0
GINGERBREAD				
(Betty Crocker) 'Classic' mix only, dry .... 1/9 pkg		200	320	6.0

Food Name	Serv. Size	Total Cal.	Sod. MGS	Fat GMS
(Betty Crocker) 'Classic,' prepared w/cholesterol-free egg product	1/9 pan	210	330	6.0
(Betty Crocker) 'Classic,' prepared w/egg	1/9 pan	220	330	7.0
(Dromedary) mix only, dry	3 tbsp	100	190	2.0
(Pillsbury) mix only, dry	1/9 pkg	180	300	5.0
(Pillsbury) prepared as directed	3-inch square	190	310	4.0
NUT				
(Pillsbury) mix only, dry	1/12 pkg	150	180	3.0
(Pillsbury) prepared w/water, 2 tbsp oil, 1 egg	1/12 loaf	170	190	6.0
(Pillsbury) prepared w/water, 2 tbsp oil, 1/4 cup egg substitute	1/12 loaf	170	190	6.0
OATMEAL RAISIN				
(Pillsbury) mix only, dry	1/12 pkg	140	170	2.0
(Pillsbury) prepared w/water, 1/4 cup oil, 1 egg	1/12 loaf	190	180	7.0
(Pillsbury) prepared w/water, 1/4 cup oil, 1/4 cup egg substitute	1/12 loaf	190	180	7.0
BREAD CRUMBS				
Italian style *(Devonsheer)*	1 oz	104	408	1.3
Italian style *(Progresso)*	2 tbsp	60	240	<1.0
Italian style, whole-wheat *(Jaclyn's)*	.5 oz	28	5	1.0
plain	1 cup	427	931	5.8
plain	1 oz	112	244	1.5
plain *(Devonsheer)*	1 oz	108	272	1.4
plain *(Progresso)*	2 tbsp	60	110	<1.0
seasoned	1 cup	440	3180	3.1
seasoned	1 oz	104	751	0.7
seasoned *(Contadina)*	1 cup	426	2970	3.6
seasoned *(Contadina)*	1 tbsp	35	250	<1.0
BREAD DOUGH				
cornbread twists, refrigerated *(Pillsbury)*	1 twist	70	150	4.0
French, crusty, refrigerated *(Pillsbury)*	1-inch slice	60	120	<1.0
honey walnut, frozen *(Bridgford)*	1 oz	76	152	0.9
refrigerated *(Roman Meal)*	1 oz	85	199	2.8
wheat, refrigerated *(Pipin' Hot)*	1-inch slice	70	170	2.0
white, frozen *(Bridgford)*	1 oz	76	156	1.2
white, frozen *(Rich's)*	2 slices	120	300	1.0
white, refrigerated *(Pipin' Hot)*	1-inch slice	70	170	2.0
BREADFRUIT				
raw	1 cup	227	4	0.5
raw	1/4 small	99	2	0.2
trimmed	1/2 cup	114	2	0.3

Food Name	Serv. Size	Total Cal.	Sod. MGS	Fat GMS
trimmed	1 oz	29	1	0.1
untrimmed	1 lb	365	6	0.8
BREADFRUIT SEEDS				
boiled	1 oz	48	7	0.7
Pacific, in soft shell, boiled	1 lb	274	na	3.8
Pacific, shelled, boiled	1 oz	48	na	0.7
raw	1 oz	54	7	1.6
roasted	1 oz	59	8	0.8
shelled, raw	1 oz	54	na	1.6
South American, in shell, raw	1 lb	590	na	17.2
South American, shelled, roasted	1 oz	59	na	0.8
BREADSTICK				
garlic, Italian style *(Barbara's Bakery)*	1 oz	120	170	3.0
onion *(Stella D'oro)*	1 stick	40	(mq)	1.3
pizza *(Fattorie & Pandea)*	3 sticks	59	100	1.0
pizza *(Stella D'oro)*	1 stick	43	(mq)	1.2
plain *(Stella D'oro)*	1 stick	41	(mq)	1.2
plain, dietetic *(Stella D'oro)*	1 stick	46	10	1.4
regular *(Barbara's Bakery)*	1 oz	120	170	3.0
sesame *(Fattorie & Pandea)*	3 sticks	65	100	2.0
sesame *(Stella D'oro)*	1 stick	51	(mq)	2.2
sesame, dietetic *(Stella D'oro)*	1 stick	49	10	2.1
sesame, Italian style *(Barbara's Bakery)*	1 oz	120	170	3.0
soft, refrigerated *(Pillsbury)*	1 stick	100	230	2.0
soft, refrigerated *(Roman Meal)*	1 stick	117	274	3.9
wheat *(Stella D'oro)*	1 stick	42	(mq)	1.4
whole wheat *(Fattorie & Pandea)*	3 sticks	57	100	1.0
BREAKFAST BAR. See SNACK BAR.				
BREAKFAST DRINK MIX, INSTANT				
CHOCOLATE FLAVOR				
(Carnation) 'Instant Breakfast' dry mix	1 pouch	130	160	2.0
(Carnation) 'Instant Breakfast' dry mix, no sugar added	1 pouch	70	90	1.0
(Pillsbury) 'Instant Breakfast' from variety pack, dry mix	1/10 pkg	130	135	0.0
(Pillsbury) 'Instant Breakfast' from variety pack, prepared w/8 oz 2% milk	1 cup	250	250	5.0
(Pillsbury) 'Instant Breakfast' from variety pack, prepared w/8 oz whole milk	1 cup	290	310	9.0
CHOCOLATE MALT FLAVOR				
(Carnation) 'Instant Breakfast' dry mix	1 pouch	130	160	2.0
(Carnation) 'Instant Breakfast' dry mix, no sugar added	1 pouch	70	135	2.0
(Pillsbury) 'Instant Breakfast' dry mix	1 pouch	130	190	0.0

Food Name	Serv. Size	Total Cal.	Sod. MGS	Fat GMS
COFFEE FLAVOR				
(Carnation) 'Instant Breakfast' dry mix	1 pouch	130	150	0.2
VANILLA FLAVOR				
(Carnation) 'Instant Breakfast' dry mix	1 pouch	130	135	0.2
(Carnation) 'Instant Breakfast' dry mix, no sugar added	1 pouch	70	120	0.0
(Pillsbury) 'Instant Breakfast' dry mix	1 pouch	140	210	0.0
(Pillsbury) 'Instant Breakfast' prepared w/whole milk	1 cup	300	330	9.0
(Pillsbury) 'Instant Breakfast' from variety pack, dry mix	1/10 pkg	130	100	0.0
(Pillsbury) 'Instant Breakfast' from variety pack, prepared w/8 oz 2% milk	1 cup	260	220	5.0
BREAKFAST JUICE. See also individual listings.				
(Health Valley)	1/2 cup	26	24	0.0
(Knudsen & Sons) 'Natural'	8 oz	90	na	0.0
(Smucker's) orange banana, 'Naturally 100%'	8 oz	120	10	0.0
BREAKFAST STRIPS. See also BACON; BACON, ALTERNATIVE.				
beef, cured, cooked	6 oz	763	3830	58.5
beef, cured, cooked	3 slices	153	766	11.7
beef, cured, raw	3 slices	276	649	26.4
beef, cured, unheated	3 slices	276	649	26.4
BROAD BEAN				
boiled, drained	4 oz	64	47	0.6
immature, boiled, drained	100 gm	56	41	0.5
immature, raw	1 cup	78	54	0.7
mature, boiled	1/2 cup	94	4	0.3
mature, raw	1/2 cup	256	10	1.1
raw, trimmed	1 oz	20	14	0.2
raw, untrimmed	1 lb	317	220	2.6
BROAD BEAN, DRIED				
mature, boiled	1/2 cup	93	4	0.3
mature, boiled	4 oz	125	6	0.5
mature, raw	1/2 cup	256	9	1.2
mature, raw	1 oz	97	4	0.4
BROCCOLI				
boiled, drained	4 oz	32	29	0.4
boiled, drained, chopped	1/2 cup	22	20	0.3
florets, raw, chopped	1/2 cup	12	12	0.2
fresh (Dole)	1 med spear	40	75	1.0
leaves, raw, chopped	1/2 cup	12	12	0.2
raw, chopped	1/2 cup	12	12	0.2
raw, trimmed	1 oz	8	8	0.1
raw, untrimmed	1 lb	77	73	1.0

Food Name	Serv. Size	Total Cal.	Sod. MGS	Fat GMS
BROCCOLI, FROZEN. See also BROCCOLI DISHES, FROZEN; BROCCOLI ENTRÉE, FROZ				
chopped (A&P)	3.3 oz	25	25	<1.0
chopped (Birds Eye)	3.3 oz	25	15	0.0
chopped (Finast)	3.3 oz	25	20	0.0
chopped (Frosty Acres)	3.3 oz	25	18	0.0
chopped (Seabrook)	3.3 oz	25	18	0.0
chopped (Southern)	3.5 oz	28	25	0.3
chopped, boiled, drained	4 oz	32	27	0.1
chopped, boiled, drained	1/2 cup	26	22	0.1
chopped, unprepared	10-oz pkg	74	68	0.8
cuts (A&P)	3.3 oz	25	25	<1.0
cuts (Birds Eye)	3.2 oz	25	25	0.0
cuts (Frosty Acres)	3.3 oz	25	50	0.0
cuts (Seabrook)	3.3 oz	25	50	0.0
cuts, 'Harvest Fresh' (Green Giant)	1/2 cup	16	95	0.0
cuts, 'Plain Polybag' (Green Giant)	1/2 cup	18	25	0.0
cuts, 'Portion Pack' (Birds Eye)	3 oz	20	20	0.0
cuts, 'Singles' (Stokely)	3 oz	25	15	1.0
florets (Frosty Acres)	3.3 oz	30	14	0.0
florets, 'Deluxe' (Birds Eye)	3.3 oz	25	20	0.0
spears (A&P)	3.3 oz	25	20	<1.0
spears (Birds Eye)	3.3 oz	25	20	0.0
spears (Frosty Acres)	3.3 oz	25	20	0.0
spears (Seabrook)	3.3 oz	25	20	0.0
spears (Southern)	3.5 oz	30	30	0.
spears, baby (Seabrook)	3.3 oz	30	14	0.0
spears, baby, 'Deluxe' (Birds Eye)	3.3 oz	30	15	0.0
spears, boiled, drained	4 oz	32	27	0.1
spears, boiled, drained	10-oz pkg	70	60	0.
spears, boiled, drained	1/2 cup	26	22	0.1
spears, 'Harvest Fresh' (Green Giant)	1/2 cup	20	115	0.0
spears, mini, 2 1/2 inch x 1/4 inch, approx .6 oz (Green Giant)	1/5 pkg	18	25	0.0
spears, unprepared	10-oz pkg	82	48	1.0
spears, whole, 'Farm Fresh' (Birds Eye)	4 oz	30	25	0.0
spears and florets, 'Deluxe' (Birds Eye)	3.3 oz	25	20	0.0
BROCCOLI DISHES, FROZEN				
cuts, in butter sauce, 'One Serving' (Green Giant)	4.5 oz	45	420	2.0
cuts, in cheese sauce, (Finast)	3.3 oz	45	310	0.0
cuts, in cheese sauce, 'One Serving' (Green Giant)	5 oz	80	700	2.0
cuts, in cheese sauce, 'Singles' (Stokely)	4 oz	80	200	4.0

Food Name	Serv. Size	Total Cal.	Sod. MGS	Fat GMS
fanfare, 'Valley Combinations' (Green Giant)	1/2 cup	80	340	2.0
in cheese flavored sauce (Green Giant)	1/2 cup	60	530	2.0
in cheese sauce, 'Family Side Dishes' (Freezer Queen)	4.5 oz	48	280	1.0
spears, 'Butter Sauce' (Green Giant)	1/2 cup	40	350	2.0
spears, 'Butter Sauce Combinations' (Birds Eye)	3.3 oz	45	320	2.0
w/baby carrots and water chestnuts, 'Farm Fresh' (Birds Eye)	4 oz	45	35	0.0
w/cauliflower (A&P)	3.2 oz	25	20	<1.0
w/cauliflower, 'Valley Combinations' medley (Green Giant)	1/2 cup	30	80	1.0
w/cauliflower, 'Singles' (Stokely)	3 oz	20	15	1.0
w/cauliflower, 'Swiss Mix' (Frosty Acres)	3 oz	25	36	0.0
w/red peppers, 'Select' (Green Giant)	1/2 cup	25	15	0.0
w/whole baby carrots and chestnuts, 'Singles' (Stokely)	3 oz	30	22	1.0

BROCCOLI ENTRÉE, FROZEN

and baked potato wedges w/cheese sauce, 9.5-oz pkg (Healthy Choice)	1 serving	240	510	5.0
au gratin w/rice, 'For One' (Birds Eye)	5.75 oz	180	430	6.0
in pastry, w/cheese (Pepperidge Farm)	1 pastry	230	380	16.0
pot pie w/cheddar cheese, organic (Amy's Kitchen)	8 oz	390	500	18.0

BRUSSELS SPROUTS

boiled, drained	4 oz	44	24	0.6
boiled, drained	1/2 cup	30	16	0.4
boiled, drained	1 sprout	8	4	0.1
fresh (Dole)	1/2 cup	19	11	0.1
'Plain Polybag' (Green Giant)	1/2 cup	25	10	0.0
raw	1/2 cup	19	11	0.1
raw	1 sprout	8	5	0.1
raw, trimmed	1 oz	12	7	0.1
raw, untrimmed	1 lb	174	101	1.2

BRUSSELS SPROUTS, FROZEN

boiled, drained	4 oz	48	26	0.4
boiled, drained	1/2 cup	33	18	0.3
(A&P)	3.3 oz	35	15	<1.0
(Birds Eye)	3.3 oz	35	15	0.0
(Birds Eye) baby, 'Cheese Sauce Combinations'	4.5 oz	130	500	7.0
(Frosty Acres)	3.3 oz	35	12	0.0
(Green Giant) in butter sauce	1/2 cup	40	280	1.0
(Seabrook)	3.3 oz	35	12	0.0
(Seabrook) baby	3.3 oz	40	5	0.0
(Southern)	3.5 oz	37	20	0.0

Food Name	Serv. Size	Total Cal.	Sod. MGS	Fat GMS
(Stokely) in butter sauce, 'Singles'	4 oz	50	325	1.0
(Stokely) 'Singles'	3 oz	35	10	0.0
BUBBLE GUM. See CANDY.				
BUCKWHEAT				
whole-grain	1/2 cup	292	1	2.9
whole-grain	1 oz	97	<1	1.0
BUCKWHEAT FLOUR				
whole-grain	1 cup	402	na	3.7
whole-grain	1 oz	95	na	0.9
whole-grain (Arrowhead Mills)	2 oz	190	0	1.0
whole-groat	1/2 cup	201	7	1.9
BUCKWHEAT GROATS/kasha				
brown (Arrowhead Mills)	2 oz	190	1	1.0
roasted, cooked	1/2 cup	91	4	0.6
roasted, cooked	4 oz	104	5	0.7
roasted, dry	1/2 cup	284	9	2.2
roasted, dry	1 oz	98	3	0.8
white (Arrowhead Mills)	2 oz	190	1	1.0
BULGUR. See also TABBOULEH MIX.				
cooked	4 oz	94	6	0.3
cooked	1/2 cup	76	5	0.2
dry	1/2 cup	239	12	0.9
dry	1 oz	97	5	0.4
BUN. See also BISCUIT; CROISSANT; ENGLISH MUFFIN; ROLL.				
brown and serve, partially baked	2.5-inch roll	85	146	2.0
brown and serve, partially baked, unbrowned	2.5-inch roll	78	133	1.8
enriched, browned	2.5-inch roll	85	146	2.0
enriched, unbrowned	2.5-inch roll	84	144	1.9
hard, enriched, ready to cook	3.75-inch roll	156	313	1.6
hard, enriched, ready to cook	2.5-inch roll	78	156	0.8
hard, unenriched, ready to cook	3.75-inch roll	156	313	1.6
hard, unenriched, ready to cook	2.5-inch roll	78	156	0.8
Kaiser, 'Big' (Holsum)	1 bun	200	320	3.0
sesame seed, 'Big BBQ Buns' (Holsum)	1 bun	200	320	3.0
'Sof-Buns' (Holsum)	1 bun	120	190	2.0
BUN, FRANKFURTER				
Dijon (Pepperidge Farm)	1 bun	160	230	5.0
'Light' (Wonder)	1 bun	80	210	1.0
mixed grain	1 bun	113	197	2.6
'New England Style' (Arnold)	1 bun	108	178	2.0
oat bran (Awrey's)	1 bun	110	210	2.0

Food Name	Serv. Size	Total Cal.	Sod. MGS	Fat GMS
'Original' (Roman Meal)	1 bun	104	210	1.9
plain	1 bun	123	241	2.2
plain (Arnold)	1 bun	100	162	1.8
plain (Country Grain)	1 bun	100	230	1.0
plain (Pepperidge Farm)	1 bun	140	270	3.0
plain (Wonder)	1 bun	80	150	1.0
potato (Aunt Hattie's)	1 bun	150	260	4.0
reduced calorie	1 bun	84	190	0.9
reduced calorie	1 oz	56	125	0.6
whole grain (Roman Meal)	1 bun	120	210	3.0
BUN, HAMBURGER				
'Light' (Wonder)	1 bun	80	210	1.0
mixed grain	1 bun	113	197	2.6
mixed grain	1 oz	75	130	1.7
'Original' (Roman Meal)	1 bun	113	228	1.9
plain	1 bun	123	241	2.2
plain	1 oz	81	159	1.5
plain (Arnold)	1 bun	115	223	2.2
plain (Pepperidge Farm)	1 bun	130	240	2.0
plain (Wonder)	1 bun	120	230	2.0
potato (Aunt Hattie's)	1 bun	150	260	4.0
reduced calorie	1 bun	84	190	0.9
reduced calorie	1 oz	56	125	0.6
whole grain (Roman Meal)	1 bun	130	230	3.0
BUN, SWEET				
apple honey, multi pak, 1.5 oz (Break Cake)	1 bun	170	90	10.0
cheese-topped (Entenmann's)	1 bun	240	240	12.0
cinnamon (Entenmann's)	1 bun	230	200	10.0
cinnamon, frozen 'Ever Fresh' 2.5 oz (Rich's)	1 bun	293	(mq)	14.6
cinnamon, frozen '2/pkg' (Pepperidge Farm)	1 bun	280	190	14.0
cinnamon, homestyle (Awrey's)	1 bun	240	200	7.0
cinnamon, iced, refrigerated (Hungry Jack)	2 buns	290	570	14.0
cinnamon swirl 'Grande' (Awrey's)	1 bun	340	370	16.0
honey (Aunt Fanny's)	3 oz	360	150	30.0
honey (Break Cake) 3 oz	1 bun	420	160	28.0
honey, apple bear (Aunt Fanny's)	4 oz	460	220	26.0
honey, birdie, jelly-filled (Aunt Fanny's)	4 oz	450	210	24.0
honey, bogie, creme-filled (Aunt Fanny's)	4 oz	460	200	27.0
honey, frozen, mini, 'Ever Fresh', 1.36 oz (Rich's)	1 bun	133	(mq)	6.6
honey, lemon bear (Aunt Fanny's)	4 oz	440	200	23.0
honey, multi pak (Break Cake)	1 bun	380	150	24.0

Food Name	Serv. Size	Total Cal.	Sod. MGS	Fat GMS
honey, snow bear *(Aunt Fanny's)*	4 oz	480	220	24.0
honey glazed *(Tastykake)*	3.25 oz	362	219	20.4
honey glazed *(Hostess)*	1 bun	360	230	21.0
honey iced *(Tastykake)*	3.25 oz	348	254	14.9
honey iced *(Hostess)*	1 bun	430	240	22.0
pecan-caramel swirl *(Hostess)*	1 bun	240	160	15.0
BURDOCK ROOT/gobo				
boiled, drained	4 oz	100	5	0.2
boiled, drained	1 root	146	7	0.2
boiled, drained	1 cup	110	5	0.2
raw	1 root	112	8	0.2
raw, 1-inch pieces	1 cup	85	6	0.2
raw, trimmed	1 oz	20	1	<.1
raw, untrimmed	1 lb	245	17	0.5
BURGER, VEGETARIAN				
canned 'Vegetarian Burger' *(Worthington)*	1/2 cup	150	780	4.0
canned 'Vegetarian Burger No Salt Added' *(Worthington)*	1/2 cup	160	500	6.0
frozen 'FriPats' *(Worthington)*	2.25-oz piece	180	350	12.0
frozen 'Grillers' *(Morningstar Farms)*	2.25-oz patty	180	350	12.0
frozen 'Harvest Burger' original flavor *(Green Giant)*	1 burger	140	380	4.0
frozen 'Harvest Burger' southwest style *(Green Giant)*	1 burger	140	370	4.0
frozen, organic *(Amy's Kitchen)*	2.5 oz	173	181	4.0
BURGER MIX, VEGETARIAN				
(Fantastic Foods) w/tofu, prep, excluding cooking fat	3.4-oz burger	133	320	5.0
(Love Natural Foods) 'Loveburger' prepared	4-oz burger	245	224	11.0
(Nature's Burger) barbecue, prepared, excluding cooking fat	3-oz burger	117	423	0.8
(Nature's Burger) 'Original' prepared, excluding cooking fat	3-oz burger	152	228	4.0
(Nature's Burger) pizza, prep, excluding cooking fat	3-oz burger	121	406	1.0
(Worthington) 'Granburger' prepared, excluding cooking fat	1 burger	110	700	1.0
BURRITO, FROZEN				
(Amy's Kitchen) bean and rice	6 oz	251	364	5.0
(Don Miguel) cheese, no beans	1 burrito	410	950	14.0
(Don Miguel) cheese and green chili	1 burrito	390	910	11.0
(Las Campanas) bean and cheese, no lard	1 burrito	272	480	7.0
(Las Campanas) beef and bean, no lard	1 burrito	304	504	12.0
(Maria's) jalapeño bean and cheese	1 burrito	360	620	11.0
(Marquez) beef, green chili, and cheese, 'Primera'	1 burrito	330	950	11.0
(Old El Paso) bean and cheese	1 burrito	330	740	11.0

Food Name	Serv. Size	Total Cal.	Sod. MGS	Fat GMS
(Swanson) hot and spicy 'Great Starts'	1 burrito	220	490	7.0
(Swanson) original, w/cheese and chili peppers 'Great Starts'	1 burrito	200	510	8.0
(Swanson) w/egg, bacon, cheese 'Great Starts'	1 burrito	250	540	11.0
(Swanson) w/egg, ham, cheese 'Great Starts'	1 burrito	210	350	6.0
(Swanson) w/egg, pizza sauce, cheese, pepperoni 'Great Starts'	1 burrito	240	410	9.0
BURRITO DINNER MIX				
(Amy's Kitchen) beans, rice, and cheese, organic	6 oz	279	370	8.0
(Hormel) beef	1 burrito	205	780	8.0
(Old El Paso) prepared, w/filling	1 burrito	299	430	13.0
(Patio)	12 oz	517	1643	16.0
(Tio Sancho) 'Dinner Kit'	1 burrito	125	569	1.9
BURRITO DINNER, FROZEN				
beef and bean *(Patio)*	5 oz	370	830	16.0
beef and bean 'Britos' *(Patio)*	3.63 oz	250	340	10.0
beef and bean 'Festive Dinners' *(Old El Paso)*	11 oz	470	1180	9.0
beef and bean, green chili *(Patio)*	5 oz	330	770	12.0
beef and bean, hot *(Old El Paso)*	1 burrito	310	710	11.0
beef and bean, medium *(Old El Paso)*	1 burrito	330	630	13.0
beef and bean, mild *(Old El Paso)*	1 burrito	320	500	11.0
beef and bean, nacho 'Britos' *(Patio)*	3.63 oz	270	420	13.0
beef and bean 'Quick Meals' 1 serving *(Healthy Choice)*	5.2 oz	270	520	7.0
beef and bean, red chili *(Patio)*	5 oz	340	810	13.0
beef steak fajita, 'Supreme' 5-oz pkg *(Ruiz)*	1 burrito	290	240	9.0
cheese *(Hormel)*	1 burrito	210	792	5.0
cheese, nacho, 'Britos' *(Patio)*	3.63 oz	250	330	10.0
chicken, spicy, 'Britos' *(Patio)*	3.63 oz	250	330	10.0
chicken and rice *(Hormel)*	1 burrito	200	594	4.0
chicken con queso 'Quick Meals' *(Healthy Choice)*	5.4 oz	280	500	8.0
chicken fajita, 'Supreme,' 5-oz pkg *(Ruiz)*	1 burrito	260	500	1.0
chili, hot *(Hormel)*	1 burrito	240	619	8.0
green chili 'Britos' *(Patio)*	3.63 oz	250	420	10.0
red chili 'Britos' *(Patio)*	3.63 oz	240	370	10.0
red hot *(Patio)*	5 oz	360	800	15.0
BURRITO FILLING FIX, beans *(Del Monte)*	1/2 cup	110	900	1.0
BURRITO SEASONING MIX				
(Lawry's) 'Seasoning Blends' dry mix	1 pkg	132	2516	1.7
(Old El Paso)	1/8 pkg	17	275	0.0
(Tio Sancho) 'Dinner Kit'	3.25 oz	265	5031	2.1

BUSH NUT. See MACADAMIA NUT.

Food Name	Serv. Size	Total Cal.	Sod. MGS	Fat GMS
BUTTER, CLARIFIED. See GHEE.				
BUTTER, REGULAR				
lightly salted *(Breakstone's)*	1 tbsp	100	90	11.0
lightly salted *(Darigold)*	1 tsp	25	25	3.0
lightly salted *(Hotel Bar)*	1 tsp	35	35	4.0
lightly salted *(Kellers)*	1 tsp	35	35	4.0
lightly salted *(Land O'Lakes)*	1 tbsp	35	40	4.0
salted	4-oz stick	813	937	92.0
salted	1 tbsp	100	115	11.4
salted	1 tsp	34	39	3.8
salted *(Challenge)*	1 tbsp	100	90	11.0
salted *(Darigold)*	1 tsp	35	40	4.0
salted *(Hotel Bar)*	1 tsp	35	35	4.0
salted *(Kellers)*	1 tsp	35	35	4.0
salted *(Land O'Lakes)*	1 tsp	35	40	4.0
salted *(Seal of Arizona)*	1 tbsp	100	90	11.0
salted, packed 90 pats per 1 lb	1 pat	36	41	4.1
unsalted	4-oz stick	813	12	92.0
unsalted	1 tbsp	100	1	11.4
unsalted	1 pat	36	1	4.1
unsalted	1 tsp	34	<1	3.8
unsalted *(Breakstone's)*	1 tbsp	100	0	11.0
unsalted *(Challenge)*	1 tbsp	100	2	11.0
unsalted *(Land O'Lakes)*	1 tbsp	35	0	4.0
BUTTER, WHIPPED				
lightly salted *(Breakstone's)*	1 tbsp	70	65	7.0
lightly salted *(Land O'Lakes)*	1 tsp	25	25	3.0
salted	1 tbsp	67	78	7.6
salted	1 tsp	23	26	2.6
salted *(Land O'Lakes)*	1 tsp	25	25	3.0
salted, packed 120 pats per 1 lb	1 pat	27	31	3.1
unsalted	1 tbsp	67	1	7.6
unsalted	1 tsp	23	<1	2.6
unsalted *(Breakstone's)*	1 tbsp	70	0	7.0
unsalted *(Darigold)*	1 tsp	25	2	3.0
unsalted *(Land O'Lakes)*	1 tsp	25	0	3.0
BUTTER FLAVORED OIL *(Wesson)*	1 tbsp	122	0	13.6
BUTTER FLAVORED TOPPING *(Molly McButter)*	1/2 tsp	4.0	60	0.0
BUTTER OIL				
	1 oz	248	na	28.2
anhydrous	1 cup	1796	3	204.0

Food Name	Serv. Size	Total Cal.	Sod. MGS	Fat GMS
anhydrous	1 tbsp	112	0	12.7
BUTTERBEAN. See LIMA BEAN.				
BUTTERBUR/Fuki				
boiled, drained	4 oz	9	5	<.1
raw	1 cup	13	7	0.0
raw, approx .2 oz	1 stalk	1	tr	tr
raw, trimmed	1/2 cup	7	4	<.1
raw, trimmed	1 oz	4	2	<.1
raw, untrimmed	1 lb	57	28	0.2
BUTTERBUR, CANNED				
	4 oz	12	5	0.1
chopped	1 cup	4	5	0.2
stalks	3 stalks	1	2	0.1
BUTTERFISH				
dry-heat cooked	3 oz	159	97	8.7
raw	1 lb	663	401	36.4
raw	3 oz	124	76	6.8
raw	1 oz	41	25	2.3
BUTTERMILK				
blend, cultured, dry *(Saco Foods)*	3.5 tbsp	79	168	0.7
cultured	1 cup	99	257	2.2
cultured	1 oz	11	30	0.2
cultured *(A&P)*	1 cup	90	260	1.0
cultured *(Crowley)*	1 cup	110	390	4.0
cultured, 1.5% 'Golden Churn' *(Borden)*	1 cup	120	250	4.0
cultured, 1.5% 'Unsalted' *(Friendship)*	1 cup	120	125	4.0
cultured, 2% *(Knudsen)*	1 cup	120	140	5.0
cultured, 'Unsalted' *(Crowley)*	1 cup	110	130	4.0
sweet cream, dry	1 cup	464	621	6.9
sweet cream, dry	1 oz	110	147	1.6
sweet cream, dry	1 tbsp	25	34	0.4
BUTTERNUT. See BRAZIL NUT.				
BUTTERSCOTCH TOPPING				
	2 tbsp	103	143	0.0
(Kraft)	1 tbsp	60	70	1.0
(Mrs. Richardson's) caramel	2 tbsp	130	90	2.0
(Mrs. Richardson's) caramel fudge, microwavable	2 tbsp	130	90	2.0
(Smucker's)	2 tbsp	140	75	1.0
(Smucker's) caramel flavor 'Special Recipe'	2 tbsp	160	40	3.0

C

Food Name	Serv. Size	Total Cal.	Sod. MGS	Fat GMS
CABBAGE				
boiled, drained	1 head	278	101	5.4
boiled, drained	4 oz	24	22	0.3
boiled, drained, shredded	1/2 cup	16	6	0.3
raw, approx 2.5 lbs	1 head	227	163	2.5
raw, medium size *(Dole)*	1/12 head	18	30	0.0
raw, shredded	1/2 cup	9	6	0.1
raw, trimmed	1 oz	7	5	0.1
raw, untrimmed	1 lb	86	65	0.7
CABBAGE, DANISH				
fresh	1 head	218	163	1.6
fresh, shredded	1/2 cup	8	6	0.1
CABBAGE, NAPA/Chinese cabbage				
boiled, drained	1 leaf	2	1	0.0
boiled, drained, shredded	1/2 cup	10	29	0.1
bok-choy, boiled, drained	4 oz	14	39	0.2
bok-choy, boiled, drained, shredded	1/2 cup	10	29	0.1
bok-choy, raw, shredded	1/2 cup	5	23	0.1
bok-choy, raw, trimmed	1 oz	4	19	0.1
bok-choy, raw, untrimmed	1 lb	52	257	0.8
pe-tsai, boiled, drained	4 oz	16	10	0.2
pe-tsai, boiled, drained, shredded	1/2 cup	8	6	0.1
pe-tsai, raw, trimmed	1 oz	5	3	0.1
pe-tsai, raw, untrimmed	1 lb	68	38	0.8
raw, shredded	1/2 cup	5	23	0.1
CABBAGE, RED				
boiled, drained	4 oz	24	9	0.2
boiled, drained, shredded	1/2 cup	16	6	0.2
raw, shredded	1/2 cup	9	4	0.1
raw, trimmed	1 oz	8	3	0.1
CABBAGE, SAVOY				
boiled, drained	4 oz	27	27	0.1
boiled, drained, shredded	1/2 cup	18	18	0.1
raw, shredded	1/2 cup	9	10	0.0
raw, trimmed	1 oz	8	8	<.1
raw, untrimmed	1 lb	100	102	0.4
CABBAGE, SKUNK/swamp cabbage/water convolvulus				
boiled, drained	4 oz	23	138	0.3

Food Name	Serv. Size	Total Cal.	Sod. MGS	Fat GMS
boiled, drained, chopped	1/2 cup	10	60	0.1
raw	1 shoot	2	15	0.0
raw, chopped	1/2 cup	10	60	0.1
raw, trimmed, chopped	1/2 cup	6	32	0.1
raw, untrimmed	1 lb	67	395	0.7
CABBAGE ENTRÉE, FROZEN				
w/meat, and tomato sauce (Lean Cuisine)	9.5 oz	210	560	6.0
CABBAGE TURNIP. See KOHLRABI.				
CAESAR SALAD, 'Easy Caesar Kit' (Saco)	.75 oz	98	246	7.0
CAJUN SEASONING (Tone's)	1 tsp	9	215	0.2
CAJUN STYLE MARINADE, barbecue sauce (Golden Dipt)	1 oz	90	360	8.0
CAKE. See also BREAD, QUICK.				
'Best Wishes' 6 inch (Awrey's)	1/4 cake	150	170	9.0
'Four-in-One Occasion' (Awrey's)	1.3 oz	150	170	8.0
Banana				
loaf (Entenmann's)	1.3 oz	90	125	0.0
single-layer, iced, frozen (Sara Lee)	1/8 cake	170	160	6.0
Black forest				
torte (Awrey's)	1/14 cake	350	330	21.0
two-layer, frozen (Sara Lee)	1/8 cake	190	100	8.0
Blueberry crunch (Entenmann's)	1 oz	70	85	0.0
Boston cream 'Supreme' frozen (Pepperidge Farm)	2.875 oz	290	190	14.0
Carrot				
cream cheese icing 'Old Fashioned' frozen				
(Pepperidge Farm)	1.5 oz	150	160	9.0
frozen (Weight Watchers)	3 oz	170	280	5.0
single-layer, iced, frozen (Sara Lee)	1/8 cake	250	240	13.0
supreme, iced (Awrey's)	1 piece	210	170	12.0
three-layer, cream cheese icing (Awrey's)	1/12 cake	390	310	23.0
Cheesecake				
brownie 'Sweet Celebrations' frozen (Weight Watchers)	3.5 oz	200	260	5.0
cream cheese, cherry, frozen (Sara Lee)	1/6 cake	243	184	8.0
cream cheese, frozen (Sara Lee)	1/6 cake	230	153	11.0
cream cheese, strawberry, frozen (Sara Lee)	1/6 cake	222	171	8.0
French 'Classics' frozen (Sara Lee)	1/8 cake	250	120	16.0
frozen (Weight Watchers)	3.9 oz	210	230	7.0
nondairy 'Better Than Cheesecake' frozen (Tofutti)	1/10 cake	160	110	10.0
strawberry, French 'Classics' frozen (Sara Lee)	1/8 cake	240	125	13.0
strawberry 'Sweet Celebrations' frozen				
(Weight Watchers)	3.9 oz	180	210	4.0

Food Name	Serv. Size	Total Cal.	Sod. MGS	Fat GMS
triple chocolate 'Sweet Celebrations' frozen (Weight Watchers)	1 cake	190	220	4.0
Cherry, and cream, frozen (Weight Watchers)	3 oz	190	200	6.0
Chocolate				
(Awrey's)	.8 oz	70	110	3.0
devil's food, fudge icing (Entenmann's)	1.2 oz	130	120	5.0
devil's food, layer, frozen (Pepperidge Farm)	1 5/8 oz	180	135	9.0
devil's food, white icing (Awrey's)	1 piece	150	160	8.0
double, iced (Awrey's)	1 piece	130	150	6.0
double, three-layer (Awrey's)	1/12 cake	310	290	14.0
double, three-layer, frozen (Sara Lee)	1/8 cake	220	130	11.0
double, torte (Awrey's)	1/14 cake	340	300	15.0
double, two-layer (Awrey's)	1/12 cake	250	260	11.0
double, fudge, frozen (Weight Watchers)	2.75 oz	200	190	5.0
'Free & Light' frozen (Sara Lee)	1/8 cake	110	140	0.0
frozen (Weight Watchers)	2.5 oz	180	250	5.0
fudge, layer, frozen (Pepperidge Farm)	1 5/8 oz	180	140	10.0
fudge stripe, layer, frozen (Pepperidge Farm)	1 5/8 oz	170	140	9.0
German, frozen (Weight Watchers)	2.5 oz	200	220	7.0
German, iced (Awrey's)	2-inch sq.	160	150	9.0
German, single-layer, frozen (Pepperidge Farm)	1 5/8 oz	180	170	10.0
German, three-layer (Awrey's)	1/12 cake	350	300	18.0
'Happy Birthday' (Awrey's)	1.4 oz	150	150	8.0
milk, and yellow, two-layer (Awrey's)	1/12 cake	290	320	17.0
mousse 'Classics' frozen (Sara Lee)	1/8 cake	260	100	17.0
'Supreme' frozen (Pepperidge Farm)	2 7/8 oz	300	140	16.0
two-layer, white icing (Awrey's)	1/12 cake	270	290	15.0
Cinnamon swirl, refrigerated (Pillsbury)	1/8 cake	180	170	9.0
Coconut				
butter cream (Awrey's)	1 piece	160	180	9.0
layer, frozen (Pepperidge Farm)	1 5/8 oz	180	120	8.0
and yellow, three-layer (Awrey's)	1/12 cake	350	340	21.0
Coffeecake				
all butter, cheese, frozen (Sara Lee)	1/8 cake	210	220	11.0
all butter, pecan, frozen (Sara Lee)	1/8 cake	160	180	8.0
all butter, streusel, frozen (Sara Lee)	1/8 cake	160	160	7.0
caramel nut (Awrey's)	1/12 cake	140	150	8.0
cheese (Entenmann's)	1.6 oz	150	140	7.0
cinnamon swirl, iced (Pillsbury)	1 piece	230	240	11.0
crumb (Entenmann's)	1.3 oz	160	160	7.0
crumb, cheese-filled (Entenmann's)	1.4 oz	130	140	6.0

Food Name	Serv. Size	Total Cal.	Sod. MGS	Fat GMS
'Long John' (Awrey's)	1/12 cake	160	130	8.0
pecan crumb, iced (Pillsbury)	1 piece	230	240	12.0
French crumb, all butter (Entenmann's)	1.6 oz	180	220	8.0
Golden				
layer, frozen (Pepperidge Farm)	1 5/8 oz	180	110	9.0
thick fudge icing (Entenmann's)	1.2 oz	130	120	6.0
Lemon				
coconut 'Supreme' frozen (Pepperidge Farm)	3 oz	280	220	13.0
cream 'Supreme' frozen (Pepperidge Farm)	1 5/8 oz	170	120	9.0
three-layer (Awrey's)	1/12 cake	320	310	19.0
yellow, two-layer (Awrey's)	1/12 cake	290	310	17.0
Louisiana crunch (Entenmann's)	1.7 oz	180	180	8.0
Neapolitan torte (Awrey's)	1/14 cake	380	370	22.0
Orange				
frosty, iced (Awrey's)	1 piece	150	170	8.0
three-layer (Awrey's)	1/12 cake	320	320	17.0
Peanut butter torte (Awrey's)	1/14 cake	380	340	22.0
Pecan streusel, refrigerated (Pillsbury)	1/8 cake	180	170	9.0
Pineapple				
cream 'Supreme' frozen (Pepperidge Farm)	2 oz	190	130	7.0
crunch (Entenmann's)	1 oz	70	85	0.0
Pistachio torte (Awrey's)	1/12 cake	370	370	22.0
Pound				
(Drake's)	1/10 cake	110	70	5.0
all butter 'Family Size Original' frozen (Sara Lee)	1/15 cake	130	85	7.0
all butter, loaf (Entenmann's)	1 oz	110	150	5.0
all butter 'Original' frozen (Sara Lee)	1/10 cake	130	85	7.0
'Free & Light' frozen (Sara Lee)	1/10 cake	70	105	0.0
golden (Awrey's)	1/14 loaf	130	150	5.0
'Old Fashioned Cholesterol Free' frozen (Pepperidge Farm)	1 oz	110	85	6.0
sour cream, loaf (Entenmann's)	1 oz	120	90	7.0
Raisin spice, iced (Awrey's)	1 piece	160	120	8.0
Raspberry nut (Awrey's)	1/16 cake	310	220	16.0
Shortcake				
strawberry 'Dessert Lights' frozen, 3 oz (Pepperidge Farm)	1 piece	170	50	5.0
strawberry, frozen (Sara Lee)	1/8 cake	190	90	8.0
Sponge (Awrey's)	2-inch sq.	80	125	3.0
Strawberry				
cream 'Supreme' frozen (Pepperidge Farm)	2 oz	190	120	7.0

Food Name	Serv. Size	Total Cal.	Sod. MGS	Fat GMS
stripe, layer, frozen *(Pepperidge Farm)*	1.5 oz	160	120	8.0
supreme, torte *(Awrey's)*	1/14 cake	270	310	12.0
Vanilla, layer, frozen *(Pepperidge Farm)*	1 5/8 oz	190	120	8.0
Walnut torte *(Awrey's)*	1/14 cake	320	290	19.0
Yellow				
(Awrey's)	.9 oz	80	135	3.0
white icing *(Awrey's)*	2-inch sq.	150	180	9.0
CUPCAKE				
Creme, 'Kreme Kup' *(Tastykake)*	1 cupcake	86	113	2.8
White *(Break Cake)*	1 cupcake	130	115	3.0
SNACK CAKE				
bar *(Sunbelt)*	1.31 oz	130	130	2.0
'Be My Valentine' *(Little Debbie)*	2.5 oz	330	125	17.0
'Best Wishes, Miniature' *(Awrey's)*	3 oz	320	280	22.0
'Caravella' *(Little Debbie)*	1.2 oz	200	95	9.0
'Christmas Tree' *(Little Debbie)*	1.6 oz	220	80	11.0
coconut covered 'Sno Balls' *(Hostess)*	1 piece	150	160	4.0
dessert cup *(Hostess)*	1 piece	90	170	2.0
dessert cup *(Little Debbie)*	.79 oz	80	170	1.0
'Doodle Dandies' *(Little Debbie)*	2.5 oz	320	140	16.0
'Easter Bunny' *(Little Debbie)*	2.5 oz	320	135	15.0
fancy *(Little Debbie)*	2.6 oz	340	150	16.0
filled twins, 3 oz *(Break Cake)*	2 pieces	310	260	10.0
filled twins, multi pak, 1.5 oz *(Break Cake)*	1 piece	150	130	5.0
'Funny Bones' *(Drake's)*	1.25 oz	150	110	8.0
'Lil' Angels' *(Hostess)*	1 piece	90	95	2.0
'Poppets' *(Erewhon)*	1 oz	110	10	1.0
'Star Crunch' *(Little Debbie)*	1.08 oz	150	95	6.0
Swiss roll *(Little Debbie)*	2.25 oz	280	135	12.0
'Tasty Twist' *(Tastykake)*	1 piece	18	(mq)	0.6
'Tiger Tail' *(Hostess)*	1 piece	240	290	8.0
'Zoinks' *(Drake's)*	1.25 oz	130	130	5.0
Apple streusel *(Awrey's)*	1 piece	160	120	9.0
Banana, iced *(Awrey's)*	1 piece	140	120	8.0
Brownie				
À la mode 'Sweet Celebrations' frozen *(Weight Watchers)*	1 serving	180	150	4.0
chocolate 'Sweet Celebrations' frozen *(Weight Watchers)*	1/3 pkg	100	150	3.0
chocolate chip 'Toll House Ready to Bake' frozen *(Nestlé)*	1.4 oz	150	60	7.0
chocolate nut, mini *(Break Cake)*	.5 oz	70	60	4.0
Dutch chocolate 'Cake' *(Awrey's)*	1/16 cake	340	260	20.0
fudge *(Break Cake)*	2.8 oz	370	260	18.0

Food Name	Serv. Size	Total Cal.	Sod. MGS	Fat GMS
fudge *(Little Debbie)*	3 oz	350	180	12.0
fudge *(Little Debbie)*	2 oz	240	140	8.0
fudge nut *(Frito-Lay's)*	3 oz	360	225	14.0
fudge nut, iced 'Sheet Cake' *(Awrey's)*	2.5 oz	300	210	17.0
fudge nut 'Sheet Cake' *(Awrey's)*	1.25 oz	150	115	9.0
fudge walnut *(Tastykake)*	3 oz	335	222	14.2
hot fudge 'Newport' frozen *(Pepperidge Farm)*	1 ramekin	400	160	20.0
low-fat, fudge, chocolate icing 'Lights' *(Hostess)*	1 brownie	140	95	2.6
mint frosting 'Sweet Celebrations' frozen				
(Weight Watchers)	1.23 oz	100	130	2.0
peanut butter fudge 'Sweet Celebrations' frozen				
(Weight Watchers)	1.23 oz	100	140	3.0
Swiss mocha fudge 'Sweet Celebrations' frozen				
(Weight Watchers)	1.23 oz	90	140	2.0
Caramel				
fudge, À la mode, frozen *(Weight Watchers)*	1 serving	180	170	3.0
peanut filled, chocolate coated *(Little Debbie)*	1 piece	230	120	12.0
Carrot				
(Break Cake)	2 pieces	370	380	12.0
'Classic' frozen, 2.5 oz *(Pepperidge Farm)*	1 piece	260	280	16.0
'Deluxe' frozen, 1.8 oz *(Sara Lee)*	1 piece	180	200	7.0
'Lights' frozen, 2.5 oz *(Sara Lee)*	1 piece	170	75	4.0
multi pak, 1.2 oz *(Break Cake)*	1 piece	120	115	4.0
Cheesecake				
brownie 'Sweet Celebrations' frozen *(Weight Watchers)*	3.5 oz	200	260	5.0
classic, frozen, 2 oz *(Sara Lee)*	1 piece	200	150	14.0
French 'Lights' frozen, 3.2 oz *(Sara Lee)*	1 piece	150	90	4.0
French, strawberry 'Lights' frozen, 3.5 oz *(Sara Lee)*	1 piece	150	65	2.0
strawberry 'Manhattan' frozen *(Pepperidge Farm)*	1 piece	300	250	9.0
strawberry 'Sweet Celebrations' frozen				
(Weight Watchers)	3.9 oz	180	210	4.0
Cinnamon, twirl *(Aunt Fanny's)*	1 oz	110	85	4.0
Coffeecake				
(Little Debbie)	2.1 oz	250	210	9.0
apple cinnamon, individually wrapped, frozen				
(Sara Lee)	1 piece	290	270	13.0
butter streusel, individually wrapped, frozen				
(Sara Lee)	1 piece	230	270	12.0
cinnamon crumb *(Drake's)*	1.33 oz	150	110	6.0
cinnamon streusel 'Microwave' frozen				
(Weight Watchers)	1 piece	190	250	7.0

Food Name	Serv. Size	Total Cal.	Sod. MGS	Fat GMS
cream filled 'Koffee Kake' (Tastykake)	1 oz	110	81	4.0
crumb (Hostess)	1 piece	120	80	5.0
crumb 'Light' (Hostess)	1 piece	80	95	1.0
'Jr.' (Drake's)	1.1 oz	140	90	6.0
'Koffee Kake Juniors' (Tastykake)	2.5 oz	261	212	8.5
pecan, individually wrapped, frozen (Sara Lee)	1 piece	280	270	16.0
'Small' (Drake's)	2 oz	220	160	9.0
Oatmeal, creme pie, individually wrapped (Little Debbie)	1.35 oz	170	140	8.0
Shortcake				
strawberry, À la mode, frozen (Weight Watchers)	1 piece	170	150	2.0
strawberry 'Dessert Lights' frozen (Pepperidge Farm)	1 piece	170	50	5.0
CAKE, MICROWAVE				
apple streusel, prepared (MicroRave)	1/12 cake	240	190	11.0
banana, w/vanilla frosting 'Snack' prepared (Pillsbury)	1/9 cake	170	160	7.0
carrot, w/cream cheese frosting 'Snack' prepared (Pillsbury)	1/9 cake	170	200	7.0
cinnamon pecan, prepared (MicroRave)	1/6 cake	290	210	13.0
cinnamon streusel, prepared (Streusel Swirl)	1/8 cake	240	180	11.0
chocolate, prepared (Pillsbury)	1/8 cake	210	260	13.0
chocolate, w/chocolate frosting, prepared (Pillsbury)	1/8 cake	300	310	17.0
chocolate, w/vanilla frosting, prepared (Pillsbury)	1/8 cake	300	300	17.0
chocolate supreme, double, prepared (Pillsbury)	1/8 cake	330	340	19.0
devil's food, w/chocolate frosting, dry mix (MicroRave)	1/6 pkg	210	240	7.0
German chocolate, w/coconut pecan frosting, dry mix (MicroRave)	1/6 pkg	230	240	8.0
lemon, prepared (Pillsbury)	1/8 cake	220	180	13.0
lemon, w/lemon frosting, prepared (MicroRave)	1/6 cake	300	250	16.0
lemon, w/lemon frosting, prepared (Pillsbury)	1/8 cake	300	220	17.0
lemon supreme, double, prepared (Pillsbury)	1/8 cake	300	210	15.0
yellow, w/chocolate frosting, prepared (Pillsbury)	1/8 cake	300	220	17.0
yellow, w/chocolate frosting 'Singles' dry mix (MicroRave)	1/6 pkg	210	210	7.0
SNACK CAKE				
Brownie				
caramel 'Supreme' prepared (Betty Crocker)	1 brownie	110	110	2.0
caramel 'Supreme' prepared (General Mills)	1 brownie	110	110	2.0
caramel fudge chunk, prepared (Pillsbury)	1 brownie	170	105	7.0
carrot, dry mix (Pillsbury)	1/9 pkg	110	170	5.0
chocolate chip 'Supreme' prepared (Betty Crocker)	1 brownie	110	85	3.0

Food Name	Serv. Size	Total Cal.	Sod. MGS	Fat GMS
chocolate chip 'Supreme' prepared (General Mills)	1 brownie	110	85	3.0
double chocolate, prepared (Great Additions)	1 brownie	140	75	6.0
double fudge 'Brownies Plus' prepared (Duncan Hines)	1 brownie	150	105	6.0
double fudge, prepared (Pillsbury)	1 brownie	160	105	6.0
frosted, prepared (MicroRave)	1 brownie	180	130	7.0
frosted 'Supreme' prepared (Betty Crocker)	1 brownie	140	100	3.0
frosted 'Supreme' prepared (General Mills)	1 brownie	140	100	3.0
fudge, mix only (Duncan Hines)	1 brownie	100	85	18.0
fudge, 21.5-oz pkg, dry mix (Pillsbury)	1/24 pkg	100	85	2.0
fudge, 15-oz pkg, dry mix (Pillsbury)	1/16 pkg	110	90	2.0
fudge 'Family Size' prepared (General Mills)	1 brownie	110	95	2.0
fudge 'Light' prepared (General Mills)	1 brownie	100	90	1.0
fudge, prepared (Pillsbury)	1 brownie	190	105	9.0
fudge, prepared (Duncan Hines)	1 brownie	130	90	5.0
fudge, prepared (Krusteaz)	1 brownie	190	135	8.0
fudge, prepared (Lovin' Lites)	1/24 pkg	100	80	2.0
fudge 'Pouch Mix' dry mix (Gold Medal)	1/16 pkg	100	85	4.0
fudge 'Pouch Mix' dry mix (Robin Hood)	1/16 pkg	100	85	4.0
fudge 'Regular Size' prepared (General Mills)	1 brownie	110	100	2.0
fudge 'Ultra Moist' dry mix (Finast)	1/16 pkg	130	120	5.0
fudge, w/fudge frosting, prepared (Pillsbury)	1/9 pkg	240	140	11.0
fudge deluxe 'Family Size' prepared (Pillsbury)	1 brownie	150	95	7.0
fudge deluxe, prepared (Pillsbury)	1 brownie	150	100	6.0
fudge deluxe, w/walnuts, prepared (Pillsbury)	1 brownie	150	90	8.0
'Funfetti Frosted' prepared (Great Additions)	1 brownie	160	100	7.0
German chocolate 'Supreme' prepared (Betty Crocker)	1 brownie	130	105	3.0
German chocolate 'Supreme' prepared (General Mills)	1 brownie	130	105	3.0
'Gourmet Turtle' prepared (Duncan Hines)	1 brownie	200	125	9.0
milk chocolate 'Brownies Plus' prepared (Duncan Hines)	1 brownie	160	95	8.0
original 'Supreme' prepared (Betty Crocker)	1 brownie	120	90	3.0
original 'Supreme' prepared (General Mills)	1 brownie	120	90	3.0
party 'Supreme' prepared (Betty Crocker)	1 brownie	140	100	3.0
party 'Supreme' prepared (General Mills)	1 brownie	140	100	3.0
peanut butter 'Brownies Plus' prepared (Duncan Hines)	1 brownie	150	105	8.0
peanut butter candies 'Supreme' prepared (Betty Crocker)	1 brownie	140	85	5.0
prepared (Estee)	1 brownie	50	0	2.0
rocky road, fudge (Pillsbury)	1 brownie	170	95	8.0
'Singles' prepared (MicroRave)	1 brownie	250	230	9.0
triple fudge, chunky (Pillsbury)	1 brownie	170	105	7.0

Food Name	Serv. Size	Total Cal.	Sod. MGS	Fat GMS
walnut 'Brownies Plus' prepared *(Duncan Hines)*	1 brownie	150	90	7.0
walnut, prepared *(MicroRave)*	1 brownie	160	95	7.0
walnut, prepared *(Great Additions)*	1 brownie	140	70	8.0
walnut 'Supreme' prepared *(Betty Crocker)*	1 brownie	110	85	4.0
walnut 'Supreme' prepared *(General Mills)*	1 brownie	110	85	4.0
walnut 'Ultra Moist' prepared *(Finast)*	1 brownie	130	110	6.0
w/hot fudge topping 'Singles' prepared *(MicroRave)*	1 brownie	340	270	12.0
CAKE MIX				
Angel food				
chocolate, dry mix *(General Mills)*	1/12 pkg	150	300	0.0
confetti, dry mix *(General Mills)*	1/12 pkg	150	300	0.0
dry mix *(Duncan Hines)*	1/12 pkg	140	130	0.0
dry mix *(Lovin' Loaf)*	1/8 pkg	90	210	0.0
lemon custard, dry mix *(General Mills)*	1/12 pkg	150	300	0.0
lemon pudding, dry mix *(General Mills)*	1/12 pkg	150	300	0.0
strawberry, dry mix *(General Mills)*	1/12 pkg	150	260	0.0
'Traditional' dry mix *(Betty Crocker)*	1/12 pkg	130	170	0.0
white, one-step, dry mix *(General Mills)*	1/12 pkg	150	300	0.0
Apple cinnamon, prepared *(SuperMoist)*	1/12 cake	250	280	10.0
Banana				
dry mix *(Duncan Hines)*	1/12 pkg	190	280	4.0
dry mix *(Pillsbury Plus)*	1/12 pkg	180	270	4.0
Black forest				
cherry 'Bundt Ring Cake' dry mix *(Pillsbury)*	1/16 pkg	200	310	4.0
mousse 'Tiarra' prepared *(Duncan Hines)*	1/12 cake	260	270	13.0
Blueberry streusel, dry mix *(Streusel Swirl)*	1/16 pkg	210	190	5.0
Boston cream, chocolate Eclair 'Bundt Ring Cake' dry mix *(Pillsbury)*	1/16 pkg	210	280	4.0
Butter brickle, prepared *(SuperMoist)*	1/12 cake	250	280	10.0
Butter pecan, dry mix *(SuperMoist)*	1/12 pkg	180	300	4.0
Butter recipe				
chocolate, dry mix *(Pillsbury Plus)*	1/12 pkg	170	330	4.0
chocolate, dry mix *(SuperMoist)*	1/12 pkg	190	300	5.0
dry mix *(Pillsbury Plus)*	1/12 pkg	170	270	3.0
fudge, dry mix *(Duncan Hines)*	1/12 pkg	190	240	4.0
golden, dry mix *(Duncan Hines)*	1/12 pkg	190	160	4.0
yellow, dry mix *(SuperMoist)*	1/12 pkg	170	250	2.0
Carrot				
dry mix *(SuperMoist)*	1/12 pkg	180	280	3.0
'n spice, dry mix *(Pillsbury Plus)*	1/12 pkg	180	280	5.0

Food Name	Serv. Size	Total Cal.	Sod. MGS	Fat GMS
prepared *(Dromedary)*	1/12 cake	232	292	15.0
prepared *(Estee)*	1/10 cake	100	65	2.0
Cheesecake				
lemon 'No Bake' dry mix *(Jell-O)*	1 pkg	170	300	3.0
lite 'No-Bake' prepared *(Royal)*	1/8 cake	210	380	10.0
New York style 'No Bake' dry mix *(Jell-O)*	1 pkg	180	320	3.0
'No Bake' dry mix *(Jell-O)*	1 pkg	160	250	4.0
real 'No-Bake' prepared *(Royal)*	1/8 cake	280	370	9.0
Cherry and cream 'Tiarra' prepared *(Duncan Hines)*	1/12 cake	250	265	11.0
Cherry chip, dry mix *(SuperMoist)*	1/12 pkg	180	250	3.0
Chocolate				
caramel 'Bundt Ring Cake' dry mix *(Pillsbury)*	1/16 pkg	220	350	5.0
chocolate chip, dry mix *(SuperMoist)*	1/12 pkg	190	380	5.0
dark, dry mix *(Pillsbury Plus)*	1/12 pkg	170	330	5.0
devil's food, dry mix *(Duncan Hines)*	1/12 pkg	190	360	5.0
devil's food, dry mix *(Lovin' Lites)*	1/12 pkg	160	370	2.0
devil's food, dry mix *(Pillsbury Plus)*	1/12 pkg	170	330	4.0
devil's food, dry mix *(SuperMoist)*	1/12 pkg	190	410	5.0
devil's food 'Light' dry mix *(SuperMoist)*	1/12 pkg	180	330	3.0
devil's food, prepared *(Krusteaz)*	1/12 cake	190	330	2.0
devil's food 'Ultra Moist' prepared *(Finast)*	1/12 cake	250	360	11.0
Dutch fudge, dark, dry mix *(Duncan Hines)*	1/12 pkg	190	455	5.0
fudge, dry mix *(SuperMoist)*	1/12 pkg	180	430	4.0
fudge 'Tunnel of Fudge' dry mix *(Pillsbury)*	1/16 pkg	210	330	4.0
fudge marble, dry mix *(Duncan Hines)*	1/12 pkg	190	280	4.0
fudge marble, dry mix *(SuperMoist)*	1/12 pkg	180	270	4.0
fudge swirl, dry mix *(Pillsbury Plus)*	1/12 pkg	190	280	5.0
German, dry mix *(Pillsbury Plus)*	1/12 pkg	170	270	4.0
German, dry mix *(SuperMoist)*	1/12 pkg	180	400	4.0
macaroon 'Bundt Ring Cake' dry mix *(Pillsbury)*	1/16 pkg	210	330	7.0
milk, dry mix *(SuperMoist)*	1/12 pkg	190	320	5.0
mousse, amaretto 'Tiarra' prepared *(Duncan Hines)*	1/12 cake	270	230	16.0
mousse 'Bundt Ring Cake' dry mix *(Pillsbury)*	1/16 pkg	180	300	4.0
mousse 'Tiarra' prepared *(Duncan Hines)*	1/12 cake	270	235	16.0
prepared *(Estee)*	1/10 cake	100	100	2.0
pudding 'Classic Dessert' dry mix *(Betty Crocker)*	1/6 pkg	220	240	4.0
Swiss, dry mix *(Duncan Hines)*	1/12 pkg	190	360	5.0
Chocolate chip				
dry mix *(Pillsbury Plus)*	1/12 pkg	180	270	5.0
dry mix *(SuperMoist)*	1/12 pkg	180	280	4.0
Cinnamon streusel, dry mix *(Streusel Swirl)*	1/16 pkg	200	190	5.0

Food Name	Serv. Size	Total Cal.	Sod. MGS	Fat GMS
Coffeecake				
apple cinnamon, prepared *(Pillsbury)*	1/8 cake	240	150	7.0
'Flako' prepared *(Quaker)*	1 piece	156	279	4.4
prepared *(Aunt Jemima)*	1 piece	156	279	4.4
Lemon				
'Bundt Tunnel of Lemon' dry mix *(Pillsbury)*	1/16 pkg	210	270	4.0
chiffon 'Classic Dessert' dry mix *(Betty Crocker)*	1/12 pkg	190	190	4.0
dry mix *(Pillsbury Plus)*	1/12 pkg	170	260	3.0
dry mix *(SuperMoist)*	1/12 pkg	180	260	4.0
prepared *(Estee)*	1/10 cake	100	68	2.0
pudding 'Classic Dessert' dry mix *(Betty Crocker)*	1/6 pkg	220	260	4.0
supreme, dry mix *(Duncan Hines)*	1/12 pkg	190	280	4.0
supreme, dry mix *(Streusel Swirl)*	1/16 pkg	200	290	6.0
Orange, supreme, dry mix *(Duncan Hines)*	1/12 pkg	190	280	4.0
Pineapple				
creme 'Bundt Ring Cake' dry mix *(Pillsbury)*	1/16 pkg	200	270	3.0
supreme, dry mix *(Duncan Hines)*	1/12 pkg	190	280	4.0
upside down 'Classic Dessert' dry mix *(Betty Crocker)*	1/9 pkg	240	200	7.0
Pound				
dry mix *(Dromedary)*	5 tbsp	130	140	5.0
golden 'Classic Dessert' dry mix *(Betty Crocker)*	1/12 pkg	190	150	8.0
prepared *(Estee)*	1/8 cake	120	85	2.5
prepared *(Martha White)*	1/10 cake	120	110	4.0
Rainbow chip, party cake, dry mix *(SuperMoist)*	1/12 pkg	180	300	4.0
Sour cream				
chocolate, dry mix *(SuperMoist)*	1/12 pkg	180	410	4.0
white, dry mix *(SuperMoist)*	1/12 pkg	180	280	3.0
Spice				
dry mix *(Duncan Hines)*	1/12 pkg	190	280	4.0
dry mix *(SuperMoist)*	1/12 pkg	180	300	4.0
prepared *(Estee)*	1/8 cake	120	80	3.0
Strawberry				
dry mix *(Pillsbury Plus)*	1/12 pkg	180	290	4.0
supreme, dry mix *(Duncan Hines)*	1/12 pkg	190	280	4.0
Swirl, party cake, prepared *(SuperMoist)*	1/12 cake	260	280	11.0
Vanilla				
French, dry mix *(Duncan Hines)*	1/12 pkg	190	280	4.0
golden, dry mix *(SuperMoist)*	1/12 pkg	180	250	4.0
golden, prepared *(MicroRave)*	1/6 cake	320	230	17.0
sunshine, dry mix *(Pillsbury Plus)*	1/12 pkg	180	280	5.0

Food Name	Serv. Size	Total Cal.	Sod. MGS	Fat GMS
White				
dry mix *(Duncan Hines)*	1/12 pkg	190	250	4.0
dry mix *(Lovin' Lites)*	1/12 pkg	170	300	2.0
dry mix *(Lovin' Loaf)*	1/12 pkg	170	300	2.0
dry mix *(Pillsbury Plus)*	1/12 pkg	180	280	4.0
dry mix *(SuperMoist)*	1/12 pkg	180	300	4.0
'Funfetti' dry mix *(Pillsbury Plus)*	1/12 pkg	180	280	4.0
'Light' dry mix *(SuperMoist)*	1/12 pkg	180	320	3.0
'n fudge swirl, dry mix *(Pillsbury Plus)*	1/12 pkg	190	280	4.0
prepared *(Estee)*	1/10 cake	100	68	2.0
prepared *(Krusteaz)*	1/12 cake	190	280	3.0
Yellow				
dry mix *(Duncan Hines)*	1/12 pkg	190	280	4.0
dry mix *(Pillsbury Plus)*	1/12 pkg	180	280	5.0
dry mix *(SuperMoist)*	1/12 pkg	180	280	4.0
'Light' dry mix *(SuperMoist)*	1/12 pkg	180	290	3.0
prepared *(Krusteaz)*	1/12 cake	200	330	5.0
prepared *(Lovin' Loaf)*	1/12 cake	180	300	3.0
'Ultra Moist' prepared *(Finast)*	1/12 cake	240	280	10.0
CALAMARI. See SQUID, MIXED SPECIES.				
CALICO BASS. See SUNFISH.				
CANADIAN BACON. See BACON, CANADIAN-STYLE.				
CANDLEFISH/eulachon				
dry-heat cooked	4 oz	141	87	3.5
raw	1 lb	440	272	11.0
raw	1 oz	27	17	0.7
CANDY				
'Bridge Mix' *(Brach's)*	1 oz	140	30	7.0
'Estee-ets' *(Estee)*	5 pieces	35	10	2.0
'Home Fashioned Favorites' *(Russell Stover)*	1.4 oz	170	60	7.0
'Smoothie' 1.6 oz *(Boyer)*	2 pieces	250	na	15.0
'Smoothie' .5 oz *(Boyer)*	1 piece	75	na	7.5
'Smoothie' .275 oz *(Boyer)*	1 piece	38	na	3.8
ALMOND				
'Almond Delights' *(Russell Stover)*	1.4 oz	210	55	12.0
chocolate covered *(Estee)*	2 squares	60	10	4.5
chocolate covered *(Featherweight)*	1 section	90	20	7.0
'Golden Almond Solitaires' chocolate covered *(Hershey's)*	1.5 oz	240	25	16.0
'Golden Almond Solitaires' chocolate covered *(Hershey's)*	3 oz	455	46	31.5

Food Name	Serv. Size	Total Cal.	Sod. MGS	Fat GMS
'Jordan Almonds' candy coated (Brach's) .... 1 oz		120	0	2.0
'Kisses w/Almonds' chocolate w/almonds, 1 oz (Hershey's) .... 6 pieces		160	25	10.0
'M&M's' candy coated almonds (M&M/Mars) .... ⅛ oz		150	30	8.0
'Solitaires' chocolate covered, 1.6 oz (Hershey's) .... 1/2 bar		260	25	17.0
AMARETTO CHOCOLATE, 'Buffalo Ball' confection (Great Cakes) .... 1 ball		105	15	3.5
BAR				
'Aero' milk chocolate, dark chocolate (Nestlé) .... 1 bar		210	20	12.0
'Aero' milk chocolate, dark chocolate, bite size (Nestlé) .... 2 bars		85	10	5.0
'Almond Crunch' date sweetened, carob (Carafection) ...... 1 oz		139	26	7.0
'Almond Joy' 1.76 oz (Hershey's) .... 1 bar		232	67	13.9
'Almond Joy' miniatures (Hershey's) .... 2 pieces		120	35	7.0
'Almond Joy' snack size (Hershey's) .... 1 bar		93	27	5.5
'Alpine White' white chocolate w/almonds (Nestlé) .... 1 bar		197	4	12.9
'Alpine White' white chocolate w/almonds, 2.2 oz (Nestlé) .... 1 bar		350	7	22.9
'A-Ok' fruit juice sweetened (Natures Warehouse) .... 1 oz		130	32	6.2
'Baby Ruth' chocolate w/peanuts (Nestlé) .... 1 bar		277	14	13.3
'Baby Ruth' chocolate w/peanuts, fun size (Nestlé) .... 1 bar		110	55	5.0
'Bar None' 1.5 oz (Bar None) .... 1 bar		224	45	14.6
'Bounty' dark chocolate (M&M/Mars) .... 1 oz		140	20	8.0
'Bounty' milk chocolate (M&M/Mars) .... 1 oz		140	30	7.0
'Brazil Nut Crunch' (Yogafection) .... 1 oz		180	70	10.0
'Butterfinger' 2.16 oz (Nestlé) .... 1 bar		267	83	11.3
'Butterfinger' snack size (Nestlé) .... 1 bar		92	29	3.9
'Caramello' 5 oz (Cadbury) .... 1 bar		694	175	35.9
'Caramello' 1.6 oz (Cadbury) .... 1 bar		220	55	11.4
carob (Caroby) .... 4 sections		150	55	9.0
carob candy, plain, date sweetened (Carafection) .... 1 oz		139	26	7.0
carob coated (Tiger's Milk) .... 1 bar		160	100	6.0
carob coated 'Light' (Tiger's Milk) .... 1 bar		110	na	3.0
'Cashew Coconut Crunch' carob candy (Carafection) .... 1 oz		139	26	7.0
'Cashew Nut Crunch' (Yogafection) .... 1 oz		180	70	10.0
'Chew!' nougat, chocolate coated, all flavors (Charleston) .... 1 oz		120	40	3.0
chocolate tofu truffle w/pralines (Barat) .... 1 oz		170	10	11.0
chocolate tofu w/almonds (Barat) .... 1 oz		170	10	11.0
chocolate tofu w/almonds and raisins (Barat) .... 1 oz		160	10	11.0

Food Name	Serv. Size	Total Cal.	Sod. MGS	Fat GMS
chocolate w/almonds, w/o sugar, extra thick				
(Fifty 50)	1 section	90	20	6.0
chocolate w/coconut (Estee)	2 squares	60	15	4.0
chocolate w/crisps and honey (Cadbury)	1 oz	150	40	7.0
chocolate w/fruit and nuts (Cadbury)	1 oz	150	40	8.0
chocolate w/fruit and nuts (Estee)	2 squares	60	10	4.5
chocolate w/fruit and nuts, w/o sugar, extra thick				
(Fifty 50)	1 section	80	20	5.0
chocolate w/roasted almonds (Cadbury)	1 oz	150	40	9.0
'Chunky' 1.4 oz (Nestlé)	1 bar	198	21	11.7
'Chunky' 1.25 oz (Nestlé)	1 bar	173	19	10.2
'Chunky' w/raisins, peanuts and cashews (Nestlé)	1.4 oz	170	20	12.0
'Cookies 'N Mint' mint chocolate, cookie pieces				
(Hershey's)	1 bar	220	75	12.0
'Crispy Crunch' carob candy, date sweetened				
(Carafection)	1 oz	139	26	7.0
crunch (Estee)	2 squares	45	10	3.0
crunch, chocolate, w/o sugar, extra thick (Fifty 50)	1 section	70	20	5.0
'Crunch' milk chocolate w/crisp rice, 1.4 oz (Nestlé)	1 bar	210	35	10.0
'Crunch' milk chocolate w/crisp rice, fun size				
(Nestlé)	2 bars	100	15	5.0
'Crunch' milk chocolate w/crisp rice, snack size				
(Nestlé)	1 bar	49	15	2.6
'Dairy Milk' milk chocolate (Cadbury)	1 oz	150	45	8.0
'Dove' dark chocolate, deluxe (Estee)	2 squares	50	0	3.0
'Dove' dark chocolate, miniatures (M&M/Mars)	4 pieces	130	0	8.0
'Dove' milk chocolate, miniatures (M&M/Mars)	4 pieces	130	20	8.0
'5th Avenue' 4.2 oz (Hershey's)	1 pkg	555	221	25.2
'5th Avenue' 2.1 oz (Hershey's)	1 bar	280	112	12.7
French chocolate (Russell Stover)	1 bar	200	30	13.0
French chocolate mint (Russell Stover)	1 bar	230	25	15.5
'Golden Almond' chocolate w/almonds, 3 oz (Hershey's)	1 bar	466	54	32.1
'Golden III' 3.2 oz	1 bar	471	79	30.0
'Halvah' (Fantastic Foods)	1.5 oz	232	0	10.0
'Hershey's Milk Chocolate Bar' (Hershey's)	1.55 oz	240	40	14.0
'Hershey's Milk Chocolate Bar w/Almonds' (Hershey's)	1.45 oz	230	55	14.0
'Kit Kat' chocolate covered wafer, 3.375 oz				
(Hershey's)	1 bar	490	97	27.4
'Kit Kat' chocolate covered wafer, 1.625 oz				
(Hershey's)	1 bar	235	46	13.1

Food Name	Serv. Size	Total Cal.	Sod. MGS	Fat GMS
'Kit Kat' chocolate covered wafer, snack size				
(Hershey's)	1.12 oz	170	40	9.0
'Krackel' chocolate w/rice crisps, 2.6 oz (Hershey's)	1 bar	371	101	20.6
'Krackel' chocolate w/rice crisps, 1.65 oz				
(Hershey's)	1 bar	236	64	13.1
'Mars Almond' 1.76 oz (M&M/Mars)	1 bar	233	85	11.5
milk chocolate (Estee)	2 squares	60	15	4.0
milk chocolate, mini (Fifty 50)	4 pieces	90	20	6.0
milk chocolate w/o sugar, extra thick (Fifty 50)	1 section	80	25	6.0
'Milky Way' dark chocolate (M&M/Mars)	1.76 oz	220	115	8.0
'Milky Way' milk chocolate, 2.1 oz (M&M/Mars)	1 bar	251	144	9.1
'Milky Way' milk chocolate, minis (M&M/Mars)	1 piece	40	15	1.0
'Milky Way' milk chocolate, snack size (M&M/Mars)	1 bar	75	43	2.7
mint (Estee)	2 squares	50	0	3.0
'Mint' date sweetened, carob candy (Carafection)	1 oz	139	26	7.0
'Mint Honey Graham' carob coated (Carafection)	1 oz	139	26	7.0
'Mounds' chocolate covered coconut, 1.9 oz (Hershey's)	1 pkg	195	68	11.7
'Mounds' chocolate covered coconut, minis (Hershey's)	2 pieces	110	30	6.0
'Mounds' chocolate covered coconut, snack size				
(Hershey's)	1 bar	72	25	4.3
'Mr. GoodBar' milk chocolate w/peanuts, 2.8 oz				
(Hershey's)	1 bar	406	27	25.5
'Mr. GoodBar' milk chocolate w/peanuts, 1.75 oz				
(Hershey's)	1 bar	257	17	16.1
'Munch' (M&M/Mars)	1.42 oz	220	110	14.0
'My O My' fruit juice sweetened (Natures Warehouse)	1 oz	103	42	1.4
'No How' peanut butter, fruit juice sweetened				
(Natures Warehouse)	1 oz	140	48	10.0
'Non Stop' fruit juice sweetened (Natures Warehouse)	1 oz	122	48	5.0
'Nut Wit' carob, caramel, and peanuts				
(Natures Warehouse)	1 oz	135	32	6.3
'Oh Henry!' chocolate covered caramel w/peanuts, 2 oz				
(Nestlé)	1 bar	246	5	9.8
'100 Grand' 1.5 oz (Nestlé)	1 bar	195	4	8.5
'Original' (Cocofection)	1 oz	155	23	10.0
'Original Honey Graham' carob coated (Carafection)	1 oz	139	26	7.0
'Pay Day' (Pay Day)	1.85 oz	250	200	12.0
peanut butter (Russell Stover)	1 bar	290	130	19.0
peanut butter, carob coated (Tiger's Milk)	1 bar	160	105	7.0
peanut butter, carob coated 'Light' (Tiger's Milk)	1 bar	110	25	3.0
peanut butter and honey, carob coated (Tiger's Milk)	1 bar	160	90	5.0

ood Name	Serv. Size	Total Cal.	Sod. MGS	Fat GMS
'Peanut Crunch' carob candy, date sweetened				
(Carafection)	1 oz	139	26	7.0
'Protein Blast' high-energy, chocolate (Weider)	1 bar	270	110	6.0
'Skor' toffee, 1.4 oz (Hershey's)	1 bar	211	92	13.8
'Sky Bar' (Necco)	1.5 oz	196	57	7.1
'Snickers' 2.16 oz (M&M/Mars)	1 bar	278	163	13.6
'Snickers,' minis (M&M/Mars)	1 piece	45	25	2.0
'Snickers' snack size (M&M/Mars)	1 bar	68	40	3.3
'Soft'n Crunchy Bar' 1 3/16 oz (Heath)	2 pieces	190	85	12.0
'Special Dark' sweet chocolate bar, 2.8 oz				
(Hershey's)	1 bar	376	8	23.9
'Special Dark' sweet chocolate bar, 1.45 oz				
(Hershey's)	1 bar	195	4	12.4
'Symphony' milk chocolate, 2.4 oz (Hershey's)	1 bar	355	58	22.0
'Symphony' milk chocolate, 1.4 oz (Hershey's)	1 bar	209	34	13.0
'Symphony' milk chocolate w/almonds and toffee chips				
(Hershey's)	1.4 oz	220	40	14.0
'3 Musketeers' 2.13 oz (M&M/Mars)	1 bar	250	116	7.7
'3 Musketeers' snack size (M&M/Mars)	1 bar	75	35	2.3
'Twix' caramel, 2.0 oz (M&M/Mars)	1 pkg	272	115	13.4
'Twix' cookies-n-creme (M&M/Mars)	1 bar	120	50	7.0
'Twix' peanut butter, 1.77 oz (M&M/Mars)	1 pkg	253	148	14.5
'Whatchamacallit' 1.8 oz (Hershey's)	1 bar	257	116	13.2
BUBBLE GUM				
(Beechies) candy coated	1 piece	6	0	0.0
(Bubble Yum)				
bananaberry split	1 piece	25	0	0.0
checkermint	1 piece	25	0	0.0
cherry	1 piece	25	0	0.0
fruit	1 piece	25	0	0.0
grape	1 piece	25	0	0.0
Hawaiian punch	1 piece	25	0	0.0
luscious lime	1 piece	25	0	0.0
strawberry stripe	1 piece	25	0	0.0
sugarless, fruit	1 piece	20	0	0.0
sugarless, grape	1 piece	20	0	0.0
sugarless, peppermint	1 piece	20	0	0.0
sugarless, strawberry	1 piece	20	0	0.0
3-flavor, grape, cherry and fruit	1 piece	25	0	0.0
wet 'n wild watermelon	1 piece	25	0	0.0

Food Name	Serv. Size	Total Cal.	Sod. MGS	Fat GMS
(Bubblicious)				
....	1 piece	25	0	tr
'Sugarless'	1 piece	5	0	tr
(Care Free) sugarless				
fruit	1 piece	10	0	0.0
wild cherry	1 piece	10	0	0.0
wintergreen	1 piece	10	0	0.0
(Chiclets)				
candy coated	1 piece	6	0	tr
'Tiny' candy coated	1 pkg	8	0	tr
(Clorets) candy coated	1 piece	6	0	tr
(Extra)				
classic	1 piece	6	0	(mq)
original	1 piece	7	0	(mq)
(Fruit Stripe)				
cherry	1 piece	8	0	0.0
fruit	1 piece	8	0	0.0
grape	1 piece	8	0	0.0
lemon	1 piece	8	0	0.0
(Hubba Bubba)				
regular, all flavors except cola	1 piece	23	0	0.0
regular, cola	1 piece	23	0	0.0
'Sugar-free' grape	1 piece	13	0	0.0
sugar-free, original	1 piece	14	0	0.0
BUTTERSCOTCH, squares *(Russell Stover)*	1.4 oz	180	65	6.5
CARAMEL				
(Allen Wertz)	1 piece	37	2	2.0
(Featherweight)	1 piece	30	10	1.0
(Kraft)	1 piece	30	25	1.0
butter cream, squares *(Russell Stover)*	1.4 oz	170	95	7.5
chocolate *(Estee)*	1 piece	20	10	1.0
chocolate coated *(Pom Poms)*	1 oz	100	70	3.0
marshmallow, milk chocolate, squares *(Russell Stover)*	1.4 oz	190	85	10.0
milk chocolate coated, approx 1.93 oz *(Rolo)*	8 pieces	270	110	12.0
'Milk Maid' *(Brach's)*	1 oz	110	70	2.0
'Milk Maid' chocolate *(Brach's)*	1 oz	110	55	3.0
'Nip' *(Pearson)*	1 oz	120	70	3.0
nougat swirl *(Allen Wertz)*	1 piece	32	2	1.0
pop *(Sugar Daddy)*	1 3/8 oz	150	85	1.0
'Regular' 1 5/8 oz *(Sugar Babies)* ...	1 pkg	180	85	2.0
'Rolos' milk chocolate covered *(Hershey's)*	1.93 oz	270	110	12.0

Food Name	Serv. Size	Total Cal.	Sod. MGS	Fat GMS
'Tidbits' 1 5/8 oz (Sugar Babies)	1 pkg	180	85	2.0
vanilla (Estee)	1 piece	20	10	1.0
CHERRY				
'Cherry Cordials' (Russell Stover)	1.4 oz	170	25	7.5
chocolate cream (Brach's)	1 oz	110	20	2.0
dark chocolate coated (Brach's)	1 oz	110	20	2.0
'Nibs' (Y&S)	1 oz	106	67	0.7
squares (Russell Stover)	1.4 oz	160	40	5.5
'Villa' milk chocolate covered (Brach's)	1 oz	110	20	2.0
CHEWING GUM				
(Beech-Nut)				
cinnamon	1 piece	10	0	0.0
fruit	1 piece	10	0	0.0
peppermint	1 piece	10	0	0.0
spearmint	1 piece	10	0	0.0
(Brach's) 'Gumdinger' balls, all flavors	1 oz	110	5	2.0
(Care Free) sugarless				
cinnamon	1 piece	8	0	0.0
peppermint	1 piece	8	0	0.0
spearmint	1 piece	8	0	0.0
(Chewels) all flavors	1 piece	8	0	tr
(Clorets) stick, all flavors	1 piece	9	0	tr
(Dentyne)				
all flavors	1 piece	6	0	tr
'Sugarless' all flavors	1 piece	5	0	tr
(Estee) gumdrops	4 pieces	25	0	0.0
(Extra)				
cinnamon	1 stick	8	0	(mq)
peppermint	1 stick	8	0	(mq)
spearmint	1 stick	8	0	(mq)
winter fresh	1 stick	8	0	(mq)
(Freedent)				
cinnamon	1 stick	10	0	(mq)
peppermint	1 stick	10	0	(mq)
spearmint	1 stick	10	0	(mq)
(Freshen-Up) all flavors	1 piece	13	0	tr
(Fruit Stripe)				
cherry	1 piece	10	0	0.0
lemon	1 piece	10	0	0.0
lime	1 piece	10	0	0.0
orange	1 piece	10	0	0.0

Food Name	Serv. Size	Total Cal.	Sod. MGS	Fat GMS
(Sticklets) all flavors	1 piece	7	0	tr
(Wrigley's)				
'Big Red'	1 piece	10	0	0.0
'Doublemint'	1 piece	10	0	0.0
'Juicy Fruit'	1 piece	10	0	0.0
'Spearmint'	1 piece	10	0	0.0
CHOCOLATE				
assorted, wrapped, 1-lb bag *(Brach's)*	1 oz	110	25	2.0
'Bits' tofu pastilles *(Barat)*	.75 oz	120	10	8.0
chewy roll *(Tootsie Roll)*	1 oz	112	6	2.5
'Choc'Oh's' *(Saco Foods)*	1.5 oz	111	14	6.6
chunks *(Saco Foods)*	3.5 oz	466	26	26.4
coated, creme center *(Spangler)*	1 piece	80	40	2.0
coated, creme center caramel, w/nuts *(Spangler)*	1 piece	100	30	6.0
coated, creme center cherry, w/nuts *(Spangler)*	1 piece	110	20	5.0
coated, creme center fudge, w/nuts *(Spangler)*	1 piece	140	25	6.0
coated, creme center fudge, w/pecans *(Spangler)*	1 piece	140	40	7.0
coated, creme center maple, w/nuts *(Spangler)*	1 piece	110	15	5.0
coated, creme center vanilla, w/nuts *(Spangler)*	1 piece	110	20	5.0
cream *(Callard & Bowser)*	1 oz	120	na	3.7
creamy milk, w/almonds and toffee chips *(Hershey's)*	.75 oz	280	50	17.0
crunch *(Featherweight)*	1 section	80	20	6.0
'Gift Box' dark and milk mix *(Russell Stover)*	1.4 oz	180	45	8.5
'Gourmet' assortment *(Allen Wertz)*	11.9 grams	55	13	2.0
'Jots' *(Brach's)*	1 oz	130	30	5.0
'Kisses' *(Hershey's)*	6 pieces	150	25	9.0
'M&M's' plain *(M&M/Mars)*	10 pieces	33	7	1.5
'M&M's' plain, 1.69 oz *(M&M/Mars)*	1 pkg	228	49	10.7
'Malted Milk Balls' milk coated *(Brach's)*	1 oz	130	40	5.0
malted milk balls, milk coated *(Whoppers)*	1 oz	136	na	6.0
milk *(Featherweight)*	1 section	80	20	6.0
milk, assortment *(Russell Stover)*	1.4 oz	190	50	8.5
'Passionettes' tofu *(Barat)*	1 piece	70	5	5.0
'Stars' *(Brach's)*	1 oz	150	30	8.0
'Stars' approx 13 pieces *(Nabisco)*	1 oz	160	35	8.0
trail mix, premium *(Cocofection)*	1 oz	130	14	9.0
COCONUT				
'Macaroo' chocolate coated *(Sunbelt)*	2 oz	288	75	16.0
Neapolitan *(Brach's)*	1 oz	120	40	2.0
COFFEE				
(Brach's)	1 oz	120	35	2.0

Food Name	Serv. Size	Total Cal.	Sod. MGS	Fat GMS
'Coffee Time' *(Allen Wertz)*	1 piece	20	2	1.0
'Coffee Time' assorted *(Allen Wertz)*	1 piece	28	2	1.0
'Coffee Time' decaffeinated *(Allen Wertz)*	1 piece	20	2	1.0
'Nip' *(Pearson)*	1 oz	120	70	3.0
FONDANT, candy corn	1 cup	728	424	4.0
FRUIT				
(Bonkers!) chews, all flavors	1 piece	20	0	0.0
(Brach's)				
orange sticks, chocolate coated	1 oz	110	25	2.0
'Orangettes'	1 oz	100	20	0.0
(Featherweight)				
berry patch	1 piece	12	0	0.0
drops, all flavors	.33 oz	30	15	0.0
orchard	1 piece	12	0	0.0
tropical blend	1 piece	12	0	0.0
(Glenny's) 'Drops'				
black cherry	1 drop	6	<1	<1.0
Mandarin orange	1 drop	6	<1	<1.0
mixed fruit	1 drop	6	<1	<1.0
twist of lemon	1 drop	6	<1	<1.0
(Jujyfruits)	11 pieces	100	0	<1.0
(Rascals) chews, all flavors	1 piece	4	0	tr
(Russell Stover) lemon squares	1.4 oz	160	35	5.5
'Skittles' *(M&M/Mars)*				
candy coated, bite size	1 oz	120	15	1.0
candy coated, bite size, 2.3 oz	1 pkg	255	30	2.0
'Starburst' *(M&M/Mars)*				
original fruit chews	2 oz	240	30	5.0
tropical fruit chews	2 oz	240	30	5.0
(Soda-Licious) all flavors	1 pouch	100	20	1.0
(SweeTARTS) chewy	1 oz	113	na	1.0
'Twizzlers' *(Y&S)*				
strawberry sticks, 5 oz	1 pkg	525	393	2.3
strawberry sticks, 2.5 oz	1 pkg	263	197	1.1
FUDGE				
chocolate, w/walnuts *(Woodys)*	1 oz	120	25	4.0
'Fudgies' *(Kraft)*	1 piece	35	25	1.0
maple walnut *(Woodys)*	1 oz	120	25	4.0
mint, w/walnuts *(Woodys)*	1 oz	120	25	4.0
w/walnuts *(Woodys)*	1 oz	120	25	4.0

Food Name	Serv. Size	Total Cal.	Sod. MGS	Fat GMS
HARD CANDY				
(Brach's)				
'Cut Rock'	1 oz	110	10	0.0
'Disks' butterscotch	1 oz	110	220	0.0
'Disks' cinnamon	1 oz	110	15	0.0
filled, assorted	1 oz	110	15	0.0
'Imperials' cinnamon	1 oz	110	5	0.0
lemon drops	1 oz	110	5	0.0
raspberry filled	1 oz	110	15	0.0
ribbon, crimp	1 oz	110	15	0.0
'Royals'	1 oz	100	60	2.0
sour balls	1 oz	110	15	0.0
'Spicettes'	1 oz	100	15	0.0
(Breath Savers)				
cores, mint-cinnamon	1 piece	2	0	0.0
cores, peppermint	1 piece	2	0	0.0
cores, spearmint	1 piece	2	0	0.0
cores, wintergreen	1 piece	2	0	0.0
mint-cinnamon	1 piece	8	0	0.0
peppermint	1 piece	8	0	0.0
spearmint	1 piece	8	0	0.0
wintergreen	1 piece	8	0	0.0
(Callard & Bowser) butterscotch	1 oz	115	na	1.9
(Ce De) 'Smarties'	1 roll	25	0	0.0
(Certs)				
sugar-free, mini	1 piece	1	tr	tr
sugar-free, mints	1 piece	6	0	tr
(Clorets)				
clear mint	1 piece	8	0	tr
pressed mints	1 piece	6	0	tr
(Estee)	2 pieces	25	0	0.0
(Featherweight)				
butterscotch	1 piece	25	25	0.0
'Sweet Pretenders' tropical blend	1 piece	12	0	0.0
(Fruit Juicers)				
citrus fruits	1 piece	8	0	0.0
fruit punch	1 piece	8	0	0.0
grape	1 piece	8	0	0.0
mixed berries	1 piece	8	0	0.0
strawberry	1 piece	8	0	0.0

od Name	Serv. Size	Total Cal.	Sod. MGS	Fat GMS
(Glenny's)				
fruit	1 piece	19	<1	<1.0
peppermint	1 piece	19	<1	<1.0
(Jolly Joes)	1 piece	9	1	tr
(Jolly Rancher)				
apple	1 piece	23	5	0.0
butterscotch	1 piece	25	37	<1.0
cherry	1 piece	23	3	0.0
fire cinnamon	1 piece	23	5	0.0
fruit punch	1 piece	23	5	0.0
grape	1 piece	23	5	0.0
lemon	1 piece	23	5	0.0
orange	1 piece	23	4	0.0
peach	1 piece	23	3	0.0
peppermint	1 piece	23	3	0.0
pink lemonade	1 piece	23	5	0.0
raspberry	1 piece	23	5	0.0
strawberry	1 piece	23	3	0.0
watermelon	1 piece	23	5	0.0
(Jurassic Park)				
'Raptor Bites' wild cherry	13 pieces	60	0	0.0
'Spitters' tropical flavors	13 pieces	60	0	0.0
(Life Savers)				
butter creme mint	1 piece	8	5	0.0
butter rum	1 piece	8	10	0.0
butterscotch	1 piece	8	10	0.0
'Cin-O-Mon'	1 piece	8	0	0.0
'Cryst-O-Mint'	1 piece	8	0	0.0
fancy fruits	1 piece	8	0	0.0
five flavor	1 piece	8	0	0.0
holes, butter rum	1 piece	2	0	0.0
holes, five flavor	1 piece	2	0	0.0
holes, pep-o-mint	1 piece	2	0	0.0
candy coated, bite size	10 pieces	43	5	0.3
holes, sunshine fruits	1 piece	2	0	0.0
holes, tangerine	1 piece	2	0	0.0
holes, 'Wint-O-Green'	1 piece	2	0	0.0
'Pep-O-Mint'	1 piece	8	0	0.0
root beer	1 piece	8	0	0.0
'Spear-O-Mint'	1 piece	8	0	0.0
sunshine fruits	1 piece	8	0	0.0

Food Name	Serv. Size	Total Cal.	Sod. MGS	Fat GMS
tropical fruits	1 piece	8	0	0.0
wild cherry	1 piece	8	0	0.0
'Wint-O-Green'	1 piece	8	0	0.0
(Mike & Ike)	1 piece	9	1	tr
(Pearson) 'Nip' butter rum	1 oz	120	70	3.0
(Russell Stover) sugar-free, mix	3 pieces	70	5	0.0
(Spree) fruit	1 oz	110	na	0.0
(SweeTARTS) fruit	1 oz	110	na	0.0
HOLIDAY				
assorted, chocolate (Brach's)	1 oz	110	25	2.0
autumn leaves (Brach's)	1 oz	100	15	0.0
bell, chocolate, in foil (Brach's)	1 oz	150	25	8.0
holiday mints (Brach's)	1 oz	110	0	1.0
holiday mix (Brach's)	1 oz	110	10	0.0
Christmas				
candy cane (Brach's)	1 oz	110	10	0.0
candy cane (Spangler)	1 piece	60	0	<1.0
jellies (Brach's)	1 oz	100	10	0.0
jellies, snowbase (Brach's)	1 oz	100	5	0.0
'Jots' (Brach's)	1 oz	130	30	5.0
nougat (Brach's)	1 oz	110	20	2.0
ornaments (Brach's)	1 oz	150	50	8.0
'Pearls' mint (Brach's)	1 oz	110	5	1.0
'Perkys' (Brach's)	1 oz	90	20	0.0
Santa, chocolate, in foil (Brach's)	1 oz	140	40	7.0
Santa, marshmallow (Brach's)	1 oz	120	35	3.0
snowmen, marshmallow, large pieces (Just Born)	1 piece	111	8	0.1
snowmen, marshmallow, small pieces (Just Born)	1 piece	37	3	<.1
'Starlight' mint (Brach's)	1 oz	110	15	0.0
trees, marshmallow, large pieces (Just Born)	1 piece	111	8	0.1
trees, marshmallow, small pieces (Just Born)	1 piece	37	3	<.1
Easter				
'Chicks & Rabbits' assorted (Brach's)	1 oz	100	10	0.0
corn (Brach's)	1 oz	100	66	0.0
'Easter Fun' assorted (Brach's)	1 oz	100	10	0.0
eggs, chocolate, in foil (Brach's)	1 oz	150	25	8.0
eggs, chocolate malted milk (Brach's)	1 oz	130	40	5.0
eggs, creme (Cadbury)	1.37 oz	190	0	8.0
eggs, creme, chocolate coated buttercream (Brach's)	1 oz	120	50	3.0
eggs, creme, chocolate coated cherry (Brach's)	1 oz	110	20	2.0
eggs, creme, chocolate coated coconut (Brach's)	1 oz	110	40	3.0

od Name	Serv. Size	Total Cal.	Sod. MGS	Fat GMS
eggs, creme, chocolate coated fruit and nut *(Brach's)*	1 oz	110	35	2.0
eggs, creme, chocolate coated maple *(Brach's)*	1 oz	110	30	2.0
eggs, creme, chocolate coated vanilla *(Brach's)*	1 oz	110	25	2.0
eggs, creme, mini *(Cadbury)*	1 oz	140	na	7.0
eggs, 'Fiesta' pastel *(Brach's)*	1 oz	120	25	3.0
eggs 'Hide'n Seek' *(Brach's)*	1 oz	110	5	0.0
eggs, jelly *(Brach's)*	1 oz	100	15	0.0
eggs, jelly, speckled *(Brach's)*	1 oz	110	40	0.0
eggs, jelly, spiced *(Brach's)*	1 oz	90	10	0.0
eggs, jelly 'Tiny' *(Brach's)*	1 oz	100	10	0.0
eggs, marshmallow *(Brach's)*	1 oz	100	5	0.0
eggs, 'Robin's Eggs' *(Brach's)*	1 oz	140	30	6.0
nougats *(Brach's)*	1 oz	100	25	1.0
peeps, marshmallow *(Just Born)*	1 piece	27	2	<.1
rabbits, 'Jube' *(Brach's)*	1 oz	100	15	0.0
rabbits, marshmallow *(Brach's)*	1 oz	120	55	3.0
'Starlight' mint *(Brach's)*	1 oz	110	15	0.0
Halloween				
cats, marshmallow *(Just Born)*	1 piece	28	2	<.1
cats 'Scary Cats' *(Brach's)*	1 oz	100	85	0.0
corn, Indian *(Brach's)*	1 oz	100	75	0.0
corn, three color *(Brach's)*	1 oz	100	95	0.0
jelly beans *(Brach's)*	1 oz	100	15	0.0
lollipops 'Picture Pops' *(Brach's)*	1 oz	110	10	0.0
'Mellowcremes' *(Brach's)*	1 oz	100	40	0.0
pumpkin heads, crazy *(Brach's)*	1 oz	100	15	1.0
pumpkins *(Brach's)*	1 oz	100	65	0.0
pumpkins, marshmallow, large pieces *(Just Born)*	1 piece	111	8	0.1
pumpkins, marshmallow, small pieces *(Just Born)*	1 piece	14	1	<.1
'Trick or Treat Party Pack' *(Brach's)*	1 oz	110	20	0.0
witches' teeth *(Brach's)*	1 oz	100	75	0.0
Valentine's Day				
'Heart Box, 1-lb' *(Brach's)*	1 oz	110	30	2.0
'Heart Box, 1/2-lb' *(Brach's)*	1 oz	110	35	2.0
'Heart Box, 1/3-lb' *(Brach's)*	1 oz	110	25	2.0
hearts 'Conversation' large *(Brach's)*	1 oz	110	5	0.0
hearts 'Conversation' small *(Brach's)*	1 oz	110	0	0.0
hearts, fruity *(Brach's)*	1 oz	100	5	0.0
hearts 'Imperial' cinnamon *(Brach's)*	1 oz	110	5	0.0
hearts, 'Jube' cherry *(Brach's)*	1 oz	100	20	0.0
hearts, red jelly *(Brach's)*	1 oz	100	10	0.0

Food Name	Serv. Size	Total Cal.	Sod. MGS	Fa GM
hearts 'Sassy Hearts' (Brach's)	1 oz	100	0	0.
'I Luv U' chocolate (Brach's)	1 oz	150	25	8
kisses, nougat (Brach's)	1 oz	110	15	2.
lollipop, pastels (Life Savers)	1 lollipop	40	0	0.
'Love' (Brach's)	1 oz	150	25	8
'Mellowcremes' (Brach's)	1 oz	100	75	0
JELLIED AND GUMMED				
cinnamon bears (Brach's)	1 oz	80	10	0.
eggs (Rodda)	1 piece	7	1	
'Fruit Bunch' (Brach's)	1 oz	100	10	0
gummi bears (Brach's)	1 oz	100	15	0.
gummi dinosaurs, tropical (Jurassic Park)	15 pieces	140	na	0.
gummi savers (Life Savers)	1 piece	12	0	0
gummi worms (Brach's)	1 oz	100	15	0
gummy bears (Estee)	4 pieces	20	0	0.
gummy bears 'Amazin Fruit' approx 12 pieces (Hershey's)	1 oz	90	20	<1
gummy bears, tropical 'Amazin Fruit' (Hershey's)	1 oz	90	20	<1
hot cinnamon (Hot Tamales)	1 piece	9	1	
jelly beans (Brach's)	1 oz	100	5	0
jelly nougat (Brach's)	1 oz	100	35	1
'Jels' sour cherry (Brach's)	1 oz	100	10	0
'Jube Jels' (Brach's)	1 oz	100	10	0
juicy (Callard & Bowser)	1 oz	90	0	0
mint, assorted (Brach's)	1 oz	100	0	0
'Petite' eggs (Just Born)	1 piece	4	<1	
'Rainbow Bears' (Brach's)	1 oz	100	10	0
'Spearmint Leaves' (Brach's)	1 oz	100	5	0
spicettes (Brach's)	1 oz	100	15	0
'Teenee Beanee Gourmet' (Just Born)	1 piece	4	<1	
LICORICE				
candy coated (Good & Fruity)	1 oz	106	8	0
candy coated (Good & Plenty)	1 oz	106	52	<
'Cherry Nibs' (Y&S)	1 oz	100	80	<1
'Nip' (Pearson)	1 oz	120	70	3
'Red Laces' (Brach's)	1 oz	100	10	0
'Twin Twists' (Brach's)	1 oz	100	10	0
'Twists' (Brach's)	1 oz	100	50	1
'Twizzlers Bites' cherry (Y&S)	1 oz	100	85	<1
'Twizzlers' strawberry (Y&S)	1 oz	100	95	1

Food Name	Serv. Size	Total Cal.	Sod. MGS	Fat GMS
LOLLIPOP				
all flavors *(Estee)*	1 lollipop	30	0	0.0
all flavors *(Life Savers)*	1 lollipop	45	10	0.0
all flavors bubble gum center *(Spangler)*	1 lollipop	57	5	<1.0
all flavors 'Dum Dums' *(Spangler)*	1 lollipop	25	0	<1.0
all flavors except chocolate *(Tootsie Pop)*	1 oz	111	1	0.6
all fruit flavors *(Sorbee)*	1 lollipop	22	0	0.0
all flavors 'Pops' *(Brach's)*	1 oz	110	10	0.0
all flavors 'Saf-T-Pops' *(Spangler)*	1 lollipop	45	0	<1.0
black raspberry *(Fruit Juicers)*	1 lollipop	40	0	0.0
chocolate *(Tootsie Pop)*	1 oz	110	2	0.6
fruit *(Glenny's)*	1 lollipop	21	<1	<1.0
fruit punch *(Fruit Juicers)*	1 lollipop	40	0	0.0
pineapple *(Fruit Juicers)*	1 lollipop	40	0	0.0
strawberry *(Fruit Juicers)*	1 lollipop	40	0	0.0
swirled *(Life Savers)*	1 lollipop	45	10	0.0
vitamin 'C' *(Glenny's)*	1 lollipop	35	<1	<1.0
MARSHMALLOW				
'Circus Peanuts' approx 1 oz *(Spangler)*	4 pieces	110	5	<1.0
'Mallow Cup' 1.6 oz *(Boyer)*	2 pieces	224	na	11.0
'Mallow Cup' .5 oz *(Boyer)*	1 piece	71	na	5.0
'Mallow Cup' .275 oz *(Boyer)*	1 piece	36	na	2.5
'Perkys Circus Peanuts' *(Brach's)*	1 oz	100	10	0.6
toasted coconut *(Just Born)*	1 piece	30	6	0.6
MINT				
'After Dinner' tofu, chocolate *(Barat)*	1 piece	40	0	2.0
'After Eight' dark chocolate *(Rowntree)*	1 mint	35	0	1.0
all flavors except cocoamint *(Velamints)*	1 mint	7	0	0.0
'Bits' tofu, chocolate *(Barat)*	.75 oz	120	15	8.0
butter *(Kraft)*	1 piece	8	0	0.0
cocoamint *(Velamints)*	1 mint	7	0	0.3
'Cool Blue' *(Featherweight)*	1 piece	25	0	0.0
'Coolers/Starlight' *(Brach's)*	1 oz	110	15	0.0
creme, chocolate covered, regular *(Brach's)*	1 oz	110	10	2.0
'Creme de Menthe' *(Brach's)*	1 oz	150	20	9.0
'Creme de Menthe' chocolate *(Andes)*	6 pieces	150	20	9.0
dark chocolate coated *(Spangler)*	1 piece	80	25	2.0
'Dessert Mints' assorted *(Brach's)*	1 oz	110	0	0.0
'Drops' *(Glenny's)*	1 drop	6	<1	<1.0
filled straws *(Brach's)*	1 oz	110	10	1.0
'Jots/Pearls' *(Brach's)*	1 oz	120	10	2.0

Food Name	Serv. Size	Total Cal.	Sod. MGS	Fat GMS
'Junior Mints' chocolate covered, 1 oz	12 pieces	120	10	3.0
'Kentucky Mints' (Brach's)	1 oz	110	0	0.0
'Meltaway' .33 oz (Mint)	1 piece	50	10	3.0
'Nip' chocolate (Pearson)	1 oz	120	70	3.0
'Mint Oh's' (Saco Foods)	1.5 oz	111	14	6.6
parfait (Brach's)	1 oz	150	35	9.0
party (Kraft)	1 piece	8	0	0.0
peppermint kisses (Brach's)	1 oz	100	25	1.0
'Peppermint Pattie' large patties (York)	1 piece	149	17	3.9
'Peppermint Pattie' small patties (York)	1 piece	38	4	1.0
peppermint swirls (Featherweight)	1 piece	20	0	0.0
squares (Russell Stover)	1.4 oz	160	35	5.0
thin, chocolate covered, regular (Brach's)	1 oz	110	10	2.0
NONPAREILS				
dark chocolate (Brach's)	1 oz	140	20	6.0
'Sno-Caps' (Nestlé)	1 oz	140	0	6.0
PEANUT				
'Bits' chocolate tofu, dipped (Barat)	1 oz	120	15	8.0
candy coated (Estee)	10 pieces	70	10	4.0
caramel cluster (Brach's)	1 oz	150	50	8.0
chocolate coated (Cocofection)	1 oz	140	12	12.0
chocolate coated (Estee)	2 squares	60	10	4.5
chocolate coated, approx 14 pieces (Nabisco)	1 oz	160	15	9.0
chocolate coated 'Small' (Brach's)	1 oz	140	40	7.0
filled (Brach's)	1 oz	110	20	1.0
French, burnt (Brach's)	1 oz	130	5	5.0
'Goobers' chocolate covered (Nestlé)	10 pieces	51	4	3.3
'Goobers' chocolate covered, 1 3/8 oz (Nestlé)	1 pkg	200	15	13.0
'Jots' (Brach's)	1 oz	140	25	6.0
'M&M's' candy coated chocolate peanuts (M&M/Mars)	10 pieces	99	19	5.4
'M&M's' candy coated chocolate peanuts, fun size (M&M/Mars)	1 pkg	110	20	5.0
milk chocolate coated (Brach's)	1 oz	150	30	9.0
'Nut Goodies' (Brach's)	1 oz	130	10	4.0
parfait (Brach's)	1 oz	160	60	10.0
'Peanut Clusters' (Brach's)	1 oz	150	25	9.0
'Peanut Delights' (Russell Stover)	1.4 oz	210	130	12.0
PEANUT BRITTLE				
(Estee)	.5 oz	60	20	2.0
(Estee)	.25 oz	35	30	1.0
(Kraft)	1 oz	130	135	5.0

Food Name	Serv. Size	Total Cal.	Sod. MGS	Fat GMS
(Sophie Mae)	1.4 oz	170	130	5.0
PEANUT BUTTER				
'Bar None' *(Hershey's)*	1.5 oz	240	50	14.0
cup *(Estee)*	1 cup	40	20	3.0
cup, 1.6 oz *(Boyer)*	2 pieces	250	na	15.0
cup, .5 oz *(Boyer)*	1 piece	75	na	7.5
cup, .275 oz *(Boyer)*	1 piece	38	na	3.8
kisses *(Brach's)*	1 oz	110	135	2.0
'Kudos' chocolate covered *(M&M/Mars)*	1.3 oz	200	80	12.0
'M&M's' candy coated *(M&M/Mars)*	1.63 oz	240	60	12.0
'M&M's' candy coated *(M&M/Mars)*	1 oz	150	60	7.0
'PB Max' chocolate covered cookie *(M&M/Mars)*	1 piece	240	150	15.0
'Reese's Crunchy Peanut Butter Cups' *(Hershey's)*	1.8 oz	280	130	18.0
'Reese's Peanut Butter Cups' *(Hershey's)*	1.6 oz	250	160	15.0
'Reese's Peanut Butter Cups' *(Hershey's)*	1.8 oz	247	148	15.9
'Reese's Peanut Butter Cups' miniatures *(Hershey's)*	6 cups	204	122	13.1
'Reese's Peanut Butter Cups' snack size *(Hershey's)*	1 cup	100	60	6.0
'Reese's Pieces' candy coated *(Hershey's)*	1.63 oz	230	80	10.0
'Reese's Pieces' candy coated *(Hershey's)*	10 pieces	38	12	1.7
'Reese's Pieces' candy coated, 1.95 oz *(Hershey's)*	1 pkg	258	83	11.4
toffee *(Flavor House)*	1 oz	150	90	7.0
PECAN				
'Demet's Turtles' milk chocolate, pecans, caramel *(Demet's)*	1 piece	82	16	4.7
'Pecan Crowns' *(Russell Stover)*	1.4 oz	200	60	13.0
'Pecan Delights' *(Russell Stover)*	1.4 oz	220	55	14.5
POWDER CANDY				
(Lik-m-aid Fun Dip)	1 oz	110	na	0.0
(Pixy Stix)	1 oz	100	na	0.0
RAISIN				
'Bits' chocolate tofu covered *(Barat)*	1 oz	120	10	7.0
chocolate coated *(Brach's)*	1 oz	130	30	5.0
chocolate coated *(Cocofection)*	1 oz	120	14	5.0
chocolate coated *(Estee)*	8 pieces	30	5	1.0
chocolate coated, approx 29 pieces *(Nabisco)*	1 oz	130	15	5.0
'Raisinets' chocolate covered *(Nestlé)*	1 3/8 oz	180	10	6.0
'Raisinets' chocolate covered *(Nestlé)*	10 pieces	41	4	1.6
'Raisinets' chocolate covered *(Nestlé)*	1.58 oz	185	16	7.2
TAFFY				
all flavors 'Salt Water Taffy' *(Brach's)*	1 oz	100	30	1.0
apple flavor 'Laffy Taffy' 1 oz *(Beich's)*	2 pieces	110	55	1.0

Food Name	Serv. Size	Total Cal.	Sod. MGS	Fat GMS
banana flavor 'Laffy Taffy' 1 oz (Beich's)	2 pieces	120	55	1.0
cherry flavor 'Laffy Taffy' 1 oz (Beich's)	2 pieces	110	55	1.0
grape flavor 'Laffy Taffy' 1 oz (Beich's)	2 pieces	110	60	1.0
honey flavor (Bit-O-Honey)	1.7 oz	200	125	4.0
passion punch flavor 'Laffy Taffy' 1 oz (Beich's)	2 pieces	120	50	1.0
strawberry flavor 'Laffy Taffy' 1 oz (Beich's)	2 pieces	110	55	1.0
tangy flavor (Tangy Taffy)	1 oz	120	na	2.5
watermelon flavor 'Laffy Taffy' 1 oz (Beich's)	2 pieces	110	55	1.0
TOFFEE				
(Brach's)	1 oz	110	80	2.0
(Callard & Bowser)	1 oz	135	0	6.5
'Bits'O Brickle' (Heath)	3 oz	448	472	28.0
English (Bits'O Heath)	3.5 oz	520	390	31.0
English, 'Heath Bar' 1 3/16 oz (Heath)	2 pieces	180	130	11.0
CANDY APPLE. See APPLE KIT.				
CANE SYRUP				
table blends	1/2 cup	397	6	0.0
table blends	1 tbsp	50	tr	0.0
CANNELLINI BEAN, canned, white (Pathmark)	1/2 cup	100	390	0.0
CANNELLONI, CANNED, mini (Chef Boyardee)	7.5 oz	230	1050	7.0
CANNELLONI ENTRÉE, frozen				
beef, w/tomato sauce (Lean Cuisine)	9 5/8 oz	200	490	3.0
cheese (Dining Lite)	9 oz	310	650	9.0
cheese, w/tomato sauce (Lean Cuisine)	9 1/8 oz	270	590	8.0
Florentine (Celentano)	12 oz	350	620	8.0
CANOLA AND VEGETABLE OIL, 'Best Blend' (Wesson)	1 tbsp	120	0	14.0
CANOLA OIL				
	1/2 cup	964	0	109.0
	1 oz	251	0	28.4
	1 tbsp	124	0	14.0
(Country Pure)	1 tbsp	120	0	14.0
(Hain)	1 tbsp	120	0	14.0
(Kroger)	1 tbsp	122	0	13.6
(Nucoa) 'Heart Beat'	1 tbsp	120	0	14.0
(Spectrum Naturals)	1 tbsp	120	0	14.0
(Spectrum Naturals) organic	1 tbsp	120	0	14.0
(Wesson)	1 tbsp	120	0	14.0
(Wesson) 'Food Service'	1 tbsp	122	0	13.6
CANOLA OIL SPRAY. See COOKING SPRAY.				
CANTALOUPE /muskmelon				
approx 5 inch diam	1/2 fruit	93	24	0.8

Food Name	Serv. Size	Total Cal.	Sod. MGS	Fat GMS
cubed	1/2 cup	29	7	0.2
pulp	1 oz	10	3	0.1
untrimmed	1 lb	82	20	0.6
untrimmed *(Dole)*	1/4 fruit	50	35	0.0
CAPOCOLLA. See LUNCHEON MEAT.				
CAPPUCCINO. See COFFEE, FLAVORED.				
CARAMEL TOPPING				
(Kraft)	1 tbsp	60	45	0.0
(Mrs. Richardson's) fat-free	2 tbsp	130	55	0.0
(Smucker's) hot	2 tbsp	150	75	4.0
CARAWAY SEED				
whole	1 oz	94	5	4.1
whole	1 tbsp	22	1	1.0
whole	1 tsp	7	0	0.3
whole *(Durkee)*	1 tsp	9	0	<0.1
whole *(Laurel Leaf)*	1 tsp	9	0	<0.1
whole *(Spice Islands)*	1 tsp	8	<1	0.4
CARDAMOM				
ground	1 oz	88	5	1.9
ground	1 tbsp	18	1	0.4
ground	1 tsp	6	0	0.1
ground *(Durkee)*	1 tsp	7	0	tr
ground *(Laurel Leaf)*	1 tsp	7	0	tr
CARDAMOM SEED *(Spice Islands)*	1 tsp	6	tr	0.1
CARDOON/cardoni				
boiled, drained	4 oz	25	200	0.1
raw, shredded	1 cup	36	303	0.2
raw, shredded	1/2 cup	18	151	0.1
raw, trimmed	1 oz	6	48	<.1
raw, untrimmed	1 lb	44	378	0.2
CAROB FLAVOR DRINK				
mix, powder	1 oz	105	29	0.1
mix, powder	3 tsp	45	12	0.0
mix, prepared w/1 cup whole milk	1 cup	195	132	8.2
mix, prepared w/1 cup 2% milk	1 cup	166	134	4.7
mix, prepared w/1 cup 1% milk	1 cup	147	135	2.6
mix, prepared w/1 cup skim milk	1 cup	131	138	0.4
CAROB FLOUR				
	1 cup	394	36	0.7
	1 oz	51	10	0.2
	1 tbsp	31	3	0.1

Food Name	Serv. Size	Total Cal.	Sod. MGS	Fat GMS
CARP				
dry-heat cooked	3 oz	138	54	6.1
dry-heat cooked, approx 7.7 oz raw wt	1 fillet	275	107	12.2
raw	1 lb	574	223	25.4
raw	3 oz	108	42	4.8
raw	1 oz	36	14	1.6
raw, approx 7.7 oz	1 fillet	277	107	12.2
CARROT				
baby, raw	1 large	6	5	0.1
baby, raw	1 med	4	4	0.1
boiled, drained	4 oz	51	75	0.2
boiled, drained	1 med	21	30	0.1
boiled, drained, sliced	1/2 cup	35	51	0.1
raw	1 med	31	25	0.1
raw (Dole)	1 med	40	40	1.0
raw, shredded	1/2 cup	24	19	0.1
raw, trimmed	1 oz	12	10	0.1
raw, untrimmed	1 lb	174	139	0.8
CARROT, CANNED				
Crinkle sliced				
(A&P)	1/2 cup	30	300	<1.0
(Freshlike)	1/2 cup	30	300	0.0
(Veg•All)	1/2 cup	30	300	0.0
Diced				
(Allens)	1/2 cup	30	190	<1.0
'Fancy' (S&W)	1/2 cup	30	240	0.0
julienne 'Fancy' (S&W)	1/2 cup	30	240	0.0
'No Salt Added' (A&P)	1/2 cup	25	40	<1.0
'No Salt or Sugar Added' (Stokely)	1/2 cup	35	35	0.0
w/liquid (Del Monte)	1/2 cup	30	265	0.0
Sliced				
(Featherweight)	1/2 cup	30	30	0.0
(Finast)	1/2 cup	35	370	0.0
(IGA)	1/2 cup	30	300	0.0
(Pathmark)	1/2 cup	35	310	0.0
(S&W Nutradiet)	1/2 cup	30	50	0.0
(Stokely)	1/2 cup	35	300	0.0
'Fancy' (S&W)	1/2 cup	30	240	0.0
large (Allens)	1/2 cup	30	250	<1.0
medium (Allens)	1/2 cup	30	250	<1.0
'No Salt Added' (Finast)	1/2 cup	35	30	0.0

Food Name	Serv. Size	Total Cal.	Sod. MGS	Fat GMS
'No Salt Added' (Pathmark)	1/2 cup	35	35	0.0
regular pack, drained	1/2 cup	17	176	0.1
regular pack, w/liquid	1/2 cup	28	297	0.2
regular pack, w/liquid, low-sodium	1/2 cup	28	48	0.2
small (Allens)	1/2 cup	30	250	<1.0
special dietary pack, drained	1/2 cup	17	31	0.1
special dietary pack, w/liquid	1/2 cup	28	48	0.2
water-packed, w/o salt (Freshlike)	1/2 cup	30	40	0.0
water-packed, w/o sugar or salt (Freshlike)	1/2 cup	30	40	0.0
w/liquid (Del Monte)	1/2 cup	30	265	0.0
Whole				
baby (Allens)	1/2 cup	30	240	<1.0
tiny 'Fancy' (S&W)	1/2 cup	30	240	0.0
w/liquid	1/2 cup	26	273	0.2
CARROT, FROZEN				
	10 oz	112	167	0.6
(A&P)	3.3 oz	40	45	<1.0
(Seabrook)	3.3 oz	40	44	0.0
baby, whole 'Deluxe' (Bird's Eye)	3.3 oz	40	45	0.0
baby, whole, 'Harvest Fresh' (Green Giant)	1/2 cup	18	75	0.0
baby, whole 'Select' (Green Giant)	1/2 cup	20	35	0.0
baby, whole, 'Singles' (Stokely)	3 oz	35	50	0.0
boiled, drained	4 oz	41	67	0.1
Parisienne 'Deluxe' (Deluxe)	2.6 oz	30	35	0.0
sliced (Birds Eye)	3.2 oz	35	40	0.0
sliced (Frosty Acres)	3.3 oz	40	44	0.0
sliced, boiled, drained	1/2 cup	26	43	0.1
sliced, unprepared	1/2 cup	25	38	0.1
whole (Southern)	3.5 oz	42	60	0.2
w/sweet peas, pearl onions 'Deluxe' (Birds Eye)	3.3 oz	50	60	0.0
CARROT JUICE				
canned	6 oz	74	53	0.3
canned	1/2 cup	49	36	0.2
canned (Biotta)	6 oz	51	158	0.1
canned (Hain)	6 oz	80	170	0.0
canned (Hollywood)	6 oz	80	170	0.0
CASABA MELON				
cubed	1 cup	44	20	0.2
1/10 of 7.75-inch melon	2-in. slice	43	20	0.2
pulp	1 oz	7	3	<.1
untrimmed	1 lb	71	33	0.3

Food Name	Serv. Size	Total Cal.	Sod. MGS	Fat GMS
CASHEW/heart nut				
(Beer Nuts)	1 oz	170	65	13.0
Dry roasted				
halves (Fisher)	1 oz	160	na	13.0
lightly salted (Planters)	1 oz	160	115	13.0
salted	1 oz	163	182	13.2
salted (Pathmark)	1 oz	170	150	13.0
salted (Planters)	1 oz	160	230	13.0
salted, 'No Frills' (Pathmark)	1 oz	170	220	13.0
salted, wholes and halves	1 cup	787	877	63.5
unsalted	1 oz	163	5	13.2
'Unsalted' (Planters)	1 oz	160	0	13.0
unsalted, approx 14 large or 26 small kernels	1 oz	163	4	13.2
unsalted, wholes and halves	1 cup	787	21	63.5
wholes (Fisher)	1 oz	160	100	13.0
Honey roasted				
(Frito-Lays)	1 oz	170	115	14.0
(Planters)	1 oz	170	170	12.0
halves (Fisher)	1 oz	150	na	13.0
wholes (Fisher)	1 oz	150	90	13.0
w/peanuts (Planters)	1 oz	170	170	12.0
Oil roasted				
halves (Fisher)	1 oz	170	155	14.0
lightly salted (Planters)	1 oz	160	80	14.0
pieces (Fisher)	1 oz	170	135	14.0
salted	1 oz	164	178	13.7
salted (Flavor House)	1 oz	180	125	16.0
salted (Pathmark)	1 oz	170	150	14.0
salted, approx 14 large or 18 medium kernels	1 oz	163	177	13.7
salted, 'Fancy' (Planters)	1 oz	170	135	14.0
salted, halves (Planters)	1 oz	170	135	14.0
salted, 'No Frills' (Pathmark)	1 oz	170	150	14.0
salted, wholes (Guy's)	1 oz	170	140	14.0
salted, wholes and halves	1 cup	749	814	62.7
unsalted	1 oz	164	5	13.7
unsalted, approx 14 large or 18 medium kernels	1 oz	163	5	13.7
unsalted, 'Fancy' (Planters)	1 oz	170	0	14.0
unsalted, halves	1 cup	749	22	62.7
'Unsalted' halves (Planters)	1 oz	170	0	14.0
wholes (Fisher)	1 oz	170	110	14.0
w/almonds (Fisher)	1 oz	170	95	15.0

Food Name	Serv. Size	Total Cal.	Sod. MGS	Fat GMS
CASHEW BUTTER				
gourmet *(Roaster Fresh)*	1 oz	165	4	14.0
peanut date *(Maranatha Natural)*	2 tbsp	190	8	14.0
peanut date 'Natural' *(Westbrae)*	2 tbsp	200	2	15.0
plain	1 oz	167	4	14.0
plain	1 tbsp	94	2	7.9
raw *(Hain)*	2 tbsp	190	(mq)	15.0
raw 'Natural' *(Westbrae)*	2 tbsp	300	0	28.0
raw, unsalted *(Hain)*	2 tbsp	210	10	19.0
roasted *(Maranatha Natural)*	2 tbsp	190	5	14.0
roasted 'Natural' *(Westbrae)*	2 tbsp	190	0	17.0
toasted *(Hain)*	2 tbsp	210	15	17.0
CASSAVA/manioc/yuca				
trimmed	1 lb	544	36	1.8
trimmed	1 oz	34	2	0.1
raw	100 gm	120	8	0.4
CATFISH, CHANNEL				
Farmed				
dry-heat cooked	3 oz	129	68	6.8
frozen, fillets *(Delta Pride)*	4 oz	132	<1	4.9
raw	3 oz	115	45	6.4
raw	1 oz	33	18	1.2
Wild				
dry-heat cooked	3 oz	89	43	2.4
raw	3 oz	81	37	2.4
CATFISH, OCEAN. See WOLF FISH.				
CATSUP/ketchup	1 oz	29	336	0.1
	1 tbsp	16	178	0.1
	.2-oz pkt	6	71	0.0
(Del Monte)	1/4 cup	60	675	0.0
(Estee)	1 tbsp	6	20	0.0
(Featherweight)	1 tbsp	6	5	0.0
(Healthy Choice)	.5 oz	9	97	0.1
(Heinz)	1 tbsp	16	213	0.0
(Hunt's)	1 tbsp	16	158	0.1
(Smucker's)	1 tsp	8	45	0.0
(Snider's)	1 tbsp	16	158	0.1
(Stokely)	1 tbsp	20	190	0.0
(Weight Watchers)	2 tsp	8	110	0.0
'All Natural' *(Life)*	1 tbsp	17	10	0.0
'Food Service' *(Hunt's)*	1 tbsp	15	158	0.1

Food Name	Serv. Size	Total Cal.	Sod. MGS	Fat GMS
fruit-sweetened *(Westbrae)*	1 tbsp	12	110	0.0
fruit-sweetened, no salt *(Westbrae)*	1 tbsp	12	10	0.0
hot *(Heinz)*	1 tbsp	16	195	0.0
'Lite' *(Heinz)*	1 tbsp	8	115	0.0
low-sodium	1 oz	29	6	0.1
low-sodium	1 tbsp	16	3	0.1
low-sodium	.2-oz pkt	6	1	0.0
'Natural' *(Hain)*	1 tbsp	16	155	0.0
'Natural No Salt Added' *(Hain)*	1 tbsp	16	5	0.0
'No Salt Added' *(Del Monte)*	1/4 cup	60	25	0.0
'No Salt Added' *(Hunt's)*	1 tbsp	20	0	0.0
organic *(Millina's Finest)*	1 oz	17	143	0.1
portion pack *(Hunt's)*	.3175 oz	10	75	0.1
w/onions *(Heinz)*	1 tbsp	19	289	(tr)
CAULIFLOWER				
boiled, drained	4 oz	27	7	0.2
boiled, drained, approx 1.9 oz	3 flowerets	12	8	0.2
boiled, drained, 1-inch pieces	1/2 cup	14	9	0.3
fresh, medium size *(Dole)*	1/6 head	18	45	0.0
green, fresh *(Dole)*	1/5 head	35	30	0.0
raw, approx 5 oz	3 flowerets	14	17	0.1
raw, 1-inch pieces	1/2 cup	13	15	0.1
raw, trimmed	1 oz	7	4	0.1
raw, untrimmed	1 lb	42	26	0.3
Frozen				
	10 oz	68	68	0.8
(A&P)	3.3 oz	25	20	<1.0
(Birds Eye)	3.3 oz	25	20	0.0
(Finast)	3.3 oz	25	15	0.0
(Frosty Acres)	3.3 oz	25	16	0.0
(Kohl's)	3 oz	20	15	<1.0
(Seabrook)	3.3 oz	25	16	0.0
(Southern)	3.5 oz	26	30	0.2
boiled, drained	4 oz	22	20	0.2
boiled, drained, 1-inch pieces	1/2 cup	17	16	0.2
cuts *(Green Giant)*	1/2 cup	12	25	0.0
florets 'Plain Polybag' *(Green Giant)*	1/2 cup	12	25	0.0
in cheddar cheese sauce 'Side Dish' *(Budget Gourmet)*	5 oz	110	300	5.0
in cheese flavored sauce *(Green Giant)*	1/2 cup	60	500	2.0
in cheese sauce *(Finast)*	3.3 oz	40	240	0.0
in cheese sauce 'One Serving' *(Green Giant)*	5.5 oz	80	690	2.0

Food Name	Serv. Size	Total Cal.	Sod. MGS	Fat GMS
in cheese sauce 'Singles' (Stokely)	4 oz	70	170	3.0
'Singles' (Stokely)	3 oz	20	20	0.0
unprepared, 1-inch pieces	1/2 cup	16	16	0.2
Pickled				
'Hot & Spicy' (Vlasic)	1 oz	4	435	0.0
sweet (Vlasic)	1 oz	35	225	0.0
CAVIAR				
black, granular	1 oz	71	420	5.0
black, granular	1 tbsp	40	240	2.9
red, granular	1 oz	71	420	5.0
red, granular	1 tbsp	40	240	2.9
CAYENNE PEPPER				
ground	1 oz	90	9	4.9
ground	1 tbsp	17	2	0.9
ground	1 tsp	6	1	0.3
ground (Spice Islands)	1 tsp	9	<1	0.3
CECI. See GARBANZO BEAN.				
CELERIAC/celery root				
boiled, drained	4 oz	28	69	0.2
boiled, drained	100 gm	25	61	0.2
raw	1/2 cup	30	78	0.2
raw (Frieda's)	3.5 oz	40	100	0.3
raw, trimmed	1 oz	11	28	0.1
raw, untrimmed	1 lb	154	390	1.2
CELERY				
boiled, drained	4 oz	20	103	0.1
boiled, drained, diced	1/2 cup	14	68	0.1
fresh, medium size (Dole)	2 stalks	20	140	0.0
raw, diced	1/2 cup	10	52	0.1
raw, trimmed	1 oz	5	25	<1
raw, untrimmed	1 lb	65	352	0.6
CELERY FLAKES (Tone's)	1 tsp	9	4	0.5
CELERY ROOT. See CELERIAC.				
CELERY ROOT JUICE, bottled (Biotta)	6 oz	67	195	0.2
CELERY SALT (Tone's)	1 tsp	6	1584	0.4
CELERY SEED				
whole	1 oz	111	45	7.2
whole	1 tbsp	25	10	1.6
whole	1 tsp	8	3	0.5
whole (Durkee)	1 tsp	9	0	<0.1
whole (Laurel Leaf)	1 tsp	9	0	<0.1

Food Name	Serv. Size	Total Cal.	Sod. MGS	Fat GMS
whole *(Spice Islands)*	1 tsp	11	4	0.5
CELLOPHANE NOODLES. See NOODLE, CHINESE.				
CEREAL, HOT				
(NOTE: All of the following hot cereals are dry unless otherwise noted.)				
BARLEY *(Erewhon)* organic plus	1 oz	110	0	1.0
BRAN *(H-O Brand)* 'Super Bran'	1/3 cup	110	0	2.0
BULGUR WHEAT				
(Arrowhead Mills)	2 oz	200	0	1.0
(Krusteaz) 'Ala'	1/4 cup	150	0	0.0
CORN GRITS. See GRITS.				
FARINA				
(H-O Brand) cream	3 tbsp	120	0	0.0
(H-O Brand) instant	1 pkt	110	235	0.0
(Krusteaz)	1 oz	100	1	0.0
(Malt•O•Meal) 'Maple Brown Sugar' 30% formulation	1 oz	100	0	0.0
GRAIN, MIXED				
(Arrowhead Mills) four grain	1 oz	94	1	1.0
(Arrowhead Mills) seven grain	1 oz	100	<1	1.0
(Breadshop) 'Triple Bran'	1 oz	100	5	2.0
(Maltex) wheat and barley	1 oz	105	0	1.0
(Malt•O•Meal) wheat and barley, chocolate flavor	1 tbsp	38	1	0.1
(Malt•O•Meal) wheat and barley, plain	1 tbsp	38	1	0.1
(Pritikin) hearty multi-grain, microwave instant	1 pkt	150	0	na
(Quaker) multi-grain	1/2 cup	130	0	1.5
(Roman Meal) multi-grain, apple, and cinnamon	2/3 cup	112	14	2.8
(Roman Meal) oat, wheat, dates, raisins, and almonds	1.3 oz	140	0	3.0
(Roman Meal) oat, wheat, honey, coconut, and almonds	1.3 oz	150	5	6.0
(Roman Meal) oat and wheat, rye, bran, and flax	1.2 oz	116	5	1.7
OAT BRAN				
(Arrowhead Mills)	1 oz	110	1	1.0
(Breadshop) 'Oat Bran Müesli'	1 oz	100	5	2.0
(Breadshop) 'Oat Bran' 100% pure	1 oz	100	5	2.0
(Erewhon) toasted wheat germ	1 oz	115	15	2.0
(Health Valley) 'Natural' apple and cinnamon	1 oz	100	10	1.0
(Health Valley) 'Natural' raisins and spice	1 oz	110	10	1.0
(Malt•O•Meal) 'Plus 40% Oat Bran'	1.3 oz	130	0	2.0
(Mother's)	1/3 cup	92	1	2.1
(Quaker)	1 oz	92	1	2.1
(3-Minute Brand) instant	1 oz	90	0	2.0
(3-Minute Brand) 'Regular'	1 oz	90	0	2.0
(Wholesome 'N Hearty)	1 oz	100	0	2.0

Food Name	Serv. Size	Total Cal.	Sod. MGS	Fat GMS
(Wholesome 'N Hearty) instant, apple cinnamon	1 3/8 oz	130	160	2.0
(Wholesome 'N Hearty) instant, honey	1.25 oz	110	160	2.0

OATMEAL AND OATS

Food Name	Serv. Size	Total Cal.	Sod. MGS	Fat GMS
(Arrowhead Mills) instant	1 oz	100	0	2.0
(Arrowhead Mills) instant, apple, date, and almond	1 oz	130	3	3.0
(Arrowhead Mills) instant, apple spice	1 oz	130	1	2.0
(Arrowhead Mills) instant, cinnamon, raisin, and almond	1 oz	140	3	3.0
(Erewhon) instant, apple and cinnamon	1.25 oz	145	100	3.0
(Erewhon) instant, apple and raisin	1.3 oz	150	100	3.0
(Erewhon) instant, maple spice	1.2 oz	140	100	3.0
(Erewhon) instant, oat bran	1.25 oz	125	0	3.0
(Erewhon) instant, raisins, dates, and walnuts	1.2 oz	130	60	3.0
(General Mills) instant, apple and cinnamon	1.5 oz	150	105	2.0
(General Mills) instant, cinnamon raisin	1.8 oz	170	130	2.0
(General Mills) 'Oatmeal Swirlers' instant, apple and cinnamon	1.7 oz	160	120	2.0
(General Mills) 'Oatmeal Swirlers' instant, cherry	1.7 oz	150	130	2.0
(General Mills) 'Oatmeal Swirlers' instant, cinnamon and spice	1.6 oz	160	100	2.0
(General Mills) 'Oatmeal Swirlers' instant, maple and brown sugar	1.6 oz	160	100	2.0
(General Mills) 'Oatmeal Swirlers' instant, milk chocolate	1.7 oz	170	100	2.0
(General Mills) 'Oatmeal Swirlers' instant, strawberry	1.6 oz	150	120	2.0
(H-O Brand) 'Gourmet'	1/3 cup	100	0	2.0
(H-O Brand) instant	1 pkt	110	230	2.0
(H-O Brand) instant, apple and cinnamon	1 pkt	130	220	2.0
(H-O Brand) instant, box	1/2 cup	130	5	2.0
(H-O Brand) instant, maple and brown sugar	1 pkt	160	285	2.0
(H-O Brand) instant, raisins and spice	1 pkt	150	240	2.0
(H-O Brand) instant, sweet 'n mellow	1 pkt	150	270	2.0
(H-O Brand) 'Quick'	1/2 cup	130	5	2.0
(H-O Brand) w/fiber, instant	1 pkt	110	140	2.0
(H-O Brand) w/fiber, instant, apple and bran	1 pkt	130	140	2.0
(H-O Brand) w/fiber, instant, box	1/3 cup	100	5	2.0
(H-O Brand) w/fiber, instant, raisin and bran	1 pkt	150	140	2.0
(Maypo)	1 cup	362	18	5.0
(Maypo) '30 Second' quick	1 oz	100	0	1.0
(Maypo) 'Vermont Style' maple flavor	1 oz	105	0	1.0
(Mother's) instant	1 oz	110	0	2.0

Food Name	Serv. Size	Total Cal.	Sod. MGS	Fat GMS
(Quaker)	1/3 cup	99	1	2.0
(Quaker) 'Extra'	1 pkt	95	219	2.0
(Quaker) 'Extra' apples and spice	1 pkt	133	191	1.9
(Quaker) 'Extra' raisins and cinnamon	1 pkt	129	119	1.9
(Quaker) instant	1 pkt	94	270	2.0
(Quaker) instant, apple and cinnamon	1 pkt	118	128	1.5
(Quaker) instant, cinnamon and spice	1 pkt	164	322	2.1
(Quaker) instant, maple and brown sugar	1 pkt	152	320	2.1
(Quaker) instant, peaches and cream	1 pkt	129	179	2.2
(Quaker) instant, raisins and spice	1 pkt	149	266	2.0
(Quaker) instant, raisins, dates, and walnuts	1 pkt	141	216	3.8
(Quaker) instant, strawberries and cream	1 pkt	129	204	2.0
(Quaker) 'Kids' Choice' instant, cinnamon graham cookie	1 pkt	140	170	2.0
(Quaker) 'Kids' Choice' instant, maple and brown sugar	1 pkt	140	240	2.0
(Quaker) 'Kids' Choice' instant, radical raspberry	1 pkt	150	170	3.0
(Quaker) 'Kids' Choice' instant, strawberries and stuff	1 pkt	140	170	2.0
(Quaker) 'Old Fashioned'	1 oz	99	1	2.0
(Quaker) plus fiber	1/2 cup	130	0	2.5
(Quaker) plus fiber, oatmeal raisin bran	1 pkt	150	65	2.0
(Quaker) 'Quick'	1 oz	99	1	2.0
(Ralston)	1 cup	402	13	2.5
(Roman Meal)	1 cup	340	20	4.0
(3-Minute Brand) oat bran and raisins	1 oz	100	0	2.0
(3-Minute Brand) 'Old Fashioned'	1 oz	100	0	2.0
(3-Minute Brand) 'Quick'	1 oz	100	0	2.0
(3-Minute Brand) 'Quick' oat bran	1 oz	100	0	2.0
(3-Minute Brand) raisins	1 oz	100	0	2.0
(Total) instant	1.2 oz	110	220	2.0
(Total) instant, maple and brown sugar	1.6 oz	160	150	2.0
(Total) 'Quick'	1 oz	90	0	2.0
QUINOA (Ancient Harvest) steam-rolled flakes	1/3 cup	105	5	1.0
RICE				
(Cream of Rice)	1 tbsp	38	1	0.1
(Lundberg Family) 'Hot'n Creamy' cooked	1 oz	110	20	1.0
(Lundberg Family) 'Hot'n Creamy' almonds and dates, cooked	1 oz	110	25	1.0
RICE, BROWN				
(Arrowhead Mills) 'Rise & Shine'	1.5 oz	160	<1	1.0
(Erewhon) cream of brown rice	1 oz	110	20	1.0
RYE				
(Breadshop) 'Rye Date Müesli'	1 oz	100	5	2.0
(Roman Meal) cream of rye	1.3 oz	110	0	<1.0

Food Name	Serv. Size	Total Cal.	Sod. MGS	Fat GMS
WHEAT				
(Arrowhead Mills) 'Bear Mush'	1 oz	100	<1	0.0
(Arrowhead Mills) cracked wheat	2 oz	180	1	1.0
(Cream of Wheat)	1 tbsp	39	1	0.2
(Cream of Wheat) instant	1 oz	100	0	<1.0
(Cream of Wheat) instant	1 tbsp	42	2	0.2
(Cream of Wheat) 'Mix'n Eat' instant	1 oz	100	170	0.0
(Cream of Wheat) 'Mix'n Eat' instant, apple and cinnamon	1 oz	130	250	0.0
(Cream of Wheat) 'Mix'n Eat' instant, apple, banana, and maple	1 pkt	132	241	0.4
(Cream of Wheat) 'Mix'n Eat' instant, brown sugar and cinnamon	1 oz	130	230	0.0
(Cream of Wheat) 'Mix'n Eat' instant, maple and brown sugar	1 oz	130	180	0.0
(Cream of Wheat) 'Quick'	1 tbsp	38	41	0.1
(General Mills) 'Wheat Hearts'	1 oz	110	0	1.0
(Krusteaz) 'Zoom'	1/3 cup	120	0	0.0
(Maltex)	1 cup	532	26	3.2
(Mother's)	1/3 cup	92	1	0.6
(Quaker)	1/3 cup	92	1	0.6
(Wheatena)	1 oz	100	0	1.0
CEREAL, READY-TO-SERVE				
(NOTE: All of the following ready-to-serve cereals are in their dry form.)				
'Addam's Family' *(Ralston)*	1 oz	110	65	1.0
'All Bran' extra fiber *(Kellogg's)*	1 oz	50	140	0.0
'All Bran' wheat bran *(Kellogg's)*	1 oz	71	320	0.5
'Almond Flavor O's' fat-free *(Health Valley)*	1 oz	90	5	0.0
'Almond Raisin' low fat *(Golden Temple)*	1 oz	110	57	1.5
'Almond Raisin' nectarsweet premium *(Breadshop)*	1 oz	120	2	4.0
'Alpha Bits' oat and other grains *(Post)*	1 oz	111	180	0.7
'Alpha Bits' super swirl marshmallows *(Post)*	1 oz	150	220	1.0
'Apple Almond Müesli' *(Ralston)*	1.45 oz	150	140	2.0
'Apple & Cinnamon Toasted Oat' *(Malt•O•Meal)*	1 oz	110	180	2.0
'Apple Cinnamon Cheerios' *(General Mills)*	1 oz	110	180	2.0
'Apple Cinnamon Corn Flakes' *(Wonder)*	1 oz	110	200	0.0
'Apple Cinnamon' low fat *(Golden Temple)*	1 oz	110	59	1.5
'Apple Cinnamon O's' fat-free *(Health Valley)*	1 oz	90	5	0.0
'Apple Cinnamon Squares' *(Kellogg's)*	1 oz	90	5	0.0
'Apple Jacks' corn and other grains *(Kellogg's)*	1 oz	110	125	0.1
'Apple Raisin Crisp' *(Kellogg's)*	1 oz	130	230	0.0
'Aztec' *(Erewhon)*	1 oz	100	85	0.0

Food Name	Serv. Size	Total Cal.	Sod. MGS	Fat GMS
'Banana Nut Crunch' (Post)	1 oz	120	95	3.0
'Banana O's' (Erewhon)	1 oz	110	15	0.0
'Banana Walnut Müesli' (Ralston)	1.45 oz	150	150	3.0
'Basic 4' (General Mills)	3/4 cup	130	210	2.0
'Batman Returns' (Ralston)	1 oz	110	190	0.0
'Berry Berry Kix' (General Mills)	1 oz	110	170	1.0
'Blueberry 'N Cream' nectarsweet gourmet (Breadshop)	1 oz	115	2	3.0
'Blueberry Squares' (Kellogg's)	1 oz	90	5	0.0
'Body Buddiesnatural Fruit' (General Mills)	1 oz	110	280	1.0
'Booberry' (General Mills)	1 oz	110	210	1.0
'Bran Buds' wheat bran (Kellogg's)	1 oz	73	174	0.7
'Bran Chex' wheat bran and corn (Kellogg's)	1 oz	91	264	0.8
'Bran Flakes' (Arrowhead Mills)	1 oz	100	100	1.0
'Bran Flakes' (Kellogg's)	1 oz	90	220	0.0
'Bran Flakes' (Malt•O•Meal)	1 oz	90	210	1.0
'Bran Flakes' (Post)	1 oz	90	210	0.0
'Breakfast O's' (Barbara's Bakery)	1 oz	120	90	2.0
Brown rice, crisp (Erewhon)	1 oz	110	185	1.0
Brown rice, crisp, low sodium (Erewhon)	1 oz	110	5	0.0
'Brown Rice Crisps' (Barbara's Bakery)	1 oz	120	105	1.0
'Buñuelitos' (General Mills)	1 oz	120	120	2.0
'C.W. Post Hearty Granola Cereal' (Post)	1 oz	130	80	4.0
'C.W. Post' oats and other grains (Post)	1 oz	126	49	4.4
'C.W. Post' oats and other grains, raisins (Post)	1 oz	123	44	4.1
'California Orange Crunch' honeysweet premium (Breadshop)	1 oz	130	1	5.0
'Captain Crunch' corn and other grains (Quaker)	1 oz	120	213	2.6
'Captain Crunch Crunchberries' corn and oat (Quaker)	1 oz	118	198	2.4
'Captain Crunch Peanut Butter' corn (Quaker)	1 oz	125	217	3.7
'Cashew Almond Granola' (Golden Temple)	1 oz	129	3	3.5
'Cheerios' oat and wheat (General Mills)	1 oz	111	308	1.8
'Cinnamon & Raisin' 100% natural (Nature Valley)	1 oz	120	50	4.0
'Cinnamon & Spice Crunch' psyllium and chia seed (Golden Temple)	1 oz	132	26	4.5
'Cinnamon Apple Raisin Granola' (Golden Temple)	1 oz	125	3	3.5
'Cinnamon Mini Buns' (Kellogg's)	1 oz	110	220	1.0
'Cinnamon Toast Crunch' (General Mills)	1 oz	120	210	3.0
'Cinnamon Toast Crunch' breakfast pack (General Mills)	1 oz	140	240	4.0
'Cinnapple Spice' honeysweet premium (Breadshop)	1 oz	125	2	4.5
'Clusters' (General Mills)	1 oz	110	140	2.0
'Cocoa Krispies' rice (Kellogg's)	1 oz	110	217	0.4

Food Name	Serv. Size	Total Cal.	Sod. MGS	Fat GMS
'Cocoa Pebbles' rice *(Post)*	1 oz	116	136	1.5
'Cocoa Puffs' *(General Mills)*	1 oz	110	180	1.0
'Coconut Almond Granola' *(Golden Temple)*	1 oz	145	26	7.0
'Common Sense Oat Bran' *(Kellogg's)*	1 oz	100	250	1.0
'Common Sense Oat Bran' raisins *(Kellogg's)*	3/4 cup	130	250	1.0
'Complete' bran flakes, beta carotene *(Kellogg's)*	1 oz	90	220	<1.0
'Cookie-Crisp' chocolate chip and vanilla *(Ralston)*	1 oz	114	196	1.0
'Corn Bran' corn bran and other grains *(Ralston)*	1 oz	98	244	1.0
'Corn Chex' *(Ralston)*	1 oz	111	272	0.1
'Corn Flakes' *(Arrowhead Mills)*	1 oz	100	100	0.0
'Corn Flakes' *(Barbara's Bakery)*	1 oz	110	70	0.0
'Corn Flakes' *(Kellogg's)*	1 oz	110	291	0.1
'Corn Flakes' *(Krusteaz)*	1 oz	110	280	1.0
'Corn Flakes' *(Malt•O•Meal)*	1 oz	110	290	0.0
'Corn Flakes' *(Ralston)*	1 oz	111	272	0.1
'Corn Flakes' sugar frosted *(Kellogg's)*	1 oz	108	230	0.1
'Corn Flakes' sugar frosted *(Ralston)*	1 oz	111	184	0.4
'Corn Pops' *(Kellogg's)*	1 oz	110	90	0.0
'Count Chocula' *(General Mills)*	1 oz	110	180	1.0
'Country Corn Flakes' *(General Mills)*	1 oz	110	270	1.0
'Cracklin' Bran' wheat bran and other grains *(Kellogg's)*	1 oz	108	230	4.2
'Cracklin' Oat Bran' *(Kellogg's)*	1 oz	110	140	3.0
'Cranberry Walnut Müesli' *(Ralston)*	1.45 oz	150	95	3.0
'Crisp 'N Crackling Rice' *(Malt•O•Meal)*	1 oz	110	240	0.0
'Crisp Rice' *(Krusteaz)*	1 oz	110	270	0.0
'Crispix' *(Kellogg's)*	1 oz	110	220	0.0
'Crispy Wheats 'N Raisins' wheat *(General Mills)*	1 oz	99	135	0.5
'Crunch Graham Oat Rings' *(Wonder)*	1 oz	110	125	1.0
'Crunchies' brown rice *(Lundberg Family)*	1 cup	171	7	0.8
'Crunchy Oat Bran' nectarsweet gourmet *(Breadshop)*	1 oz	120	2	5.0
'Date Almond Müesli' *(Ralston)*	1.45 oz	140	95	2.0
'Dino Pebbles' *(Post)*	1 oz	110	150	1.0
'Double Chex' *(Ralston)*	1 oz	100	260	0.0
'Double Dip Crunch' *(Kellogg's)*	1 oz	120	160	2.0
'Fiber One' aspartame *(General Mills)*	1 oz	60	140	1.0
'Fiberwise' *(Kellogg's)*	1 oz	90	140	1.0
'Fingos' cinnamon *(General Mills)*	1 oz	110	170	3.0
'Fingos' honey toasted oat *(General Mills)*	1 oz	110	210	3.0
'40% Bran Flakes' wheat bran *(Kellogg's)*	1 oz	93	220	0.5
'40% Bran Flakes' wheat bran *(Post)*	1 oz	92	260	0.5
'40% Bran Flakes' wheat bran *(Ralston)*	1 oz	92	264	0.4

Food Name	Serv. Size	Total Cal.	Sod. MGS	Fat GMS
'Frankenberry' *(General Mills)*	1 oz	110	210	1.0
'Froot Loops' corn and other grains *(Kellogg's)*	1 oz	111	145	0.5
'Frosted Chex Juniors' *(Ralston)*	1 oz	110	200	0.0
'Frosted Flakes' *(Kellogg's)*	1 oz	110	200	0.0
'Frosted Funnies' *(Barbara's Bakery)*	1 cup	110	100	0.0
'Frosted Krispies' *(Kellogg's)*	1 oz	110	220	0.0
'Frosted Mini Wheats' *(Kellogg's)*	1 oz	100	0	0.0
'Frosted Mini Wheats' bite size *(Kellogg's)*	1 oz	100	0	0.0
'Frosted Mini Wheats' brown sugar and cinnamon *(Kellogg's)*	1 oz	102	8	0.3
'Frosted Rice Krinkles' rice	1 oz	109	179	0.1
'Frosted Rice Krispies' rice *(Kellogg's)*	1 oz	109	240	0.1
'Fruit & Fibre' oat, dates, raisins, and walnuts *(Post)*	1.25 oz	120	170	2.0
'Fruit & Fibre' oat, peaches, raisins, and almonds *(Post)*	1.25 oz	120	170	2.0
'Fruit & Fibre' oat, pineapple, banana, and coconut *(Post)*	1.25 oz	120	170	3.0
'Fruit & Fibre' oat, tropical fruit *(Post)*	1.25 oz	120	170	3.0
'Fruit & Frosted O's' mixed grain *(Malt•O•Meal)*	1 oz	110	120	1.0
'Fruit & Nut' 100%natural *(Nature Valley)*	1 oz	130	45	5.0
'Fruit 'N Nut Granola' *(Golden Temple)*	1 oz	129	26	4.5
'Fruit 'n Wheat' *(Erewhon)*	1 oz	100	75	1.0
'Fruit Wheats' apple *(Nabisco)*	1 oz	90	15	0.0
'Fruit Whirls' *(Krusteaz)*	1 oz	110	120	1.0
'Fruitful Bran' fruit *(Kellogg's)*	1 oz	120	240	0.0
'Fruity Marshmallow Krispies' *(Kellogg's)*	1 1/4 cups	140	210	0.0
'Fruity Pebbles' rice *(Post)*	1 oz	115	158	1.5
'Golden Crisp' *(Post)*	1 oz	110	45	0.0
'Golden Grahams' corn and wheat *(General Mills)*	1 oz	109	281	1.1
'Golden Granola' *(Golden Temple)*	1 oz	138	25	6.0
'Golden Maple Nut' honeysweet premium *(Breadshop)*	1 oz	130	2	5.0
'Gone Nuts!' nectarsweet premium *(Breadshop)*	1 oz	125	2	5.0
'Graham Chex' *(Ralston)*	1 oz	110	220	1.0
'Graham Crackos' wheat	1 oz	103	185	0.2
Granola, banana almond *(Sunbelt)*	1 oz	130	25	4.0
Granola, date and almond, fat-free *(Health Valley)*	1 oz	90	20	0.0
Granola, fruit and nut *(Sunbelt)*	1 oz	120	20	5.0
Granola, raisin cinnamon, fat-free *(Health Valley)*	1 oz	90	20	0.0
Granola, tropical fruit, fat-free *(Health Valley)*	1 oz	90	20	0.0
'Granola' toasted oat mix *(Nature Valley)*	1 oz	126	58	4.9
'Grape-Nuts' wheat and barley *(Post)*	1 oz	101	197	0.1
'Grape-Nuts Flakes' wheat and barley *(Post)*	1 oz	102	160	0.3
'Great Grains' double pecan *(Post)*	1 oz	120	60	3.0

Food Name	Serv. Size	Total Cal.	Sod. MGS	Fat GMS
'Great Grains' raisins, dates, and pecans *(Post)*	1.25 oz	140	70	3.0
'Hawaiian Granola' *(Golden Temple)*	1 oz	126	3	4.0
'Hazelnut Boysenberry' organic oats *(Golden Temple)*	1 oz	135	2	5.5
'Heritage O's' *(Natures Path)*	1 cup	165	140	<1.0
'High Fiber O's' fat-free *(Health Valley)*	1 oz	90	5	0.0
'High 5' *(Barbara's Bakery)*	3/4 cup	100	180	0.5
'High Protein Granola' *(Golden Temple)*	1 oz	124	6	3.5
'Honey Almond Delight' *(Ralston)*	1 oz	110	200	2.0
'Honey Almond Granola' *(Golden Temple)*	1 oz	130	25	3.5
'Honey & Nut Toasted Oat' *(Malt•O•Meal)*	1 oz	110	190	1.0
'Honey Apple Blueberry' honeysweet premium *(Breadshop)*	1 oz	125	1	5.0
'Honey Blueberry Apple Granola' *(Golden Temple)*	1 oz	128	2	3.5
'Honey Bunches of Oats' almonds *(Post)*	1 oz	120	160	3.0
'Honey Bunches of Oats' honey roasted *(Post)*	1 oz	110	180	2.0
'Honey Gone Nuts!' honeysweet premium *(Breadshop)*	1 oz	130	2	5.5
'Honey Nut' toasted oatmeal *(Quaker)*	1 oz	120	110	3.0
'Honey Nut Cheerios' oat and wheat *(General Mills)*	1 oz	107	257	0.7
'Honey Nut Cheerios' oat and wheat, breakfast pack *(General Mills)*	4/5 oz	100	230	1.0
'Honey Nut Crispy Rice' *(Wonder)*	1 oz	110	205	1.0
'Honey Nut O's' *(Krusteaz)*	1 oz	110	190	1.0
'HoneyComb' corn and oats *(Post)*	1 oz	111	160	0.5
'Just Right' fiber nuggets *(Kellogg's)*	1 oz	100	200	1.0
'Just Right' raisins, dates, and nuts *(Kellogg's)*	3/4 cup	140	190	1.0
'Kaboom' *(General Mills)*	1 oz	110	270	1.0
'Kamut Flakes' *(Erewhon)*	1 oz	90	60	0.0
'Kenmei Rice Bran' *(Kellogg's)*	1 oz	110	230	1.0
'King Vitaman' corn and other grains	1 oz	115	218	1.6
'Kix' corn and other grains *(General Mills)*	1 oz	110	291	0.7
'Life' oat and other grains *(Quaker)*	1 oz	105	148	0.5
'Life' oat and other grains, cinnamon *(Quaker)*	1 oz	105	148	0.5
'Lite Müesli' *(Golden Temple)*	1 oz	102	60	1.0
'Lite 'N Crunchy Granola' *(Golden Temple)*	1 oz	129	9	4.5
'Lucky Charms' oat and other grains *(General Mills)*	1 oz	111	202	1.1
'Lucky Charms' oat and other grains, breakfast pack *(General Mills)*	7/8 oz	110	180	1.0
'Maple Almond Granola' *(Golden Temple)*	1 oz	129	25	3.5
'Maple Corns' *(Arrowhead Mills)*	1 oz	100	75	1.0
'Maple Frosted Corn' mini puffs *(Glenny's)*	1 oz	109	50	<.5
'Marshmallow Alpha Bits' *(Post)*	1 oz	110	150	1.0

Food Name	Serv. Size	Total Cal.	Sod. MGS	Fat GMS
'Most' wheat bran and wheat	1 oz	96	151	0.3
'Müeslix Crispy Blend' (Kellogg's)	2/3 cup	150	150	2.0
'Müeslix Golden Crunch' (Kellogg's)	1/2 cup	120	170	2.0
'Multi Grain Cheerios' (General Mills)	1 oz	100	220	1.0
'Multi-Bran Chex' (Ralston)	1 oz	90	200	1.0
'Natural Blueberry Granola' (Golden Temple)	1 oz	132	3	5.0
'Natural Blueberry Granola' coconut-free (Golden Temple)	1 oz	131	3	4.5
'Natural Bran Flakes' (Post)	1 oz	90	240	0.0
'Natural Delite Granola' (Golden Temple)	1 oz	128	26	3.5
'Natural Foods Apple Cinnamon' low fat (Golden Temple)	1 oz	110	3	1.0
'Natural Foods Raisin Almond' low fat (Golden Temple)	1 oz	110	3	1.0
'Natural Foods Strawberry/Raspberry' low fat (Golden Temple)	1 oz	111	3	1.0
'Natural' oat and wheat germ (Heartland)	1 oz	123	72	4.4
'Natural' oat and wheat germ, coconut (Heartland)	1 oz	125	58	4.6
'Natural' oat and wheat germ, raisins (Heartland)	1 oz	121	58	4.0
'Natural Raisin Bran' (Post)	1.4 oz	120	200	1.0
'Nut & Honey Crunch' (Kellogg's)	1 oz	110	200	1.0
'Nut & Honey Crunch O's' (Kellogg's)	1 oz	110	190	2.0
'Nutri-Grain' barley (Kellogg's)	1 oz	106	192	0.2
'Nutri-Grain' corn (Kellogg's)	1 oz	108	187	0.7
'Nutri-Grain' rye (Kellogg's)	1 oz	102	193	0.2
'Nutri-Grain' wheat (Kellogg's)	1 oz	102	193	0.3
'Nutri-Grain Almond Raisin' (Kellogg's)	2/3 cup	140	220	2.0
'Nutri-Grain Raisin Bran' (Kellogg's)	1 cup	130	200	1.0
'Oat Bran Almond' (Golden Temple)	1 oz	120	3	3.5
'Oat Bran Apple' (Golden Temple)	1 oz	112	3	3.5
'Oat Bran Flakes' (Arrowhead Mills)	1 oz	100	100	2.0
'Oat Bran Granola' berries (Golden Temple)	1 oz	120	3	3.5
'Oat Bran Granola' raisins and almonds (Golden Temple)	1 oz	119	3	3.5
'Oat Bran Müesli' dates and almonds (Golden Temple)	1 oz	108	79	1.5
'Oat Bran Müesli' raisins and hazelnuts (Golden Temple)	1 oz	102	59	1.5
'Oat Bran Oregonberry' (Golden Temple)	1 oz	116	3	3.5
'Oat Flakes' (Arrowhead Mills)	2 oz	220	1	4.0
'Oat Flakes' (Post)	1 oz	110	130	1.0
'Oat Mini Puffs' (Glenny's)	1 oz	108	30	<.5
'Oat Mini Puffs' w/o salt, w/o sugar (Glenny's)	1 oz	108	7	<.5
'Oatbake Honey Bran' (Kellogg's)	1 oz	110	190	3.0
'Oatbake Raisin Nut' (Kellogg's)	1 oz	110	190	3.0
'Oatmeal Crisp' (General Mills)	1 oz	110	180	2.0
'Oatmeal Crisp With Apples' (General Mills)	1 oz	110	180	1.0

Food Name	Serv. Size	Total Cal.	Sod. MGS	Fat GMS
'Oatmeal Raisin Crisp' *(General Mills)*	1/2 cup	130	170	2.0
'100% Bran' wheat bran and barley *(Nabisco)*	1 oz	76	197	1.4
'100% Natural Almond' *(Golden Temple)*	1 oz	123	15	4.0
'100% Natural Apple/Cinnamon' *(Golden Temple)*	1 oz	120	14	4.0
'100% Natural' mixed grain *(Quaker)*	1 oz	127	14	5.5
'100% Natural' mixed grain, raisins, low fat *(Quaker)*	1 oz	110	15	2.0
'100% Natural Oat Bran' *(Golden Temple)*	1 oz	70	1	2.5
'100% Natural' oats and wheat *(Quaker)*	1 oz	133	12	6.1
'100% Natural' oats and wheat, apple and cinnamon *(Quaker)*	1 oz	130	14	5.3
'100% Natural' oats and wheat, raisins, low fat *(Quaker)*	1 oz	150	80	2.0
'100% Natural' oats and wheat, raisins and dates *(Quaker)*	1 oz	128	12	5.3
'100% Natural Raisin/Almond' *(Golden Temple)*	1 oz	120	7	4.0
'100% Organic Blue Corn Flakes' *(Health Valley)*	1 oz	90	10	<1.0
'Orange Almond' nectarsweet premium *(Breadshop)*	1 oz	120	2	4.0
'Orange Almond Granola' *(Golden Temple)*	1 oz	133	25	4.0
'Oregon Blueberry Crunch' honeysweet gourmet *(Breadshop)*	1 oz	125	2	5.0
'Organic Amaranth Flakes' *(Health Valley)*	1 oz	90	10	0.0
'Original' toasted oatmeal *(Quaker)*	1 oz	100	160	1.0
'Peach Pecan Müesli' *(Ralston)*	1.45 oz	150	150	3.0
'Peaches 'N Cream' nectarsweet gourmet *(Breadshop)*	1 oz	115	2	3.0
'Post Toasties Corn Flakes' *(Post)*	1 oz	110	310	0.0
'Product 19' corn and other grains *(Kellogg's)*	1 oz	108	325	0.2
'Puffed Corn' *(Arrowhead Mills)*	.5 oz	50	1	0.0
'Puffed Kamut' *(Arrowhead Mills)*	.5 oz	40	0	0.0
'Puffed Rice' *(Arrowhead Mills)*	.5 oz	50	1	0.0
'Puffed Rice' *(Malt•O•Meal)*	.5 oz	50	0	0.0
'Puffed Wheat' *(Arrowhead Mills)*	.5 oz	50	1	0.0
'Puffed Wheat' *(Malt•O•Meal)*	.5 oz	50	0	0.0
'Quisp' corn and oat	1 oz	118	228	2.0
'Raisin Apricot-Date Granola' *(Golden Temple)*	1 oz	127	25	3.5
'Raisin Bran' *(Barbara's Bakery)*	1 oz	170	80	1.0
'Raisin Bran' *(Erewhon)*	1 oz	100	80	0.0
'Raisin Bran' *(Krusteaz)*	3/4 cup	120	210	1.0
'Raisin Bran' wheat *(Kellogg's)*	1.3 oz	115	204	0.7
'Raisin Bran' wheat *(Post)*	1 oz	87	185	0.5
'Raisin Bran' wheat *(Ralston)*	1 1/3 oz	120	328	0.2
'Raisin Bran Flakes' *(Malt•O•Meal)*	1.4 oz	130	200	2.0
'Raisin Grape-Nuts' *(Post)*	1 oz	100	140	0.0
'Raisin Squares' *(Kellogg's)*	1 oz	90	0	0.0

Food Name	Serv. Size	Total Cal.	Sod. MGS	Fot GM
'Raspberry Almond Müesli' *(Ralston)*	1.45 oz	150	140	3.
'Raspberry 'N Cream' nectarsweet gourmet *(Breadshop)*	1 oz	115	2	3.
'Rice Chex' *(Ralston)*	1 oz	112	237	0.
'Rice Krispies' *(Kellogg's)*	1 oz	112	341	0.
'Rice Krispies Treats' *(Kellogg's)*	1 oz	110	160	1.
'Rice Mini Puffs' *(Glenny's)*	1 oz	109	30	<.
'Right Start' *(Erewhon)*	1 oz	90	80	0.
'Right Start With Raisins' *(Erewhon)*	1 oz	90	80	0.
'Ripple Crisp' *(General Mills)*	1 oz	110	280	<1.
'Ripple Crisp' honey bran *(General Mills)*	1 oz	100	210	<1.
'Shredded Wheat' *(Barbara's Bakery)*	1.4 oz	140	0	1.
'Shredded Wheat' *(Nabisco)*	1 biscuit	80	0	1.
'Shredded Wheat 'n Bran' *(Nabisco)*	1 oz	90	0	0.
'Shredded Wheat With Oat Bran' *(Nabisco)*	1 oz	100	0	1.
'6-Grain Crisp' fruit and flaxseed *(Golden Temple)*	1 oz	118	73	3.
'Smacks' *(Kellogg's)*	1 oz	110	70	1.
'Smacks' wheat *(Kellogg's)*	1 oz	106	75	0.
'S'Mores Grahams' *(General Mills)*	1 oz	120	230	2.
'Smurf-Magic Berries' *(Post)*	1 oz	120	60	1.
'Special K' rice and wheat *(Kellogg's)*	1 oz	111	266	0.
'Spelt Flakes' *(Arrowhead Mills)*	1 oz	100	60	1
'Spoon Size Shredded Wheat' *(Nabisco)*	1 oz	90	0	1.
'Sprinkle Spangles' corn puffs, sprinkles *(General Mills)*	1 oz	110	130	1.
'Sprouts 7' bananas and Hawaiian fruit *(Health Valley)*	1 oz	90	0	0
'Sprouts 7' raisins, fat-free *(Health Valley)*	1 oz	90	0	0
'Startoons' cocoa *(Barbara's Bakery)*	1 cup	110	140	0.
'Startoons' honey *(Barbara's Bakery)*	1 cup	110	50	0.
'Strawberry 'N Cream' nectarsweet gourmet *(Breadshop)*	1 oz	110	5	4
'Strawberry Squares' *(Kellogg's)*	1 oz	90	5	0
'Sugar Corn Pops' *(Kellogg's)*	1 oz	108	104	0.
'Sugar Frosted Flakes' *(Krusteaz)*	1 oz	110	230	0
'Sugar Frosted Flakes' *(Malt•O•Meal)*	1 oz	110	170	0
'Sugar Puffs' *(Malt•O•Meal)*	1 oz	110	25	0
'Sunflakes Multi-Grain' *(Ralston)*	1 oz	100	240	1
'Super Nutty Granola' *(Golden Temple)*	1 oz	135	25	5.
'Super O's' *(Erewhon)*	1 oz	110	5	0
'Super Sugar Crisp' wheat *(Post)*	1 oz	106	25	0
'Supernatural' honeysweet gourmet *(Breadshop)*	1 oz	100	2	5
'Supernatural New England' honeysweet gourmet *(Breadshop)*	1 oz	130	2	5
'Sweet Home Farm Almond' *(Golden Temple)*	1 oz	123	14	4

Food Name	Serv. Size	Total Cal.	Sod. MGS	Fat GMS
'Sweet Home Farm Crunchy Müesli' low fat *(Golden Temple)*	1 oz	105	98	2.0
'Sweet Home Farm Granola' low fat *(Golden Temple)*	1 oz	110	65	2.0
'Sweet Home Farm Raisin' *(Golden Temple)*	1 oz	120	13	4.0
'Sweetened Puffed Wheat' *(Malt•O•Meal)*	1 oz	110	25	0.0
'Swiss Style Müesli' *(Golden Temple)*	1 oz	105	15	1.5
'Tasteeos' oat and other grains	1 oz	112	216	0.8
'Team' rice and other grains *(Nabisco)*	1 oz	111	176	0.5
'Team Flakes' *(Nabisco)*	1 oz	110	180	1.0
'Teenage Mutant Ninja Turtles' *(Ralston)*	1 oz	110	190	0.0
'35% Fruit Müesli' *(Golden Temple)*	1 oz	97	16	1.0
'Toasted Oat' 100%natural *(Nature Valley)*	1 oz	130	50	5.0
'Toasted Oats' *(Krusteaz)*	1 oz	110	290	1.0
'Toasted Oats' *(Malt•O•Meal)*	1 oz	110	240	2.0
'Toasties' corn *(Post)*	1 oz	110	298	0.1
'Tootie Fruities' *(Malt•O•Meal)*	1 oz	110	120	1.0
'Total Corn Flakes' *(General Mills)*	1 oz	110	200	1.0
'Total Raisin Bran' *(General Mills)*	1.5 oz	140	190	1.0
'Total' wheat *(General Mills)*	1 oz	100	281	0.6
'Triples' *(General Mills)*	1 oz	110	200	1.0
'Triples' breakfast pack *(General Mills)*	1 oz	110	190	1.0
'Trix' corn and other grains *(General Mills)*	1 oz	109	181	0.4
'Uncle Sam' *(US Mills)*	1 oz	110	65	1.0
'Urkel-O's' *(Ralston)*	1 oz	110	160	1.0
'Waffelos' wheat and other grains	1 oz	115	118	1.2
'Wheat Chex' *(Ralston)*	1 oz	104	190	0.7
'Wheat Flakes' *(Erewhon)*	1 oz	110	75	0.0
'Wheat 'n Raisin Chex' *(Ralston)*	1 1/3 oz	130	214	0.3
'Wheaties' *(General Mills)*	1 oz	99	270	0.5
'Wheaties Honey Gold' *(General Mills)*	1 oz	100	200	1.0
'Whole-Grain Shredded Wheat' *(Kellogg's)*	1 oz	90	0	0.0
'Whole-Grain Wheat Chex' *(Ralston)*	1 oz	100	230	1.0
CEREAL SNACK. See also GRANOLA AND CEREAL BAR; GRANOLA SNACK.				
'Cheerios-to-Go' *(General Mills)*	1 pouch	80	220	2.0
'Cheerios-to-Go' apple cinnamon *(General Mills)*	1 pouch	110	180	2.0
'Cheerios-to-Go' honey nut *(General Mills)*	1 pouch	110	250	1.0
'Fingos' cinnamon *(General Mills)*	1 oz	110	170	3.0
'Fingos' honey toasted oat *(General Mills)*	1 oz	110	210	3.0
CHARD. See SWISS CHARD.				
CHAYOTE				
boiled, drained	4 oz	27	1	0.5
boiled, drained, 1-inch pieces	1/2 cup	19	1	0.4

Food Name	Serv. Size	Total Cal.	Sod. MGS	Fat GMS
raw, approx 7.2 oz	1 med	49	8	0.6
raw, 1-inch pieces	1/2 cup	16	3	0.2
raw, trimmed	1 oz	7	1	0.1
raw, untrimmed	1 lb	108	18	1.4
CHEDDARWURST				
'Bun Size' *(Hillshire Farm)*	2 oz	200	480	18.0
'Links' *(Hillshire Farm)*	2 oz	190	480	17.0

CHEESE. See also CHEESE, ALTERNATIVE; CHEESE BALL; CHEESE FOOD; CHEESE LOG; CHEESE NUGGET; CHEESE NUT; CHEESE PRODUCT; CHEESE SPREAD; CHEESE STICK.

AMERICAN

Food Name	Serv. Size	Total Cal.	Sod. MGS	Fat GMS
(Borden) fat-free, low-cholesterol	1 oz	40	380	0.0
(Borden) 'Light'	1 oz	70	420	4.0
(Borden) 'Loaf'	1 oz	110	40	9.0
(Borden) 'Slices'	1 oz	110	40	9.0
(Borden) slices 'Premium'	1 oz	110	460	9.0
(Dorman's)	1 oz	110	440	9.0
(Dorman's) 'Loaf Low Sodium'	1 oz	110	140	9.0
(Healthy Favorites)	2/3 oz	45	260	2.0
(Hoffman's)	1 oz	110	400	9.0
(Kraft) 'Deluxe Loaf'	1 oz	110	430	9.0
(Kraft) 'Deluxe Slices'	1 oz	110	450	9.0
(Land O'Lakes)	1 oz	110	405	9.0
(Land O'Lakes) sharp	1 oz	100	360	9.0
(Old English) sharp 'Loaf'	1 oz	110	400	9.0
(Old English) sharp 'Slices'	1 oz	110	440	9.0
(Sargento) hot pepper	1 oz	110	410	9.0
ASIAGO *(Frigo)* wheel	1 oz	110	400	9.0
BABYBEL				
(Laughing Cow)	1 oz	91	227	7.0
(Laughing Cow) mini	3/4 oz	74	170	6.0
BLUE				
crumbled, not packed	1 cup	477	1884	38.8
(Dorman's) 'Castello 70%'	1 oz	134	286	12.3
(Dorman's) 'Danablu 60%'	1 oz	108	200	9.7
(Dorman's) 'Danablu 50%'	1 oz	100	200	8.2
(Dorman's) 'Saga 70%'	1 oz	134	286	12.3
(Frigo)	1 oz	100	400	8.0
(Hickory Farms) 'Domestic'	1 oz	101	396	8.3
(Kraft)	1 oz	100	330	9.0
(Sargento)	1 oz	100	400	8.0

Food Name	Serv. Size	Total Cal.	Sod. MGS	Fat GMS
BONBEL				
(Laughing Cow)	1 oz	100	227	8.0
(Laughing Cow) mini, 3/4 oz	1 oz	74	170	6.0
BONBINO (Laughing Cow)	1 oz	103	227	9.0
BRICK				
(Dorman's)	1 oz	110	180	8.0
(Kraft)	1 oz	110	180	9.0
(Land O'Lakes)	1 oz	110	160	8.0
BRIE				
(Dorman's)	1 oz	81	229	6.6
(Sargento)	1 oz	100	180	8.0
BURGER (Sargento)	1 oz	110	410	9.0
BUTTERNIP (Hickory Farms)	1 oz	110	82	9.4
CAJUN (Sargento)	1 oz	110	165	9.0
CALJACK (Churny)	1 oz	100	(mq)	8.0
CAMEMBERT				
domestic	1 oz	84	236	6.8
(Dorman's) '50%'	1 oz	89	285	7.3
(Dorman's) '45%'	1 oz	82	226	6.3
(Hickory Farms)	1 oz	90	239	7.0
(Sargento)	1 oz	90	240	7.0
CARAWAY	1 oz	105	193	8.2
CHEDDAR				
American domestic	1 oz	113	174	9.3
American domestic, shredded, not packed	1 cup	455	701	37.5
(Alpine Lace) 'Cheddar Flavored'	1 oz	100	95	8.0
(Alpine Lace) shredded 'Ched-R-Lo' milk cheese	1 oz	80	95	5.0
(Alta•Dena) mild	1 oz	110	200	9.0
(Alta•Dena) sharp	1 oz	110	200	9.0
(Axelrod) extra sharp	1 oz	110	200	9.0
(Boar's Head) sliced	1 oz	110	100	9.0
(Darigold)	1 oz	110	170	9.0
(Dorman's)	1 oz	110	200	9.0
(Dorman's) 'Chedda-Delite'	1 oz	90	100	7.0
(Dorman's) reduced fat 'Low Sodium'	1 oz	80	100	5.0
(Dorman's) w/Monterey Jack 'Chedda-Jack'	1 oz	90	100	7.0
(Featherweight) 'Low Sodium'	1 oz	110	5	9.0
(Frigo)	1 oz	110	200	9.0
(Golden Balance) mild, shredded 'Natural Shreds'	1 oz	90	150	6.0
(Golden Balance) sharp, shredded 'Natural Shreds'	1 oz	90	130	6.0
(Healthy Choice) shredded, fat-free	1 oz	40	200	0.0

Food Name	Serv. Size	Total Cal.	Sod. MGS	Fat GMS
(Healthy Favorites) mild, fancy shredded	1 oz	70	220	4.0
(Hickory Farms)	1 oz	110	176	9.0
(Hickory Farms) raw milk 'Light Choice Low Sodium'	1 oz	114	100	8.0
(Hoffman's) super sharp processed	1 oz	110	390	8.0
(Kraft)	1 oz	110	180	9.0
(Kraft) mild, finely shredded 'Light Naturals'	1 oz	80	220	5.0
(Kraft) mild, reduced fat 'Light Naturals'	1 oz	80	220	5.0
(Kraft) mild, shredded 'Light Naturals'	1 oz	80	220	5.0
(Kraft) sharp, shredded 'Light Naturals'	1 oz	80	220	5.0
(Land O'Lakes)	1 oz	110	175	9.0
(Land O'Lakes) 'Chedarella'	1 oz	100	180	8.0
(Laughing Cow)	1 oz	110	227	9.0
(Sargento)	1 oz	110	176	9.0
(Sargento) mild, fancy shredded 'Preferred Light'	1 oz	90	210	5.0
(Sargento) 'New York'	1 oz	110	180	9.0
(Weight Watchers) mild, 'Natural'	1 oz	80	150	5.0
(Weight Watchers) mild, 'Natural Low Sodium'	1 oz	80	70	5.0
(Weight Watchers) mild, shredded 'Natural'	1 oz	80	150	5.0
CHESHIRE	1 oz	108	196	8.6
CHUTTER *(Hickory Farms)* 'Cold Pack'	1 oz	87	213	5.8
COLBY				
(Alpine Lace) 'Colby-Lo'	1 oz	80	85	5.0
(Dorman's)	1 oz	110	190	9.0
(Hickory Farms) 'Light Choice Low Sodium'	1 oz	100	4	6.0
(Hickory Farms) 'Longhorn'	1 oz	112	171	8.6
(Hickory Farms) lowfat, calcium-enriched 'Light Choice'	1 oz	100	180	8.0
(Kraft)	1 oz	110	180	9.0
(Kraft) reduced fat 'Light Naturals'	1 oz	80	220	5.0
(Kraft) w/Monterey Jack, reduced fat 'Light Naturals'	1 oz	80	220	.0
(Land O'Lakes)	1 oz	110	170	9.0
(Sargento)	1 oz	110	170	9.0
(Sargento) Jack	1 oz	110	160	9.0
(Weight Watchers) 'Natural'	1 oz	80	130	5.0
COTTAGE CHEESE				
Creamed				
large curd	4 oz	117	457	5.1
large curd, not packed	1 cup	217	850	9.5
lowfat 1%	1 oz	20	115	0.3
lowfat 2%	1 oz	25	115	0.5
small curd	4 oz	117	457	5.1
small curd, not packed	1 cup	217	850	9.5

Food Name	Serv. Size	Total Cal.	Sod. MGS	Fat GMS
(Bison) chive	1/2 cup	120	420	5.0
(Bison) 4% fat	1/2 cup	120	420	5.0
(Bison) garden salad	1/2 cup	110	420	4.0
(Bison) lowfat 1%	1/2 cup	90	350	2.0
(Bison) w/pineapple	1/2 cup	140	340	4.0
(Borden) 4% fat	1/2 cup	120	400	5.0
(Borden) 4% fat, unsalted	1/2 cup	120	40	5.0
(Breakstone's)	4 oz	110	370	5.0
(Breakstone's) lowfat 2%	4 oz	100	510	2.0
(Carnation) 4% fat, large curd	1/2 cup	115	440	5.0
(Carnation) 4% fat, small curd	1/2 cup	115	440	5.0
(Carnation) 4% fat, w/pineapple	1/2 cup	130	430	5.0
(Crowley) 4% fat	1/2 cup	120	390	5.0
(Crowley) 4% fat, w/peaches	1/2 cup	140	340	3.0
(Crowley) 4% fat, w/pineapple	1/2 cup	140	330	4.0
(Crowley) lowfat 1%	1/2 cup	90	390	1.0
(Crowley) lowfat 1%, calcium-fortified	1/2 cup	90	390	1.0
(Crowley) lowfat 1% 'No Salt Added'	1/2 cup	90	50	1.0
(Crowley) lowfat 1%, w/pineapple	1/2 cup	110	330	1.0
(Darigold) 4% fat	4 oz	120	510	4.2
(Darigold) lowfat 2% 'Trim'	4 oz	100	510	3.2
(Friendship) 'California Style 4%'	1/2 cup	120	380	5.0
(Friendship) 4% fat, w/pineapple	1/2 cup	140	300	4.0
(Friendship) lowfat 1%	1/2 cup	90	350	1.0
(Friendship) lowfat 1%, lactose-reduced	1/2 cup	90	350	1.0
(Friendship) lowfat 1% 'No Salt Added'	1/2 cup	90	31	1.0
(Friendship) lowfat 1%, w/pineapple	1/2 cup	110	300	1.0
(Friendship) lowfat 2%, pot style, large curd	1/2 cup	100	405	2.0
(Knudsen) 4% fat, large curd	4 oz	120	340	5.0
(Knudsen) 4% fat, small curd	4 oz	120	370	5.0
(Knudsen) 4% fat, w/pineapple	4 oz	140	260	5.0
(Lite-Line) lowfat 1.5%	1/2 cup	90	400	2.0
(Weight Watchers) lowfat 1%	1/2 cup	90	460	1.0
(Weight Watchers) lowfat 2%	1/2 cup	100	460	2.0
Lowfat				
1%, not packed	1 cup	164	918	2.3
2%, not packed	1 cup	203	918	4.4
(Carnation) 1.5% 'Slender'	1/2 cup	90	440	2.0
(Knudsen) 2%	4 oz	100	370	2.0
(Knudsen) 2%, w/fruit cocktail	4 oz	130	330	2.0
(Knudsen) 2%, w/Mandarin orange	4 oz	110	320	2.0

Food Name	Serv. Size	Total Cal.	Sod. MGS	Fat GMS
(Knudsen) 2%, w/peach	6 oz	170	270	2.0
(Knudsen) 2%, w/pear	4 oz	110	320	2.0
(Knudsen) 2%, w/pineapple	6 oz	170	300	2.0
(Knudsen) 2%, w/spiced apple	6 oz	180	280	2.0
(Knudsen) 2%, w/strawberry	6 oz	170	320	2.0
(Light n' Lively) 1%	4 oz	80	370	2.0
(Light n' Lively) 1%, garden salad	4 oz	80	350	2.0
(Sealtest) 2%	4 oz	100	340	2.0
Nonfat				
(Knudsen)	4 oz	70	420	0.0
(Light n' Lively)	4 oz	90	400	0.0
Uncreamed				
dry, large curd	4 oz	96	14	0.5
dry, large curd, not packed	1 cup	123	19	0.6
dry, small curd	4 oz	96	14	0.5
dry, small curd, not packed	1 cup	123	19	0.6
dry curd, unsalted *(Borden)*	1/2 cup	80	20	1.0
dry curd, unsalted *(Darigold)*	4 oz	80	15	1.0
dry curd, unsalted, nonfat *(Breakstone's)*	4 oz	90	65	0.0
CREAM CHEESE				
natural	1 oz	98	83	9.8
(Alta•Dena) pasteurized	1 oz	100	110	10.0
(Crowley)	1 oz	110	100	9.0
(Darigold)	1 oz	99	84	9.9
(Dorman's) '70%'	1 oz	102	200	9.9
(Dorman's) '65%'	1 oz	90	200	8.4
(Healthy Choice) fat-free	1 oz	30	200	0.0
(Healthy Choice) herb and garlic, fat-free	1 oz	30	200	0.0
(Healthy Favorites)	1 oz	60	110	5.0
(Philadelphia Brand)	1 oz	100	90	10.0
(Philadelphia Brand) 'Free'	1 oz	25	170	0.0
(Philadelphia Brand) pasteurized process 'Light'	1 oz	60	160	5.0
(Philadelphia Brand) w/chives	1 oz	90	125	9.0
(Philadelphia Brand) w/olive and pimento, fat-free	1 oz	90	160	8.0
(Philadelphia Brand) w/pimento	1 oz	90	150	9.0
Soft				
(Friendship)	1 oz	103	70	10.0
(Philadelphia Brand)	1 oz	100	100	10.0
(Philadelphia Brand) w/chives and onion	1 oz	100	100	9.0
(Philadelphia Brand) w/herb and garlic	1 oz	100	160	9.0
(Philadelphia Brand) w/olives and pimento	1 oz	90	160	8.0

ood Name	Serv. Size	Total Cal.	Sod. MGS	Fat GMS
(Philadelphia Brand) w/pineapple	1 oz	90	90	8.0
(Philadelphia Brand) w/smoked salmon	1 oz	90	180	9.0
(Philadelphia Brand) w/strawberries	1 oz	90	75	8.0
Whipped				
(Philadelphia Brand)	1 oz	100	85	10.0
(Philadelphia Brand) w/chives	1 oz	90	150	8.0
(Philadelphia Brand) w/onions	1 oz	90	170	8.0
(Philadelphia Brand) w/smoked salmon	1 oz	90	170	8.0
(Temp-Tee)	1 oz	100	85	10.0
ANBO				
(Dorman's) 20%	1 oz	62	200	2.8
(Dorman's) 45%	1 oz	98	200	7.5
DAM				
(Dorman's)	1 oz	100	200	8.0
(Dorman's) 45%	1 oz	91	200	7.0
(Hickory Farms) 'Domestic'	1 oz	100	182	8.4
(Kaukauna)	1 oz	100	275	8.0
(Kraft)	1 oz	90	310	7.0
(Land O'Lakes)	1 oz	100	275	8.0
(Laughing Cow)	1 oz	100	227	8.0
(May-Bud)	1 oz	100	275	8.0
(Sargento)	1 oz	100	270	8.0
FORT, sheep's milk	1 oz	314	1538	26.0
ARMER				
(Friendship)	1/2 cup	160	356	12.0
(Friendship) 'No Salt Added'	1/2 cup	160	8	12.0
(Hickory Farms)	1 oz	90	210	7.0
(Hickory Farms) 'Light Choice'	1 oz	90	150	7.0
(Kaukauna)	1 oz	100	(mq)	8.0
(May-Bud)	1 oz	90	210	7.0
(Sargento)	1 oz	100	130	8.0
ETA				
sheep's milk	1 oz	75	316	6.0
(Churny) 'Natural'	1 oz	75	316	6.5
(Dorman's) 45%	1 oz	91	(mq)	7.3
(Sargento)	1 oz	80	320	6.0
ONTINA (Sargento)	1 oz	110	(mq)	9.0
RENCH ONION (Alouette)	1 oz	95	205	9.0
JETOST				
goat's milk, fresh	1 oz	82	180	6.8
(Sargento)	1 oz	130	170	8.0

Food Name	Serv. Size	Total Cal.	Sod. MGS	Fat GMS
GOAT				
hard type	1 oz	128	98	10.1
semisoft type	1 oz	103	146	8.5
soft type	1 oz	76	104	6.0
GOUDA				
(Dorman's)	1 oz	100	210	8.0
(Kaukauna)	1 oz	100	230	8.0
(Kaukauna) w/caraway seed	1 oz	100	230	8.0
(Kaukauna) w/hickory smoke flavor	1 oz	100	230	8.0
(Kraft)	1 oz	110	200	9.0
(Land O'Lakes)	1 oz	100	230	8.0
(Laughing Cow)	1 oz	110	227	9.0
(Laughing Cow) mini	3/4 oz	80	170	6.4
(May-Bud)	1 oz	100	230	8.0
(Sargento)	1 oz	100	230	8.0
GRATED. See also PARMESAN; ROMANO.				
(Polly-O)	1 oz	130	530	10.0
(Sargento) Italian style	1 oz	110	105	8.0
GRUYERE	1 oz	116	94	9.1
HAVARTI				
(Casino)	1 oz	120	140	11.0
(Dorman's) 45%	1 oz	91	200	7.0
(Dorman's) 60%	1 oz	118	200	10.8
(Hickory Farms) 'Danish Special'	1 oz	117	198	10.5
(Sargento)	1 oz	120	200	11.0
HORSERADISH (Kaukauna) hearty, cold pack 'Cup'	1 oz	100	250	7.0
HOT PEPPER (Hickory Farms)	1 oz	106	406	8.9
JARLSBERG				
(Hickory Farms)	1 oz	100	130	7.0
(Norseland)	1 oz	97	135	7.0
LIMBURGER				
(Mohawk Valley) 'Little Gem'	1 oz	90	250	8.0
(Sargento)	1 oz	90	230	8.0
MASCARPONE 'Imported' (Galbani)	1 oz	128	17	13.1
MONTEREY	1 oz	105	150	8.5
MONTEREY JACK				
(Alpine Lace) 'Monti-Jack-Lo'	1 oz	80	75	5.0
(Alpine Lace) 'Monti-Jack-Lo' sliced	1 oz	80	75	5.0
(Alta•Dena)	1 oz	100	180	8.0
(Alta•Dena) w/jalapeño pepper	1 oz	100	180	8.0
(Axelrod)	1 oz	100	150	8.0

Food Name	Serv. Size	Total Cal.	Sod. MGS	Fat GMS
(Axelrod) w/jalapeño pepper	1 oz	100	220	8.0
(Darigold)	1 oz	110	150	8.0
(Dorman's)	1 oz	100	180	8.0
(Dorman's) reduced fat 'Low Sodium'	1 oz	80	90	5.0
(Hickory Farms) 'Light Choice Low Sodium'	1 oz	110	100	8.0
(Kaukauna)	1 oz	110	150	9.0
(Kraft)	1 oz	110	190	9.0
(Kraft) reduced fat 'Light Naturals'	1 oz	80	220	5.0
(Kraft) reduced fat 'Light Naturals' w/peppers	1 oz	80	220	5.0
(Kraft) 'Singles'	1 oz	90	390	7.0
(Kraft) w/caraway	1 oz	100	180	8.0
(Kraft) w/jalapeño pepper	1 oz	110	190	9.0
(Land O'Lakes)	1 oz	110	150	9.0
(Land O'Lakes) hot pepper	1 oz	110	150	9.0
(Land O'Lakes) processed 'Jalapeño Jack'	1 oz	90	430	8.0
(May-Bud)	1 oz	110	150	9.0
(Sargento)	1 oz	110	150	9.0
(Weight Watchers) 'Natural'	1 oz	80	120	5.0
MOZZARELLA. See also CHEESE NUGGET.				
(Dorman's)	1 oz	90	190	6.0
(Healthy Choice) fat-free, chunk	1 oz	40	200	0.0
(Hickory Farms)	1 oz	72	132	4.5
(Hickory Farms) 'Light Choice Low Sodium'	1 oz	80	90	5.0
(Kraft)	1 oz	90	190	7.0
(Polly-O) 'Fior di Latte'	1 oz	80	20	6.0
(Polly-O) 'Lite'	1 oz	70	200	4.0
(Weight Watchers) 'Natural'	1 oz	70	150	4.0
Part skim milk				
(Alpine Lace) low moisture	1 oz	70	75	5.0
(Crowley)	1 oz	70	240	4.0
(Dorman's) low moisture 'Low Sodium'	1 oz	80	90	5.0
(Frigo) low moisture	1 oz	80	190	5.0
(Frigo) low moisture, reduced fat	1 oz	60	150	3.0
(Kraft) low moisture	1 oz	80	200	5.0
(Kraft) w/jalapeño pepper	1 oz	80	230	5.0
(Land O'Lakes) low moisture	1 oz	80	150	5.0
(Polly-O)	1 oz	80	280	5.0
(Sargento) low moisture	1 oz	80	150	5.0
Reduced fat				
(Dorman's) 'Low Sodium'	1 oz	80	90	4.0
(Kraft) 'Light Naturals'	1 oz	80	200	4.0

Food Name	Serv. Size	Total Cal.	Sod. MGS	Fat GMS
Shredded				
(Alpine Lace)	1 oz	70	75	5.0
(Alpine Lace) sliced	1 oz	70	75	5.0
(Healthy Choice) fat-free	1 oz	40	200	0.0
(Kraft) 'Light Naturals'	1 oz	80	150	4.0
(Sargento) fancy 'Preferred Light'	1 oz	60	150	3.0
(Weight Watchers) 'Natural'	1 oz	80	150	4.0
Whole milk				
(Crowley)	1 oz	90	240	7.0
(Frigo) low moisture	1 oz	90	190	7.0
(Sargento)	1 oz	90	120	7.0
(Polly-O)	1 oz	90	280	6.0
MOZZARELLA CHEDDAR				
(Precious) shredded 'Pizza Cheese'	1 oz	95	180	7.0
MUENSTER				
(Alpine Lace)	1 oz	100	85	8.0
(Alpine Lace) sliced 'Low Sodium'	1 oz	100	85	9.0
(Dorman's)	1 oz	110	190	9.0
(Dorman's) 50%	1 oz	100	200	8.2
(Dorman's) 'Low Sodium'	1 oz	110	95	9.0
(Dorman's) reduced fat 'Low Sodium'	1 oz	80	140	5.0
(Hickory Farms)	1 oz	100	180	8.5
(Hickory Farms) 'Light Choice Low Sodium'	1 oz	110	95	9.0
(Kaukauna)	1 oz	110	180	9.0
(Land O'Lakes)	1 oz	100	180	9.0
(Sargento) red rind	1 oz	100	180	9.0
NEUFCHATEL				
(Hickory Farms) chocolate	1 oz	110	90	8.0
(Hickory Farms) orange	1 oz	100	75	8.0
(Hickory Farms) peach	1 oz	90	85	8.0
(Hickory Farms) pineapple	1 oz	90	60	8.0
(Hickory Farms) rum date nut	1 oz	100	80	8.0
(Hickory Farms) strawberry	1 oz	90	70	8.0
(Kaukauna) garden vegetable	1 oz	80	200	7.0
(Kaukauna) garlic and herbs	1 oz	80	150	7.0
(Philadelphia Brand) 'Light'	1 oz	80	115	7.0
NEW HOLLAND (Hickory Farms) w/herbs 'Light Choice'	1 oz	90	100	8.0
PARMESAN				
natural, piece	1 oz	110	448	7.2
natural, shredded	1 oz	116	475	7.7
natural, shredded	1 tbsp	21	85	1.4

Food Name	Serv. Size	Total Cal.	Sod. MGS	Fat GMS
(Churny) 'Natural'	1 oz	110	455	7.0
(Hickory Farms)	1 oz	110	350	7.0
(Kraft)	1 oz	100	290	7.0
(Sargento) fresh	1 oz	110	450	7.0
Grated				
natural	1 oz	128	521	8.4
natural	1 tbsp	23	93	1.5
(Frigo)	1 oz	130	510	9.0
(Frigo) fresh	1 oz	110	350	7.0
(Kraft)	1 oz	130	430	9.0
(Polly-O)	1 oz	130	530	9.0
(Progresso)	1 tbsp	23	95	2.0
(Sargento)	1 oz	130	530	9.0
Hard	1 oz	111	454	7.3
Wheel *(Frigo)*	1 oz	110	350	7.0
W/Romano cheese, grated				
(Frigo)	1 oz	130	510	9.0
(Sargento)	1 oz	110	400	7.0
PARMESAN REGGIANO *(Galbani)* 'Imported'	1 oz	105	188	7.1
PIZZA				
(Frigo) shredded	1 oz	90	190	7.0
(Frigo) shredded, lowfat	1 oz	65	150	3.0
(Healthy Choice) fancy, shredded, fat-free	1 oz	40	200	0.0
PORT DU SALUT	1 oz	98	150	7.9
PORT WINE *(Hickory Farms)*	1 oz	97	262	6.9
POT *(Sargento)*	1 oz	25	1	0.2
PRIMAVERA *(Bel Paese)* 'Lite'	1 oz	68	165	4.0
PROVOLONE				
(Alpine Lace) 'Provo-Lo'	1 oz	70	85	5.0
(Dorman's)	1 oz	90	290	7.0
(Frigo)	1 oz	100	230	7.0
(Frigo) smoked	1 oz	100	230	7.0
(Hickory Farms) 'Light Choice Low Sodium'	1 oz	90	140	7.0
(Kraft)	1 oz	100	260	7.0
(Land O'Lakes)	1 oz	100	250	8.0
(Sargento)	1 oz	100	250	8.0
PUB *(Hickory Farms)*	1 oz	94	237	6.9
QUESO BLANCO *(Sargento)*	1 oz	100	180	9.0
QUESO DE PAPA *(Sargento)*	1 oz	110	180	9.0
QUESO DE TACO *(Hickory Farms)*	1 oz	106	450	8.9

Food Name	Serv. Size	Total Cal.	Sod. MGS	Fat GMS
RICOTTA				
Light/lowfat				
(Gardenia) '95% Fat-free'	1 oz	30	130	1.0
(Polly-O) 'Lite'	2 oz	80	65	4.0
(Precious) 'Lowfat'	1 oz	40	20	2.0
(Sargento) 'Lite'	1 oz	23	20	1.0
Part skim milk				
(Crowley)	2 oz	80	50	4.0
(Frigo)	1 oz	45	100	3.0
(Frigo) 'Truly Lite' fat-free	1 oz	20	15	0.0
(Polly-O)	2 oz	90	45	6.0
(Sargento)	1 oz	30	30	2.0
Whole milk				
(Breakstone's)	4 oz	200	95	15.0
(Crowley)	2 oz	100	50	7.0
(Frigo)	1 oz	50	100	4.0
(Polly-O)	2 oz	100	45	7.0
ROMANO				
Grated				
(Frigo)	1 oz	130	510	9.0
(Kraft)	1 oz	130	350	9.0
(Kraft) 'Natural'	1 oz	100	250	7.0
(Polly-O)	1 oz	130	530	10.0
(Progresso)	1 tbsp	23	70	2.0
(Sargento)	1 oz	110	340	8.0
Loaf (Hickory Farms)	1 oz	110	350	8.0
Wedge (Frigo)	1 oz	110	350	8.0
ROQUEFORT				
	1 oz	103	507	8.6
sheep's milk	1 oz	105	513	8.7
SLIM JACK (Dorman's)	1 oz	90	90	7.0
SMOKED				
(Hickory Farms) 'Light Choice Smoky Lyte'	1 oz	80	449	6.0
(Hoffman's) sharp, processed	1 oz	110	440	9.0
(Sargento) 'Smokestick'	1 oz	100	390	7.0
STRING				
(Frigo)	1 oz	80	190	5.0
(Kraft) low moisture	1 oz	80	230	5.0
(Polly-O)	1 oz	90	200	6.0
(Sargento)	1 oz	80	150	5.0
(Sargento) smoked	1 oz	80	150	5.0

Food Name	Serv. Size	Total Cal.	Sod. MGS	Fat GMS
SWISS				
domestic	1 oz	105	73	7.7
domestic	1-inch cube	56	39	4.1
(Boar's Head) 'Domestic'	1 oz	110	75	8.0
(Boar's Head) 'No Salt Added'	1 oz	100	12	8.0
(Casino)	1 oz	110	35	8.0
(Cracker Barrel) baby 'Natural'	1 oz	110	65	9.0
(Dorman's)	1 oz	100	80	8.0
(Dorman's) 'No Salt Added'	1 oz	100	8	8.0
(Hickory Farms) creamy 'Cold Pack'	1 oz	92	237	7.2
(Hickory Farms) 'Domestic'	1 oz	110	75	7.8
(Hickory Farms) 'Light Choice Lorraine'	1 oz	100	35	7.8
(Hickory Farms) 'Light Choice Low Sodium'	1 oz	100	8	8.0
(Kraft)	1 oz	110	40	8.0
(Kraft) aged	1 oz	110	45	8.0
(Kraft) 'Light Naturals'	1 oz	90	45	5.0
(Land O'Lakes)	1 oz	110	75	8.0
(Sargento) 'Finland'	1 oz	110	75	8.0
(Weight Watchers) 'Natural'	1 oz	90	50	5.0
Processed				
(Alpine Lace) sliced, milk cheese 'Swiss-Lo'	1 oz	90	35	6.0
(Alpine Lace) 'Swiss-Lo'	1 oz	100	35	7.0
(Borden)	1 oz	100	380	8.0
(Borden) fat-free, low-cholesterol	1 oz	40	na	0.0
(Dorman's) 'Reduced Fat'	1 oz	90	80	5.0
(Dorman's) smoked	1 oz	100	390	7.0
(Healthy Favorites) sliced, reduced fat	1 oz	80	70	4.0
(Hoffman's) smoky, w/cheddar	1 oz	110	410	8.0
(Kraft) 'Deluxe'	1 oz	90	420	7.0
(Kraft) 'Light'	1 oz	70	350	3.0
(Kraft) reduced fat 'Light Naturals'	1 oz	90	70	5.0
(Kraft) %75% Very Low Sodium'	1 oz	110	10	8.0
(Sargento)	1 oz	110	75	8.0
TACO				
(Frigo) shredded	1 oz	110	200	9.0
(Kraft) shredded	1 oz	110	190	9.0
(Sargento)	1 oz	110	160	9.0
TALEGGIO (Tal-Fino) 'Brand Imported'	1 oz	89	176	7.4
TILSIT				
whole milk	1 oz	95	211	7.3
(Sargento)	1 oz	100	210	7.0

Food Name	Serv. Size	Total Cal.	Sod. MGS	Fat GMS
TYBO				
(Dorman's) 45%	1 oz	98	200	7.5
(Sargento) red wax	1 oz	100	200	7.0
VERMONT *(Churny)*	1 oz	110	180	9.0
CHEESE, ALTERNATIVE				
(Cheeztwin)	1 oz	90	400	6.0
American cheddar style *(Soya Kaas)*	1 oz	79	250	5.4
American style *(Delicia)*	1 oz	80	300	6.0
American style *(Golden Image)*	1 oz	90	360	6.0
American style, hickory smoked *(Delicia)*	1 oz	80	470	6.0
American style, lactose-free, singles *(Formägg)*	3/4 oz	70	280	5.0
American style, 'Low Sodium Slices' *(Weight Watchers)*	1 oz	50	120	2.0
American style, 'Slices' *(Weight Watchers)*	1 oz	50	400	2.0
American style, w/caraway *(Delicia)*	1 oz	80	275	6.0
American style, w/hot pepper *(Delicia)*	1 oz	80	300	6.0
American style, w/salami *(Delicia)*	1 oz	80	370	6.0
California cheddar style 'AlmondRella' *(Sharon's Finest)*	1 oz	50	170	1.4
California cheddar style 'Zero-Fat Rella' *(Sharon's Finest)*	1 oz	45	170	0.0
cheddar style *(Frigo)*	1 oz	90	280	7.0
cheddar style *(Sargento)*	1 oz	90	350	6.0
cheddar style, fancy shredded *(Formägg)*	1 oz	70	70	5.0
cheddar style, shredded 'Ched-O-Mate' *(Fisher)*	1 oz	90	330	7.0
colby style *(Golden Image)*	1 oz	110	190	9.0
colby style 'LoChol' *(Dorman's)*	1 oz	90	140	5.0
colby style, Longhorn style *(Delicia)*	1 oz	80	550	6.0
cream cheese style *(Soya Kaas)*	1 oz	90	60	9.4
cream cheese style *(Weight Watchers)*	1 oz	35	40	2.0
cream cheese style, all flavors 'Better than Cream Cheese' *(Tofutti)*	1 oz	80	200	8.0
garlic-herb style 'AlmondRella' *(Sharon's Finest)*	1 oz	50	170	1.4
'Heart Beat' *(Nucoa)*	1 oz	50	280	2.0
jalapeño jack style 'Zero-Fat Rella' *(Sharon's Finest)*	1 oz	45	170	0.0
'Jalapeño Mexi Kaas' *(Soya Kaas)*	1 oz	77	160	5.3
'Low Cholesterol' *(Lite-Line)*	1 oz	90	430	7.0
mild cheddar style *(Golden Image)*	1 oz	110	190	9.0
mild cheddar style 'TofuRella' *(Sharon's Finest)*	1 oz	80	170	5.0
mild cheddar style 'TofuRella' slices *(Sharon's Finest)*	3/4 oz	60	280	4.0
mozzarella style *(Frigo)*	1 oz	90	240	7.0
mozzarella style *(Sargento)*	1 oz	80	310	6.0
mozzarella style *(Soya Kaas)*	1 oz	78	155	5.6
mozzarella style 'AlmondRella' *(Sharon's Finest)*	1 oz	50	170	1.4

Food Name	Serv. Size	Total Cal.	Sod. MGS	Fat GMS
mozzarella style, shredded 'Pizza-Mate' (Fisher)	1 oz	90	310	7.0
mozzarella style 'TofuRella' (Sharon's Finest)	1 oz	80	170	5.0
mozzarella style 'TofuRella' slices (Sharon's Finest)	3/4 oz	60	280	4.0
mozzarella style 'Zero-Fat Rella' (Sharon's Finest)	1 oz	45	170	0.0
Muenster style 'LoChol' (Dorman's)	1 oz	100	140	7.0
'Sandwich-Mate' (Fisher)	1 oz	90	400	6.0
sharp cheddar style 'Slices' (Weight Watchers)	1 oz	50	400	2.0
Swiss style, lactose-free, singles (Formägg)	3/4 oz	70	280	5.0
Swiss style 'LoChol' (Dorman's)	1 oz	100	140	7.0
Swiss style 'Slices' (Weight Watchers)	1 oz	50	400	2.0
CHEESE BALL				
cheddar, w/almonds and bacon (Kaukauna)	1 oz	100	250	7.0
green onion flavor, w/almonds (Kaukauna)	1 oz	100	250	7.0
Port wine, w/almonds (Kaukauna)	1 oz	100	250	7.0
sharp cheddar, w/almonds (Kaukauna)	1 oz	100	250	7.0
CHEESE BLINTZ. See BLINTZ.				
CHEESE FLAVORED SNACKS				
(Barbara's Bakery)				
'Pinta Puffs' tangy triple cheese	1 oz	70	100	2.0
puff lights	1 oz	40	55	3.0
(Bearitos) puffs, cheddar, baked, original	.5 oz	80	2	5.0
(Chee•tos)				
cheddar valley	1 oz	160	240	9.0
crunchy	1 oz	150	310	9.0
crunchy, light	1 oz	140	360	6.0
curls	1 oz	150	270	9.0
flamin' hot	1 oz	150	240	9.0
light	1 oz	140	280	6.0
paws	1 oz	160	310	10.0
puffed balls	1 oz	160	360	10.0
puffs	1 oz	160	330	9.0
(Flavor Tree) sticks, cheddar	1/4 cup	129	335	8.1
(Health Valley)				
'Cheddar Lite' puffs, w/organic corn, baked	.25 oz	40	35	2.0
puffs, fat-free	1 oz	100	75	0.0
puffs, w/chili, fat-free	1 oz	100	75	0.0
puffs, w/green onion, fat-free	1 oz	100	75	0.0
(Keebler) 'RC Ricers' zesty cheddar	1 oz	140	200	8.0
(Planter)				
'Cheez Balls'	1 oz	160	270	11.0
'Cheez Balls' nacho	1 oz	160	290	10.0

Food Name	Serv. Size	Total Cal.	Sod. MGS	Fat GMS
'Cheez Curls'	1 oz	160	290	11.0
'Cheez Curls' nacho	1 oz	160	290	10.0
(Weight Watchers) curls, crunchy	.5-oz pkg	70	45	2.0
(Wise)				
'Cheez Doodles' baked, puffed	1 oz	150	360	9.0
'Cheez Doodles' fried, crunchy	1 oz	160	230	10.0
'Cheez Waffies'	1 oz	140	420	8.0
corn spirals, nacho	1 oz	160	190	10.0
corn twists, nacho, crispy	1 oz	160	190	10.0
CHEESE FOOD				
AMERICAN				
(Darigold)	1 oz	80	381	6.0
cold pack	1 oz	94	274	6.9
colored (Hoffman's)	1 oz	100	490	7.0
grated (Kraft)	1 oz	130	740	7.0
'Light' (Kraft)	1 oz	70	420	4.0
sharp, 'Singles' (Borden)	1 oz	90	470	7.0
'Singles' (Borden)	1 oz	90	350	7.0
'Singles' (Kraft)	1 oz	90	390	7.0
'Slices' (Borden)	1 oz	100	420	7.0
white, 'Singles' (Kraft)	1 oz	90	400	7.0
w/Swiss cheese (Land O'Lakes)	1 oz	100	400	8.0
BACON				
(Cracker Barrel)	1 oz	90	280	7.0
'Chees'N Bacon' (Hoffman's)	1 oz	90	540	6.0
'Cheez'N Bacon' (Kraft)	1 oz	90	400	7.0
CARAWAY, 'Swisson Rye' (Hoffman's)	1 oz	90	400	7.0
CHEDDAR				
extra sharp (Cracker Barrel)	1 oz	90	240	7.0
extra sharp (Land O'Lakes)	1 oz	100	370	9.0
extra sharp, cold pack 'Cup' (Kaukauna)	1 oz	100	250	7.0
'La Chedda' (Land O'Lakes)	1 oz	90	335	7.0
nacho, cold pack, 'Cup' (Kaukauna)	1 oz	100	250	7.0
Port wine (Cracker Barrel)	1 oz	100	230	7.0
sharp (Cracker Barrel)	1 oz	100	230	7.0
sharp, cold pack (Wispride)	1 oz	100	210	7.0
sharp, cold pack 'Cup' (Kaukauna)	1 oz	100	250	7.0
sharp, cup 'Lite 50' (Kaukauna)	1 oz	70	190	3.0
sharp 'Lite' (Kaukauna)	1 oz	70	230	4.0
smoky 'Lite' (Kaukauna)	1 oz	70	230	4.0
w/bacon (Land O'Lakes)	1 oz	110	350	9.0

Food Name	Serv. Size	Total Cal.	Sod. MGS	Fat GMS
w/bacon and horseradish, cold pack, 'Cup' (Kaukauna)	1 oz	100	250	7.0
GARLIC (Kraft)	1 oz	90	370	7.0
ITALIAN HERB (Land O'Lakes)	1 oz	90	430	7.0
JALAPEÑO				
(Hoffman's)	1 oz	90	580	7.0
(Kraft)	1 oz	90	390	7.0
(Land O'Lakes)	1 oz	90	400	7.0
hot, 'Mexican' (Velveeta)	1 oz	100	430	7.0
mild, 'Mexican' (Velveeta)	1 oz	100	420	7.0
'Singles' (Kraft)	1 oz	90	450	7.0
MEXICAN				
hot, shredded (Velveeta)	1 oz	100	430	7.0
mild, shredded (Velveeta)	1 oz	100	420	7.0
ONION				
(Land O'Lakes)	1 oz	90	330	7.0
'Chees'N Onion' (Hoffman's)	1 oz	100	490	7.0
PEPPPERONI (Land O'Lakes)	1 oz	90	395	7.0
PIMIENTO				
'Deluxe' (Kraft)	1 oz	100	440	8.0
'Singles' (Kraft)	1 oz	90	390	7.0
PORT WINE				
cold pack (Wispride)	1 oz	100	210	7.0
cold pack, 'Cup' (Kaukauna)	1 oz	100	250	7.0
cup, 'Lite 50' (Kaukauna)	1 oz	70	190	3.0
PROCESSED				
(Land O'Lakes)	1 oz	90	350	6.0
singles, fat-free (Healthy Choice)	1 oz	40	390	0.0
singles, 'Free' (Kraft)	1 oz	45	430	0.0
slices (Land O'Lakes)	3/4 oz	70	260	5.0
slices (Land O'Lakes)	2/3 oz	60	230	4.0
SALAMI				
(Land O'Lakes)	1 oz	90	410	7.0
'Chees'N Salami' (Hoffman's)	1 oz	90	560	6.0
SHARP, 'Singles' (Kraft)	1 oz	100	400	8.0
SHREDDED (Velveeta)	1 oz	100	410	7.0
SMOKY, cold pack, 'Cup' (Kaukauna)	1 oz	100	250	7.0
SWISS				
(Velveeta)	1 oz	100	410	7.0
almond, cup, 'Lite 50' (Kaukauna)	1 oz	70	180	3.0
country, cold pack, 'Cup' (Kaukauna)	1 oz	100	250	7.0
country, 'Lite' (Kaukauna)	1 oz	70	200	4.0

Food Name	Serv. Size	Total Cal.	Sod. MGS	Fat GMS
singles (Kraft)	1 oz	90	440	7.0
singles, 'Free' (Kraft)	1 oz	45	390	0.0
slices, 'Singles' (Borden)	1 oz	100	420	7.0
CHEESE LOG				
hickory smoke/white sharp cheddar, double (Kaukauna)	1 oz	100	250	7.0
Port wine (Sargento)	1 oz	100	250	7.0
Port wine, w/almonds (Kaukauna)	1 oz	100	250	7.0
sharp cheddar (Sargento)	1 oz	100	250	7.0
sharp cheddar, w/almonds (Cracker Barrel)	1 oz	90	410	6.0
sharp cheddar, w/almonds (Kaukauna)	1 oz	100	250	7.0
smoky, w/almonds (Cracker Barrel)	1 oz	90	410	6.0
Swiss almond (Sargento)	1 oz	90	350	7.0
Swiss almond, w/almonds (Kaukauna)	1 oz	100	250	7.0
white sharp cheddar/green onion, double (Kaukauna)	1 oz	100	250	7.0
CHEESE NUGGET				
mozzarella, breaded, frozen 'Hot Bites' (Banquet)	2.63 oz	240	530	13.0
CHEESE NUT				
Port wine (Cracker Barrel)	1 oz	90	260	6.0
sharp, w/bell and jalapeño peppers (Kaukauna)	1 oz	100	250	7.0
sharp cheddar (Cracker Barrel)	1 oz	100	250	7.0
CHEESE PASTRY, pocket (Tastykake)	3 oz	325	231	16.7
CHEESE PRODUCT				
(Alpine Lace)	1 oz	90	200	7.0
'Free N' Lean' singles (Alpine Lace)	1 oz	40	260	0.0
'Free Singles' (Kraft)	1 oz	45	420	0.0
'Light' (Velveeta)	1 oz	70	470	4.0
sandwich slices (Lunch Wagon)	1 oz	90	370	7.0
'Singles' fat-free (Borden)	1 oz	40	380	0.0
'Slices' (Velveeta)	1 oz	90	400	6.0
slices, fat-free (Lite-Line)	1 slice	25	250	0.0
AMERICAN FLAVOR				
(Harvest Moon)	1 oz	70	420	4.0
(Lite-Line)	1 oz	50	410	2.0
'Light' (Borden)	1 oz	70	420	5.0
'Light Singles' (Kraft)	1 oz	70	420	4.0
'Reduced Sodium' (Lite-Line)	1 oz	70	90	4.0
'Singles' (Light n' Lively)	1 oz	70	420	4.0
'Sodium Lite' (Lite-Line)	1 oz	70	200	4.0
white 'Light Singles' (Kraft)	1 oz	70	410	4.0
white 'Singles' (Light n' Lively)	1 oz	70	410	4.0

Food Name	Serv. Size	Total Cal.	Sod. MGS	Fat GMS
CHEDDAR FLAVOR				
medium-sharp (Spreadery)	1 oz	70	250	4.0
mild (Lite-Line)	1 oz	50	380	2.0
sharp (Lite-Line)	1 oz	50	440	2.0
sharp (Spreadery)	1 oz	70	240	4.0
sharp, 'Free' (Kraft)	1 oz	45	390	0.0
sharp, 'Light' (Kraft)	1 oz	70	380	4.0
sharp, 'Singles' (Kraft)	1 oz	100	400	8.0
sharp, 'Singles' (Light n' Lively)	1 oz	70	380	4.0
sharp, slices (Lite-Line)	1 slice	35	300	2.0
Vermont white (Spreadery)	1 oz	70	230	4.0
CREAM CHEESE FLAVOR 'Light' (Philadelphia Brand)	1 oz	60	160	5.0
MEXICAN FLAVOR mild, w/jalapeños (Spreadery)	1 oz	70	260	4.0
MOZZARELLA FLAVOR (Lite-Line)	1 oz	50	340	2.0
MUENSTER FLAVOR (Lite-Line)	1 oz	50	450	2.0
NACHO FLAVOR (Spreadery)	1 oz	70	240	4.0
NEUFCHATEL				
classic ranch (Spreadery)	1 oz	70	190	7.0
French onion (Spreadery)	1 oz	70	135	6.0
garden vegetable (Spreadery)	1 oz	70	220	6.0
garlic and herb (Spreadery)	1 oz	70	140	6.0
w/strawberries (Spreadery)	1 oz	70	270	5.0
PORT WINE FLAVOR (Spreadery)	1 oz	70	250	4.0
SWISS FLAVOR				
(Lite-Line)	1 oz	50	380	2.0
'Free Singles' (Kraft)	1 oz	45	390	0.0
'Light' (Kraft)	1 oz	70	350	3.0
'Singles' (Light n' Lively)	1 oz	70	350	3.0
CHEESE SPREAD				
AMERICAN				
(Kraft)	1 oz	80	470	6.0
'Easy Cheese American' (Nabisco)	1 oz	80	350	6.0
sharp 'Cracker Snacks' (Sargento)	1 oz	110	410	9.0
w/pimiento 'Cracker Snacks' (Sargento)	1 oz	110	410	9.0
BACON				
(Kraft)	1 oz	80	560	7.0
(Squeez-A-Snak)	1 oz	80	500	7.0
BLUE (Roka)	1 oz	70	270	6.0
BRICK 'Cracker Snacks' (Sargento)	1 oz	100	430	9.0
CHEDDAR				
'Easy Cheese Cheddar' (Nabisco)	1 oz	80	370	6.0

Food Name	Serv. Size	Total Cal.	Sod. MGS	Fat GMS
'Easy Cheese Cheddar 'n Bacon' *(Nabisco)*	1 oz	80	350	6.0
'Easy Cheese Sharp Cheddar' *(Nabisco)*	1 oz	80	320	6.0
sharp, 'Cup' *(Weight Watchers)*	1 oz	70	190	3.0
FRENCH ONION *(Alouette)*	1 oz	95	205	9.0
GARLIC				
(Squeez-A-Snak)	1 oz	80	430	7.0
and herbs, soft 'Lite' *(Rondel)*	1 oz	70	170	6.0
and spices *(Alouette)*	1 oz	95	165	9.0
HERB				
and garlic, soft 'Light' *(Alouette)*	1 oz	60	130	4.5
soft, 'Fines Herbes' *(Rondel)*	1 oz	90	170	8.0
HICKORY *(Squeez-A-Snak)*	1 oz	80	440	7.0
HORSERADISH, and chive *(Alouette)*	1 oz	85	130	8.0
JALAPEÑO				
(Cheez Whiz)	1 oz	80	430	6.0
(Kraft)	1 oz	70	95	5.0
(Squeez-A-Snak)	1 oz	80	510	6.0
loaf *(Kraft)*	1 oz	80	470	6.0
LIMBURGER *(Mohawk Valley)*	1 oz	70	420	6.0
MEXICAN				
'Easy Cheese Nacho' *(Nabisco)*	1 oz	80	340	6.0
hot *(Velveeta)*	1 oz	80	520	6.0
mild *(Cheez Whiz)*	1 oz	80	430	6.0
mild *(Velveeta)*	1 oz	80	440	6.0
OLIVE, and pimiento *(Kraft)*	1 oz	60	160	5.0
PIMIENTO				
(Kraft)	1 oz	70	120	5.0
(Velveeta)	1 oz	80	400	6.0
PINEAPPLE *(Kraft)*	1 oz	70	15	5.0
PORT WINE, 'Cup' *(Weight Watchers)*	1 oz	70	190	3.0
SALMON *(Alouette)*	1 oz	70	140	6.0
SHARP				
(Old English)	1 oz	80	480	7.0
(Squeez-A-Snak)	1 oz	80	440	7.0
SPINACH, creamy *(Alouette)*	1 oz	90	125	8.0
SWISS, 'Cracker Snacks' *(Sargento)*	1 oz	100	390	7.0
VEGETABLE				
garden, soft *(Rondele)*	1 oz	90	160	8.0
spring, soft 'Light' *(Alouette)*	1 oz	60	120	4.5
CHEESE STICK				
cheddar, breaded, frozen *(Farm Rich)*	3 oz	300	740	21.0

Food Name	Serv. Size	Total Cal.	Sod. MGS	Fat GMS
cheddar, snack (Flavor Tree)	1/4 cup	129	335	8.1
hot pepper, breaded, frozen (Farm Rich)	3 oz	260	700	17.0
mozzarella, breaded, frozen (Farm Rich)	3 oz	240	570	13.0
provolone, breaded, frozen (Farm Rich)	3 oz	270	820	16.0
CHEESE STRAW				
made w/lard, 5 x 3/8 x 3/8 inches	10 straws	272	433	17.9
made w/vegetable shortening, 5 x 3/8 x 3/8 inches	10 straws	272	433	17.9
CHEESE TOPPING, cheddar, w/bacon (Tone's)	1 tsp	10	81	1.0
CHEESECAKE. See CAKE.				
CHEESECAKE FILLING				
'No-Bake' lite (Royal)	1/8 pie	130	230	3.0
'No-Bake' real (Royal)	1/8 pie	160	250	3.0
CHERRY				
SOUR, RED				
trimmed, w/pits	1 cup	52	3	0.3
trimmed, w/pits	1 oz	14	1	0.1
trimmed, w/o pits	1 cup	78	5	0.5
untrimmed	1 lb	203	13	1.2
SWEET				
trimmed, w/pits	1 cup	104	0	1.4
trimmed, w/pits	1 oz	20	tr	0.3
trimmed, w/pits, approx 2.6 oz	10 med	49	0	0.7
untrimmed	1 lb	293	2	3.9
untrimmed (Dole)	1 cup	90	0	1.0
CHERRY, CANNED				
SOUR, RED				
(A&P)	1/2 cup	50	5	<1.0
in extra heavy syrup	1/2 cup	148	9	0.1
in heavy syrup	1/2 cup	116	9	0.1
in light syrup	1/2 cup	94	9	0.1
in water	1/2 cup	44	9	0.1
Pitted				
in extra heavy syrup	1/2 cup	129	8	0.1
in heavy syrup	1/2 cup	103	8	0.1
in light syrup	1/2 cup	85	8	0.1
in water	1/2 cup	41	8	0.1
in water (Stokely)	1/2 cup	45	15	0.0
tart (Lucky Leaf)	4 oz	50	0	0.0
tart (Musselman's)	4 oz	50	0	0.0
(White House)	3.5 oz	43	5	0.0

Food Name	Serv. Size	Total Cal.	Sod. MGS	Fat GMS
SWEET				
dark *(Del Monte)*	1/2 cup	90	10	0.0
in extra heavy syrup	1/2 cup	116	3	0.2
in heavy syrup	1/2 cup	94	3	0.2
in juice	1/2 cup	61	3	<.1
in light syrup	1/2 cup	76	3	0.2
in light syrup *(Del Monte)*	1/2 cup	100	10	0.0
in water	1/2 cup	52	1	0.1
Pitted				
dark *(Del Monte)*	1/2 cup	90	10	0.0
in extra heavy syrup	1/2 cup	133	4	0.2
in heavy syrup	1/2 cup	107	4	0.2
in juice	1/2 cup	68	4	0.0
in light syrup	1/2 cup	84	4	0.2
in water	1/2 cup	57	1	0.2
CHERRY, FROZEN				
SOUR, RED				
unsweetened	4 oz	52	1	0.5
unsweetened	1/2 cup	36	1	0.3
SWEET				
sweetened	10-oz pkg	253	3	0.4
sweetened	1 cup	231	3	0.3
sweetened	4 oz	101	1	0.1
sweetened *(Lucky Leaf)*	4 oz	130	150	0.0
CHERRY, MARASCHINO, in jar, w/liquid	1 oz	33	na	0.1
CHERRY, PUERTO RICAN				
approx .2 oz	1 med	2	tr	<.1
trimmed	1/2 cup	16	4	0.1
trimmed	1 oz	9	2	0.1
untrimmed	1 lb	114	26	1.1
CHERRY CIDER *(Knudsen & Sons)*	8 oz	100	na	0.0
CHERRY DRINK				
(Hi-C) aseptic box	6 oz	100	25	0.0
(Hi-C) chilled	6 oz	100	25	0.0
(Kool-Aid) 'Koolers'	8.45 oz	140	10	0.0
(Squeezit) 'Chucklin Cherry'	6.75 oz	110	5	0.0
CHERRY DRINK MIX				
(Finast) prepared	8 oz	80	15	0.0
(Kool-Aid) sugar-sweetened, prepared	8 oz	80	0	0.0
(Kool-Aid) unsweetened, prepared w/sugar	8 oz	100	0	0.0
(Kool-Aid) unsweetened, prepared w/o sugar	8 oz	2	0	0.0

Food Name	Serv. Size	Total Cal.	Sod. MGS	Fat GMS
(Kool-Aid) w/NutraSweet, prepared	8 oz	4	0	0.0
(Pathmark) 'No Frills' prepared	8 oz	90	65	0.0
(Wyler's) 'Fruit Slush' prepared	4 oz	157	10	0.0
CHERRY JUICE				
(Dole) 'Pure and Light Mountain Cherry'	6 oz	87	8	0.1
(Juicy Juice) bottled	6 oz	90	10	0.0
(Juicy Juice) boxed	8.45 oz	130	10	0.0
(Knudsen & Sons) tart	8 oz	125	na	0.0
(Santa Cruznatural) 'Cruz' organic	8 oz	125	na	<1.0
(Welch's) 'Orchard'	6 oz	180	10	0.0
CHERRY JUICE DRINK				
(Hi-C)	8.45 oz	141	24	0.1
(Hi-C)	6 oz	100	17	0.1
(Tang) 'Fruit Box'	8.45 oz	130	10	0.0
CHERRY LEMONADE				
(Knudsen & Sons)	8 oz	105	na	0.0
(Santa Cruz natural) dark, sweet, organic	8 oz	60	na	<1.0
CHERRY PASTRY				
(Hormel) frozen 'Cherry Dulcita'	4 oz	300	345	9.0
(Tastykake) pocket	3 oz	325	231	16.7
CHERRY STRUDEL, individual *(Aunt Fanny's)*	3 oz	320	190	16.0
CHERVIL				
dried	1 oz	67	24	1.1
dried	1 tbsp	4	2	0.1
dried	1 tsp	1	1	0.0
CHESTNUT, CHINESE				
boiled or steamed	1 oz	43	1	0.2
dried	1 oz	103	1	0.5
raw	1 oz	64	1	0.3
raw, in shell	1 lb	852	13	4.2
roasted	1 oz	68	1	0.3
CHESTNUT, EUROPEAN/Italian chestnut/sweet chestnut				
boiled or steamed, shelled	1 oz	37	8	0.4
dried, in shell	1 lb	1357	135	16.1
dried, shelled, peeled	1 oz	105	11	1.1
dried, shelled, unpeeled	1 oz	106	11	1.3
raw, in shell	1 lb	714	9	7.6
raw, shelled, peeled	1 oz	56	1	0.4
raw, shelled, unpeeled	1 cup	309	4	3.3
raw, shelled, unpeeled	1 oz	60	1	0.6
roasted, in shell	1 lb	700	6	6.3

Food Name	Serv. Size	Total Cal.	Sod. MGS	Fat GMS
roasted, in shell	1 cup	350	3	3.2
roasted, in shell	1 oz	70	1	0.6
roasted, shelled	1 oz	70	1	0.6
roasted, shelled, approx 17 nuts	1 cup	350	3	3.2
CHESTNUT, ITALIAN. See CHESTNUT, EUROPEAN.				
CHESTNUT, JAPANESE				
boiled or steamed	1 oz	16	1	0.1
dried, in shell	1 lb	1078	101	3.7
dried, shelled	1 oz	102	10	0.4
dried, shelled	1 cup	558	53	1.9
raw, in shell	1 lb	462	43	1.6
raw, shelled	1 oz	44	4	0.2
roasted	1 oz	57	5	0.2
CHESTNUT, SWEET. See CHESTNUT, EUROPEAN.				
CHESTNUT FLOUR	100 gm	362	11	3.7
CHEWING GUM. See CANDY.				
CHICK PEA. See GARBANZO BEAN.				
CHICK PEA FLOUR. See GARBANZO FLOUR.				
CHICKEN. For fresh chicken see CHICKEN, BROILER-FRYER; CHICKEN, CAPON; CHICKEN ROASTER; CHICKEN, STEWING.				
CHICKEN, ALTERNATIVE				
(Heartline) 'Chicken Fillet Style'	2 oz	176	260	7.0
(Heartline) 'Chicken Fillet Style' lite	.5 oz	22	135	0.0
Canned				
(Worthington) diced, drained	1/4 cup	90	330	8.0
(Worthington) 'FriChik' 1.6-oz pieces	2 pieces	180	610	13.0
(Worthington) sliced, drained, 1.05-oz slices	2 slices	90	330	8.0
Frozen				
(Morningstar Farms) nuggets, homestyle 'Country Crisps'	3 oz	250	480	16.0
(Morningstar Farms) nuggets, zesty 'Country Crisps'	3 oz	280	740	19.0
(Morningstar Farms) patty 'Country Crisps'	2.5 oz	220	620	15.0
(Worthington) 'Crispy Chik'	3 oz	280	500	19.0
(Worthington) diced 'Meatless Chicken'	1/2 cup	190	680	13.0
(Worthington) patty 'Crispy Chik'	2.5 oz	220	620	15.0
(Worthington) roll 'Chic-ketts'	1/2 cup	160	640	7.0
(Worthington) roll 'Meatless Chicken'	2.5 oz	150	570	10.0
(Worthington) sliced 'Meatless Chicken' 1-oz slices	2 slices	130	460	9.0
(Worthington) sticks 'Chik Stiks' approx 1.7-oz pieces	1 stick	110	390	7.0
CHICKEN, BONELESS BREAST, PREPARED				
(Hillshire Farm) smoked 'Deli Select'	1 oz	31	290	0.2
(Louis Rich) hickory-smoked	1 oz	30	356	0.8

Food Name	Serv. Size	Total Cal.	Sod. MGS	Fat GMS
(Louis Rich) hickory-smoked, 97% fat-free	1 oz	30	370	<1.0
(Louis Rich) oven-roasted 'Deluxe'	1 oz	30	332	0.8
(Louis Rich) oven-roasted, 'Deluxe' 96% fat-free	1 oz	30	330	1.0
(Oscar Mayer) oven-roasted	1 oz	29	414	0.7
(Oscar Mayer) smoked	1 oz	25	397	0.4

CHICKEN, BROILER-FRYER

BACK MEAT AND SKIN

Food Name	Serv. Size	Total Cal.	Sod. MGS	Fat GMS
fried, flour-coated	4 oz	375	102	23.5
raw	1 oz	90	18	8.1
roasted	4 oz	340	99	23.8
stewed	4 oz	293	73	20.6

BACK MEAT ONLY

Food Name	Serv. Size	Total Cal.	Sod. MGS	Fat GMS
raw	1 lb	624	400	28.8
raw	1 oz	39	23	1.7
roasted	4 oz	271	109	14.9
stewed	4 oz	237	76	12.7

BREAST MEAT AND SKIN

Food Name	Serv. Size	Total Cal.	Sod. MGS	Fat GMS
fried, batter-dipped	4 oz	295	312	15.0
fried, flour-coated	4 oz	252	86	10.1
raw	1 lb	784	288	41.6
raw	1 oz	49	18	2.6
roasted	4 oz	223	81	8.8
stewed	4 oz	209	70	8.4

BREAST MEAT ONLY

Food Name	Serv. Size	Total Cal.	Sod. MGS	Fat GMS
raw	1 lb	496	288	6.4
raw	1 oz	31	18	0.4
roasted	4 oz	187	84	4.0
stewed	4 oz	171	71	3.4

DARK MEAT AND SKIN

Food Name	Serv. Size	Total Cal.	Sod. MGS	Fat GMS
fried, batter-dipped	4 oz	338	335	21.1
fried, flour-coated	4 oz	323	101	19.2
raw	1 lb	1072	336	83.2
raw	1 oz	67	21	5.2
roasted	4 oz	287	99	17.9
stewed	4 oz	264	79	16.6

DARK MEAT ONLY

Food Name	Serv. Size	Total Cal.	Sod. MGS	Fat GMS
fried, chopped or diced	1 cup	335	136	16.3
raw	1 lb	560	384	19.2
raw	1 oz	35	24	1.2
roasted	1 cup	287	130	13.6
roasted	4 oz	232	105	11.0

Food Name	Serv. Size	Total Cal.	Sod. MGS	Fat GMS
roasted, chopped or diced	1 cup	286	130	13.6
stewed	1 cup	269	104	12.6
stewed	4 oz	218	84	10.2
stewed, chopped or diced	1 cup	269	104	12.6
DRUMSTICK MEAT AND SKIN				
fried, batter-dipped	4 oz	304	305	17.9
fried, flour-coated	4 oz	278	101	15.6
raw	1 lb	736	384	40.0
raw	1 oz	46	24	2.5
roasted	4 oz	245	102	12.6
stewed	4 oz	231	86	12.1
DRUMSTICK MEAT ONLY				
raw	1 lb	544	400	16.0
raw	1 oz	34	25	1.0
roasted	4 oz	195	108	6.4
stewed	4 oz	192	91	6.5
LEG MEAT AND SKIN				
fried, batter-dipped	4 oz	310	316	18.3
fried, flour-coated	4 oz	285	99	16.2
raw	1 lb	848	352	54.4
raw	1 oz	53	22	3.4
stewed	4 oz	249	83	14.7
LEG MEAT ONLY				
raw	1 lb	544	384	17.6
raw	1 oz	34	24	1.1
roasted	4 oz	217	103	9.6
stewed	4 oz	210	88	9.1
LIGHT MEAT AND SKIN				
fried, batter-dipped	4 oz	312	324	17.4
fried, flour-coated	4 oz	279	87	13.7
raw	1 lb	848	288	49.6
raw	1 oz	53	18	3.1
roasted	4 oz	252	85	12.3
stewed	4 oz	228	71	11.3
LIGHT MEAT ONLY				
fried	8 oz	269	113	7.8
raw	1 lb	512	304	8.0
raw	1 oz	32	19	0.5
roasted	1 cup	242	108	6.3
roasted	4 oz	196	87	5.1
roasted, chopped or diced	1 cup	242	108	6.3

Food Name	Serv. Size	Total Cal.	Sod. MGS	Fat GMS
stewed, chopped or diced	1 cup	223	91	5.6
stewed	4 oz	180	74	4.5
NECK MEAT AND SKIN				
fried, batter-dipped	4 oz	374	313	26.7
fried, flour-coated	4 oz	376	93	26.8
raw	1 lb	1344	288	118.4
raw	1 oz	84	18	7.4
simmered	4 oz	280	59	20.5
NECK MEAT ONLY				
raw	1 lb	704	368	40.0
raw	1 oz	44	23	2.5
simmered	4 oz	203	73	9.3
SKIN ONLY				
fried, batter-dipped	1 oz	112	165	8.2
roasted	1 oz	129	18	11.5
stewed	1 oz	103	16	9.4
THIGH MEAT AND SKIN				
fried, batter-dipped	4 oz	314	327	18.7
fried, flour-coated	4 oz	297	100	17.0
raw	1 lb	960	352	68.8
raw	1 oz	60	22	4.3
roasted	4 oz	280	95	17.6
stewed	4 oz	263	81	16.7
THIGH MEAT ONLY				
raw	1 lb	544	384	17.6
raw	1 oz	34	24	1.1
roasted	4 oz	237	100	12.3
stewed	4 oz	221	85	11.1
WING MEAT AND SKIN				
fried, batter-dipped	4 oz	367	363	24.7
fried, flour-coated	4 oz	364	87	25.1
raw	1 lb	1008	336	72.0
raw	1 oz	63	21	4.5
roasted	4 oz	329	93	22.1
stewed	4 oz	282	76	19.1
WING MEAT ONLY				
raw	1 lb	576	368	16.0
raw	1 oz	36	23	1.0
roasted	4 oz	230	104	9.2
stewed	4 oz	205	83	8.1

Food Name	Serv. Size	Total Cal.	Sod. MGS	Fat GMS
CHICKEN, CANNED				
Chunk				
(Featherweight)	3 oz	90	60	3.0
(Hormel) breast	6.75 oz	350	855	20.0
(Hormel) breast	2.5 oz	90	310	3.0
(Hormel) breast, no salt	2.5 oz	90	25	3.0
(Hormel) dark	6.75 oz	327	933	18.0
(Hormel) white and dark	6.75 oz	340	857	20.0
(Hormel) white and dark, unsalted	6.75 oz	330	75	18.0
(Swanson) 'Mixin' Chicken'	2.5 oz	130	230	8.0
(Swanson) white and dark	2.5 oz	100	240	4.0
Loaf (Hormel)	2 oz	130	608	10.0
White (Swanson)	2.5 oz	100	235	4.0
CHICKEN, CAPON				
GIBLETS				
raw	1 lb	592	352	24.0
raw	1 oz	37	22	1.5
simmered	1 cup	238	80	7.8
simmered	4 oz	186	62	6.1
MEAT AND SKIN				
raw	1 lb	1056	208	76.8
raw	1 oz	66	13	4.8
roasted	4 oz	260	56	13.2
CHICKEN, FROZEN. See also CHICKEN DINNER/ENTRÉE, FROZEN.				
BREAST				
Boneless				
(Pilgrim's Pride)	3 oz	195	450	10.2
(Tyson)	3 oz	190	400	9.0
(Tyson) barbecue	3 oz	110	310	3.0
(Tyson) chunks	3 oz	240	430	17.0
(Tyson) grilled	2.75 oz	100	410	3.0
(Tyson) hot and spicy	2.75 oz	110	490	3.0
(Tyson) skinless, wholesale club item	3.5 oz	110	380	2.0
Halves, wholesale club item (Tyson)	3.5 oz	230	50	13.0
Pieces				
(Banquet) fried	5.75 oz	220	710	11.0
(Tyson) mesquite, wholesale club item	3.5 oz	170	540	7.0
Portions (Swanson) fried, 'Plump & Juicy'	4.5 oz	360	800	20.0
Strips (Weaver)	3.3 oz	200	500	10.0
Tenders				
(Banquet) Southern fried	2.25 oz	160	340	7.0

Food Name	Serv. Size	Total Cal.	Sod. MGS	Fat GMS
(Pilgrim's Pride)	3 oz	181	430	9.5
(Tyson) blanched, wholesale club item	3.5 oz	200	340	8.0
(Tyson) breaded, wholesale club item	3.5 oz	200	340	8.0
(Tyson) Southern fried	3 oz	220	630	11.0
(Tyson) unbreaded, wholesale club item	3.5 oz	120	55	1.0
Whole				
(Tyson) wholesale club item	3.5 oz	210	50	12.0
(Weaver)	4.5 oz	270	520	13.0
(Weaver) batter-dipped	4.4 oz	310	220	20.0
CHUNKS				
(Country Pride)	3 oz	240	560	15.0
(Country Pride) Southern fried	3 oz	280	690	20.0
(Tyson) diced	3 oz	150	50	5.0
(Tyson) mesquite flavor 'Hors D'Oeuvres'	3.5 oz	100	600	1.0
(Tyson) microwave, boneless	3.5 oz	220	na	15.0
LEG MEAT				
(Banquet) thighs and drumsticks, fried	6.25 oz	250	790	14.0
(Pilgrim's Pride) drumsters	3 oz	200	320	12.5
(Tyson) drums and thighs, wholesale club item	3.5 oz	270	110	17.0
(Tyson) 'Julienne Leg Meat' wholesale club item	3.5 oz	160	60	6.0
(Tyson) thighs, skinless, wholesale club item	3.5 oz	200	70	10.0
(Weaver) batter-dipped	3 oz	210	220	14.0
(Weaver) drums and thighs, 'Crispy Dutch Frye'	3.5 oz	290	640	19.0
NUGGETS				
(Country Pride)	3 oz	250	460	16.0
(Pilgrim's Pride)	3 oz	202	370	12.3
(Weaver)	2.6 oz	190	450	12.0
(Weight Watchers)	5.9 oz	220	500	7.0
PORTIONS				
(Pilgrim's Pride) fried	3 oz	255	480	17.7
(Swanson) 'Homestyle Recipe'	7 oz	390	1100	21.0
(Swanson) 'Take-Out Pre-Fried'	3.25 oz	270	650	16.0
ROASTER *(Tyson)* wholesale club item	3.5 oz	230	80	13.0
WINGS				
(Pilgrim's Pride) Southern fried	3 oz	228	480	17.2
(Pilgrim's Pride) 'Wing Zappers'	3 oz	187	340	12.8
(Tyson) all varieties, 'Flyers'	3.5 oz	220	400	14.0
(Tyson) drummettes, wholesale club item	3.5 oz	260	80	17.0
(Tyson) barbecue 'Hors D'Oeuvres' wholesale club item	3.5 oz	210	430	12.0
(Tyson) raw, hot, wholesale club item	3.5 oz	280	80	19.0
(Tyson) roaster 'Hors D'Oeuvres' wholesale club item	3.5 oz	210	280	12.0

Food Name	Serv. Size	Total Cal.	Sod. MGS	Fat GMS
(Weaver) batter-dipped	4 oz	400	520	28.0
(Weaver) 'Crispy Dutch Frye'	4 oz	400	520	28.0
(Weaver) hot	2.7 oz	170	670	11.0
CHICKEN, ROASTER				
DARK MEAT ONLY				
raw	1 lb	512	432	16.0
raw	1 oz	32	27	1.0
roasted	4 oz	202	108	9.9
GIBLETS, simmered	1 cup	239	87	7.6
LIGHT MEAT ONLY				
raw	1 lb	496	224	8.0
raw	1 oz	31	14	0.5
roasted	1 cup	214	71	5.7
roasted	4 oz	174	58	4.6
MEAT AND SKIN				
raw	1 lb	976	304	72.0
raw	1 oz	61	19	4.5
roasted	4 oz	253	83	15.2
CHICKEN, STEWING				
DARK MEAT ONLY				
raw	1 lb	720	464	36.8
raw	1 oz	45	29	2.3
stewed	1 cup	361	133	21.4
stewed	4 oz	293	108	17.3
GIBLETS				
raw	1 lb	560	352	20.8
raw	1 oz	35	22	1.3
simmered	1 cup	281	81	13.5
LIGHT MEAT ONLY				
raw	1 lb	624	240	19.2
raw	1 oz	39	15	1.2
stewed	1 cup	298	81	11.2
stewed	4 oz	242	66	9.0
MEAT AND SKIN				
raw	1 lb	1168	320	92.8
raw	1 oz	73	20	5.8
stewed	4 oz	323	83	21.4
CHICKEN DINNER/ENTRÉE, CANNED				
(Featherweight) and dumplings	7.5 oz	160	115	5.0
(LaChoy)				
chow mein	3/4 cup	240	1420	2.0

Food Name	Serv. Size	Total Cal.	Sod. MGS	Fat GMS
chow mein 'Bi-Pack'	8.642 oz	97	1199	3.8
chow mein 'Bi-Pack'	3/4 cup	80	980	3.0
Oriental 'Bi-Pack'	3/4 cup	240	1400	2.0
Oriental w/noodles 'Bi-Pack'	9 oz	160	1163	3.8
sweet and sour	3/4 cup	240	1420	2.0
sweet and sour 'Bi-Pack'	8.959 oz	161	745	2.5
sweet and sour 'Bi-Pack'	3/4 cup	120	440	2.0
teriyaki 'Bi-Pack'	8.642 oz	110	1226	3.0
teriyaki 'Bi-Pack'	3/4 cup	85	850	2.0
(Luck's) and dumplings	7.25 oz	240	605	11.0
(Swanson)				
à la king	5 1/4 oz	190	690	12.0
and dumplings	7.5 oz	220	980	11.0
CHICKEN DINNER/ENTRÉE, FROZEN				
(Armour)				
à la king 'Classics Lite'	11.25 oz	290	630	7.0
and noodles 'Classics'	11 oz	230	660	7.0
breast, Marsala 'Classics Lite'	10.5 oz	250	930	7.0
Burgundy 'Classics Lite'	10 oz	210	780	2.0
fettuccini 'Classics'	11 oz	260	660	9.0
glazed 'Classics'	10.75 oz	300	960	16.0
mesquite 'Classics'	9.5 oz	370	660	16.0
Oriental 'Classics Lite'	10 oz	180	660	1.0
parmigiana 'Classics'	11.5 oz	370	1060	19.0
sweet and sour 'Classics Lite'	11 oz	240	820	2.0
w/wine and mushroom sauce 'Classics'	10.75 oz	280	900	11.0
(Banquet)				
à la king 'Cookin' Bags'	4 oz	110	na	5.0
and dumplings	10 oz	430	940	24.0
and dumplings 'Family Entrées'	7 oz	280	(mq)	14.0
drumsnackers 'Platters'	7 oz	430	690	19.0
fettuccini 'Healthy Balance'	11.25 oz	320	650	7.0
fried	10 oz	400	1100	22.0
fried 'Extra Helping'	16 oz	570	1470	28.0
fried, white meat 'Extra Helping'	16 oz	570	1470	28.0
fried, white meat 'Platter'	9 oz	430	(mq)	22.0
fried, white meat, hot'n spicy 'Platter'	9 oz	430	(mq)	22.0
hot'n spicy 'Snack'n'	3.75 oz	140	480	9.0
nuggets, breast, Southern fried w/barbecue sauce	4.5 oz	370	930	23.0
nuggets, hot'n spicy, w/barbecue sauce	4.5 oz	360	820	21.0
nuggets, 'Platters'	6.4 oz	430	630	21.0

Food Name	Serv. Size	Total Cal.	Sod. MGS	Fat GMS
nuggets, Southern fried, w/barbecue sauce	4.5 oz	370	930	23.0
nuggets, w/barbecue sauce 'Extra Helping'	10 oz	640	1390	36.0
nuggets, w/sweet and sour sauce 'Extra Helping'	10 oz	650	(mq)	34.0
nuggets, w/sweet and sour sauce 'Microwave'	4.5 oz	360	770	21.0
parmesan, w/vermicelli 'Healthy Balance'	10.8 oz	290	710	10.0
patties, breast, Southern fried, w/biscuit	4 oz	320	980	14.0
patties 'Platters'	7.5 oz	380	760	21.0
pie	7 oz	550	860	36.0
pie 'Supreme Microwave'	7 oz	430	740	28.0
primavera and vegetable 'Cookin' Bags'	4 oz	100	(mq)	2.0
primavera and vegetable 'Family Entrées'	7 oz	140	(mq)	3.0
sweet and sour 'Cookin' Bags'	4 oz	130	na	2.0
(Budget Gourmet)				
and egg noodles, w/broccoli	10 oz	450	1110	26.0
cacciatore	11 oz	300	810	13.0
Marsala	10 oz	250	660	5.0
Mexicana	12.8 oz	510	1210	15.0
Oriental, and vegetables 'Light and Healthy'	9 oz	280	690	6.0
roast	11.2 oz	280	1110	7.0
sweet and sour, w/rice	10 oz	350	640	7.0
teriyaki	12 oz	360	610	12.0
w/fettuccini	10 oz	400	740	21.0
(Celentano)				
parmigiana	9 oz	330	560	20.0
primavera	11.5 oz	270	580	10.0
(Chun King)				
chow mein	13 oz	370	1560	6.0
imperial	13 oz	300	1540	1.0
walnut, crunchy	13 oz	310	1700	5.0
(Country Pride) primavera sticks	3 oz	240	400	15.
(Dining Lite)				
à la king	9 oz	240	780	7.
and noodles	9 oz	240	570	7.
chow mein	9 oz	180	650	2.0
glazed	9 oz	220	680	4.0
(Freezer Queen)				
à la king 'Cook-In-Pouch'	4 oz	70	460	1.
à la king, w/rice 'Single Serve'	9 oz	270	520	5.
cacciatore 'Single Serve'	9 oz	270	710	6.
croquettes, breaded, w/gravy 'Family Suppers'	7 oz	240	1000	12.
nuggets 'Deluxe Family Suppers'	3 oz	270	770	17.

Food Name	Serv. Size	Total Cal.	Sod. MGS	Fat GMS
nuggets platter	6 oz	410	950	23.0
pattie 'Platter'	7.5 oz	360	1160	17.0
primavera, sliced, w/gravy 'Cook-In-Pouch'	5 oz	80	820	3.0
sweet and sour, w/rice 'Single Serve'	9 oz	300	700	4.0
(Green Giant) and broccoli 'Entrées'	9.5 oz	340	890	15.0
(Healthy Choice)				
à l'orange	9 oz	260	340	2.0
and pasta divan	11.5 oz	300	520	4.0
and vegetables	11.5 oz	210	490	1.0
breast, glazed	8.5 oz	220	510	3.0
cacciatore 'Classics'	12.5 oz	310	430	3.0
chow mein	9 oz	240	530	5.0
chow mein, low fat, low cholesterol	9 oz	240	530	5.0
Dijon	11 oz	260	420	3.0
herb roasted	11 oz	380	470	7.0
honey mustard, low fat, low cholesterol	9.5 oz	250	480	3.0
Mandarin	10 oz	240	370	2.0
mesquite	10.5 oz	300	390	3.0
Oriental	11.25 oz	200	440	1.0
parmigiana	11.5 oz	290	340	6.0
roasted	12.3 oz	290	430	4.0
'Salsa Chicken Dinner'	11.25 oz	240	450	2.0
southwestern style, low fat, low cholesterol	12.5 oz	340	550	5.0
stir fry, w/vermicelli 'Extra Portion'	12 oz	300	550	5.0
sweet and sour	11.5 oz	280	320	2.0
teriyaki, low fat, low cholesterol	12.25 oz	290	560	4.0
w/barbecue sauce, low fat, low cholesterol	12.75 oz	410	550	6.0
(Hot Bites)				
drumsnackers	2.63 oz	220	530	15.0
nuggets	2.63 oz	210	550	14.0
nuggets, hot'n spicy	2.63 oz	250	380	19.0
nuggets, Southern fried	2.63 oz	220	530	14.0
nuggets, w/cheddar	2.63 oz	250	560	18.0
primavera sticks	2.63 oz	220	350	15.0
tenders, breast	2.25 oz	150	280	6.0
tenders, breast 'Microwave'	4 oz	260	560	10.0
(Kid Cuisine)				
fried	7.25 oz	420	1050	22.0
fried 'Mega Meal'	10.8 oz	720	1400	41.0
nuggets	6.25 oz	400	610	19.0
nuggets 'Mega Meal'	8.4 oz	470	1010	20.0

Food Name	Serv. Size	Total Cal.	Sod. MGS	Fat GMS
(LaChoy)				
almond, w/rice and vegetables 'Fresh & Lite'	9.75 oz	270	1092	8.0
imperial, w/rice 'Fresh & Lite'	11 oz	260	1269	6.0
Oriental, spicy 'Fresh & Lite'	9.75 oz	270	560	4.0
sweet and sour, w/rice and vegetables 'Fresh & Lite'	10 oz	260	601	3.0
(LeMenu)				
à la king	10.25 oz	330	830	13.0
à la king, w/seasoned rice 'LightStyle'	8.25 oz	240	670	5.0
breast, glazed 'LightStyle'	10 oz	230	430	3.0
breast, herb roasted, w/rice and vegetables	7.75 oz	260	500	6.0
cordon bleu	11 oz	460	850	20.0
Dijon, w/pasta and vegetables 'LightStyle'	8.5 oz	240	500	7.0
empress, w/seasoned rice 'LightStyle'	8.25 oz	210	690	5.0
herb-roasted 'LightStyle'	10 oz	240	400	7.0
in wine sauce	10 oz	280	680	7.0
Kiev	8 oz	530	780	39.0
parmigiana	11.75 oz	410	1030	20.0
sweet and sour	11.25 oz	400	1020	18.0
sweet and sour 'LightStyle'	10 oz	250	530	7.0
(Mrs. Paterson's) 'Aussie Pie'	5.5 oz	440	760	24.0
(Myers)				
à la gratin	3.5 oz	129	276	7.0
à la king	3.5 oz	137	357	9.0
and noodles	3.5 oz	136	399	8.0
creamed	3.5 oz	151	372	10.0
croquettes	3.5 oz	168	364	7.0
pie	3.5 oz	129	253	7.0
(Pilgrim's Pride) Cajun style	3 oz	241	480	17.0
(Pillsbury)				
and cheese casserole 'Microwave Classic'	1 pkg	480	940	29.0
casserole 'Microwave Classic'	1 pkg	400	890	22.0
(Right Course)				
Italiano, w/fettuccini and vegetables	9 5/8 oz	280	560	8.0
sesame primavera	10 oz	320	590	9.0
tenderloins in barbecue sauce	8.75 oz	270	590	6.0
tenderloins in peanut sauce	9.25 oz	330	570	10.0
(Shanghai) stir fry	10.3 oz	190	1220	3.0
(Smart Ones)				
a l'orange	8 oz	190	530	<1.0
chow mein	9 oz	170	470	1.0
fiesta, w/Spanish rice	8 oz	210	390	1.0

Food Name	Serv. Size	Total Cal.	Sod. MGS	Fat GMS
Francais, w/garlic vegetables	8.5 oz	150	400	1.0
grilled, glazed, and sauce	8 oz	130	540	1.0
honey mustard, and sauce	7.5 oz	140	220	1.0
Mirabella	9.2 oz	160	420	1.0
piccata, lemon herb	7.5 oz	160	500	1.0
(Stouffer's)				
à la king, w/rice	9.5 oz	270	800	5.0
a l'orange, w/almond rice, 'Lean Cuisine'	8 oz	280	290	4.0
and noodles, homestyle	10 oz	290	1040	13.0
and vegetables, w/vermicelli 'Lean Cuisine'	11.75 oz	240	500	5.0
breaded, baked, w/parsleyed potatoes and vegetables, 'Lean Cuisine'	8 oz	200	480	5.0
breast, baked, in gravy, w/potato, homestyle	8 7/8 oz	250	550	10.0
breast, fried, and whipped potatoes, homestyle	7 1/8 oz	350	900	18.0
breast, grilled, in barbecue sauce, homestyle	7 5/8 oz	210	550	7.0
breast, Marsala, w/vegetables, 'Lean Cuisine'	8 1/8 oz	180	430	4.0
breast, Parmesan, w/rib meat, 'Lean Cuisine'	10 7/8 oz	260	580	7.0
cacciatore, w/vermicelli, 'Lean Cuisine'	10 7/8 oz	280	570	7.0
chow mein, w/rice	10.75 oz	250	720	5.0
chow mein, w/rice, 'Lean Cuisine'	9 oz	240	530	5.0
creamed	6.5 oz	300	690	21.0
divan	8 oz	220	610	10.0
escalloped, and noodles	10 oz	420	840	24.0
fettuccini, 'Lean Cuisine'	9 oz	280	500	6.0
fettuccini, w/vegetable medley, homestyle	9.5 oz	350	780	17.0
fiesta, 'Lean Cuisine'	8.5 oz	240	560	5.0
glazed, w/vegetable rice, 'Lean Cuisine'	8.5 oz	250	590	7.0
honey mustard, 'Lean Cuisine'	7.5 oz	230	540	4.0
in barbecue sauce, w/rice pilaf, 'Lean Cuisine'	8.75 oz	260	500	6.0
Italiano, w/fettuccini 'Lean Cuisine'	9 oz	270	590	6.0
Oriental, w/vermicelli, 'Lean Cuisine'	9 oz	280	480	7.0
parmigiana and pasta Alfredo, homestyle	9 7/8 oz	360	990	15.0
pie	10 oz	440	750	27.0
sweet-n-sour, w/rice, 'Lean Cuisine'	9 oz	280	490	6.0
tenderloins in herb sauce, 'Lean Cuisine'	9.5 oz	240	490	5.0
tenderloins in peanut sauce, 'Lean Cuisine'	9 oz	290	530	7.0
tenders, breaded, w/potatoes, homestyle	8 3/8 oz	430	950	18.0
(Swanson)				
boneless 'Hungry Man'	17.75 oz	700	1530	28.0
cacciatore 'Homestyle Recipe'	10.95 oz	260	1030	8.0
fried, barbecue flavored	10 oz	540	1160	22.0

Food Name	Serv. Size	Total Cal.	Sod. MGS	Fat GMS
fried, dark meat	9.75 oz	560	1130	28.0
fried, dark meat 'Hungry Man'	1 pkg	860	1660	45.0
fried, white meat	10.25 oz	550	1460	25.0
fried, white meat 'Hungry Man'	1 pkg	870	2150	46.0
grilled, white meat in garlic sauce, almonds	10 oz	310	630	9.0
nibbles 'Homestyle Recipe'	4.25 oz	340	730	20.0
nibbles 'Plump & Juicy'	3.25 oz	300	690	19.0
nuggets	8.75 oz	470	650	23.0
nuggets 'Plump & Juicy'	3 oz	230	360	14.0
parmigiana 'Budget'	10 oz	300	780	15.0
pie 'Homestyle Recipe'	8 oz	410	1030	21.0
pie 'Hungry Man'	16 oz	630	1600	35.0
thighs/drumsticks 'Plump & Juicy'	3.25 oz	290	610	18.0
(Swift)				
cordon bleu 'International'	6 oz	360	1010	17.0
Kiev 'International'	6 oz	420	1030	24.0
(Tyson)				
a l'orange 'Gourmet Selection'	9.5 oz	300	670	8.0
and beef luau 'Gourmet Selection'	10.5 oz	330	1030	10.0
'Barbecue Chicken Meal'	12.5 oz	400	600	8.0
breast, boneless, barbecue marinated	3.75 oz	120	400	3.0
breast, boneless, butter garlic marinated	3.75 oz	160	320	7.0
breast, boneless, Italian marinated	3.75 oz	130	320	2.0
breast, boneless, lemon pepper marinated	3.75 oz	120	210	2.0
breast, boneless, teriyaki marinated	3.75 oz	130	290	2.0
breast strips, Oriental, boneless	2.75 oz	110	250	3.0
'Chick'n Cheddar' (Tyson)	2.6 oz	220	310	15.0
'Chick'n Chunks'	2.6 oz	220	500	15.0
'Chick'n Chunks' Southern fried	2.6 oz	220	540	15.0
'Chicken Marinara Meal'	13.75 oz	340	590	7.0
'Classic Colonial' wholesale club item	3.5 oz	180	190	9.0
'Cordon Bleu' wholesale club item	7 oz	480	1030	22.0
'Cordon Bleu' wholesale club item	5 oz	340	740	16.0
Dijon 'Gourmet Selection'	8.5 oz	310	840	17.0
Français 'Gourmet Selection'	9.5 oz	280	1130	14.0
glazed, w/sauce 'Gourmet Selections'	9.25 oz	240	930	4.0
grilled, 'Gourmet Selections'	7.75 oz	220	520	3.0
grilled, Italian 'Gourmet Selections'	9 oz	210	420	3.0
'Herb Chicken Meal'	13.75 oz	340	550	4.0
'Honey Mustard Chicken Meal'	13.75 oz	390	520	6.0
honey roasted 'Gourmet Selections'	9 oz	220	500	4.0

Food Name	Serv. Size	Total Cal.	Sod. MGS	Fat GMS
'Italian Style Chicken Meal'	13.75 oz	310	600	4.0
Kiev 'Gourmet Selection'	9.25 oz	520	1200	33.0
'Looney Tunes Bugs Bunny' chunks	7.7 oz	290	480	11.0
'Looney Tunes Road Runner'	6.7 oz	300	490	11.0
'Looney Tunes Tazmanian Devil' drummettes	8 oz	310	480	14.0
'Looney Tunes Yosemite Sam' barbecue glazed	7.38 oz	230	510	8.0
Marsala 'Gourmet Selection'	10.5 oz	300	900	13.0
mesquite breast tenders, boneless	2.75 oz	110	420	3.0
'Mesquite Chicken Meal'	13.25 oz	330	600	5.0
mesquite 'Gourmet Selections'	9 oz	320	660	8.0
'Mini Cordon Bleu' wholesale club item	1 piece	90	210	4.0
nuggets 'Microwave'	3.5 oz	220	(mq)	15.0
Oriental 'Gourmet Selection'	10.25 oz	270	1140	7.0
parmigiana 'Gourmet Selection'	11.25 oz	380	1100	17.0
piccata 'Gourmet Selection'	9 oz	240	680	10.0
pie, premium	9 oz	390	1065	20.0
pie, white meat, premium	9 oz	400	783	20.0
roasted 'Gourmet Selections'	9 oz	200	430	2.0
'Salsa Chicken Meal'	13.75 oz	370	470	6.0
'Sesame Chicken Meal'	13.5 oz	400	400	6.0
sesame 'Healthy Portions'	13.5 oz	390	410	5.0
stir fry w/vegetables, wholesale club item	3.5 oz	130	710	5.0
supreme 'Gourmet Selections'	9 oz	230	480	6.0
sweet and sour 'Gourmet Selection'	11 oz	420	850	15.0
tenders 'Microwave'	3.5 oz	230	(mq)	11.0
'Wings of Fire' wholesale club item	3.5 oz	220	390	12.0
(Ultimate 200)				
barbecue, glazed, w/vegetables	7 oz	200	450	6.0
cordon bleu, w/vegetables	7.7 oz	170	560	5.0
grilled, glazed	7.5 oz	150	520	2.0
imperial	8.5 oz	200	430	3.0
Kiev, w/vegetables and rice	7 oz	190	470	5.0
patty, Southern baked, w/vegetables	6.3 oz	170	520	7.0
teriyaki	7.6 oz	150	590	4.0
(Weaver)				
batter-dipped, assorted pieces	3.6 oz	290	550	18.0
crispy, light, skinless	2.9 oz	170	320	9.0
'Crispy Dutch Frye' assorted pieces	3.6 oz	290	550	18.0
'Crispy Dutch Frye' breast	4.5 oz	350	520	22.0
crispy mini drums	3 oz	210	480	12.0
croquettes	2 pieces	280	780	16.0

Food Name	Serv. Size	Total Cal.	Sod. MGS	Fat GMS
mini drums, herb and spice	3 oz	200	320	11.0
'Rondolet, Cheese'	2.6 oz	190	520	11.0
'Rondolet, Italian'	2.6 oz	190	560	11.0
'Rondolet, Original'	3 oz	190	610	10.0
'Tenders, Honey Batter'	3 oz	220	500	12.0
'Tenders, Premium'	3 oz	170	500	9.0
(Weight Watchers)				
fettuccini, w/Parmesan sauce	8.25 oz	280	590	9.0
ginger, w/vegetable, Hunan 'Stir Fry'	9 oz	160	430	2.0
grilled, Suiza, w/Spanish rice 'Mexican Style'	8.6 oz	220	590	7.0
orange glazed, w/rice 'Stir Fry'	9 oz	170	360	2.0
Polynesian 'Stir Fry'	9 oz	190	240	1.0
sesame, w/lo mein noodles 'Stir Fry'	9 oz	200	420	4.0
teriyaki, w/spring vegetables 'Stir Fry'	9 oz	140	470	3.0
'Tex Mex' w/Spanish rice 'Mexican Style'	8.3 oz	250	590	5.0

CHICKEN DINNER/ENTRÉE, PACKAGED

Food Name	Serv. Size	Total Cal.	Sod. MGS	Fat GMS
(Chicken By George)				
Cajun	5 oz	180	890	8.0
Caribbean grill	5 oz	200	610	6.0
Italian blue cheese	5 oz	180	890	8.0
lemon herb	5 oz	170	870	6.0
lemon oregano	5 oz	160	580	4.0
mesquite barbecue	5 oz	170	790	6.0
mustard dill	5 oz	180	640	7.0
roasted	5 oz	150	710	4.0
teriyaki	5 oz	180	740	5.0
tomato herb, w/basil	5 oz	190	800	7.0
(Chicken Helper) 'Skillet Dinner'				
cheesy broccoli, dry	1/5 pkg	160	700	2.0
cheesy broccoli, prepared	7 oz	310	790	9.0
creamy chicken, dry	1/5 pkg	170	720	5.0
creamy chicken, prepared	8.25 oz	330	820	13.0
creamy mushroom, dry	1/5 pkg	170	720	4.0
creamy mushroom, prepared	8 oz	320	810	11.0
fettuccini Alfredo, dry	1/5 pkg	160	690	4.0
fettuccini Alfredo, prepared	7.5 oz	320	780	12.0
stir fry, dry	1/5 pkg	170	800	<1.0
stir fry, prepared	7 oz	370	950	14.0
(Dinty Moore) and dumplings, microwave cup	7.5 oz	190	680	6.0
(LaChoy)				
sweet and sour, 'Dinner Classics' prepared	3/4 cup	310	860	6.0

ood Name	Serv. Size	Total Cal.	Sod. MGS	Fat GMS
sweet and sour, w/noodles	9.383 oz	256	697	3.1
ibby's)				
chow mein 'Diner' microwave cup	7.75 oz	130	830	4.0
w/pasta spirals 'Diner' microwave cup	7.75 oz	120	910	3.0
ipton) 'Microeasy'				
barbecue style, dry	1/4 pkg	110	980	<1.0
barbecue style, prepared	1/4 pkg	220	1020	6.0
country style, dry	1/4 pkg	80	840	<1.0
country style, prepared	1/4 pkg	190	880	6.0
Lunch Bucket)				
and dumplings, microwave cup	7.5 oz	140	880	2.0
w/beans and rice 'Light'n Healthy' micro cup	7.5 oz	170	600	3.0
Top Shelf)				
à la king	10 oz	360	890	10.0
Acapulco	1 serving	390	1320	13.0
breast, glazed	10 oz	170	780	2.0
breast, w/Spanish rice	10 oz	400	810	15.0
'Cacciatore'	10 oz	210	810	3.0
sweet and sour	1 serving	270	280	1.0
Ultra Slim Fast)				
and vegetables	12 oz	290	850	3.0
chow mein	12 oz	320	580	6.0
fettuccini	12 oz	390	980	12.0
mesquite	12 oz	350	300	1.0
roasted, in mushroom sauce	12 oz	280	830	6.0
sweet and sour	12 oz	330	340	2.0
HICKEN ENTRÉE, ALTERNATIVE				
(Worthington) pie, frozen	8 oz	380	1200	20.0
HICKEN FAT				
	1 cup	1846	0	204.6
	1 oz	178	9	19.3
	1 tbsp	115	0	12.8
HICKEN FRYING MIX, dry mix _(Golden Dipt)_	1 oz	90	1430	0.0
HICKEN GIBLETS				
fried	1 cup	402	164	19.5
simmered	1 cup	228	84	6.9
HICKEN GIZZARD				
all classes, simmered	1 cup	222	97	5.3
broiler-fryer, raw, approx 1.3 oz	1 med	44	28	1.6
broiler-fryer, simmered, approx .8 oz	1 med	34	15	0.8

Food Name	Serv. Size	Total Cal.	Sod. MGS	Fa GM
CHICKEN LIVER				
all classes, simmered	1 cup	220	71	7.
broiler-fryer, chopped, simmered	1 cup	219	71	7.
broiler-fryer, raw, approx 1.1 oz	1 liver	40	25	1.
broiler-fryer, simmered	4 oz	178	58	6.
CHICKEN POT PIE (Swanson), frozen	7 oz	380	760	22.
CHICKEN SALAD				
(Longacre)	1 oz	64	110	5.
(Longacre) 'Saladfest'	1 oz	47	150	3.
CHICKEN SALAD SPREAD, 'Spreadables' (Libby's)	1.9 oz	90	230	6.
CHICKEN SEASONING MIX				
(Featherweight) dry mix	1/4 pkg	18	30	0.
(Schilling) 'Bag 'n Season'	1 pkg	134	4771	5.
(Schilling) dry mix, for fried chicken	1/4 tsp	1	132	<.
CHICKEN SPREAD, CANNED				
(Hormel)	.5 oz	30	(mq)	2.
(Underwood) chunky	2 1/8 oz	150	440	9.
(Underwood) 'Light'	2 1/8 oz	80	330	3.
(Underwood) smoky	2 1/8 oz	150	290	8.
CHICKEN STEW				
(Dinty Moore) canned	7.5 oz	260	850	18.
(Dinty Moore) microwave cup	7.5 oz	260	850	18.
(Featherweight) w/wild rice, canned	7.5 oz	140	400	1.
(Heinz) w/dumplings, canned	7.5 oz	210	850	9.
(Mountain House) freeze-dried, prepared	1 cup	230	209	8.
(Swanson) canned	7 5/8 oz	160	990	7.
CHICORY, WITLOOF				
raw	1/2 cup	8	1	0.
raw, approx 2.1 oz	1 head	9	1	0.
trimmed	1 oz	4	2	<.
untrimmed	1 lb	61	28	0.
CHICORY GREENS				
trimmed	1 oz	7	13	0.
trimmed, chopped	1/2 cup	21	41	0.
untrimmed	1 lb	87	167	1.
CHICORY ROOT				
raw, approx 2.6 oz	1 root	44	30	0.
raw, 1-inch pieces	1/2 cup	33	23	0.
trimmed	1 oz	21	14	0.
untrimmed	1 lb	272	186	0.

ood Name	Serv. Size	Total Cal.	Sod. MGS	Fat GMS
CHILI, CANNED				
beef, w/beans *(Cimmaron)*	7.5 oz	230	na	9.0
chicken, w/beans *(Cimmaron)*	7.5 oz	180	970	5.0
chicken, w/beans *(Stagg)*	7.5 oz	200	na	6.0
'Chili Con Carne' *(Heinz)*	7.75 oz	350	1000	21.0
'Chili Mac' *(Chef Boyardee)*	7.5 oz	230	1410	11.0
'Chili Mac' *(Heinz)*	7.5 oz	250	860	12.0
country, w/beans *(Stagg)*	7.5 oz	270	na	12.0
plain *(Gebhardt)*	1 cup	530	990	41.0
vegetarian *(Gebhardt)*	4 oz	219	555	17.1
vegetarian *(Worthington)*	2/3 cup	190	550	10.0
vegetarian, plain *(Gebhardt)*	4.339 oz	232	736	18.5
vegetarian, plain *(Open Range)*	4.409 oz	176	608	12.8
vegetarian, spicy *(Hain)*	7.5 oz	160	1060	1.0
vegetarian, spicy *(Hain)* 'Reduced Sodium'	7.5 oz	170	200	1.0
vegetarian, spicy *(Natural Touch)*	2/3 cup	230	890	12.0
vegetarian, 3-bean, mild, fat-free *(Health Valley)*	5 oz	90	180	0.0
vegetarian, w/beans *(Gebhardt)*	4.444 oz	195	694	12.0
vegetarian, w/beans *(Just Rite)*	4.55 oz	190	616	13.3
vegetarian, w/beans *(Open Range)*	4.5 oz	136	645	8.0
vegetarian, w/beans, 'Longhorn' *(Gebhardt)*	4.55 oz	225	545	15.7
vegetarian, w/beans, mild *(Health Valley)*	4 oz	130	730	3.0
vegetarian, w/beans, mild *(Health Valley)* 'No Salt Added'	4 oz	130	25	3.0
vegetarian, w/beans, spicy *(Health Valley)*	4 oz	130	430	3.0
vegetarian, w/beans, spicy *(Health Valley)* 'No Salt Added'	4 oz	130	25	3.0
vegetarian, w/black beans, mild, fat-free *(Health Valley)*	5 oz	140	290	0.0
vegetarian, w/black beans, spicy, fat-free *(Health Valley)*	5 oz	70	180	0.0
vegetarian, w/lentils, mild *(Health Valley)*	4 oz	130	200	3.0
vegetarian, w/lentils, mild *(Health Valley)* 'No Salt Added'	4 oz	130	50	3.0
vegetarian, w/tempeh, spicy *(Hain)*	7.5 oz	160	1350	4.0
w/beans	1/2 cup	143	668	7.0
w/beans *(Armour)*	6 oz	320	870	22.0
w/beans *(Armour)*	7.5 oz	390	1080	26.0
w/beans *(Estee)*	7.5 oz	370	125	20.0
w/beans *(Featherweight)*	7.5 oz	280	440	10.0
w/beans *(Gebhardt)*	1 cup	495	1010	28.0
w/beans *(Just Rite)*	4 oz	200	500	11.0
w/beans *(Nalley's)*	7.5 oz	260	880	9.0
w/beans *(Van Camp's)*	1 cup	352	1215	23.2
w/beans *(Wolf Brand)*	8 oz	345	1013	22.0
w/beans '15-oz' *(Dennison's)*	7.5 oz	310	875	15.0

Food Name	Serv. Size	Total Cal.	Sod. MGS	Fa GM
w/beans '15-oz' (Hormel)	7.5 oz	310	1127	17.
w/beans '15-oz' (Libby's)	7.5 oz	270	810	13.
w/beans, '9.2 oz' (Quincy's)	1 serving	346	1380	16.
w/beans '24-oz' (Libby's)	8 oz	290	860	14.
w/beans '25-oz' (Hormel)	8 1/3 oz	350	1202	20.
w/beans '30-oz' (Dennison's)	7.5 oz	310	840	15.
w/beans '40-oz' (Dennison's)	8 oz	340	1050	17.
w/beans '40-oz' (Hormel)	8 oz	320	1135	17.
w/beans, beef (Chef Boyardee)	7.5 oz	330	1005	17.
w/beans, chunky (Dennison's)	7.5 oz	310	780	14.
w/beans, chunky (Hormel)	7.5 oz	290	780	14.
w/beans 'Cook-Off' (Dennison's)	7.5 oz	340	915	19.
w/beans, extra spicy (Wolf Brand)	7.75 oz	324	926	20.
w/beans, hot (Armour)	7.5 oz	390	1080	26
w/beans, hot (Gebhardt)	1 cup	470	1000	27.
w/beans, hot (Gebhardt)	4 oz	189	497	14
w/beans, hot (Heinz)	7.75 oz	330	1140	16.
w/beans, hot (Just Rite)	4 oz	195	495	10.
w/beans, hot (Nalley's)	7.5 oz	280	810	10
w/beans, hot '15 oz' (Hormel)	7.5 oz	310	1121	16.
w/beans, hot '15 oz' (Dennison's)	7.5 oz	310	910	16.
w/beans, hot '40 oz' (Dennison's)	8 oz	350	950	19.
w/beans, hot, jalapeño (Nalley's)	7.5 oz	260	920	10
w/beans 'Laredo' (Stagg)	7.5 oz	260	na	12
w/beans 'Micro-Cup' (Hormel)	7.5 oz	250	980	11.
w/beans 'Premium Lite' (Armour)	7.5 oz	260	1110	10
w/beans 'Thick' (Nalley's)	7.5 oz	260	840	9
w/chicken, spicy (Hain)	7.5 oz	130	1030	2
w/o beans (Armour)	7.5 oz	390	1150	31
w/o beans (Hormel)	10.5 oz	540	1384	41
w/o beans (Just Rite)	4 oz	180	515	11
w/o beans (Libby's)	7.5 oz	390	800	30
w/o beans (Van Camp's)	1 cup	412	1499	33
w/o beans (Wolf Brand)	8 oz	387	1042	26
w/o beans 'Big Chunk' (Nalley's)	7.5 oz	270	810	16
w/o beans 'Chili-Mac' (Wolf Brand)	7.75 oz	317	854	19
w/o beans '15 oz' (Dennison's)	7.5 oz	300	1380	19
w/o beans '15 oz' (Hormel)	7.5 oz	370	1012	28
w/o beans, 15 oz (Libby's)	7.5 oz	390	800	30
w/o beans '19 oz' (Dennison's)	9.5 oz	380	1335	24
w/o beans 'Steak House' (Stagg)	7.5 oz	300	na	19

Food Name	Serv. Size	Total Cal.	Sod. MGS	Fat GMS
w/o beans '25 oz' (Hormel)	8 1/3 oz	430	1070	33.0
w/o beans, extra spicy (Wolf Brand)	7.5 oz	363	962	24.9
w/o beans, hot '15 oz' (Hormel)	7.5 oz	370	985	28.0
w/o beans, w/franks 'Chilee Weenee' (Van Camp's)	1 cup	309	1057	15.7
CHILI, FREEZE-DRIED				
w/beans, prepared (Mountain House)	1 cup	390	153	16.0
w/beef 'Chili Mac' prepared (Mountain House)	1 cup	250	115	8.0
CHILI, FROZEN				
con carne 'Homestyle Recipe' (Swanson)	8.25 oz	270	740	10.0
con carne, w/beans (Stouffer's)	8.75 oz	260	1270	10.0
vegetarian (Right Course)	9.75 oz	280	590	7.0
CHILI, MICROWAVE				
'Chili Mac' micro cup (Hormel)	7.5 oz	192	977	9.0
w/beans (Armour)	7.5 oz	300	1120	14.0
w/beans, 'Diner' microwave cup (Libby's)	7.75 oz	280	820	12.0
w/beans, hot, micro cup (Hormel)	7.38 oz	250	977	11.0
w/beans, microwave cup (Lunch Bucket)	7.5 oz	300	1120	14.0
w/o beans, micro cup (Hormel)	7.38 oz	290	830	17.0
CHILI BEAN, CANNED. See also KIDNEY BEAN, CANNED; PINTO BEAN.				
(Gebhardt)	4.586 oz	134	630	1.0
(Hunt's)	4 oz	102	488	0.0
(Hunt's)	4.48 oz	87	597	1.0
(S&W)	1/2 cup	130	520	1.0
baked style, hot (Campbell's)	7.75 oz	180	870	4.0
caliente style (Green Giant)	1/2 cup	100	700	1.0
caliente style (Joan of Arc)	1/2 cup	100	700	1.0
extra spicy (Green Giant)	1/2 cup	100	580	1.0
extra spicy (Joan of Arc)	1/2 cup	100	580	1.0
50% less salt (Green Giant)	1/2 cup	100	310	1.0
50% less salt (Joan of Arc)	1/2 cup	100	310	1.0
hot (A&P)	1/2 cup	140	440	1.0
hot (Allens)	1/2 cup	90	420	<1.0
hot (Bush's Best)	1/2 cup	70	420	0.0
in chili gravy (Dennison's)	7.5 oz	180	770	1.0
in sauce (Hormel)	5 oz	130	453	3.0
Mexican style (Allens)	1/2 cup	135	430	<1.0
Mexican style (Van Camp's)	1 cup	210	730	2.4
spiced (Gebhardt)	4 oz	113	590	1.1
spicy 'Dry Beans in Sauce' (Green Giant)	1/2 cup	100	620	1.0
spicy 'Dry Beans in Sauce' (Joan of Arc)	1/2 cup	100	620	1.0

Food Name	Serv. Size	Total Cal.	Sod. MGS	Fat GMS
CHILI MIX				
'Chili Quick' dry (Gebhardt)	1.5-oz pkt	82	2784	1.1
'Chili con Carne' prepared (Old El Paso)	1 cup	162	510	7.0
'Homestyle Chili Fixins' (Hunt's)	4.656 oz	84	858	1.2
vegetarian, w/beans, prepared (Fantastic Foods)	1/2 cup	104	180	0.8
w/beans, prepared (Old El Paso)	1 cup	217	480	10.0
CHILI POWDER				
(Durkee)	1 tsp	11	0	0.01
(Laurel Leaf)	1 tsp	11	0	0.01
CHILI SAUCE. See SAUCE.				
CHILI SEASONING				
(Gebhardt)	1 tsp	6	30	0.0
(Gebhardt)	.0106 oz	1	0	0.0
(Gebhardt) mix 'Chili Quick'	1 tsp	10	165	<1.0
(Hain) hot	1/4 pkg	30	370	1.0
(Hain) medium	1/4 pkg	30	300	1.0
(Hain) mild	1/2 pkg	30	330	1.0
(Lawry's) 'Seasoning Blends'	1 pkg	143	2291	1.8
(Old El Paso)	1/5 pkg	21	717	1.0
(Schilling)	1/4 pkg	27	290	0.5
(Tio Sancho)	1.23 oz	109	832	2.2
CHIMICHANGA				
beef 'Primera' (Marquez)	1 chimichanga	380	890	17.0
CHIMICHANGA DINNER, FROZEN				
bean and cheese (Old El Paso)	1 pkg	380	610	19.0
beef (Old El Paso)	1 piece	370	470	21.0
beef and cheese 'Festive Dinners' (Old El Paso)	11 oz	510	1400	23.0
beef and pork (Old El Paso)	1 pkg	340	700	16.0
beef 'Festive Dinners' (Old El Paso)	11 oz	540	1200	21.0
chicken (Old El Paso)	1 piece	360	470	20.0
CHINESE APPLE. See POMEGRANATE.				
CHINESE CABBAGE. See CABBAGE, NAPA.				
CHINESE DATE				
dried	1 oz	81	3	0.3
raw, seeded	1 oz	22	1	0.1
raw, w/seeds	1 lb	331	11	0.8
CHINESE FUNGUS/Jew's ear				
approx .2 oz	1 piece	2	0	(tr)
sliced	1/2 cup	13	5	(tr)
trimmed	1 oz	7	3	na
untrimmed	1 lb	111	41	0.2

Food Name	Serv. Size	Total Cal.	Sod. MGS	Fat GMS
CHINESE GOOSEBERRY. See KIWI FRUIT.				
CHINESE NOODLE. See NOODLE, CHINESE.				
CHINESE PARSLEY. See CORIANDER.				
CHINESE RADISH				
boiled, drained	4 oz	19	15	0.3
boiled, drained, sliced	1/2 cup	13	10	0.2
dried	1/2 cup	157	161	0.4
dried	1 oz	77	79	0.2
raw, 7 inches long, 2 1/4 inches diam, approx 15.1 oz	1 med	62	71	0.3
raw, trimmed	1 oz	5	6	<.1
raw, trimmed (Frieda's)	1 lb	86	(mq)	0.5
raw, trimmed (Frieda's)	1 oz	5	(mq)	<.1
raw, trimmed, sliced	1/2 cup	8	9	<.1
raw, untrimmed	1 lb	65	75	0.4
CHINESE WATERMELON				
boiled, drained	4 oz	15	121	0.2
boiled, drained, cubes	1/2 cup	11	93	0.2
raw, cubes	1 cup	17	147	0.3
raw, trimmed	1 oz	4	31	0.1
raw, untrimmed	1 lb	42	358	0.6
CHINESE YAM. See JICAMA.				
CHIVES				
	1 oz	7	2	0.2
freeze-dried	1 tbsp	1	0	0.0
freeze-dried	1/4 cup	2	1	0.0
raw, chopped	1 tbsp	1	0	0.0
raw, chopped	1 tsp	0	0	0.0
CHOCOLATE, BAKING				
Bar				
semi-sweet (Baker's)	1 oz	140	0	9.0
semi-sweet (Nestlé)	1 oz	160	0	9.0
semi-sweet 'Premium' (Hershey's)	1 oz	140	0	8.0
sweet 'German' (Baker's)	1 oz	140	0	10.0
unsweetened (Baker's)	1 oz	140	0	15.0
unsweetened (Hershey's)	1 oz	190	5	16.0
unsweetened (Nestlé)	1 oz	180	0	14.0
unsweetened 'Premium' (Hershey's)	1 oz	190	5	16.0
white 'Premier' (Nestlé)	1 oz	150	15	9.0
Chips				
milk chocolate (Baker's)	1 oz	140	25	8.0
milk chocolate (Hershey's)	1/4 cup	220	55	12.0

Food Name	Serv. Size	Total Cal.	Sod. MGS	Fat GMS
milk chocolate *(Hershey's)*	1 oz	150	55	12.0
milk chocolate 'Big Chips' *(Baker's)*	1/4 cup	240	40	13.0
mint chocolate *(Hershey's)*	1.5 oz	230	<1	12.0
semi-sweet *(Baker's)*	1/4 cup	200	30	9.0
semi-sweet 'Big Chips' *(Baker's)*	1/4 cup	220	0	13.0
semi-sweet, mini, approx 1/4 cup *(Hershey's)*	1.5 oz	220	5	12.0
semi-sweet, real chocolate *(Baker's)*	1/4 cup	200	0	11.0
semi-sweet, regular *(Hershey's)*	1.5 oz	220	0	12.0
vanilla 'White' milk *(Hershey's)*	1.5 oz	240	65	14.0
Chunks				
milk chocolate, 12 pieces *(Hershey's)*	1 oz	160	25	9.0
semi-sweet *(Hershey's)*	1 oz	140	na	8.0
white 'Premier Treasures' *(Nestlé)*	1 oz	160	25	10.0
Grated, bitter	1 cup	667	5	70.0
Powder				
cocoa, 100% *(Nestlé)*	1 oz	80	5	5.0
cocoa 'Premium' *(Saco Foods)*	1 tbsp	15	51	0.9
Premelted, unsweetened 'Choco Bake' *(Nestlé)*	1 oz	190	na	16.0
Squares				
unsweetened, grated	1 cup	689	18	73.0
unsweetened, 1 oz	1 square	148	4	15.7
CHOCOLATE FLAVOR DRINK. See also DIET DRINK.				
Canned				
(Frostee)	8 oz	200	160	8.0
Dutch 'Lite' *(Sego)*	10 oz	150	480	3.0
liquid food, nutritionally complete *(Sustacal)*	8 oz	240	220	5.5
liquid nutrition *(Ensure)*	8 oz	250	200	8.8
liquid nutrition 'Plus' *(Ensure)*	8 oz	355	250	12.6
liquid nutrition, w/fiber *(Ensure)*	8 oz	260	200	8.8
'Lite' *(Sego)*	10 oz	150	480	3.0
malt 'Very Chocolate' *(Sego)*	10 oz	225	450	1.0
'Very Chocolate' *(Sego)*	10 oz	225	450	1.0
Mix/powder				
approx 2-3 heaping tsp	.8 oz	75	45	0.7
approx 2-3 heaping tsp, prepared w/1 cup 1% milk	1 cup	177	168	3.3
approx 2-3 heaping tsp, prepared w/1 cup 2% milk	1 cup	196	167	5.4
approx 2-3 heaping tsp, prepared w/1 cup skim milk	1 cup	161	171	1.1
'Chocolate Milk Maker' *(Swiss Miss)*	.6702 oz	73	55	0.3
classic chocolate chip *(Nestlé)*	1.13 oz	90	170	2.0
classic chocolate chip, prepared *(Nestlé)*	8 oz	180	300	2.0
creamy milk chocolate *(Nestlé)*	1.13 oz	90	150	2.0

Food Name	Serv. Size	Total Cal.	Sod. MGS	Fat GMS
creamy milk chocolate, prepared *(Nestlé)*	8 oz	180	280	2.0
dairy, reduced calorie, w/aspartame	.75-oz pkt	63	166	0.6
'Hershey's Chocolate Milk Mix' *(Hershey's)*	3 heaping tsp	90	40	<1.0
protein powder, prepared w/lowfat milk *(Turbo Nutrition)*	8 oz	330	450	6.0
'Quik' *(Nestlé)*	1 heaping tsp	90	25	1.0
'Quik' prepared w/skim milk *(Nestlé)*	1 cup	170	150	1.0
'Quik' prepared w/2% milk *(Nestlé)*	1 cup	210	150	5.0
'Quik' prepared w/whole milk *(Nestlé)*	1 cup	230	150	9.0
'Quik' sugar-free, approx 1 heaping tsp *(Nestlé)*	.2 oz	18	35	<1.0
'Quik' sugar-free, prepared w/2% milk *(Nestlé)*	1 cup	140	150	5.0
weight gain protein powder *(Turbo Nutrition)*	2 oz	210	320	1.0
Refrigerated				
'Hershey's Genuine' *(Hershey's)*	8 oz	150	85	2.0
(Yoo-Hoo)	9 oz	140	130	1.0
CHOCOLATE MILK				
whole	1 cup	208	149	8.5
whole	1 oz	26	19	1.1
whole *(Hershey's)*	1 cup	210	120	9.0
whole *(Nestlé Quik)*	1 cup	230	120	9.0
3.5% fat *(Hershey's)*	1 cup	210	120	8.0
2% fat	1 cup	179	150	5.0
2% fat *(Darigold)*	1 cup	190	210	5.0
2% fat *(Lucerne)*	1 cup	200	200	5.0
2% fat *(Hershey's)*	1 cup	190	130	5.0
2% fat 'Dutch Brand' *(Borden)*	1 cup	180	180	5.0
1% fat	1 cup	158	152	2.5
CHOCOLATE SAUCE. See SAUCE.				
CHOCOLATE SYRUP				
chocolate-flavored *(Hershey's)*	2 tbsp	103	19	.4
'Choco-Syp' *(Estee)*	1 tbsp	20	5	0.0
fudge-type	1 cup	1176	442	45.6
fudge type	1 oz	124	33	5.1
fudge-type	1 tbsp	73	27	2.8
'Quik' *(Nestlé)*	1.22 oz	100	45	1.0
unsweetened, 1 oz	1 pkt	134	3	13.5
w/added nutrients	1 cup	735	459	3.9
w/added nutrients	1 oz	92	57	0.5
w/added nutrients	1 tbsp	46	29	0.2
w/o added nutrients	1 cup	654	288	2.7
w/o added nutrients	1 oz	82	36	0.3

Food Name	Serv. Size	Total Cal.	Sod. MGS	Fat GMS
CHOCOLATE TOPPING				
(Kraft)	1 tbsp	50	15	0.0
(Mrs. Richardson's) dark chocolate fudge	2 tbsp	130	55	6.0
(Mrs. Richardson's) dark, fudge, microwavable	2 tbsp	130	55	6.0
(Nestlé) milk chocolate, w/almonds 'Candytops'	1.25 oz	230	15	18.0
(Nestlé) milk chocolate, w/crisps 'Crunch Candytops'	2 tbsp	220	40	17.0
(Nestlé) white chocolate, w/almonds 'Candytops'	1.25 oz	230	20	19.0
(Smucker's) chocolate fudge 'Magic Shell'	2 tbsp	190	50	15.0
(Smucker's) dark chocolate 'Special Recipe'	2 tbsp	130	45	1.0
(Smucker's) flavored syrup	2 tbsp	130	35	2.0
(Smucker's) 'Magic Shell'	2 tbsp	190	25	15.0
(Smucker's) milk chocolate fudge, Swiss	2 tbsp	140	70	1.0
(Smucker's) nut 'Magic Shell'	2 tbsp	200	40	16.0
CHORIZO				
	1 oz	129	350	10.9
4 inches	1 link	273	741	23.0
(Carmelita) beef	2.5 oz	250	510	23.0
(Carmelita) pork	2.5 oz	250	500	23.0
CHOW MEIN				
chicken, w/o noodles, can	1 cup	95	725	0.3
vegetarian, Mandarin, prepared w/tofu (Tofu Classics)	1/2 cup	110	390	6.0
CHOW MEIN NOODLE				
with almonds (Chun King)	1/3 cup	140	380	7.0
with sesame bits (Chun King)	1/3 cup	140	460	7.0
CHUB/cisco				
raw	1 lb	446	249	8.7
raw	1 oz	28	16	0.5
smoked	1 oz	50	135	3.3
smoked	1 oz	50	135	3.3
CILANTRO				
approx .8 oz	9 plants	4	6	0.1
trimmed	1 oz	6	8	0.2
trimmed	1/4 cup	1	1	<.1
untrimmed	1 lb	77	108	2.3
CILANTRO LEAF				
dried	1 oz	79	60	1.3
dried	1 tbsp	5	4	0.1
dried	1 tsp	2	1	<.1
CILANTRO SEED				
whole	1 oz	84	10	5.0
whole	1 tbsp	15	2	0.9

Food Name	Serv. Size	Total Cal.	Sod. MGS	Fat GMS
whole	1 tsp	5	1	0.3
whole (Spice Islands)	1 tsp	6	<1	0.3
CINNAMON				
ground	1 oz	74	7	0.9
ground	1 tbsp	18	2	0.2
ground	1 tsp	6	1	0.1
ground (Durkee)	1 tsp	8	0	tr
ground (Laurel Leaf)	1 tsp	8	0	tr
ground (Spice Islands)	1 tsp	6	<1	<.1
CISCO. See CHUB.				
CITRON, candied	1 oz	88	81	0.1
CITRUS COOLER DRINK (Gatorade) 'Thirst Quencher'	8 oz	50	110	0.0
CITRUS DRINK				
(Five Alive) chilled	6 oz	90	20	0.0
(Fruitopia) 'Citrus Consciousness' real fruit	8 oz	120	25	0.0
CITRUS DRINK MIX				
(Crystal Light) blend, sugar-free, w/NutraSweet	8 oz	4	0	0.0
(Five Alive) frozen, diluted	6 oz	90	na	0.0
CITRUS FRUIT JUICE DRINK				
frozen concentrate	12-oz can	685	13	0.4
frozen concentrate, diluted	1 cup	114	7	0.0
(Five Alive) aseptic box	8.45 oz	123	32	0.0
(Five Alive) chilled or frozen, berry, diluted	6 oz	88	21	0.1
(Five Alive) chilled or frozen, diluted	6 oz	87	23	0.0
(Five Alive) chilled or frozen, tropical, diluted	6 oz	85	19	0.1
(Hi-C) 'Citrus Cooler'	6 oz	95	17	<.1
CITRUS GRILL MARINADE (Lawry's)	2 tbsp	34	3350	0.4
CITRUS JUICE (Santa Cruz Natural) organic 'Cruz'	8 oz	125	na	<1.0
CITRUS PUNCH				
(Minute Maid) can or bottle 'Juices To Go'	6 oz	90	20	0.0
(Minute Maid) chilled	6 oz	90	20	0.0
(Tampico) 2% orange, tangerine, and lemon juice	8 oz	120	10	0.0
CITRUS PUNCH DRINK				
(Sunny Delight) 'California Style'	8 oz	100	95	0.0
(Sunny Delight) 'Florida Citrus Punch'.	8 oz	120	125	<1.0
(Sunny Delight) 'Florida Citrus Punch' plus calcium	8 oz	130	125	<1.0
CITRUS PUNCH MIX (Minute Maid) frozen, concentrate	6 oz	90	0	0.0
CITRUS SALAD (Florigold)	8 oz	120	3	0.0
CLAM, CANNED				
chopped (Gorton's)	3.25 oz	40	5.90	<1.0
chopped (Progresso)	1/2 cup	70	140	<1.0

Food Name	Serv. Size	Total Cal.	Sod. MGS	Fat GMS
chopped, w/liquid *(Doxsee)*	6.5 oz	100	1160	<1.0
chopped, w/liquid *(Orleans)*	6.5 oz	100	1160	<1.0
minced *(Gorton's)*	3.25 oz	40	5.90	<1.0
minced *(Progresso)*	1/2 cup	70	140	<1.0
minced, w/liquid *(Doxsee)*	6.5 oz	100	1160	<1.0
minced, w/liquid *(Orleans)*	6.5 oz	100	1160	<1.0
mixed species, drained	1 cup	237	179	3.1
mixed species, drained	4 oz	168	127	2.2
mixed species, drained	3 oz	126	95	1.7
mixed species, liquid only	1 cup	5	516	0.1
mixed species, liquid only	3 oz	2	183	0.0
CLAM, MIXED SPECIES				
boiled	4 oz	168	127	2.2
breaded and fried	20 small	380	684	21.0
breaded and fried	4 oz	229	413	12.6
breaded and fried	3 oz	172	309	9.5
moist-heat cooked	20 small	133	101	1.8
moist-heat cooked	3 oz	126	95	1.7
poached	4 oz	168	127	2.2
raw	1 lb	335	253	4.4
raw	1 oz	21	16	0.3
raw	20 small	133	101	1.8
raw	9 large	133	101	1.8
raw	3 oz	63	48	0.8
steamed	4 oz	168	127	2.2
CLAM, STUFFED, New England style *(Matlaw's)*	2 clams	180	730	8.0
CLAM JUICE				
(Doxsee)	3 oz	4	110	0.0
(Snow's)	3 oz	4	110	0.0
CLAM SAUCE. See SAUCE.				
CLAM TOMATO JUICE, canned	5.5 oz	76	664	0.2
CLARIFIED BUTTER. See GHEE.				
CLEARMALT. See ALCOHOLIC BEVERAGES.				
CLOVES				
ground	1 tbsp	21	16	1.3
ground	1 tsp	7	5	0.4
ground *(Durkee)*	1 tsp	9	0	<0.1
ground *(Laurel Leaf)*	1 tsp	9	0	<0.1
ground *(Spice Islands)*	1 tsp	7	4	0.2
CLUB SODA. See SOFT DRINKS AND MIXERS.				
COATING MIX. See SEASONING AND COATING MIX.				

Food Name	Serv. Size	Total Cal.	Sod. MGS	Fat GMS
COBBLER				
Fresh				
apple *(Stilwell)*	4 oz	200	225	4.0
apple, deep dish *(Awrey's)*	1/8 pie	320	300	14.0
blueberry, deep dish *(Awrey's)*	1/8 pie	310	360	14.0
Frozen				
apple, 4.33 oz *(Pet-Ritz)*	1/6 pkg	290	(mq)	9.0
blackberry *(Stilwell)*	4 oz	280	220	8.0
blackberry, 4.33 oz *(Pet-Ritz)*	1/6 pkg	250	(mq)	10.0
blueberry, 4.33 oz *(Pet-Ritz)*	1/6 pkg	370	(mq)	12.0
cherry *(Stilwell)*	4 oz	250	205	6.0
cherry, 4.33 oz *(Pet-Ritz)*	1/6 pkg	280	(mq)	10.0
peach *(Stilwell)*	4 oz	270	200	5.0
peach, 4.33 oz *(Pet-Ritz)*	1/6 pkg	260	(mq)	10.0
strawberry, 4.33 oz *(Pet-Ritz)*	1/6 pkg	290	(mq)	9.0
COBNUT, SHELLED. See HAZELNUT, SHELLED.				
COCOA BUTTER OIL				
	1 cup	1927	0	218.0
	1 oz	251	0	28.4
	1 tbsp	120	0	13.6
COCOA MIX				
Amaretto creme flavor *(Swiss Miss)*	1.25 oz	150	220	3.0
Bavarian chocolate, hot cocoa *(Swiss Miss)*	1 oz	110	170	3.0
chocolate, w/marshmallows *(Carnation)*	1 oz	110	120	1.2
chocolate almond mocha *(Swiss Miss)*	1.235 oz	144	207	2.7
chocolate and mint 'Cocoa Classics' *(Land O'Lakes)*	1 envelope	160	160	5.0
chocolate and raspberry 'Cocoa Classics' *(Land O'Lakes)*	1 envelope	160	160	5.0
chocolate Bavarian mint *(Swiss Miss)*	1.235 oz	142	231	2.3
chocolate English toffee *(Swiss Miss)*	1.235 oz	142	223	2.3
chocolate flavor *(Pathmark)*	1 oz	110	110	1.0
chocolate flavor *(Swiss Miss)*	1 oz	110	125	1.0
chocolate flavor 'Sugar-free' *(Swiss Miss)*	.5 oz	50	130	1.0
chocolate fudge flavor *(Carnation)*	1-oz pkt	110	135	1.3
chocolate praline and creme *(Swiss Miss)*	1.235 oz	142	223	2.3
chocolate raspberry truffle *(Swiss Miss)*	1.235 oz	144	220	2.8
chocolate supreme 'Cocoa Classics' *(Land O'Lakes)*	1 envelope	160	160	5.0
dark chocolate truffle *(Swiss Miss)*	1.235 oz	142	225	2.5
diet *(Swiss Miss)*	.26 oz	20	180	<1.0
diet 'Hot Cocoa Mix' *(Swiss Miss)*	.26 oz	22	205	0.2
double rich chocolate flavor *(Swiss Miss)*	1 oz	110	125	1.0

Food Name	Serv. Size	Total Cal.	Sod. MGS	Fat GMS
fat-free 'Hot Cocoa Mix' (Swiss Miss)	.5 oz	50	197	0.3
lite (Swiss Miss)	.75 oz	70	160	<1.0
lite 'Hot Cocoa Mix' (Swiss Miss)	.7407 oz	74	197	0.5
marshmallow lovers 'Hot Cocoa Mix' (Swiss Miss)	1.199 oz	132	167	1.5
milk chocolate flavor (Alba '66)	.68 oz	60	160	0.0
milk chocolate flavor (Saco Foods)	1 oz	110	150	1.0
milk chocolate flavor (Swiss Miss)	1-oz pkt	110	170	3.0
milk chocolate flavor 'Sugar-free' (Swiss Miss)	.5 oz	60	125	1.0
milk chocolate flavor, w/marshmallows (Alba '66)	.68 oz	60	160	0.0
milk chocolate 'Hot Cocoa Mix' (Swiss Miss)	1.199 oz	133	169	1.5
milk chocolate 'Hot Cocoa Mix' (Swiss Miss)	1 oz	110	139	1.3
milk chocolate w/mini marshmallows 'Hot Cocoa Mix' (Swiss Miss)	1.199 oz	132	181	1.5
milk chocolate w/mini marshmallows 'Hot Cocoa Mix' (Swiss Miss)	1 oz	109	149	1.3
milk flavor (Carnation)	1-oz pkt	110	130	1.1
mini (Pathmark)	1 oz	110	140	1.0
mint flavor (Featherweight)	.44 oz	50	110	1.0
mocha flavor 'Sugar-free' (Carnation)	1 pkt	50	140	0.3
reduced calorie, aspartame sweetened	1 oz	8	(mq)	0.1
regular (Finast)	6 oz	110	150	1.0
rich, sugar-free 'Hot Cocoa Mix' (Swiss Miss)	.5 oz	50	165	0.3
rich chocolate 'Hot Cocoa Mix' (Swiss Miss)	1 oz	110	166	1.2
rich milk flavor (Carnation)	1-oz pkt	110	120	1.1
rich milk flavor 'Sugar-free' (Carnation)	1 pkt	50	160	0.4
rich milk flavor, w/marshmallows (Weight Watchers)	1 pkt	60	160	0.0
'70-Calorie' (Carnation)	1 pkt	70	135	0.4
'Sugar-free' (Hills Bros)	3 tbsp	60	145	2.0
sugar-free 'Hot Cocoa Mix' (Swiss Miss)	.7055 oz	67	242	0.3
sugar-free 'Hot Cocoa Mix' (Swiss Miss)	.5 oz	49	179	0.2
sugar-free, sweetened w/NutraSweet (Saco Foods)	1 pkt	50	150	1.0
sugar-free, w/mini marshmallows 'Hot Cocoa Mix' (Swiss Miss)	.7055 oz	68	210	0.8
sugar-free, w/mini marshmallows 'Hot Cocoa Mix' (Swiss Miss)	.5 oz	51	159	0.6
vending 'Hot Cocoa Mix' (Swiss Miss)	1.34 oz	146	185	1.7
white chocolate 'Hot Cocoa Mix' (Swiss Miss)	1 oz	111	130	1.4
w/added nutrients	1-oz pkt	120	201	3.0
w/added nutrients, prepared	1 pkt	119	207	2.9
w/aspartame	.53-oz pkt	48	104	0.4
w/aspartame, w/added calcium and potassium	.53-oz pkt	48	98	0.5

Food Name	Serv. Size	Total Cal.	Sod. MGS	Fat GMS
w/aspartame, w/added sodium and vitamin A	.53-oz pkt	48	168	0.5
w/marshmallows *(Carnation)*	1-oz pkt	110	120	1.0
w/mini marshmallows *(Finast)*	6 oz	110	150	1.0
w/mini marshmallows *(Swiss Miss)*	1 oz	110	140	1.0
w/mini marshmallows 'Sugar-free' *(Swiss Miss)*	.5-oz pkt	50	120	<1.0
w/o added nutrients	1-oz pkt	103	143	1.1
w/o added nutrients, prepared	3-4 heaping tsp	103	148	1.2

COCOA POWDER. See also CHOCOLATE, BAKING.

Food Name	Serv. Size	Total Cal.	Sod. MGS	Fat GMS
(Bensdorp)	1 oz	130	5	7.0
(Hershey's) approx 1/3 cup	1 oz	120	10	4.0
(Hershey's) 'European'	1 oz	90	15	3.0
(Hershey's) unsweetened, European style	1 cup	170	52	8.3
(Hershey's) unsweetened, European style	1 tbsp	10	3	0.5
(Nestlé)	1.5 oz	180	6	6.0

COCONUT

Food Name	Serv. Size	Total Cal.	Sod. MGS	Fat GMS
mature kernel, in shell	1 lb	834	47	79.0
mature kernel, shelled	1 oz	100	6	9.5
mature kernel, shelled, grated, packed	1 cup	460	26	43.5
meat, raw, 2 x 2 x 1/2 inch	1 piece	159	9	15.1
meat, raw, shredded	1 cup	283	16	26.8

COCONUT, DRIED

Food Name	Serv. Size	Total Cal.	Sod. MGS	Fat GMS
creamed	1 oz	194	11	19.6
sweetened, flaked, canned	4 oz	505	23	36.1
sweetened, flaked, canned	1 cup	341	15	24.4
sweetened, flaked, canned	1 oz	126	6	9.0
sweetened, flaked, canned 'Angel Flake' *(Baker's)*	1/3 cup	110	5	9.0
sweetened, flaked, packaged	7-oz pkg	943	509	64.0
sweetened, flaked, packaged	1 cup	351	189	23.8
sweetened, flaked, packaged	1 oz	134	73	9.1
sweetened, flaked, packaged 'Angel Flake' *(Baker's)*	1/3 cup	120	75	8.0
sweetened, flaked, packaged 'Snowflake' *(Finast)*	1 oz	137	<1	9.0
sweetened, flaked, packaged, toasted *(Baker's)*	1/3 cup	200	85	17.0
sweetened, shredded	7-oz pkg	997	521	70.6
sweetened, shredded	1 cup	466	244	33.0
sweetened, shredded	1 oz	142	74	10.1
sweetened, shredded 'Premium Shred' *(Baker's)*	1/3 cup	140	85	9.0
sweetened, shredded, toasted	1 oz	168	11	13.4
sweetened, shredded, toasted 'Angel Flake' *(Baker's)*	1/3 cup	200	85	17.0
unsweetened	1 oz	187	11	18.3

Food Name	Serv. Size	Total Cal.	Sod. MGS	Fat GMS
COCONUT CREAM				
Canned				
liquid expressed from grated meat	1 cup	568	148	52.5
liquid expressed from grated meat	1 tbsp	36	10	3.4
sweetened	1 oz	54	14	5.0
sweetened (Coco Lopez)	2 tbsp	120	10	5.0
sweetened (Holland House)	1 oz	81	21	(mq)
Raw				
liquid expressed from grated meat	1 cup	792	10	83.2
liquid expressed from grated meat	1 tbsp	49	1	5.2
liquid expressed from grated meat	1 oz	94	1	9.8
COCONUT MILK				
canned	1 cup	445	29	48.2
canned	1 oz	56	4	6.0
canned	1 tbsp	30	2	3.2
frozen	1 cup	485	29	49.9
frozen	1 oz	57	3	5.9
frozen	1 tbsp	30	2	3.1
raw	1 cup	552	36	57.2
raw	1 oz	65	4	6.8
raw	1 tbsp	35	2	3.6
COCONUT NECTAR (Knudsen & Sons)	8 oz	150	na	0.0
COCONUT OIL				
	1/2 cup	964	0	109.0
	1 oz	251	0	28.4
	1 tbsp	120	0	13.6
(Hain)	1 tbsp	120	0	14.0
COCONUT PINEAPPLE NECTAR, can or bottle (Kern's)	6 oz	140	25	4.0
COCONUT VEGETABLE OIL				
	1 cup	1879	0	218.0
	1 tbsp	117	0	13.6
COCONUT WATER				
	1 cup	46	252	0.5
	1 oz	5	30	0.1
	1 tbsp	3	16	0.0
COD, ALASKAN				
raw	1 oz	55	16	4.3
raw, 6.8 oz	1/2 fillet	377	108	29.5
smoked	4 oz	291	836	22.8
COD, ATLANTIC				
baked	4 oz	119	88	1.0

Food Name	Serv. Size	Total Cal.	Sod. MGS	Fat GMS
broiled	4 oz	119	88	1.0
dried and salted	3 oz	247	5973	2.0
dried and salted	1 oz	81	1968	0.7
dry-heat cooked	3 oz	89	66	0.7
microwaved	4 oz	119	88	1.0
raw	1 lb	372	246	3.1
raw	3 oz	70	46	0.6
raw	1 oz	23	15	0.2
COD, BLACK				
raw	1 lb	886	254	69.4
raw	1 oz	55	16	4.3
smoked	1 oz	73	209	5.7
COD, FROZEN				
breaded 'Light' *(Mrs. Paul's)*	1 piece	240	430	11.0
breaded 'Light' *(Van de Kamp's)*	1 piece	250	510	11.0
breaded, lemon thyme crumb 'Select' *(Gorton's)*	1 fillet	90	240	2.0
fillet *(Booth)*	4 oz	89	350	1.0
fillet *(Finast)*	4 oz	80	200	1.0
fillet *(SeaPak)*	4 oz	90	135	1.0
fillet 'Fishmarket Fresh' *(Gorton's)*	5 oz	110	90	1.0
fillet 'Individually Wrapped' *(Booth)*	4 oz	90	80	1.0
fillet, light *(Van de Kamp's)*	1 piece	250	510	11.0
fillet, natural *(Van de Kamp's)*	4 oz	90	90	1.0
natural *(Van de Kamp's)*	4 oz	90	90	1.0
COD, PACIFIC				
dry-heat cooked	3 oz	89	77	0.7
fillets, raw *(Peter Pan Seafoods)*	3.5 oz	80	71	0.6
raw	1 lb	372	322	2.9
raw	3 oz	70	60	0.5
raw	1 oz	23	20	0.2
COD CAKE, CANNED, 2 cakes *(Gorton's)*	4 oz	100	640	<1.0
COD ENTRÉE, FROZEN				
fillet, au gratin *(Booth)*	9.5 oz	280	1160	11.0
fillet, Florentine *(Booth)*	9.5 oz	244	880	6.0
fillet, w/lemon butter sauce and rice *(Booth)*	9.5 oz	567	1330	38.0
fillet, w/mushroom sauce and rice *(Booth)*	9.5 oz	280	1010	11.0
COD LIVER OIL				
cherry *(Hain)*	1 tbsp	120	0	14.0
mint *(Hain)*	1 tbsp	120	0	14.0
regular	1 cup	1966	0	218.0
regular	1 tbsp	123	0	13.6

Food Name	Serv. Size	Total Cal.	Sod. MGS	Fat GMS
regular *(Hain)*	1 tbsp	120	0	14.0
COD NUGGETS, FROZEN				
minced, crunchy 'Bunch O'Crunch' 4 oz *(Frionor)*	8 pieces	320	411	21.0
COFFEE				
brewed	6 oz	4	2	0.0
brewed 'Regular' *(Chock Full o'Nuts)*	6 oz	2	0	0.0
freeze-dried, prepared, dark roast 'Maragor' *(Taster's Choice)*	8 oz	4	0	<1.0
freeze-dried, prepared 'Colombian Select' *(Taster's Choice)*	8 oz	4	0	<1.0
freeze-dried, prepared 'Original' *(Taster's Choice)*	8 oz	4	0	<1.0
COFFEE, ALTERNATIVE				
cereal grain beverage, powder *(Pero)*	1 serving	4	2	0.0
cereal grain beverage, powder *(Pionier)*	1 serving	6	0	0.0
cereal grain beverage, powder, dry	1 tsp	9	2	0.1
cereal grain beverage, powder,'Instant,' prepared *(Postum)*	6 oz	12	0	0.0
cereal grain beverage, prepared w/water	1 tsp	9	7	0.0
cereal grain beverage, prepared w/skim milk	6 oz	74	97	0.4
cereal grain beverage, prepared w/1% milk	6 oz	86	94	2.0
cereal grain beverage, prepared w/2% milk	6 oz	100	94	3.6
cereal grain beverage, prepared w/whole milk	6 oz	120	91	6.1
cereal grain beverage, w/o added ingredients *(Kaffree Roma)*	8 oz	6	(mq)	0.0
COFFEE, DECAFFEINATED				
(Chock Full o'Nuts)	6 oz	2	0	0.0
freeze-dried, prepared, dark roast 'Maragor' *(Taster's Choice)*	8 oz	4	0	<1.0
freeze-dried, prepared 'Original' *(Taster's Choice)*	8 oz	4	0	<1.0
instant, powder	1 round tsp	4	0	0.0
instant, powder, prepared	6 oz	4	5	0.0
instant, prepared 'Decaf' *(Nescafé)*	8 oz	4	0	<1.0
instant, w/chicory, prepared *(Mountain Blend)*	8 oz	6	0	<1.0
'Suisse Mocha International' *(General Foods)*	6 oz	50	30	3.0
'Suisse Mocha International' sugar-free *(General Foods)*	6 oz	30	30	2.0
COFFEE, FLAVORED				
'Cafe Amaretto International' prepared *(General Foods)*	6 oz	50	20	2.0
'Cafe Français International' prepared *(General Foods)*	6 oz	60	25	3.0
'Cafe Français International' sugar-free prepared *(General Foods)*	6 oz	35	30	2.0
'Cafe Irish Creme International' prepared *(General Foods)*	6 oz	50	15	2.0
cafe vienna 'Cafe Coffees' prepared *(Hills Bros)*	6 oz	60	35	2.0
'Cafe Vienna International' prepared *(General Foods)*	6 oz	60	110	2.0
'Cafe Vienna International' sugar-free, prepared *(General Foods)*	6 oz	30	80	2.0

Food Name	Serv. Size	Total Cal.	Sod. MGS	Fat GMS
'Cappio Cinnamon Iced Cappuccino' (Maxwell House)	8 oz	130	70	3.0
'Cappio Coffee Iced Cappuccino' (Maxwell House)	8 oz	120	75	3.0
'Cappio Mocha Iced Cappuccino' (Maxwell House)	8 oz	130	65	2.0
'Cinnamon Hot Cappuccino' (Maxwell House)	6 oz	60	100	1.0
'Coffee Hot Cappuccino' (Maxwell House)	6 oz	60	110	1.0
'Double Dutch Chocolate International' prepared (General Foods)	6 oz	50	15	2.0
'Dutch Chocolate Mint International' prepared (General Foods)	6 oz	50	80	2.0
'French Vanilla Cafe International' prepared (General Foods)	6 oz	60	50	3.0
'Hazelnut Belgian Cafe International' prepared (General Foods)	6 oz	60	55	2.0
mocha, banana nut 'sugar-free' prepared (MJB)	6 oz	39	60	1.8
mocha, cherry, prepared (MJB)	6 oz	53	17	1.4
mocha, fudge 'sugar-free' prepared (MJB)	6 oz	39	88	1.8
mocha, mint, prepared (MJB)	6 oz	53	16	1.3
mocha, mint 'sugar-free' prepared (MJB)	6 oz	37	43	1.3
mocha, prepared (MJB)	6 oz	52	54	1.3
mocha, Swiss 'Cafe Coffees' prepared (Hills Bros)	6 oz	60	10	2.0
mocha, Swiss 'Cafe Coffees Sugar-free' prepared (Hills Bros)	6 oz	40	25	2.0
mocha, vanilla 'sugar-free' prepared (MJB)	6 oz	39	50	1.7
'Mocha Hot Cappuccino' (Maxwell House)	6 oz	70	80	2.0
orange, Capri 'Cafe Coffees' prepared (Hills Bros)	6 oz	60	30	2.0
'Orange Cappuccino International' prepared (General Foods)	6 oz	60	100	2.0
'Orange Cappuccino International' sugar-free, prepared (General Foods)	6 oz	30	60	2.0
'Suisse Mocha International' prepared (General Foods)	6 oz	50	15	3.0
'Suisse Mocha International' sugar-free, prepared (General Foods)	6 oz	30	15	2.0
'Viennese Chocolate Cafe International' prepared (General Foods)	6 oz	50	20	2.0
COFFEE, INSTANT				
'Brava' prepared (Nescafé)	8 oz	4	0	<1.0
'Classic' prepared (Nescafé)	8 oz	4	0	<1.0
powder (Kava)	1 tsp	2	5	0.0
prepared (Nescafé)	8 oz	4	0	<1.0
regular powder	1 oz	68	10	0.1
regular, powder	1 round tsp	4	1	0.0

Food Name	Serv. Size	Total Cal.	Sod. MGS	Fat GMS
regular, prepared	6 oz	4	5	0.0
'Silka' prepared *(Nescafé)*	8 oz	4	0	<1.0
w/chicory, powder	1 round tsp	6	5	0.0
w/chicory, prepared	6 oz	7	11	0.0
w/chicory, prepared *(Sunrise)*	8 oz	6	0	<1.0
w/chicory 'Mountain Blend' prepared *(Nescafé)*	8 oz	6	0	<1.0
w/sugar, cappuccino flavor, powder	2 round tsp	62	98	2.1
w/sugar, cappuccino flavor, prepared	6 oz	61	104	2.1
w/sugar, French flavor, powder	2 round tsp	57	24	3.4
w/sugar, French flavor, prepared	6 oz	57	30	3.4
w/sugar, mocha flavor, powder	2 round tsp	51	31	1.9
w/sugar, mocha flavor, prepared	6 oz	51	36	1.9
COFFEE FLAVOR DRINK, canned, liquid nutrition *(Ensure)*	8 oz	250	na	8.8

COFFEE LIQUEUR. See ALCOHOLIC BEVERAGES.

COLA BEVERAGE. See SOFT DRINKS AND MIXERS.

COLD CUTS. See LUNCHEON MEATS.

COLE. See KALE.

COLESLAW

fresh	4 oz	78	26	3.0
fresh	1/2 cup	41	14	1.6
fresh	1 tbsp	6	2	0.2

COLESLAW DRESSING

(Kraft)	1 tbsp	70	200	6.0
(Kraft) 'Miracle Whip'	1 tbsp	70	105	6.0
(Litehouse) refrigerated	1 tbsp	80	41	8.0
(T. Marzetti) light	1 tbsp	50	240	3.0
(T. Marzetti) original	1 tbsp	79	180	7.0
(T. Marzetti) 'South Recipe'	1 tbsp	66	93	5.0

COLEWORT. See KALE.

COLLARDS

boiled, drained	4 oz	31	18	0.2
boiled, drained, chopped	1/2 cup	17	161	0.1
raw, chopped	1/2 cup	6	4	0.0
raw, trimmed	1 oz	9	6	0.1
raw, untrimmed	1 lb	80	51	0.6
Canned				
chopped *(Allens)*	1/2 cup	20	15	<1.0
chopped, greens *(Bush's Best)*	1/2 cup	30	320	0.0
chopped, w/pork *(Luck's)*	7.5 oz	90	420	7.0
Frozen				
boiled, drained	4 oz	41	57	0.5

Food Name	Serv. Size	Total Cal.	Sod. MGS	Fat GMS
chopped *(Seabrook)*	3.3 oz	25	45	0.0
chopped *(Southern)*	3.5 oz	30	60	0.4
chopped, boiled, drained	1/2 cup	31	43	0.4
chopped, unprepared	10-oz pkg	94	136	1.0
COLORADO PINYON PINE NUT. See PINE NUT.				
CONCORD PUNCH, 'Juices To Go' *(Minute Maid)*	6 oz	90	20	0.0
CONDIMENTS. See individual listings.				
COOKIE				
ALMOND				
(Health Valley) date 'Fruit Jumbos'	1 cookie	70	30	3.0
(Mother's) shortbread	2 cookies	120	50	7.0
(Natures Warehouse) butter, approx 1 oz	2 cookies	122	41	4.1
(Stella D'oro) 'Breakfast Treats'	1 cookie	101	(mq)	3.6
(Stella D'oro) 'Chinese Dessert'	1 cookie	169	(mq)	8.9
(Stella D'oro) toast 'Mandel'	1 cookie	58	(mq)	1.4
AMARANTH *(Health Valley)*	1 cookie	90	30	3.0
ANGEL WINGS *(Stella D'oro)*	1 cookie	74	(mq)	4.7
ANIMAL CRACKERS				
(FFV)	1.25-oz pkg	160	150	6.0
(Finast) 15 pieces	1 oz	120	110	3.0
(Grandma's) candied, 5 cookies	1 oz	140	80	6.0
(Keebler) approx .5 oz	5 cookies	70	75	2.0
(Mother's) circus animal	4 cookies	110	40	6.0
(Nabisco) 'Barnum's Animals' 5 1/2 pieces	.5 oz	60	70	2.0
(Sunshine)	13 cookies	130	160	4.0
ANISE				
(Stella D'oro) 'Anisette Sponge'	1 cookie	51	(mq)	0.8
(Stella D'oro) 'Anisette Toast'	1 cookie	46	(mq)	0.6
(Stella D'oro) 'Anisette Toast Jumbo'	1 cookie	109	(mq)	1.0
APPLE				
(Archway) n' raisin	1 cookie	120	169	3.0
(Bakery Wagon) cinnamon	1 cookie	100	100	3.0
(Bakery Wagon) filled oatmeal	1 cookie	90	115	4.0
(Bakery Wagon) walnut raisin	1 cookie	100	110	3.0
(Break Cake) sandwich	1 cookie	90	70	3.0
(Estee) cinnamon 'Snack Crisps' new blue pkg	.66 oz	80	75	2.0
(Frookie) cinnamon oat bran	1 cookie	45	35	2.0
(Frookie) 'Fruitins'	1 cookie	60	25	1.0
(Frookie) spice, fat-free	1 cookie	50	80	0.0
(Great Cakes)	4.5 oz	260	20	6.0
(Health Valley) cinnamon 'Mini Fruit Centers' fat-free	3 cookies	75	60	0.0

Food Name	Serv. Size	Total Cal.	Sod. MGS	Fat GMS
(Health Valley) 'Fruit Centers' fat-free	1 cookie	80	80	0.0
(Health Valley) raisin 'Fruit Chunks'	3 cookies	85	80	0.0
(Health Valley) raisin 'Jumbos' fat-free	1 cookie	80	80	0.0
(Health Valley) spice, fat-free	3 cookies	80	80	0.0
(Healthy Times) 'Hugga Bears' organic	1 oz	120	38	3.0
(Nabisco) 'Newtons' 1.25 oz	1 cookie	120	110	3.0
(Nabisco) 'Newtons' .75 oz	1 cookie	70	70	2.0
(Nabisco) 'Newtons' fat-free, .75 oz	1 cookie	70	45	0.0
(Stella D'oro) bar, Dutch	1 cookie	112	(mq)	3.3
(Stella D'oro) pastry, dietetic	1 cookie	86	10	3.3
(Weight Watchers) fruit filled	1 cookie	80	35	<1.0
(Weight Watchers) raisin bar	1 cookie	100	115	3.0
APRICOT				
(Health Valley) almond 'Fancy Fruit Chunks'	2 cookies	90	45	4.0
(Health Valley) apple 'Fruit Chunks'	3 cookies	85	80	0.0
(Health Valley) delight, fat-free	3 cookies	80	80	0.0
(Health Valley) 'Fruit Centers' fat-free	1 cookie	80	80	0.0
(Pepperidge Farm) raspberry 'Fruit Cookies'	2 cookies	100	50	4.0
(Pepperidge Farm) raspberry 'Zurich'	1 cookie	60	30	2.0
ARROWROOT (Nabisco) 'National Arrowroot Biscuit' 6 pieces	1 oz	130	85	4.0
ASSORTED				
(Archway) 'Select Assortment'	1 cookie	50	40	2.0
(Fifty 50) wafers, creme filled, w/o sugar	1 wafer	35	10	2.0
(Stella D'oro) 'Hostess'	1 cookie	42	(mq)	2.0
(Stella D'oro) 'Lady Stella'	1 cookie	42	(mq)	2.0
BANANA				
(Break Cake) creme	1 cookie	240	200	9.0
(Frookie) fat-free	1 cookie	45	90	0.0
(Health Valley) spice 'Fruit Chunks'	3 cookies	85	80	0.0
(Natures Warehouse) wheat-free, fat-free	1 oz	90	84	0.7
BLUEBERRY (Great Cakes)	4.5 oz	260	20	6.0
BROWNIE				
(Break Cake) creme	1 cookie	240	150	8.0
(Pepperidge Farm) chocolate nut 'Old Fashioned'	2 pieces	110	45	7.0
(Pepperidge Farm) cream sandwich 'Capri'	1 cookie	80	45	5.0
BUTTER				
(Barbara's Bakery) pecan bites 'Small Indulgences'	1 oz	140	95	8.0
(Delicious) frosted, made w/Land O'Lakes butter	1 cookie	88	44	5.0
(Fifty 50) fructose sweetened, low sodium	1 cookie	40	20	2.0
(Keebler) flavor, chocolate coated 'Baby Bear' .5 oz	3 cookies	70	55	2.0
(Keebler) flavor, chocolate coated 'E.L. Fudge' .5 oz	2 cookies	80	40	4.0

Food Name	Serv. Size	Total Cal.	Sod. MGS	Fat GMS
(Lu) 'Little Schoolboy'	1 cookie	70	35	4.0
(Lu) 'Petite Beurre'	1 cookie	40	45	1.0
(Mother's) flavored	5 cookies	140	130	6.0
(Pepperidge Farm) flavor 'Chessmen'	2 cookies	90	60	4.0
(Stella D'oro) 'Como Delight'	1 cookie	145	(mq)	7.2
CANDY (Oven Lovin')	1 cookie	70	40	3.0
CARAMEL				
(FFV) patties, approx 1 oz	2 cookies	150	125	7.0
(Keebler) apple oatmeal 'Elfin Delights'	1 cookie	65	55	2.0
(Natures Warehouse) crisp, wheat-free, fat-free	1 oz	90	84	0.7
CAROB				
(Health Valley) 'Healthy Chips' fat-free	3 cookies	80	80	0.0
(Natures Warehouse) fudge, approx 1 oz	2 cookies	116	78	3.1
(Westbrae) 'Rice Malt Snap'	1 oz	140	70	7.0
CARROT WALNUT 'Wholesome Choice' (Pepperidge Farm)	1 piece	60	45	1.0
CHERRY				
(Great Cakes) carob	4.5 oz	280	20	8.0
(Natures Warehouse) wheat-free, fat-free	1 oz	90	84	0.7
CHIPS AND CREME				
(Break Cake)	1 cookie	140	130	6.0
(Frookie) and vanilla sandwich 'Frookwich'	1 cookie	50	30	2.0
CHOCOLATE				
(Barbara's Bakery) raspberry 'Cookies & Creme'	2 cookies	120	80	5.0
(Barbara's Bakery) vanilla 'Cookies & Creme'	2 cookies	120	80	5.0
(Betty Crocker) w/peanut butter creme 'Dunkaroos'	1 tray	140	140	8.0
(Drake's) approx 1 oz	2 cookies	130	85	5.0
(Estee) 'Snack Crisps'	.66 oz	80	65	2.0
(Featherweight) creme wafer	1 cookie	20	0	1.0
(Frookie) 'Animal Frackers'	6 cookies	60	70	2.0
(Frookie) 'Funky Monkeys'	8 cookies	60	60	2.0
(Grandma's) 'Chocolate Cookie Bits' 8 cookies	1 oz	140	180	6.0
(Lu) 'Chocolatiers'	2 cookies	85	10	4.0
(Lu) 'Chocolatiers' dipped	2 cookies	105	15	6.0
(Nabisco) 'Chocolate Snap' 4 pieces	.5 oz	70	80	2.0
(Nabisco) 'Pure Chocolate Middles'	.5 oz cookie	80	35	5.0
(Pepperidge Farm) walnut 'Beacon Hill'	1 cookie	120	65	7.0
(Stella D'oro) 'Castelets'	1 cookie	64	(mq)	2.8
(Stella D'oro) 'Margherite'	1 cookie	72	(mq)	3.1
(Tastykake) 'Soft 'n Chewy'	1.4 oz	171	111	7.0
(Weight Watchers)	3 cookies	80	70	3.0

Food Name	Serv. Size	Total Cal.	Sod. MGS	Fat GMS
CHOCOLATE CHIP				
(Almost Home)	.5 oz	60	45	3.0
(Archway)	1 cookie	50	40	3.0
(Barbara's Bakery)	1 oz	130	60	6.0
(Barbara's Bakery) crisp 'Small Indulgences'	1 oz	140	105	7.0
(Break Cake) approx 1 oz	5 cookies	140	115	6.0
(Chips Ahoy!)	.5 oz	50	35	2.0
(Chips Ahoy!) 'Chewy'	.5 oz	60	40	3.0
(Chips Ahoy!) 'Mini'	.5 oz	70	50	3.0
(Chips Ahoy!) pecan 'Selections'	.5 oz	100	65	6.0
(Chips Ahoy!) 'Rockers'	1 cookie	60	40	3.0
(Chips Ahoy!) 'Sprinkled'	.5 oz	60	40	3.0
(Chips Ahoy!) 'Striped'	.5 oz	90	45	5.0
(Chips Ahoy!) walnut 'Selections'	.5 oz	100	70	6.0
(Chips Ahoy!) white fudge chunk	1 cookie	90	75	5.0
(Drake's) approx 1 oz	2 cookies	140	110	6.0
(Duncan Hines)	2 cookies	110	85	5.0
(Entenmann's)	3 cookies	140	85	7.0
(Estee)	3 cookies	110	20	5.0
(Featherweight)	1 cookie	45	0	2.0
(Fifty 50) fructose sweetened	1 cookie	35	10	2.0
(Finast)	1 oz	90	60	7.0
(Frookie)	1 cookie	45	35	2.0
(Frookie) Mandarin	1 cookie	45	35	2.0
(Frookie) mint	1 cookie	45	35	2.0
(Grandma's) 'Big Cookies' 2.75 oz	2 cookies	370	270	17.0
(Grandma's) 'Rich'N Chewy' 3 cookies	1 oz	140	80	6.0
(Keebler) bakery crisp 'Chips Deluxe'	1 cookie	60	45	3.0
(Keebler) chewy 'Elfin Delights'	1 cookie	65	55	2.0
(Keebler) 'Chips Deluxe' approx .5 oz	1 cookie	80	75	4.0
(Keebler) 'Coconut Chocolate Drop'	1 cookie	80	60	5.0
(Keebler) deluxe 'Bakery Crisp'	1 cookie	60	45	3.0
(Keebler) 'Rainbow Chips Deluxe' .5 oz	1 cookie	80	45	3.0
(Keebler) 'Soft Batch' approx .5 oz	1 cookie	80	70	4.0
(Mother's)	1 cookie	70	55	3.0
(Mother's) angel	2 cookies	120	45	8.0
(Nabisco) bite size 'Snack Wells'	.5 oz	60	85	1.0
(Nabisco) 'Chocolate Chip Snaps' 3 pieces	.5 oz	70	50	2.0
(Oven Lovin')	1 cookie	70	50	3.0
(Pepperidge Farm) 'Family Request'	2 cookies	90	55	5.0
(Pepperidge Farm) 'Old Fashioned'	2 cookies	100	45	5.0

Food Name	Serv. Size	Total Cal.	Sod. MGS	Fat GMS
(Pepperidge Farm) w/macadamia nuts 'Big, Soft and Chewy'	1 cookie	130	45	7.0
(Pepperidge Farm) w/macadamia nuts 'Sausalito'	1 cookie	120	65	7.0
(Tastykake) bar, 1.5 oz	1 cookie	193	97	8.4
(Tastykake) 'Soft 'n Chewy'	1.4 oz	174	168	7.3
(Weight Watchers)	2 cookies	90	65	2.0
CHOCOLATE CHOCOLATE CHIP				
(Barbara's Bakery)	1 oz	125	50	5.0
(Natures Warehouse) approx 1 oz	2 cookies	130	69	6.1
(Pepperidge Farm) walnut, big, soft & chewy	1 cookie	130	45	6.0
(Pillsbury's Best)	1 cookie	70	35	3.0
CHOCOLATE CHUNK				
(Chips Ahoy!) 'Chunky'	1 cookie	80	60	4.0
(Chips Ahoy!) 'Selections'	.5 oz	90	65	5.0
(Dunkin' Donuts) 1.5 oz	1 cookie	200	110	10.0
(Dunkin' Donuts) w/nuts, 1.5 oz	1 cookie	210	100	11.0
(Pepperidge Farm) 'Big, Soft and Chewy'	1 cookie	130	45	6.0
CHOCOLATE-FILLED SANDWICH				
(Keebler) 'E.L. Fudge'	1 cookie	60	35	3.0
(Pepperidge Farm) 'Brussels'	2 cookies	110	65	5.0
(Pepperidge Farm) 'Brussels Mint'	2 cookies	130	40	7.0
(Pepperidge Farm) 'Double Chocolate Milano'	2 cookies	150	45	8.0
(Pepperidge Farm) 'Hazelnut Milano'	2 cookies	130	30	8.0
(Pepperidge Farm) 'Lido'	1 cookie	90	30	5.0
(Pepperidge Farm) 'Milano'	2 cookies	120	45	6.0
(Pepperidge Farm) 'Mint Milano'	2 cookies	150	60	7.0
(Pepperidge Farm) 'Orange Milano'	2 cookies	150	60	7.0
(Pepperidge Farm) 'Orleans'	2 cookies	120	40	8.0
CHOCOLATE GRAHAM				
(Keebler) 'Thin Bits' approx .5 oz	12 cookies	70	75	3.0
(Nabisco) approx .5 oz	11 cookies	60	90	2.0
(Nabisco) 'Bugs Bunny'	.5 oz	60	80	2.0
(Nabisco) 'Chocolate Grahams'	.5 oz	150	80	7.0
(Teddy Grahams) 'Bearwichs'	.5 oz	70	60	3.0
(Teddy Grahams) w/vanilla creme 'Bearwichs'	4 cookies	70	60	3.0
CHOCOLATE SANDWICH				
(Estee)	1 cookie	50	15	2.0
(Frookie) 'Frookwich'	1 cookie	50	30	2.0
(Keebler) 'Chocolate Creme Sandwich'	.5 oz	80	70	4.0
(Keebler) 'E.L. Fudge'	1 cookie	70	50	3.0
(Keebler) fudge creme 'Elfin Delights'	1 cookie	55	50	2.0

Food Name	Serv. Size	Total Cal.	Sod. MGS	Fat GMS
(Keebler) peanut butter 'E.L. Fudge'	1 cookie	50	50	3.0
(Little Debbie)	1.8 oz	250	260	12.0
(Oreo) 'Big Stuf'	.25 oz	200	200	9.0
(Oreo) 'Double Stuf' 2 cookies	1 oz	70	75	4.0
(Oreo) fudge covered	.75 oz	110	80	6.0
(Oreo) 'Halloween Treats' 1 oz	2 cookies	140	150	7.0
(Oreo) 2 1/2 cookies	1 oz	140	170	6.0
(Oreo) white fudge covered	.75 oz	110	75	6.0
(Weight Watchers)	2 cookies	90	90	3.0
CHUNK				
(Pepperidge Farm) 'Nantucket'	1 cookie	120	60	6.●
(Pepperidge Farm) pecan 'Chesapeake'	1 cookie	120	60	7.●
(Pepperidge Farm) pecan 'Special Collection'	1 cookie	70	25	4.0
CINNAMON				
(Frookie) 'Animal Frackers'	6 cookies	60	45	2.●
(Mother's) dinosaur, mini	7 cookies	70	40	2.●
(Mother's) dinosaur grahams	1 cookie	80	50	3.●
CINNAMON GRAHAM				
(Honey Maid) approx .5 oz	2 cookies	60	85	1.●
(Keebler) 'Alpha Grahams'	6 cookies	70	55	2.●
(Keebler) 'Cinnamon Crisp' .5 oz	4 cookies	70	85	2.●
(Keebler) fudge covered 'Deluxe' .5 oz	2 cookies	90	60	4.●
(Keebler) 'Thin Bits' approx .5 oz	12 cookies	70	50	3.●
(Nabisco) 'Bugs Bunny'	.5 oz	60	80	2.●
(Nabisco) fat-free 'Snack Wells'	.5 oz	50	45	0.
(Nabisco) w/fudge 'Cookies'N Fudge'	1 cookie	45	35	2.
(Natures Warehouse) approx 1 oz	2 cookies	113	71	3.●
(Pepperidge Farm) sugar 'Family Request'	2 cookies	80	40	4.
(Sunshine)	1 cookie	70	95	3.
(Teddy Grahams) 'Bearwichs'	.5 oz	70	60	3.
COCOA				
(Westbrae) chip 'Rice Malt Snap'	1 oz	130	60	7.
(Westbrae) 'Rice Malt Snap'	1 oz	140	70	7.●
COCONUT				
(Break Cake) macaroons	2 cookies	270	160	14.
(Drake's) approx 1 oz	2 cookies	130	95	5.
(Estee)	3 cookies	110	15	5.
(Glenny's) almonds, raisins 'Nookie Bar'	1.15 oz	138	na	3.
(Mother's) cocadas	4 cookies	120	150	6.
(Mother's) macaroons	1 cookie	80	40	5.
(Natures Warehouse) approx 1 oz	2 cookies	130	20	7.

Food Name	Serv. Size	Total Cal.	Sod. MGS	Fat GMS
(Pepperidge Farm) chocolate-filled 'Tahiti'	1 cookie	90	25	6.0
(Stella D'oro) dietetic	1 cookie	52	10	2.4
(Stella D'oro) macaroon	1 cookie	60	(mq)	3.4
COFFEE				
(Barbara's Bakery) coffee cake crunch 'Small Indulgences'	1 oz	130	140	6.0
(Pepperidge Farm)	1 cookie	50	20	3.0
CRANBERRY				
(Frookie) orange, fat-free	1 cookie	45	75	0.0
(Nabisco) 'Newtons' fat-free	1 cookie	70	70	0.0
(Pepperidge Farm) honey, soft 'Wholesome Choice'	1 cookie	60	50	2.0
CROKINE *(Lu)*	2 cookies	35	70	0.0
DATE				
(Bakery Wagon) filled oatmeal	1 cookie	90	100	3.0
(Break Cake) creme	1 cookie	140	140	5.0
(Health Valley) delight, fat-free	3 cookies	80	80	0.0
(Health Valley) 'Fruit Centers' fat-free	1 cookie	70	35	0.0
(Health Valley) pecan 'Fancy Fruit Chunks'	2 cookies	90	45	4.0
(Pepperidge Farm) pecan 'Kitchen Hearth'	2 cookies	110	40	5.0
DEVIL'S FOOD				
(Break Cake) creme	1 cookie	130	120	5.0
(FFV) 'Trolley Cakes' 2 oz	2 cookies	120	80	2.0
(Nabisco) cakes	1 cookie	70	40	1.0
DUPLEX SANDWICH *(Mother's)*	2 cookies	105	70	5.0
EGG BISCUIT				
(Estee) 'Original Sandwich'	1 cookie	45	5	2.0
(FFV) 'Kreem Pilot Bread'	1 cookie	60	60	2.0
(FFV) 'Royal Dainty' .7 oz	2 cookies	120	90	6.0
(FFV) 'T.C. Rounds' approx 1 oz	2 cookies	160	65	8.0
(FFV) 'Tango' 1.2 oz	2 cookies	160	50	5.0
(Stella D'oro)	1 cookie	43	(mq)	1.1
(Stella D'oro) 'Anginetti'	1 cookie	31	(mq)	1.0
(Stella D'oro) dietetic	1 cookie	43	10	1.1
(Stella D'oro) dietetic 'Kitchen'	1 cookie	8	10	0.5
(Stella D'oro) 'Jumbo'	1 cookie	47	(mq)	0.7
(Stella D'oro) 'Roman'	1 cookie	137	(mq)	5.0
(Stella D'oro) sugared	1 cookie	75	(mq)	1.4
ENGLISH TEA *(Mother's)* sandwich	1 cookie	100	60	4.0
FIG				
(Estee) bar	2 cookies	90	60	1.0
(FFV) bar, vanilla	1 cookie	70	55	1.0
(FFV) bar, whole wheat	1 cookie	70	50	2.0

Food Name	Serv. Size	Total Cal.	Sod. MGS	Fat GMS
(Frookie) 'Fruitins'	1 cookie	60	25	1.0
(Frookie) 'Fruitins' fat-free	2 cookies	90	75	0.0
(Keebler) bar	1 cookie	60	70	2.0
(Mother's) bar	2 cookies	110	85	2.0
(Mother's) whole wheat	2 cookies	120	105	2.0
(Nabisco) 'Newtons'	.5 oz	60	6	1.0
(Nabisco) 'Newtons'	1.25 oz	120	110	3.0
(Nabisco) 'Newtons Cookie Variety'	1 oz	120	110	3.0
(Nabisco) 'Newtons' fat-free, 1 piece	.75 oz	70	80	0.0
(Natures Warehouse) bar, apple cinnamon, wheat-free	1 oz	98	18	2.0
(Natures Warehouse) bar, raspberry, wheat-free	1 oz	98	18	2.0
(Natures Warehouse) bar, wheat-free	1 oz	98	18	2.0
(Natures Warehouse) bar, whole wheat	1 oz	98	18	2.0
(Stella D'oro) pastry, dietetic	1 cookie	89	10	3.7
FORTUNE				
(LaChoy)	1 oz	112	11	0.2
(LaChoy)	1 cookie	15	1	<1.0
FRUIT				
(Barbara's Bakery) and nut	1 oz	140	55	6.0
(Health Valley) 'Fruit & Fitness'	5 cookies	200	249	6.0
(Health Valley) Hawaiian, fat-free	3 cookies	80	80	0.0
(Health Valley) tropical 'Fancy Fruit Chunks'	2 cookies	80	45	3.0
(Health Valley) tropical 'Fruit Centers' fat-free	1 cookie	80	80	0.0
(Health Valley) tropical 'Fruit Jumbos'	1 cookie	70	26	2.0
(Stella D'oro) slices	1 cookie	60	(mq)	2.2
FUDGE				
(Almost Home)	.5 oz	70	50	3.0
(Almost Home) chocolate chip	.5 oz	70	50	3.0
(Chips Ahoy!) mini bites 'Little Fudgies'	1 oz	230	105	12.0
(Estee)	1 cookie	30	0	1.0
(Fifty 50) brownie, fructose sweetened	1 cookie	35	0	2.0
(Grandma's) 'Big Cookies' 2.75 oz	2 cookies	350	380	13.0
(Keebler) mint 'Grasshopper' approx .5 oz	2 cookies	70	35	3.0
(M&M/Mars) 'Twix'	1 bar	100	35	6.0
(Mother's) double fudge sandwich	2 cookies	100	75	4.0
(Mother's) wafer 'Flaky Flix'	2 cookies	130	30	9.0
(Nabisco) caramel, peanut 'Heyday Bars' 1 piece	.75 oz	110	40	6.0
(Nabisco) middles	.5 oz	80	35	5.0
(Nabisco) wafer 'Famous Wafers' 2 1/2 pieces	.5 oz	70	110	2.0
(Nabisco) snaps, approx .5 oz	4 cookies	70	75	2.0
(Stella D'oro) 'Swiss Fudge Cookie'	1 cookie	68	(mq)	3.4

ood Name	Serv. Size	Total Cal.	Sod. MGS	Fat GMS
(Tastykake) bar	1.8 oz	205	155	6.8
GINGER				
(FFV) boys	1.25-oz pkg	150	210	5.0
(Frookie) spice	1 cookie	45	35	2.0
(Pepperidge Farm) 'Gingerman'	2 cookies	70	50	3.0
(Westbrae) 'Rice Malt Snap'	1 oz	130	140	5.0
GINGERSNAPS				
(Archway) '80/pkg'	1 cookie	25	20	<1.0
(Archway) '54/pkg'	1 cookie	35	30	1.0
(Break Cake) approx 1 oz	5 cookies	130	110	5.0
(Delicious)	.5 oz	64	78	1.7
(FFV) approx 1 oz	5 cookies	130	140	4.0
(Nabisco) 'Old Fashioned'	.25 oz	30	45	1.0
(Sunshine)	5 cookies	100	120	3.0
GRAHAM. See also HONEY GRAHAM.				
(Betty Crocker) w/chocolate frosting 'Dunkaroos'	1 tray	130	70	5.0
(Betty Crocker) w/vanilla frosting 'Dunkaroos'	1 tray	130	60	5.0
(Keebler) chocolate 'Selects'	4 cookies	60	55	3.0
(Keebler) honey nut 'Selects'	4 cookies	60	70	3.0
(Mother's) dinosaur, original	1 cookie	70	50	2.0
(Mother's) dinosaur, mini	7 cookies	60	40	1.0
(Nabisco) 'Bugs Bunny' 5 pieces	.5 oz	60	70	2.0
(Pepperidge Farm) cinnamon 'Goldfish'	1 oz	130	130	7.0
(Pepperidge Farm) 'Goldfish'	1 oz	140	140	7.0
(Teddy Grahams) snacks, chocolate	.5 oz	60	80	2.0
(Teddy Grahams) snacks, cinnamon	.75-oz bag	100	120	3.0
(Teddy Grahams) snacks, honey, 11 pieces	.5 oz	60	90	2.0
(Teddy Grahams) vanilla honey 'Bearwichs'	4 cookies	70	65	3.0
GRANOLA				
(Betty Crocker) chocolate filling 'Incredibites'	1 pouch	170	150	7.0
(Betty Crocker) peanut butter 'Incredibites'	1 pouch	170	160	8.0
(Betty Crocker) vanilla creme 'Incredibites'	1 pouch	170	180	7.0
(Health Valley) 'Healthy'	3 cookies	75	60	0.0
HERMIT *(Break Cake)*	1 cookie	230	280	7.0
HOB-NOBS' *(Carr's)*	1 cookie	72	78	3.2
HONEY				
(Bakery Wagon) fruit bar	1 cookie	100	70	3.0
(Health Valley) cinnamon, crisp 'Honey Jumbos'	1 cookie	70	35	2.0
(Health Valley) oat bran, fancy 'Honey Jumbos'	1 cookie	70	22	2.0
(Health Valley) peanut butter, crisp 'Honey Jumbos'	1 cookie	70	24	2.0
(Stella D'oro) 'Royal Nuggets'	1 cookie	2	na	0.1

Food Name	Serv. Size	Total Cal.	Sod. MGS	Fa GM
HONEY GRAHAM				
(Carafection) 'Original' carob coated	1 oz	139	26	7.
(Carr's) wheat 'Home Wheat Graham'	1 cookie	74	<1	3.
(Health Valley) 'Fancy'	7 cookies	130	89	5.
(Health Valley) oat bran	7 cookies	130	47	2.
(Honey Maid) .5 oz	2 pieces	60	90	1.
(Honey Maid) honey'n oat bran 'Graham Bites'	.5 oz	60	55	2.
(Keebler) approx .5 oz	4 cookies	70	85	2.
(Nabisco) vanilla, approx .5 oz	11 cookies	60	75	2.
(Pepperidge Farm) hazelnut 'Old Fashioned'	2 cookies	110	75	6.
(Sunshine)	1 piece	60	90	2.
JELLY				
(Delicious) top	.8 oz	112	34	5.
(FFV) tarts	1 cookie	60	55	2.
LEMON				
(Barbara's Bakery) almond delights 'Small Indulgences'	1 oz	140	135	6.
(Delicious) sugar wafer	1 wafer	35	3	2.
(Estee)	3 cookies	100	15	5.
(Estee) 'Snack Crisps'	.66 oz	80	75	2.
(Featherweight)	1 cookie	45	0	2.
(Frookie) sandwich 'Frookwich'	1 cookie	50	30	2.
(Pepperidge Farm) nut crunch 'Old Fashioned'	2 cookies	110	50	7.
(Westbrae) 'Rice Malt Snap'	1 oz	130	70	6.
MARSHMALLOW				
(Nabisco) cake 'Mallomars'	1 cookie	60	20	3.
(Nabisco) fudge cake 'Puffs'	.75 oz	90	45	4.
(Nabisco) fudge cake 'Twirls'	1 oz	140	70	6.
(Nabisco) fudge graham 'Suddenly S'Mores'	.75 oz	100	90	4.
(Nabisco) 'Pinwheels'	1 cookie	130	35	5.
(Pinwheels) chocolate cake	1 oz	130	40	5.
MINI-CREME (Delicious)	1 wafer	24	2	1.
MINT				
(Carafection) honey graham, carob coated	1 oz	139	26	7.
(FFV) sandwich, approx 1.1 oz	2 cookies	160	50	7
(Girl Scout Cookies) thin mints	4 cookies	160	140	9
(Keebler) 'Soft Batch'	1 cookie	80	70	4
(Nabisco) sandwich 'Mystic Mint'	.5 oz	90	65	4.
MOLASSES				
(Archway)	1 cookie	100	155	2
(Bakery Wagon) iced	1 cookie	100	120	4.
(Grandma's) 'Old Time Big Cookies'	2 cookies	320	520	9.

Food Name	Serv. Size	Total Cal.	Sod. MGS	Fat GMS
(Nabisco) 'Pantry'	.5 oz	80	75	3.0
(Pepperidge Farm) crisps 'Old Fashioned'	2 cookies	70	50	3.0
MÜESLI (Carr's)	1 cookie	84	30	4.1
OAT BRAN				
(Awrey's) raisin	1 cookie	100	115	4.0
(Frookie) muffin	1 cookie	45	35	2.0
(Health Valley) animal cookies	7 cookies	110	50	4.0
(Health Valley) fruit and nut	2 cookies	110	70	4.0
(Health Valley) fruit 'Oat Bran Fruit Jumbos'	1 cookie	70	22	2.0
(Health Valley) raisin 'Fancy Fruit Chunks'	2 cookies	90	95	3.0
(Natures Warehouse) chocolate chip, approx 1 oz	2 cookies	139	55	6.0
(Natures Warehouse) wheat-free, approx 1 oz	2 cookies	129	54	6.2
OATMEAL				
(Almost Home) raisin	.5 oz	70	40	3.0
(Archway)	1 cookie	110	90	3.0
(Archway) apple filled	1 cookie	90	115	1.0
(Archway) date filled	1 cookie	100	105	2.0
(Archway) iced	1 cookie	140	107	5.0
(Archway) 'Ruth's Golden'	1 cookie	120	122	4.0
(Bakers Bonus)	.5 oz	80	65	3.0
(Bakery Wagon) chocolate chunk	1 cookie	100	80	3.0
(Bakery Wagon) soft	1 cookie	100	105	5.0
(Bakery Wagon) walnut raisin	1 cookie	100	80	4.0
(Barbara's Bakery) raisin	1 oz	100	50	2.0
(Break Cake) approx 1 oz	5 cookies	140	60	6.0
(Chips Ahoy!) chocolate chip 'Selections'	.5 oz	90	60	5.0
(Drake's) approx 1 oz	2 cookies	120	50	4.0
(Dunkin' Donuts) pecan, raisin	1 cookie	200	100	9.0
(Duncan Hines) raisin	2 cookies	110	85	5.0
(Entenmann's) chocolatey chip 'Fat-Free Cholesterol-Free'	2 cookies	80	110	0.0
(Entenmann's) raisin	2 cookies	30	120	0.0
(Estee) raisin	3 cookies	100	15	4.0
(FFV) approx 1 oz	5 cookies	130	150	4.0
(Fifty 50) hearty oatmeal, fructose sweetened	1 cookie	35	15	1.0
(Frookie) raisin	1 cookie	45	35	2.0
(Frookie) raisin, fat-free	1 cookie	50	75	0.0
(Frookie) 7-grain oatmeal	1 cookie	45	35	2.0
(Glenny's) wheat-free 'Noah 'N Friends Animal'	.5 oz	65	20	2.0
(Grandma's) apple spice 'Big Cookies' 2.75 oz	2 cookies	330	570	12.0
(Health Valley) raisin cinnamon 'Fruit Chunks'	3 cookies	85	80	0.0
(Keebler) 'Old Fashion' approx .5 oz	1 cookie	80	110	3.0

Food Name	Serv. Size	Total Cal.	Sod. MGS	Fat GMS
(Keebler) w/chocolate 'Magic Middles' .5 oz	1 cookie	80	30	5.0
(Keebler) w/raisins, chewy 'Raisin Ruckus'	1 cookie	70	45	3.0
(Little Debbie)	2.75 oz	340	440	12.0
(Mother's)	1 cookie	60	80	3.0
(Mother's) chocolate chip	1 cookie	70	85	3.0
(Mother's) iced	1 cookie	70	70	3.0
(Mother's) walnut chocolate chip	1 cookie	70	60	3.0
(Nabisco) raisin, 'Snack Wells'	1 cookie	60	65	1.0
(Natures Warehouse) raisin, approx 1 oz	2 cookies	135	44	6.4
(Pepperidge Farm) chocolate chunk 'Dakota'	1 cookie	110	70	6.0
(Pepperidge Farm) 'Family Request'	2 cookies	90	70	4.0
(Pepperidge Farm) Irish 'Old Fashioned'	2 cookies	90	80	5.0
(Pepperidge Farm) raisin, soft, low-fat 'Wholesome Choice'	1 cookie	60	50	1.0
(Weight Watchers) raisin	2 cookies	90	75	<1.0
(Weight Watchers) spice	3 cookies	80	75	2.0
(Westbrae) 'Rice Malt Snap'	1 oz	130	130	5.0
ORANGE-PINEAPPLE				
(Health Valley) 'Mini Fruit Centers' fat-free	3 cookies	75	60	0.0
PEACH (Great Cakes)	4.5 oz	260	20	6.0
PEACH-APRICOT				
(FFV) bar, vanilla	1 cookie	70	50	1.0
(FFV) bar, whole wheat	1 cookie	70	50	2.0
(Health Valley) 'Mini Fruit Centers' fat-free	3 cookies	75	60	0.0
(Stella D'oro) pastry	1 cookie	93	(mq)	3.8
(Stella D'oro) pastry, dietetic	1 cookie	87	10	3.7
PEANUT (Health Valley) 'Fancy Peanut Chunks'	2 cookies	100	585	3.0
PEANUT BUTTER				
(Bakery Wagon) oatmeal	1 cookie	110	150	7.0
(Break Cake)	1 cookie	140	110	7.0
(Break Cake) wafer	1 wafer	180	75	9.0
(Delicious) and jelly sandwich 'Skippy & Welchs'	1 cookie	120	90	6.0
(Delicious) made w/Skippy peanut butter	1 cookie	80	65	5.0
(Estee) sandwich	1 cookie	50	35	3.0
(Featherweight)	1 cookie	40	10	2.0
(Featherweight) creme wafer	1 cookie	25	0	1.0
(FFV) sandwich, approx 1.1 oz	2 cookies	170	110	8.0
(Fifty 50) fructose sweetened	1 cookie	40	10	2.0
(Frookie) sandwich 'Frookwich'	1 cookie	50	30	2.0
(Glenny's) 'Noah 'N Friends Animal Cookies'	.5 oz	65	35	3.0
(Grandma's) 'Big Cookies' 2.75 oz	2 cookies	410	410	30.0
(Grandma's) cookie bits, 8 cookies	1 oz	140	125	6.0

ood Name	Serv. Size	Total Cal.	Sod. MGS	Fat GMS
(Great Cakes) and jelly	4.5 oz	280	20	8.0
(Keebler) chocolate chip 'Soft Batch' .5 oz	1 cookie	80	55	5.0
(Keebler) nut 'Soft Batch' approx .5 oz	1 cookie	80	60	4.0
(Mother's) sandwich 'Gaucho'	1 cookie	90	75	5.0
(Nabisco) 'Ideal Bars'	.5 oz cookie	90	80	5.0
(Nabisco) 'Nutter Butter Peanut Sandwich'	.5 oz	70	50	3.0
(Natures Warehouse) approx 1 oz	2 cookies	128	29	6.1
(Natures Warehouse) chocolate chip; approx 1 oz	2 cookies	139	50	8.5
(Pepperidge Farm) chocolate chunk 'Cheyenne'	1 cookie	110	80	6.0
(Pepperidge Farm) chocolate filled 'Nassau'	1 cookie	80	45	5.0
(Pepperidge Farm) 'Family Request'	2 cookies	80	65	5.0
(Pitter Patter) cream filled, approx .5 oz	1 cookie	90	115	4.0
(Planters) crispy cookie 'P.B. Crisps'	1 oz	140	125	7.0
EANUT CREME (Nabisco) 'Nutter Butter Patties'	.5 oz	80	45	4.0
ECAN				
(Archway) crunch	1 cookie	60	45	3.0
(Dunkin' Donuts) raisin cookie, 1.6 oz	1 cookie	200	100	9.0
RALINE PECAN (FFV)	1 cookie	40	40	2.0
RUNE, pastry, dietetic (Stella D'oro)	1 cookie	95	10	3.4
AISIN				
(Almost Home)	.5 oz	70	40	3.0
(Archway)	1 cookie	100	107	3.0
(Archway) bran	1 cookie	100	95	3.0
(Archway) oatmeal	1 cookie	50	20	2.0
(Break Cake) creme	1 cookie	140	120	5.0
(Entenmann's)	2 cookies	80	120	0.0
(Featherweight)	1 cookie	45	0	2.0
(Grandma's) soft 'Big Cookies' approx 2.75 oz	2 cookies	320	280	10.0
(Health Valley) apple 'Fruit Centers' fat-free	1 cookie	70	35	0.0
(Health Valley) 'Jumbos' fat-free	1 cookie	80	80	0.0
(Health Valley) nut 'Fruit Jumbos'	1 cookie	70	35	3.0
(Health Valley) oatmeal, fat-free	3 cookies	80	80	0.0
(Keebler) bar, iced	1 cookie	80	85	4.0
(Keebler) 'Soft Batch' approx .5 oz	1 cookie	70	65	3.0
(Mother's) iced	1 cookie	80	45	4.0
(Nabisco) nut 'Newtons'	.5 oz	60	50	2.0
(Pepperidge Farm) bran 'Kitchen Hearth'	2 cookies	110	55	5.0
(Pepperidge Farm) 'Old Fashioned'	2 cookies	110	115	5.0
(Pepperidge Farm) 'Santa Fe'	1 cookie	100	70	4.0
(Stella D'oro) 'Golden Bars'	1 cookie	109	(mq)	4.3
(Sunshine)	2 cookies	110	125	5.0
(Tastykake) bar	1.8 oz	212	255	8.3

Food Name	Serv. Size	Total Cal.	Sod. MGS	F G
(Tastykake) 'Soft'n Chewy'	1.4 oz	161	158	5
(Weight Watchers) spice	3 cookies	80	75	2
RASPBERRY				
(Bakery Wagon) filled	1 cookie	90	125	3
(Frookie) 'Fruitins' fat-free	2 cookies	90	75	0
(Great Cakes)	4.5 oz	260	20	6
(Health Valley) apple 'Fruit Chunks'	3 cookies	85	80	0
(Health Valley) apple 'Mini Fruit Centers' fat-free	3 cookies	75	60	0
(Health Valley) 'Fruit Centers' fat-free	1 cookie	80	80	0
(Health Valley) 'Jumbos' fat-free	1 cookie	80	80	0
(Lu) 'Pims'	2 cookies	95	25	2
(Nabisco) 'Newtons' .75 oz	1 cookie	80	70	2
(Nabisco) 'Newtons' fat-free	1 cookie	60	75	0
(Natural Nectar) swirl 'Incredible Edible Novelties'	1 cookie	220	115	8
(Natures Warehouse) wheat-free, fat-free	1 oz	90	84	0
(Pepperidge Farm) filled 'Chantilly'	1 cookie	80	35	2
(Pepperidge Farm) filled, chocolate 'Chantilly'	1 cookie	90	35	3
(Pepperidge Farm) filled 'Linzer'	1 cookie	120	55	4
(Pepperidge Farm) tart, low fat 'Wholesome Choice'	1 cookie	60	35	1
(Weight Watchers) fruit filled	1 cookie	80	45	<1
REESE'S PIECES *(Oven Lovin')*	1 cookie	70	50	3
SESAME				
(Glenny's) 'Nookie' bite size	.5 oz	60	8	4
(Stella D'oro) dietetic 'Regina'	1 cookie	41	10	2
(Stella D'oro) 'Regina'	1 cookie	48	(mq)	2
SHORTBREAD				
(Break Cake) approx 1 oz	5 cookies	140	70	•
(Estee)	3 cookies	100	100	
(FFV) country	1 cookie	70	45	
(Keebler) covered 'Fudge'n Caramel'	1 cookie	60	30	3
(Keebler) fudge covered 'Toffee Toppers'	2 cookies	60	50	4
(Keebler) fudge striped 'Fudge Stripes' .5 oz	1 cookie	50	55	
(Keebler) 'Pecan Sandies' approx .5 oz	1 cookie	80	75	
(Keebler) 'Pecan Sandies' bite size	4 cookies	90	50	5
(Keebler) w/chocolate center 'Magic Middles' .5 oz	1 cookie	80	25	
(Keebler) w/toffee pieces 'Toffee Sandies'	1 cookie	70	45	
(Lorna Doone) .5 oz	3 cookies	70	65	
(Mother's) striped	2 cookies	100	55	
(Nabisco) fudge striped 'Cookies 'n Fudge' .5 oz		60	50	5
(Nabisco) pecan supreme, low cholesterol	1 cookie	80	45	5
(Pepperidge Farm) 'Old Fashioned'	2 cookies	150	85	

Food Name	Serv. Size	Total Cal.	Sod. MGS	Fat GMS
(Pepperidge Farm) pecan 'Old Fashioned' .... 1 cookie	70	15	5.0	
(Weight Watchers) .... 3 cookies	80	95	2.0	
SNACK, for weight control *(Spicer's)* .... 1 oz	100	70	4.0	
SPICE *(Stella D'oro)* 'Pfeffernusse' .... 1 piece	35	(mq)	0.8	
STRAWBERRY				
(Healthy Times) 'Hugga Bears' organic .... 1 oz	120	38	3.0	
(Health Valley) 'Mini Fruit Centers' fat-free .... 3 cookies	75	60	0.0	
(Nabisco) 'Newtons' .... 1.25 oz	120	110	3.0	
(Nabisco) 'Newtons' .75 oz .... 1 cookie	70	70	2.0	
(Nabisco) 'Newtons' fat-free .... 1 cookie	60	80	0.0	
(Nabisco) 'Suddenly S'Mores' .... .75 oz	100	90	4.0	
(Natural Nectar) swirl 'Incredible Edible Novelties' ...... 1 cookie	220	115	8.0	
(Pepperidge Farm) 'Fruit Cookies' .... 2 cookies	100	50	5.0	
SUGAR				
(Almost Home) .... .5 oz	70	80	3.0	
(Almost Home) 'Old Fashioned' .... .5 oz	70	80	3.0	
(Mother's) .... 1 cookie	70	35	4.0	
(Pepperidge Farm) 'Old Fashioned' .... 2 cookies	100	55	5.0	
(Stella D'oro) 'Holiday Trinkets' .... 1 cookie	38	(mq)	1.9	
TAFFY *(Mother's)* sandwich .... 1 cookie	100	60	6.0	
TEA BISCUIT *(Nabisco)* 'Social Tea Biscuit' 3 pieces .... .5 oz	60	60	2.0	
TOFFEE				
(Chips Ahoy!) chunk, Heath 'Selections' .... 1 cookie	90	85	5.0	
(Delicious) w/Heath English toffee .... 1 cookie	90	45	5.0	
(Pepperidge Farm) 'Old Fashioned' .... 2 cookies	100	75	5.0	
TOFU *(Health Valley)* 'The Great Tofu Cookie' .... 2 cookies	90	29	3.0	
VANILLA				
(Barbara's Bakery) animal cookies .... 1 oz	145	85	7.0	
(Barbara's Bakery) 'Cookies & Creme' .... 2 cookies	120	75	5.0	
(Barbara's Bakery) raspberry 'Cookies & Creme' ...... 2 cookies	120	75	5.0	
(Estee) .... 3 cookies	100	15	5.0	
(Estee) sandwich .... 2 cookies	110	20	4.0	
(Featherweight) .... 1 cookie	45	0	2.0	
(Frookie) 'Funky Monkeys' .... 8 cookies	60	60	2.0	
(Frookie) sandwich 'Frookwich' .... 1 cookie	50	30	2.0	
(Frookie) 'Trolls' .... 11 cookies	60	65	2.0	
(Glenny's) 'Noah 'N Friends Animal Cookies' .... .5 oz	65	35	2.0	
(Grandma's) cookie bits, artificially flavored .... 1 oz	140	75	6.0	
(Keebler) creme sandwich 'French' .5 oz .... 1 cookie	80	80	4.0	
(Lu) 'Marie Lu' .... 1 cookie	50	45	2.0	
(Lu) 'Marie Lu' mini .... 5 cookies	50	45	2.0	

Food Name	Serv. Size	Total Cal.	Sod. MGS	Fa GM
(Nabisco) creme sandwich 'Cameo'	.5 oz	70	50	3.
(Nabisco) creme sandwich 'Cookie Break'	1 cookie	50	35	2.
(Nabisco) creme sandwich 'Giggles' 2 pieces	1 oz	60	20	3
(Nabisco) reduced fat 'Snack Wells'	.5 oz	50	50	1.
(Pepperidge Farm) 'Bordeaux'	2 cookies	70	40	3
(Pepperidge Farm) chocolate coated 'Orleans'	3 cookies	90	30	6.
(Pepperidge Farm) chocolate laced 'Pirouettes'	2 cookies	70	20	4.
(Pepperidge Farm) chocolate nut coated 'Geneva'	2 cookies	130	50	6
(Pepperidge Farm) 'Goldfish'	1 oz	140	50	7
(Pepperidge Farm) 'Pirouettes'	2 cookies	70	35	4
(Stella D'oro) 'Angelica Goodies'	1 cookie	106	(mq)	4.
(Stella D'oro) 'Castelets'	1 cookie	72	(mq)	3
(Stella D'oro) 'Margherite'	1 cookie	72	(mq)	2
(Tastykake) creme sandwich, shortbread	.4 oz	55	31	3
(Weight Watchers) sandwich	2 cookies	90	50	3
WAFER				
(Archway) vanilla	1 wafer	30	30	<1
(Biscos) sugar, 4 pieces	.5 oz	70	20	3
(Biscos) waffle creme	1 wafer	45	10	2
(Break Cake) chocolate, sugar	4 wafers	200	95	9
(Break Cake) strawberry, sugar	4 wafers	220	100	11
(Break Cake) 'Striper Wafer'	1 wafer	190	80	10
(Break Cake) vanilla, sugar	4 wafers	220	105	11
(Delicious) chocolate strawberry, sugar	1 wafer	35	4	2
(Delicious) chocolate, sugar	1 wafer	34	5	2
(Delicious) strawberry, sugar	1 wafer	35	3	2
(Delicious) sugar, assorted	.25 oz	38	<1	2
(Delicious) vanilla	.5 oz	70	41	2
(Delicious) vanilla, sugar	.25 oz	37	<1	2
(Delicious) vanilla, sugar	1 wafer	35	3	2
(Estee) chocolate creme	4 wafers	90	0	5
(Estee) strawberry	3 wafers	100	0	5
(Estee) vanilla	3 wafers	100	0	5
(Estee) vanilla creme	4 wafers	90	0	4
(Featherweight) strawberry creme	1 wafer	20	0	1
(Featherweight) vanilla creme	1 wafers	20	0	1
(FFV) vanilla, approx 1 oz	8 wafers	130	100	5
(Fifty 50) chocolate creme filled, w/o sugar	1 wafer	35	10	2
(Fifty 50) vanilla, creme filled, w/o sugar	1 wafer	35	5	2
(Keebler) vanilla, golden	4 wafers	80	60	3
(Lu) cream	3 cookies	110	50	7

Food Name	Serv. Size	Total Cal.	Sod. MGS	Fat GMS
(Mother's) checkerboard	5 wafers	85	15	4.0
(Mother's) vanilla, 'Flaky Flix'	2 wafers	115	na	5.0
(Nabisco) 'Brown Edge Wafers' 2 1/2 wafers	.5 oz	70	45	4.0
(Nabisco) 'Famous Chocolate Wafers' 2 1/2 wafers	.5 oz	60	100	2.0
(Nabisco) striped wafer 'Cookies 'N Fudge'	1 wafer	70	25	4.0
(Nabisco) vanilla, cinnamon 'Nilla Wafers' .5 oz	3 1/2 wafers	60	45	2.0
(Nabisco) vanilla, 'Nilla Wafers' approx .5 oz	3 1/2 wafers	60	45	2.0
(Tastykake) vanilla, sugar	10 wafers	34	11	1.9
(Weider) 'Victory Explosive Workout'	6 wafers	30	60	0.0
(Westbrae) 5-spice	4 1/2 wafers	40	30	0.0
WALNUT				
(Keebler) 'Soft Batch' approx .5 oz	1 cookie	80	70	4.0
(Lu) whole wheat and cinnamon 'Marie Lu'	1 cookie	45	55	1.0
(Mother's) fudge	1 cookie	70	50	4.0
COOKIE DOUGH, PREPARED				
chocolate chip	1 oz	126	59	5.8
chocolate chip	1 cookie	71	33	3.3
chocolate chip (Pillsbury)	1 cookie	70	55	3.0
chocolate chip, baked	1 oz	139	66	6.4
chocolate chip, baked	1 cookie	59	28	2.7
chocolate chip 'Ready To Bake' (Toll House)	1.2 oz	150	115	7.0
chocolate chip 'Ready To Bake' w/nuts (Toll House)	1.2 oz	160	90	8.0
double chocolate chip 'Ready To Bake' 1.2 oz (Toll House)	2 cookies	150	60	7.0
oatmeal	1 oz	120	83	5.4
oatmeal	1 cookie	68	47	3.0
oatmeal, baked	1 oz	134	93	5.9
oatmeal, baked	1 cookie	57	39	2.5
oatmeal raisin (Pillsbury)	1 cookie	60	55	3.0
oatmeal raisin 'Ready To Bake' 2 cookies (Toll House)	1.2 oz	130	55	5.0
peanut butter (Pillsbury)	1 cookie	70	75	3.0
sugar	1 oz	124	120	5.9
sugar	1 cookie	70	68	3.3
sugar (Pillsbury)	1 cookie	70	70	3.0
sugar, baked	1 oz	137	133	6.6
COOKIE MIX				
chocolate chip (Duncan Hines)	2 cookies	130	85	5.0
chocolate chip (Finast)	2 cookies	110	290	5.0
chocolate chip, 2-inch diam each (Estee)	2 cookies	90	80	4.0
chocolate chip 'Big Batch' (Betty Crocker)	2 cookies	120	100	6.0
'Deluxe' 2-inch diam (Krusteaz)	1 cookie	120	126	5.0

Food Name	Serv. Size	Total Cal.	Sod. MGS	Fat GMS
golden sugar *(Duncan Hines)*	2 cookies	130	70	6.0
oatmeal raisin *(Duncan Hines)*	2 cookies	130	70	6.0
peanut butter *(Duncan Hines)*	2 cookies	140	120	7.0
COOKING SPRAY				
(Mazola) corn oil 'No Stick'	2.5-sec spray	6	0	1.0
(Pam) for 1/3 of 10-inch skillet	1 spray	2	0	1.0
(Weight Watchers) 'Buttery Spray' butter flavor	1-sec spray	2	0	<1.0
(Weight Watchers) canola oil spray	.33 grams	2	0	<1.0
(Weight Watchers) 'Cooking Spray'	1-sec spray	2	0	1.0
(Wesson) lite	.27 grams	<1	0	<1.0
(Wesson) no-stick	.25 gram	2	0	0.3
COOL WHIP. See CREAM TOPPING, NONDAIRY.				
CORIANDER/Chinese parsley				
raw	1 tbsp	5	4	0.1
raw	1 tsp	2	1	0.0
raw, approx .8 oz	9 plants	4	6	0.1
trimmed	1 oz	6	8	0.2
untrimmed	1 lb	77	108	2.3
CORIANDER LEAF/Chinese parsley leaf				
dried	1 oz	79	60	1.3
dried	1 tbsp	5	4	0.1
dried	1 tsp	2	1	<.1
CORIANDER SEED/Chinese parsley seed				
whole	1 oz	84	10	5.0
whole	1 tbsp	15	2	0.9
whole	1 tsp	5	1	0.3
whole *(Durkee)*	1 tsp	8	0	<0.1
whole *(Laurel Leaf)*	1 tsp	8	0	<0.1
whole *(Spice Islands)*	1 tsp	6	<1	0.3
CORN				
cooked	1/2 cup	88	0	0.5
dry	1 cup	375	3	2.2
dry	2 oz	203	2	1.2
sweet, boiled, drained	4 oz	122	19	1.5
sweet, raw, trimmed	1 oz	24	4	0.3
sweet, raw, untrimmed	1 lb	140	25	1.9
sweet, white, boiled, drained, cut	1/2 cup	89	14	1.0
sweet, white, kernels, boiled, drained	1 ear	83	13	1.0
sweet, white, kernels from cob, raw	1 ear	77	14	1.1
sweet, white, raw, cut	1/2 cup	66	12	0.9
sweet, yellow, boiled, drained, cut	1/2 cup	89	14	1.0

Food Name	Serv. Size	Total Cal.	Sod. MGS	Fat GMS
sweet, yellow, kernels, boiled, drained	1 ear	83	13	1.0
sweet, yellow, kernels from cob, raw	1 ear	77	14	1.1
sweet, yellow, raw, cut	1/2 cup	66	12	0.9
white	1/2 cup	303	29	3.9
yellow	1/2 cup	303	29	3.9
CORN, CANNED				
cream style	1/2 cup	93	365	0.5
cream style	4 oz	82	323	0.5
cream style (A&P)	1/2 cup	100	330	1.0
cream style (Finast)	1/2 cup	105	350	1.0
cream style (Green Giant)	1/2 cup	100	390	<1.0
cream style (S&W Nutradiet)	1/2 cup	100	0	1.0
cream style, golden (Del Monte)	1/2 cup	80	355	1.0
cream style, golden (Pathmark)	1/2 cup	100	350	1.0
cream style, golden (Stokely)	1/2 cup	100	380	0.0
cream style, golden, low-sodium	4 oz	82	3	0.5
cream style, golden 'No Salt Added' (Del Monte)	1/2 cup	80	10	1.0
cream style, golden, white (Stokely)	1/2 cup	100	380	0.0
cream style 'No Frills' (Pathmark)	1 cup	210	700	1.0
cream style 'Premium Homestyle No Starch Added' (S&W)	1/2 cup	120	285	1.0
cream style 'Premium Homestyle Starch Added' (S&W)	1/2 cup	105	435	1.0
cream style, white (Del Monte)	1/2 cup	90	355	0.0
'Crisp 'N Sweet' vacuum packed (Freshlike)	1/2 cup	80	5	1.0
'Delicorn' (Green Giant)	1/2 cup	80	350	<1.0
golden (Pathmark)	1/2 cup	90	330	1.0
golden (Stokely)	1/2 cup	90	300	0.0
golden, cream style (Freshlike)	1/2 cup	110	290	1.0
golden, cream style (Veg•All)	1/2 cup	110	290	1.0
golden, cream style, no salt added (Freshlike)	1/2 cup	110	15	1.0
golden, 50% less salt (Green Giant)	1/2 cup	70	175	<1.0
golden 'No Salt Added' (Del Monte)	1/2 cup	80	10	1.0
golden 'No Salt or Sugar Added' (Green Giant)	1/2 cup	80	0	<1.0
golden 'No Salt or Sugar Added' (Stokely)	1/2 cup	80	5	0.0
golden 'Pantry Express' (Green Giant)	1/2 cup	80	210	<1.0
golden, sweet (IGA)	1/2 cup	70	10	1.0
golden, vacuum pack (Green Giant)	1/2 cup	80	330	0.0
golden, vacuum pack (Stokely)	1/2 cup	90	300	0.0
golden, whole kernel (Veg•All)	1/2 cup	80	320	1.0
golden, whole kernel, vacuum packed (Freshlike)	1/2 cup	100	260	1.0
golden, whole kernel, vacuum packed (Veg•All)	1/2 cup	100	260	1.0
golden, whole kernel, water packed, w/o salt (Freshlike)	1/2 cup	80	5	1.0

Food Name	Serv. Size	Total Cal.	Sod. MGS	Fat GMS
golden, whole kernel, water packed, w/o sugar and salt				
(Freshlike)	1/2 cup	80	5	1.0
golden, w/liquid (Del Monte)	1/2 cup	70	355	1.0
in brine, w/liquid (Green Giant)	1/2 cup	70	350	0.0
kernel, w/liquid	4 oz	69	287	0.5
kernel, w/liquid (A&P)	1/2 cup	80	350	1.0
kernel, w/liquid (Featherweight)	1/2 cup	80	10	1.0
kernel, w/liquid (Finast)	1/2 cup	90	390	1.0
kernel, w/liquid (Green Giant)	1/2 cup	80	280	0.0
kernel, w/liquid (S&W Nutradiet)	1/2 cup	80	0	1.0
kernel, w/liquid, drained	4 oz	92	(mq)	1.1
kernel, w/liquid, 50% less salt, no sugar (Green Giant)	1/2 cup	50	140	1.0
kernel, w/liquid, low-sodium	4 oz	69	3	0.5
kernel, w/liquid 'No Frills' (Pathmark)	1 cup	160	550	1.0
kernel, w/liquid 'No Salt Added' (A&P)	1/2 cup	80	10	<1.0
kernel, w/liquid 'No Salt Added' (Finast)	1/2 cup	80	10	1.0
kernel, w/liquid 'No Salt Added' (Pathmark)	1/2 cup	70	10	1.0
niblets (Green Giant)	1/2 cup	80	310	0.0
niblets, no salt, no sugar added (Green Giant)	1/2 cup	80	0	<1.0
sweet, select (Green Giant)	1/2 cup	60	280	<1.0
sweet, white, brine pack, drained solids	1/2 cup	66	265	0.8
sweet, white, brine pack, regular, w/liquid	1/2 cup	78	324	0.6
sweet, white, brine pack, dietary, w/liquid	1/2 cup	78	4	0.6
sweet, white, cream style, regular pack	1/2 cup	92	365	0.5
sweet, white, cream style, special dietary pack	1/2 cup	92	4	0.5
sweet, white, vacuum pack, regular pack	1/2 cup	83	286	0.5
sweet, white, vacuum pack, special dietary pack	1/2 cup	83	3	0.5
sweet, yellow, brine pack, drained solids	1/2 cup	66	265	0.8
sweet, yellow, brine pack, regular, w/liquid	1/2 cup	78	324	0.6
sweet, yellow, brine pack, dietary, w/liquid	1/2 cup	78	4	0.6
sweet, yellow, cream style, regular pack	1/2 cup	92	365	0.5
sweet, yellow, cream style, special dietary pack	1/2 cup	92	4	0.5
sweet, yellow, vacuum pack, regular pack	1/2 cup	83	286	0.5
sweet, yellow, vacuum pack, special dietary pack	1/2 cup	83	3	0.5
vacuum pack, w/liquid (Del Monte)	1/2 cup	90	355	1.0
vacuum pack, w/liquid 'No Salt Added' (Del Monte)	1/2 cup	90	10	1.0
white (Green Giant)	1/2 cup	80	310	0.0
white (Stokely)	1/2 cup	90	290	0.0
white, vacuum pack (A&P)	1/2 cup	100	300	1.0
white, vacuum pack (Finast)	4 oz	90	150	1.0
white, vacuum pack (Green Giant)	1/2 cup	80	290	0.0

Food Name	Serv. Size	Total Cal.	Sod. MGS	Fat GMS
white, vacuum pack *(Pathmark)*	1/2 cup	120	350	1.0
white, vacuum pack 'Niblets' *(Green Giant)*	1/2 cup	80	280	1.0
white, w/liquid *(Del Monte)*	1/2 cup	70	355	0.0
white, young, tender 'Premium' *(S&W)*	1/2 cup	90	295	1.0
whole kernel, golden, sweet *(Green Giant)*	1/2 cup	70	360	0.0
whole kernel, golden, sweet,50% less salt *(Green Giant)*	1/2 cup	70	180	<1.0
w/peppers 'Mexicorn' *(Green Giant)*	1/2 cup	80	450	<1.0
CORN, FROZEN				
(Health Valley)	1/2 cup	76	4	0.0
cream style *(Green Giant)*	1/2 cup	110	370	1.0
freeze-dried, prepared *(Mountain House)*	1/2 cup	90	<1	1.0
golden, in butter sauce *(Green Giant)*	1/2 cup	100	310	2.0
in butter sauce *(Finast)*	1/2 cup	170	390	4.0
in butter sauce 'Niblets' *(Green Giant)*	1/2 cup	100	280	2.0
in butter sauce 'Niblets One Serving' *(Green Giant)*	4.5 oz	120	350	2.0
in butter sauce 'Side Dish' *(Budget Gourmet)*	5.5 oz	190	310	6.0
in butter sauce 'Singles' *(Stokely)*	4 oz	110	230	1.0
in sauce, country style 'Side Dish' *(Budget Gourmet)*	5.75 oz	140	290	5.0
kernel *(A&P)*	3.3 oz	80	0	<1.0
kernel *(Finast)*	3.3 oz	80	5	1.0
kernel, cut *(Frosty Acres)*	3.3 oz	80	3	1.0
kernel, cut *(Seabrook)*	3.3 oz	80	3	1.0
kernel, cut *(Southern)*	3.5 oz	98	20	0.7
kernel, cut, petite 'Deluxe' *(Birds Eye)*	2.6 oz	70	0	1.0
kernel, cut 'Portion Pack' *(Birds Eye)*	3 oz	70	0	1.0
kernel, cut 'Singles' *(Stokely)*	3 oz	75	5	1.0
kernel 'Harvest Fresh Niblets' *(Green Giant)*	1/2 cup	80	40	1.0
kernel 'Niblets' *(Green Giant)*	1/2 cup	90	5	<1.0
kernel 'Niblets Supersweet' *(Green Giant)*	1/2 cup	60	5	1.0
kernel 'Sweet' *(Birds Eye)*	3.3 oz	80	0	1.0
kernel 'Tender Sweet Deluxe' *(Birds Eye)*	3.3 oz	80	0	1.0
niblets 'Butter Sauce' *(Green Giant)*	1/2 cup	100	310	2.0
niblets 'Plain Polybag' *(Green Giant)*	1/2 cup	90	5	<1.0
on the cob *(A&P)*	1 ear	120	0	1.0
on the cob *(Birds Eye)*	1 ear	120	0	1.0
on the cob *(Frosty Acres)*	1 ear	120	0	1.0
on the cob *(Seabrook)*	5-inch ear	120	4	1.0
on the cob *(Southern)*	5-inch ear	140	na	1.0
on the cob, baby 'Deluxe' *(Birds Eye)*	2.6 oz	25	10	0.0
on the cob 'Big Ears' *(Birds Eye)*	1 ear	160	0	1.0
on the cob, boiled, drained, kernels from ear	4 oz	59	3	0.5

Food Name	Serv. Size	Total Cal.	Sod. MGS	Fat GMS
on the cob 'Cob Treats' (A&P)	2 ears	130	5	1.0
on the cob, 5.3 oz edible portion (Ore-Ida)	1 ear	180	40	2.0
on the cob, in butter sauce 'Singles' (Stokely)	1 ear	70	200	1.0
on the cob, kernels from ear	8 oz	123	6	1.0
on the cob 'Little Ears' (Birds Eye)	2 ears	130	0	1.0
on the cob, miniature 'Mini-Gold' (Ore-Ida)	2 ears	180	40	2.0
on the cob 'Nibblers, 6-ear pkg' (Green Giant)	2 ears	120	10	1.0
on the cob 'Nibblers Supersweet' (Green Giant)	2 ears	90	10	2.0
on the cob 'Niblet Ears' (Green Giant)	1 ear	120	10	1.0
on the cob 'Niblet Ears Supersweet' (Green Giant)	1 ear	90	10	2.0
on the cob 'One Serving' (Green Giant)	2 half ears	120	10	1.■
on the cob 'Sweet Select' (Green Giant)	1 ear	90	10	2.■
on the cob 'Sweet Select' half ears (Green Giant)	2 half ears	90	10	2.■
sweet (Birds Eye)	3.3 oz	80	0	1.0
sweet, select 'Plain Polybag' (Green Giant)	1/2 cup	60	5	1.■
sweet, tender 'Butter Sauce Combination' (Birds Eye)	3.3 oz	90	250	2.■
sweet, tender 'Deluxe' (Birds Eye)	3.3 oz	80	0	1.■
sweet, white, kernels, boiled, drained	1 ear	59	3	0.■
sweet, white, kernels, boiled, drained	1/2 cup	76	3	0.■
sweet, white, kernels, unprepared	1/2 cup	72	2	0.■
sweet, yellow, kernels, boiled, drained	1 ear	59	3	0.
sweet, yellow, kernels, boiled, drained	1/2 cup	76	3	0.■
sweet, yellow, kernels, unprepared	1/2 cup	72	2	0.■
white (Green Giant)	1/2 cup	90	5	1.■
white (Seabrook)	3.3 oz	80	3	1.■
white, in butter sauce (Green Giant)	1/2 cup	100	280	2.■
white, shoepeg 'Butter Sauce' (Green Giant)	1/2 cup	100	280	2.
white, shoepeg 'Harvest Fresh' (Green Giant)	1/2 cup	90	60	1.■
white, shoepeg 'Select' (Green Giant)	1/2 cup	90	5	<1.■
whole kernel, 'Portion Pack' (Birds Eye)	3 oz	70	0	1.■

CORN AND PEPPERS, CANNED

Food Name	Serv. Size	Total Cal.	Sod. MGS	Fat GMS
red and green peppers, solid and liquid	1/2 cup	86	396	0.
vacuum packed (Freshlike)	1/2 cup	90	300	1.
vacuum packed (Veg•All)	1/2 cup	90	300	1.

CORN BRAN

Food Name	Serv. Size	Total Cal.	Sod. MGS	Fat GMS
crude	1 cup	170	5	0.
crude	1 oz	64	2	0.

CORN CAKE

Food Name	Serv. Size	Total Cal.	Sod. MGS	Fat GMS
apple cinnamon flavor (Roman Meal)	1 cake	49	<5	<1.
caramel, fat-free (Quaker)	1 cake	50	30	0.
caramel flavor, fat free (Roman Meal)	1 cake	50	5	0.

Food Name	Serv. Size	Total Cal.	Sod. MGS	Fat GMS
cheddar flavor *(Roman Meal)*	1 cake	43	14	<1.0
natural butter flavor, fat free *(Roman Meal)*	1 cake	40	35	0.0
plain	1 cake	35	44	0.2
popcorn	1 cake	38	29	0.3
popcorn, butter flavor *(Chico-San)*	1 cake	40	45	0.0
popcorn, caramel *(Chico-San)*	1 cake	50	55	0.0
popcorn, lightly salted *(Chico-San)*	1 cake	40	45	0.0
popcorn, white cheddar cheese *(Chico-San)*	1 cake	50	65	1.0
popped, butter flavor *(Quaker)*	1 cake	35	55	0.0
popped, white cheddar flavor *(Quaker)*	1 cake	40	110	0.0
very low sodium	1 cake	24	5	0.0
white cheddar flavor, fat free *(Roman Meal)*	1 cake	45	15	0.0
CORN CHIPS AND SNACKS. See also TORTILLA CHIPS.				
barbecue *(Bachman)*	1 oz	150	230	9.0
barbecue 'Rowdy Rustlers' 34 chips *(Fritos)*	1 oz	150	300	9.0
'Bar-B-Q Fritos' 34 pieces *(Fritos)*	1 oz	150	320	9.0
bare bean 'Garden Vegetable Chips' *(Harry's)*	1 oz	144	<1	7.0
bare bean 'Offbeat Originals' *(Peddlers)*	1 oz	144	<1	7.0
beet garlic 'Garden Vegetable Chips' *(Harry's)*	1 oz	134	43	5.0
beet garlic 'Offbeat Originals' *(Peddlers)*	1 oz	134	43	5.0
bell pepper 'Garden Vegetable Chips' *(Harry's)*	1 oz	140	40	6.0
bell pepper 'Offbeat Originals' *(Peddlers)*	1 oz	140	40	6.0
blue corn 'Corn Curls' *(Arrowhead Mills)*	1 oz	120	54	2.0
blue corn 'Corn Curls Unsalted' *(Arrowhead Mills)*	1 oz	120	1	2.0
blue corn, no salt added *(Barbara's Bakery)*	1 oz	140	15	7.0
blue corn, regular *(Barbara's Bakery)*	1 oz	140	120	7.0
blue garlic 'Garden Vegetable Chips' *(Harry's)*	1 oz	129	28	4.0
blue garlic 'Offbeat Originals' *(Peddlers)*	1 oz	129	28	4.0
caramel corn puffs, apple cinnamon, fat-free *(Health Valley)*	1 oz	100	50	0.0
caramel corn puffs, original style, fat-free *(Health Valley)*	1 oz	100	45	0.0
caramel corn puffs, peanut flavor, fat-free *(Health Valley)*	1 oz	100	65	0.0
carrot caraway 'Garden Vegetable Chips' *(Harry's)*	1 oz	131	31	4.0
carrot caraway 'Offbeat Originals' *(Peddlers)*	1 oz	131	31	4.0
cheddar cheese *(Health Valley)*	1 oz	160	120	10.0
cheese 'Baked' *(Jax)*	1 oz	140	290	7.0
cheese 'Baked, Corn Puffs' *(Cheez Doodles)*	1 oz	150	360	8.0
cheese 'Cheese Curls Low Salt' *(Featherweight)*	1 oz	150	81	9.0
cheese 'Crunchy' *(Jax)*	1 oz	160	250	11.0

Food Name	Serv. Size	Total Cal.	Sod. MGS	Fat GMS
cheese curls 'Great Tasting' (Ultra Slim Fast)	1 oz	110	360	3.0
cheese 'Fried Corn Puffs' (Cheez Doodles)	1 oz	160	220	10.0
chili cheese, 34 chips (Fritos)	1 oz	160	300	10.0
cones, nacho-flavor	1 oz	152	270	9.0
cones, plain	1 oz	145	290	7.6
cool ranch (Doritos)	1 oz	140	115	7.0
corn chips (Wise)	1 oz	160	180	10.0
corn crunchies (Wise)	1 oz	160	180	10.0
corn nuggets, toasted (Fritos)	1.38 oz	170	265	5.0
corn ridgies (Wise)	1 oz	160	180	10.0
corn spirals, toasted (Wise)	1 oz	160	125	10.0
corn twists, crispy (Wise)	1 oz	160	125	10.0
'Crisp 'N Thin' 18 chips (Fritos)	1 oz	160	210	10.0
curls, barbecue flavored (Weight Watchers)	.5 oz	60	110	2.0
curls, pizza flavored (Weight Watchers)	.5 oz	60	130	2.0
curls, ranch flavored (Weight Watchers)	.5 oz	60	170	2.0
'Dip Size Fritos' 13 pieces (Fritos)	1 oz	150	210	9.0
'Fritos' 34 pieces (Fritos)	1 oz	150	230	9.0
'Low Salt' (Featherweight)	1 oz	170	3	11.0
mild bean 'Garden Vegetable Chips' (Harry's)	1 oz	144	74	7.0
mild bean 'Offbeat Originals' (Peddlers)	1 oz	144	74	7.0
nacho cheese (Bugles)	1 oz	160	250	9.0
nacho cheese (Corn Snackers)	.5-oz pkg	60	240	2.0
nacho cheese flavor (Doritos)	1 oz	140	150	7.0
nacho cheese 'Non-Stop' 34 chips (Fritos)	1 oz	150	220	9.0
'No Salt Added' (Health Valley)	1 oz	160	1	11.0
onion-flavor	1 oz	142	278	6.4
'Pinta Blues' picante (Barbara's Bakery)	1 oz	130	250	6.0
'Pinta Blues' regular (Barbara's Bakery)	1 oz	140	110	6.0
'Pinta Puffs' salsa (Barbara's Bakery)	1 oz	70	130	2.0
'Pinta' regular (Barbara's Bakery)	1 oz	138	100	6.0
plain	1 oz	153	179	9.5
plain (Bachman)	1 oz	160	160	10.0
plain (Bugles)	1 oz	150	290	8.0
plain (Corn Snackers)	.5-oz pkg	60	190	2.0
plain (Health Valley)	1 oz	160	90	11.0
plain (Planters)	1 oz	160	160	10.0
plain (Snyder's)	1 oz	160	150	11.0
'Potilla' chipotle chili (Barbara's Bakery)	1 oz	140	180	8.0
'Potilla' regular (Barbara's Bakery)	1 oz	140	120	8.0
puffs, cheese-flavor	1 oz	157	298	9.8

Food Name	Serv. Size	Total Cal.	Sod. MGS	Fat GMS
puffs, cheese-flavor, enriched	1 oz	110	8	0.7
ranch *(Bugles)*	1 oz	150	290	9.0
'Rippled Corn Chips' *(Dipsy Doodles)*	1 oz	160	180	10.0
toasted corn, crunchy, barbecue *(Cornuts)*	2 oz	247	553	8.1
toasted corn, crunchy, barbecue *(Cornuts)*	1 oz	124	277	4.1
toasted corn, crunchy, chili picante *(Cornuts)*	1 oz	120	260	4.0
toasted corn, crunchy, nacho *(Cornuts)*	2 oz	248	359	8.1
toasted corn, crunchy, nacho *(Cornuts)*	1 oz	124	180	4.0
toasted corn, crunchy, original *(Cornuts)*	2 oz	249	311	8.0
toasted corn, crunchy, original *(Cornuts)*	1 oz	124	156	4.0
toasted corn, crunchy, ranch *(Cornuts)*	1 oz	120	190	4.0
toasted corn, crunchy, unsalted *(Cornuts)*	1 oz	120	30	4.0
'Unsalted' *(Azteca)*	1 oz	140	110	7.0
veggie 'Garden Vegetable Chips' *(Harry's)*	1 oz	141	40	7.0
veggie 'Offbeat Originals' *(Peddlers)*	1 oz	141	40	7.0
wild bean 'Garden Vegetable Chips' *(Harry's)*	1 oz	141	51	6.0
wild bean 'Offbeat Originals' *(Peddlers)*	1 oz	141	51	6.0
'Wild 'N Mild' 32 chips *(Fritos)*	1 oz	160	240	9.0
yellow 'Corn Chips' *(Arrowhead Mills)*	.75 oz	90	31	1.0
yellow, w/cheese 'Corn Chips' *(Arrowhead Mills)*	.75 oz	90	30	2.0
CORN FLAKE CRUMBS *(Kellogg's)*	1 oz	100	290	0.0
CORN FLOUR				
masa	1 oz	103	1	1.1
masa, enriched, white	1 cup	416	6	4.3
masa, enriched, yellow	1 cup	416	6	4.3
'Masa Harina De Maiz' approx 1/3 cup *(Quaker)*	1.3 oz	137	5	1.5
'Masa Trigo' approx 1/3 cup *(Quaker)*	1.3 oz	149	794	4.0
whole-grain	1 oz	102	1	1.1
whole-grain, white	1/2 cup	209	3	2.2
whole-grain, yellow	1/2 cup	209	3	2.2
CORN FRITTER, frozen *(Mrs. Paul's)*	2 pieces	240	560	9.0
CORN GRITS. See GRITS.				
CORN NUGGETS, FROZEN				
breaded, fried 'Quickkrisp' *(Stilwell)*	3 oz	210	420	8.0
CORN OIL				
	1/2 cup	964	0	109.0
	1 oz	251	0	28.4
	1 tbsp	120	0	13.6
(Crisco)	1 tbsp	120	0	14.0
(Crisco) 'Puritan'	1 tbsp	120	0	14.0
(Hain)	1 tbsp	120	0	14.0

Food Name	Serv. Size	Total Cal.	Sod. MGS	Fat GMS
(Kroger)	1 tbsp	122	0	13.6
(Mazola)	1 tbsp	120	0	14.0
(Pathmark)	1 tbsp	130	0	14.0
(Pathmark) 'No Frills'	1 tbsp	130	0	14.0
(Spectrum Naturals)	1 tbsp	120	0	14.0
(Wesson)	1 tbsp	120	0	14.0
CORN OIL SPRAY. See COOKING SPRAY.				
CORN OIL SPREAD				
(Fleischmann's) 60% oil 'Light'	1 tbsp	80	70	8.0
(Fleischmann's) 40% oil 'Extra Light'	1 tbsp	50	55	6.0
CORN SALAD, raw	1/2 cup	6	1	0.1
CORN SOUFFLÉ, FROZEN, 1 pkg (Stouffer's)	6 oz	240	760	11.0
CORN SYRUP				
dark	1 cup	925	508	0.0
dark	1 tbsp	56	31	0.0
dark (Karo)	1 tbsp	60	40	0.0
high-fructose	1 cup	871	6	0.0
high-fructose	1 tbsp	53	0	0.0
light	1 cup	925	397	0.0
light	1 tbsp	56	24	0.0
light (Karo)	1 tbsp	60	30	0.0
table blends, refiner, and sugar	1 cup	1008	224	0.0
table blends, refiner, and sugar	1 tbsp	64	14	0.0
CORNBREAD. See BREAD.				
CORNMEAL				
	1 cup	605	58	7.9
	1 oz	103	10	1.3
blue, whole-grain (Arrowhead Mills)	2 oz	210	1	3.0
degermed	1 oz	104	1	0.5
degermed, enriched, white	1 cup	505	4	2.3
degermed, enriched, yellow	1 cup	505	4	2.3
degermed, unenriched, white	1 cup	505	4	2.3
degermed, unenriched, yellow	1 cup	505	4	2.3
white, bolted (Aunt Jemima)	1 oz	99	337	0.7
white, bolted, enriched (Aunt Jemima)	1 oz	99	382	0.9
white, dry (Albers)	1 oz	100	0	1.0
white, enriched, approx 3 tbsp (Aunt Jemima)	1 oz	102	1	0.5
white, whole-grain	1 cup	442	43	4.4
whole-grain	1 oz	103	10	1.0
whole-grain, hi-lysine (Arrowhead Mills)	2 oz	210	1	2.0
yellow, dry (Albers)	1 oz	100	0	1.0

Food Name	Serv. Size	Total Cal.	Sod. MGS	Fat GMS
yellow, enriched *(Aunt Jemima)*	1 oz	102	1	0.5
yellow, whole-grain	1 cup	442	43	4.4
yellow, whole-grain *(Arrowhead Mills)*	2 oz	210	1	2.0
CORNMEAL, SELF-RISING				
bolted	1 oz	95	353	1.0
bolted, w/wheat flour	1 oz	99	374	0.8
degermed	1 oz	101	382	0.5
white *(Aunt Jemima)*	1 oz	98	381	0.5
white, bolted *(Aunt Jemima)*	1 oz	98	381	0.5
white, bolted, enriched *(Aunt Jemima)*	1 oz	99	382	0.9
white, bolted, plain, enriched	1 cup	407	1521	4.2
white, bolted, wheat flour added, enriched	1 cup	592	2242	4.8
white, buttermilk *(Aunt Jemima)*	3 tbsp	101	439	1.1
white, degermed, enriched	1 cup	490	1860	2.4
yellow *(Aunt Jemima)*	3 tbsp	100	490	1.0
yellow, bolted, plain, enriched	1 cup	407	1521	4.2
yellow, bolted, wheat flour added, enriched	1 cup	592	2242	4.8
yellow, degermed, enriched	1 cup	490	1860	2.4
CORNED BEEF. See BEEF, CORNED.				
CORNISH GAME HEN				
frozen *(Tyson)*	3.5 oz	240	70	14.0
frozen, w/skin *(Tyson)*	3.5 oz	250	80	15.0
w/wild rice, wholesale club item *(Tyson)*	3.5 oz	190	125	11.0
CORNSTARCH				
	1 cup	488	12	0.1
	1 oz	108	3	<.1
	1 tbsp	30	1	tr
(Argo)	1 tbsp	30	0	0.0
(Cream)	1 tbsp	29	tr	tr
(Kingsford)	1 tbsp	30	0	0.0
COTTAGE CHEESE. See CHEESE.				
COTTONSEED FLOUR				
lowfat	1 oz	94	10	0.4
partially defatted	1 cup	337	33	5.8
partially defatted	1 oz	102	10	1.8
partially defatted	1 tbsp	18	2	0.3
COTTONSEED KERNELS				
roasted	1 cup	754	37	54.1
roasted	1 oz	143	7	10.3
roasted	1 tbsp	51	3	3.6
COTTONSEED MEAL, partially defatted	1 oz	104	11	1.4

Food Name	Serv. Size	Total Cal.	Sod. MGS	Fat GMS
COTTONSEED OIL				
....	1 cup	1927	0	218.0
....	1/2 cup	964	0	109.0
....	1 tbsp	120	0	13.6
(Wesson)	1 tbsp	122	0	13.6
COUSCOUS				
cooked	1/2 cup	101	4.5	.1
cooked	4 oz	127	6	0.2
dry	1/2 cup	346	9	0.6
dry	1 oz	107	3	0.2
mix, dry (Near East)	1.25 oz	120	5	0.0
mix, prepared w/2 tbsp salted butter (Fantastic Foods)	1/2 cup	122	35	3.0
mix, prepared w/o added ingredients (Fantastic Foods)	1/2 cup	105	1	0.0
mix, whole-wheat (Fantastic Foods)	1/2 cup	94	0	0.0
mix, whole-wheat, prepared w/2 tbsp salted butter (Fantastic Foods)	1/2 cup	111	23	2.0
COUSCOUS PILAF MIX				
(Casbah) dry	1 oz	100	na	0.0
(Casbah) prepared w/o added ingredients	1/2 cup	100	na	0.0
(Quick Pilaf) savory, prepared w/2 tbsp salted butter	1/2 cup	124	254	3.0
(Quick Pilaf) savory, prepared w/o added ingredients	1/2 cup	94	215	0.0
COWPEA. See BLACK-EYED PEAS.				
CRAB				
ALASKAN KING				
boiled	4 oz	110	1216	1.7
boiled, approx 4.7 oz	1 leg	129	1436	1.7
moist-heat cooked	3 oz	82	911	1.3
poached	4 oz	110	1216	1.7
poached, approx 4.7 oz	1 leg	129	1436	1.7
raw	1 lb	379	3792	2.7
raw	3 oz	71	711	0.5
raw	1 oz	24	237	0.2
steamed	4 oz	110	1216	1.7
steamed, approx 4.7 oz	1 leg	129	1436	1.7
BLUE				
boiled	4 oz	116	316	2.0
boiled, approx 4.75 oz	1 cup	138	376	2.4
cake, fried	4 oz	176	374	8.5
cake, fried, approx 2.1 oz	1 med	93	198	4.5
canned	1 cup	134	450	1.7
canned	4 oz	112	378	1.4

Food Name	Serv. Size	Total Cal.	Sod. MGS	Fat GMS
canned	3 oz	84	283	1.0
moist-heat cooked	1 cup	138	377	2.4
moist-heat cooked	3 oz	87	237	1.5
poached	4 oz	116	316	2.0
poached, approx 4.75 oz	1 cup	138	376	2.4
raw	1 lb	395	1329	4.9
raw	3 oz	74	249	0.9
raw	1 oz	25	83	0.3
steamed	4 oz	116	316	2.0
steamed, approx 4.75 oz	1 cup	138	376	2.4
DUNGENESS				
canned *(S&W)*	3.25 oz	81	920	2.0
moist-heat cooked	3 oz	94	321	1.0
raw	1 lb	391	1340	4.4
raw	3 oz	73	251	0.8
raw	1 oz	24	84	0.3
IMPERIAL	1 cup	323	1602	16.7
QUEEN				
moist-heat cooked	100 gm	115	691	1.5
moist-heat cooked	3 oz	98	587	1.3
raw	1 lb	407	2445	5.4
raw	3 oz	77	458	1.0
raw	1 oz	26	153	0.3
SNOW				
frozen *(Wakefield)*	3 oz	60	270	1.0
raw, Opilio, clusters *(Peter Pan Seafoods)*	3.5 oz	91	539	1.2
raw, Opilio, 'Snap 'n' Eat' scored *(Peter Pan Seafoods)*	3.5 oz	91	539	1.2
SOFTSHELL				
boiled	4 oz	116	316	2.0
boiled, approx 4.75 oz	1 cup	138	376	2.4
cake, fried	4 oz	176	374	8.5
cake, fried, approx 2.1 oz	1 med	93	198	4.5
poached	4 oz	116	316	2.0
poached, approx 4.75 oz	1 cup	138	376	2.4
raw	1 lb	395	1329	4.9
raw	1 oz	25	83	0.3
raw, approx .7 oz	1 crab	18	62	0.2
steamed	4 oz	116	316	2.0
steamed, approx 4.75 oz	1 cup	138	376	2.4
CRAB, ALTERNATIVE				
	1 lb	463	3815	5.9

Food Name	Serv. Size	Total Cal.	Sod. MGS	Fat GMS
....	1 oz	29	238	0.4
Alaskan King, made from surimi	3 oz	87	715	1.1
(Icicle Brand)	3.5 oz	99	900	0.1
CRAB, DEVILED				
....	1 cup	451	2081	22.6
breaded, frozen, cake (Mrs. Paul's)	3 oz	180	480	9.0
breaded, frozen, miniature (Mrs. Paul's)	3.5 oz	240	540	12.0
CRAB AND SHRIMP, frozen (Wakefield)	3 oz	60	210	1.0
CRAB CAKE				
....	100 gm	147	504	2.1
....	1 cake	88	302	1.3
blue crab	1 cake	93	198	4.5
CRABAPPLE				
raw	100 gm	76	1	0.3
raw, slices, w/skin	1 cup	84	1	0.3
trimmed, w/skin	1 oz	22	<1	0.1
trimmed, w/skin, sliced	1/2 cup	42	1	0.2
untrimmed	1 lb	316	4	1.3
CRABAPPLE, CANNED				
spiced (Lucky Leaf)	4 oz	110	(mq)	0.0
spiced (Musselman's)	4 oz	110	(mq)	0.0
CRACKER				
apple cinnamon 'Orchard Crisps' (Nabisco)	.5 oz	60	40	2.0
bacon flavor (Delicious)	.5 oz	70	190	3.0
bacon flavor 'Bacon Flavored Thins' .5 oz (Nabisco) ...	7 crackers	70	210	4.0
bacon flavor 'Toasteds' approx .5 oz (Keebler)	4 crackers	60	125	3.0
banana walnut 'Orchard Crisps' (Nabisco)	.5 oz	60	40	2.0
barbecue wheat, for weight control (Spicer's)	1 oz	100	75	5.0
bar-b-que, tater crisps (Mr. Phipps)	.5 oz	60	160	2.0
bite size (Delicious)	.5 oz	70	90	3.0
bite size, low sodium (Delicious)	.5 oz	70	55	3.0
'Bits' approx .5 oz (Triscuit)	15 crackers	60	85	3.0
bran (FiberRich)	1 cracker	18	10	<1.0
bran, toasted 'Bran Thins' (Nabisco)	7 crackers	60	70	3.0
butter, country flavor (McCrakens)	1 oz	140	170	8.0
butter flavor (Ritz)	4 crackers	70	140	4.0
butter flavor, approx .5 oz (Escort)	3 crackers	70	115	4.0
butter flavor 'Club Low Salt' approx .5 oz (Keebler)	4 crackers	60	75	3.0
butter flavor, dairy, .5 oz (American Classic)	4 crackers	70	140	3.0
butter flavor 'Flutters' (Pepperidge Farm)	.75 oz	100	150	4.0
butter flavor 'Ritz Bits' 22 pieces (Ritz)	.5 oz	70	120	4.0

Food Name	Serv. Size	Total Cal.	Sod. MGS	Fat GMS
butter flavor 'Ritz Bits Low Salt' 22 pieces (Ritz)	.5 oz	70	60	4.0
butter flavor 'Ritz Low Salt' approx .5 oz (Ritz)	4 crackers	70	60	4.0
butter flavor 'Ritz' approx .5 oz (Ritz)	4 crackers	70	120	4.0
butter flavor 'Toasteds Buttercrisp' .5 oz (Keebler)	4 crackers	60	125	3.0
butter flavor 'Town House Low Salt' .5 oz (Keebler)	4 crackers	70	60	4.0
butter flavor 'Town House' approx .5 oz (Keebler)	4 crackers	70	120	4.0
butter flavor, thins 'Distinctive' (Pepperidge Farm)	4 crackers	70	115	3.0
cheese (Combos)	1.8 oz	240	580	10.0
cheese (Delicious)	.5 oz	70	135	3.0
cheese 'Better Cheddars' (Nabisco)	.5 oz	70	130	4.0
cheese 'Better Cheddars' low salt (Nabisco)	.5 oz	70	65	4.0
cheese, bite size (Delicious)	.5 oz	70	135	3.0
cheese, cheddar, approx 13-16 crackers (Frito-Lay's)	.5 oz	70	150	4.0
cheese, cheddar, baked, cracker chips 'Zings' (Nabisco)	.5 oz	70	140	3.0
cheese, cheddar 'Crackups' (Nabisco)	.5 oz	70	100	3.0
cheese, cheddar 'Goldfish' (Pepperidge Farm)	1 oz	120	230	4.0
cheese, cheddar 'Goldfish Thins' (Pepperidge Farm)	4 crackers	50	160	2.0
cheese, cheddar 'Guppies' 12 pieces (Pepperidge Farm)	.5 oz	40	95	2.0
cheese, cheddar 'Original Goldfish' (Pepperidge Farm)	1 oz	130	190	5.0
cheese, cheddar 'Snorkels' (Nabisco)	.5 oz	70	150	2.0
cheese, cheddar, tangy (McCrakens)	1 oz	140	170	8.0
cheese, cheddar 'Town House Jrs.' 8 pieces (Keebler)	.5 oz	80	95	4.0
cheese 'Cheddar Wedges' 31 pieces (Nabisco)	.5 oz	70	150	3.0
cheese 'Cheese Nips' 13 pieces (Nabisco)	.5 oz	70	130	3.0
cheese 'Cheese Peanut Butter Sandwich' 4 pieces (Nabisco)	1 oz	130	320	7.0
cheese 'Cheese Ritz Bits Mini Ritz' 22 pieces (Ritz)	.5 oz	70	130	4.0
cheese 'Cheez-Its' (Sunshine)	12 crackers	70	135	4.0
cheese 'Cheez-Its Low Salt' (Sunshine)	12 crackers	70	65	4.0
cheese, Parmesan 'Goldfish' (Pepperidge Farm)	1 oz	120	330	4.0
cheese, reduced fat 'Snack Wells' 18 pieces (Nabisco)	.5 oz	60	160	1.0
cheese 'Ritz Bits Sandwiches' approx .5 oz (Ritz)	6 crackers	80	135	5.0
cheese, sandwich-type w/peanut butter filling	.5 oz	68	141	3.3
cheese, Swiss 'Naturally Flavored' .5 oz (Nabisco)	7 crackers	70	170	3.0
cheese 'Tid-Bits' 15 pieces (Nabisco)	.5 oz	70	200	4.0
cheese, white cheddar 'Cheez-Its' (Sunshine)	.5 oz	76	160	4.0
cheese flavor (Hain)	1 oz	130	180	6.0
cheese flavor, organic, fat-free (Health Valley)	.5 oz	40	80	0.0
cheese flavor, 25 pieces (Rokeach)	1 oz	140	(mq)	8.0
cheese sandwich, and cheese 'Handi-Snacks' (Kraft)	1 pkg	120	360	8.0
cheese sandwich, and peanut butter, .5 oz (Keebler)	2 crackers	70	150	3.0

Food Name	Serv. Size	Total Cal.	Sod. MGS	Fat GMS
cheese sandwich, cheddar 'Town House' .5 oz (Keebler)	1 cracker	70	105	4.0
cheese sandwich, wheat and American cheese, .5 oz (Keebler)	1 cracker	70	85	4.0
cheese-filled, 6 crackers (Frito-Lay's)	1.5 oz	210	470	10.0
chicken flavor 'Chicken in a Biskit' 7 pieces (Nabisco)	.5 oz	80	130	5.0
cinnamon graham (Delicious)	.5 oz	60	50	2.0
cinnamon graham, fat-free 'Snack Wells' (Nabisco)	.5 oz	50	45	0.0
cracked pepper, fat-free 'Snack Wells' (Nabisco)	.5 oz	60	160	0.0
cracked pepper 'Gourmet' fat-free (Frookie)	4 crackers	35	40	0.0
cracked wheat, approx .5 oz (American Classic)	4 crackers	70	140	4.0
cracked wheat 'Distinctive' (Pepperidge Farm)	3 crackers	100	180	4.0
cracked wheat 'Wafers' (Hickory Farms)	8 crackers	100	290	3.0
'Crackerbread' (Crisp & Light)	1 slice	17	25	<1.0
'Crackerbread Salt Free' (Crisp & Light)	1 slice	17	<1	<1.0
'Crackerdiles' (Delicious)	.5 oz	70	135	3.0
crispbread (Dar-Vida)	1 cracker	20	40	<1.0
crispbread 'Breakfast' (Wasa)	1 cracker	50	65	1.0
crispbread, dark (Finn Crisp)	2 crackers	38	130	<1.0
crispbread 'Extra Crisp' (Wasa)	1 cracker	25	40	0.0
crispbread 'Fiber Plus' (Wasa)	1 cracker	35	65	1.0
crispbread, garlic flavor (Weight Watchers)	2 crackers	30	55	0.0
crispbread, high fiber 'Crisp Bread' (Ryvita)	1 cracker	23	10	<1.0
crispbread, high fiber 'Snackbread' (Ryvita)	1 cracker	14	25	<1.0
crispbread, regular (Finn Crisp)	2 crackers	38	130	<1.0
crispbread, thick (Kavli Norwegian)	1 slice	35	31	0.3
crispbread, thin (Kavli Norwegian)	2 slices	40	32	0.3
crispbread, w/caraway (Finn Crisp)	2 slices	38	130	<1.0
5-spice wafer (Westbrae)	4.5 wafers	40	30	0.0
garlic 'Discos' (Delicious)	.5 oz	78	184	5.0
garlic 'Garlic Tams' (Manischewitz)	10 crackers	153	165	8.0
garlic and herb 'Gourmet' fat-free (Frookie)	8 crackers	70	170	0.0
graham, chocolate 'Selects' (Keebler)	4 crackers	60	55	3.0
graham, honey nut 'Selects' (Keebler)	4 crackers	60	70	3.0
graham cracker 'Amaranth Graham Crackers' (Health Valley)	7 crackers	110	110	3.0
graham cracker, apple cinnamon 'Graham Bites' (Honey Maid)	11 crackers	60	80	2.0
graham cracker, approx .5 oz (Keebler)	4 crackers	70	85	2.0
graham cracker, approx 1 oz (Regal)	2 crackers	140	120	7.0
graham cracker, approx 1 oz (Rokeach)	8 crackers	120	(mq)	3.0

Food Name	Serv. Size	Total Cal.	Sod. MGS	Fat GMS
graham cracker, brown sugar 'Graham Bites' .5 oz (Honey Maid) .... 11 crackers		60	80	2.0
graham cracker 'Grahamy Bears' (Sunshine) .... 9 crackers		130	160	5.0
graham cracker, 2 pieces (Nabisco) .... .5 oz		60	90	1.0
grain, 6 pieces (Harvest Crisps) .... .5 oz		60	135	2.0
hearty wheat 'Distinctive' (Pepperidge Farm) .... 4 crackers		100	140	5.0
herb, garden 'Flutters' (Pepperidge Farm) .... .75 oz		100	190	4.0
herb, organic, fat-free (Health Valley) .... .5 oz		40	80	0.0
herb 'Stoned Wheat' (Health Valley) .... 13 crackers		120	160	6.0
herb 'Stoned Wheat No Salt Added' (Health Valley) ... 13 crackers		120	30	6.0
honey graham (Delicious) .... .5 oz		60	50	2.0
hot and spicy 'Cheez-Its' approx 12 crackers (Sunshine) ..... .5 oz		70	160	4.0
'Low Salt' (Featherweight) .... 2 crackers		30	1	1.0
matzo, American board (Manischewitz) .... 1 oz		115	na	1.9
matzo 'Daily Unsalted' board (Manischewitz) .... 1 oz		110	1	0.3
matzo, dietetic, thin board (Manischewitz) .... .8 oz		91	<1	0.4
matzo, egg .... .5 oz		55	3	0.3
matzo, egg, 1 oz .... 1 matzo		111	6	0.6
matzo, egg, miniature 'Passover' approx 1 oz (Manischewitz) .... 10 crackers		108	10	2.0
matzo, egg 'Passover' board (Manischewitz) .... 1.2 oz		132	5	2.0
matzo, egg and onion .... .5 oz		55	40	0.6
matzo, egg and onion, 1 oz .... 1 matzo		111	81	1.1
matzo, egg n' onion, board (Manischewitz) .... 1 oz		112	180	1.0
matzo, miniature (Manischewitz) .... 10 crackers		90	10	<1.0
matzo 'Passover' board (Manischewitz) .... 1.1 oz		129	5	0.4
matzo, plain .... .5 oz		56	0	0.2
matzo, plain, 1 oz .... 1 matzo		112	1	0.4
matzo, tea 'Daily' thin board (Manischewitz) .... .9 oz		103	1	0.3
matzo, thin board (Manischewitz) .... .9 oz		100	0	0.3
matzo, whole-wheat .... .5 oz		50	0	0.2
matzo, whole-wheat, 1 oz .... 1 matzo		100	1	0.4
matzo, whole wheat, w/bran, board (Manischewitz) .... 1 oz		110	1	0.6
melba toast, bacon 'Rounds' (Old London) .... .5 oz		53	126	1.0
melba toast, garlic 'Rounds' (Old London) .... .5 oz		56	132	1.2
melba toast, honey bran (Devonsheer) .... 1 cracker		16	25	0.4
melba toast, honey bran 'Rounds' (Devonsheer) .... .5 oz		52	98	0.9
melba toast, oat, .5 oz (Harvest Crisps) .... 6 crackers		60	135	2.0
melba toast, onion 'Rounds' (Devonsheer) .... .5 oz		51	120	0.6
melba toast, onion 'Rounds' (Old London) .... .5 oz		52	121	0.8
melba toast, plain .... .5 oz		55	118	0.5

Food Name	Serv. Size	Total Cal.	Sod. MGS	Fat GMS
melba toast, plain *(Devonsheer)*	1 cracker	16	30	0.4
melba toast, plain 'Rounds' *(Devonsheer)*	.5 oz	53	111	0.6
melba toast, plain 'Unsalted' *(Devonsheer)*	1 cracker	16	5	0.4
melba toast, plain 'Unsalted Rounds' *(Devonsheer)*	.5 oz	52	5	0.6
melba toast, plain, w/o salt	.5 oz	55	3	0.5
melba toast, pumpernickel *(Old London)*	.5 oz	54	156	0.6
melba toast, rye	.5 oz	55	127	0.5
melba toast, rye *(Devonsheer)*	1 cracker	16	30	0.4
melba toast, rye *(Old London)*	.5 oz	52	132	0.7
melba toast, rye, .5 oz *(Devonsheer)*	1 cracker	16	30	0.4
melba toast, rye 'Rounds' *(Devonsheer)*	.5 oz	53	130	0.6
melba toast, rye 'Rounds' *(Old London)*	.5 oz	52	132	0.7
melba toast, rye 'Unsalted' *(Devonsheer)*	1 cracker	16	5	0.4
melba toast, sesame *(Devonsheer)*	1 cracker	16	25	0.5
melba toast, sesame *(Old London)*	.5 oz	55	148	1.8
melba toast, sesame 'Rounds' *(Devonsheer)*	.5 oz	57	131	1.8
melba toast, sesame 'Rounds' *(Old London)*	.5 oz	56	149	1.8
melba toast, sesame 'Unsalted' *(Old London)*	.5 oz	55	5	1.8
melba toast, vegetable *(Devonsheer)*	1 cracker	16	25	0.4
melba toast, wheat	.5 oz	53	119	0.3
melba toast, wheat *(Old London)*	.5 oz	51	121	0.7
melba toast, wheat '6-calorie' *(Estee)*	1 cracker	6	5	<1.0
melba toast, wheat 'Snax' *(Estee)*	1 oz	100	15	<1.0
melba toast, white *(Old London)*	.5 oz	51	111	0.6
melba toast, white 'Rounds' *(Old London)*	.5 oz	48	111	0.6
melba toast, white 'Unsalted' *(Old London)*	.5 oz	51	4	0.6
melba toast, whole grain *(Old London)*	.5 oz	52	116	0.9
melba toast, whole grain 'Rounds' *(Old London)*	.5 oz	54	102	1.2
melba toast, whole grain 'Unsalted' *(Old London)*	.5 oz	53	4	1.0
melba toast, whole wheat *(Devonsheer)*	1 cracker	16	30	0.4
melba toast, whole wheat 'Unsalted' *(Devonsheer)*	1 cracker	16	5	0.4
milk	.5 oz	65	84	2.2
multi-grain *(Premium)*	.5 oz	60	140	2.0
multi-grain 'Wheat Thins' *(Nabisco)*	.5 oz	60	135	2.0
nacho cheese flavor *(Delicious)*	.5 oz	89	150	5.0
natural, for weight control *(Spicer's)*	1 oz	100	65	4.0
nutty wheat 'Wheat Thins' approx .5 oz *(Nabisco)*	7 crackers	70	170	4.0
oat 'Oat Krisp' *(Ralston)*	.5 oz	50	140	2.0
oat 'Oat Thins' approx .5 oz *(Nabisco)*	8 crackers	70	90	3.0
oat, .5 oz *(Harvest Crisps)*	6 crackers	60	135	2.0
oat bran 'Oat Bran Krisps' *(Ralston)*	.5 oz	60	140	3.0

Food Name	Serv. Size	Total Cal.	Sod. MGS	Fat GMS
'Old Fashioned' (Hickory Farms)	10 crackers	90	170	3.0
onion (Delicious)	.5 oz	70	180	3.0
onion 'Discos' (Delicious)	.5 oz	76	156	5.0
onion, minced, approx .5 oz (American Classic)	4 crackers	70	120	3.0
onion, organic, fat-free (Health Valley)	.5 oz	40	80	0.0
onion flavor (Hain)	1 oz	130	160	6.0
onion flavor 'No Salt Added' (Hain)	1 oz	130	5	6.0
onion flavor 'Onion Tams' (Manischewitz)	10 crackers	150	157	8.0
onion flavor 'Toasteds' approx .5 oz (Keebler)	4 crackers	60	140	3.0
onion garlic wafer (Westbrae)	4.5 crackers	40	50	0.0
oyster	.5 oz	62	185	1.7
oyster (OTC)	1 cracker	25	65	1.0
oyster (Premium)	20 crackers	60	210	1.0
oyster (Sunshine)	16 crackers	60	190	1.0
oyster, approx .5 oz (Dandy)	20 crackers	60	220	2.0
oyster, low salt	.5 oz	62	90	1.7
oyster 'Oysterettes' approx .5 oz (Nabisco)	18 crackers	60	140	1.0
oyster, unsalted tops	.5 oz	62	109	1.7
peanut butter (Combos)	1.8 oz	240	360	10.0
peanut butter, cheese (Little Debbie)	1.4 oz	190	390	9.0
peanut butter, cheese (Little Debbie)	.93 oz	130	260	6.0
peanut butter, cheese sandwich (Handi-Snacks)	1 pkg	190	180	14.0
peanut butter 'Ritz Bits Sandwiches' 1 oz (Ritz)	12 crackers	80	80	4.0
peanut butter, toast, approx .5 oz (Keebler)	2 crackers	70	120	3.0
peanut butter 'Toast Sandwich' 4 pieces (Nabisco)	1 oz	130	300	7.0
peanut butter, toasty (Little Debbie)	1.4 oz	200	380	12.0
peanut butter, toasty (Little Debbie)	.93 oz	140	250	7.0
peanut butter bar (Frito-Lay's)	1.75 oz	270	65	16.0
peanut butter-filled, 6 crackers (Frito-Lay's)	1.5 oz	210	450	10.0
pizza 'Goldfish' (Pepperidge Farm)	1 oz	130	220	5.0
poppy, toasted, approx .5 oz (American Classic)	4 crackers	70	140	3.0
pumpernickel (Delicious)	.5 oz	70	160	3.0
pumpernickel 'Snack Sticks' (Pepperidge Farm)	8 crackers	140	330	6.0
ranch, baked, cracker chips 'Zings' (Nabisco)	.5 oz	70	140	3.0
ranch 'Snack Crisps' (Estee)	.66 oz	80	135	2.0
'Regency' (Delicious)	.5 oz	70	100	<3.0
rice, approx .5 oz (Harvest Crisps)	6 crackers	60	135	2.0
rice, harvest 'Crispbread' (Weight Watchers)	2 crackers	30	55	0.0
rice bran (Health Valley)	7 crackers	130	64	4.0
'Rich' (Hain)	1 oz	130	160	5.0
'Rich, No Salt Added' (Hain)	1 oz	130	15	5.0

Food Name	Serv. Size	Total Cal.	Sod. MGS	Fat GMS
'Royal Lunch Milk Crackers' .5 oz *(Nabisco)*	1 cracker	60	80	2.0
rusk toast	.5 oz	58	36	1.0
rye	.5 oz	52	37	0.2
rye *(Hain)*	1 oz	120	200	4.0
rye, BBQ 'Rounds O' Rye' *(Hickory Farms)*	1 oz	153	60	10.6
rye, dark 'Crisp Bread' *(Ryvita)*	1 cracker	26	35	<1.0
rye, garlic 'Rounds O' Rye' *(Hickory Farms)*	1 oz	147	126	8.9
rye, golden 'Crispbread' *(Wasa)*	1 cracker	35	55	0.0
rye, hearty 'Crispbread' *(Wasa)*	1 cracker	45	70	0.0
rye, light 'Crisp Bread' *(Ryvita)*	1 cracker	26	20	<1.0
rye, light 'Crispbread Lite' *(Wasa)*	1 cracker	25	40	0.0
rye, light 'Hi-Fiber' *(Finn Crisp)*	1 cracker	35	60	1.0
rye, natural 'Rounds O' Rye' *(Hickory Farms)*	1 oz	156	93	10.9
rye 'No Salt Added' *(Hain)*	1 oz	120	10	4.0
rye, original 'Hi-Fiber' *(Finn Crisp)*	1 cracker	40	95	0.0
rye 'RyKrisp' *(Ralston)*	.5 oz	40	75	0.0
rye 'Rykrisp Twindividuals' 2 triple pieces *(Ralston)*	.5 oz	45	105	1.0
rye 'Salt Free' *(Hickory Farms)*	8 crackers	90	na	1.0
rye, sandwich-type w/cheese filling	.5 oz	68	148	3.2
rye, seasoned 'Rykrisp' *(Ralston)*	.5 oz	45	105	1.0
rye, sesame 'Rykrisp' 2 triple pieces *(Ralston)*	.5 oz	50	105	2.0
rye, sesame, toasted 'Crisp Bread' *(Ryvita)*	1 cracker	31	10	<1.0
rye, sour cream 'Rounds O'Rye' *(Hickory Farms)*	1 oz	155	130	10.7
rye 'Toasteds' approx .5 oz *(Keebler)*	4 crackers	60	140	3.0
rye 'Wafers' *(Hickory Farms)*	8 crackers	90	250	3.0
rye wafers, plain	.5 oz	47	113	0.1
rye wafers, seasoned	.5 oz	54	126	1.3
salsa 'Crackups' *(Nabisco)*	.5 oz	70	100	3.0
salt sticks, Vienna bread type, 6.5 inches long	1 stick	106	548	1.1
saltine, approx .5 oz *(Zesta)*	5 crackers	60	190	2.0
saltine 'Bits Mini Saltine Crackers' .5 oz *(Premium)*	16 crackers	70	160	3.0
saltine, crumbs, not packed	1 cup	303	770	8.4
saltine 'Fat-Free' .5 oz *(Premium)*	4 crackers	50	115	0.0
saltine 'Krispy' *(Sunshine)*	5 crackers	60	210	1.0
saltine 'Krispy Unsalted Tops' *(Sunshine)*	5 crackers	60	120	1.0
saltine, low salt	.5 oz	62	90	1.7
saltine 'Low Salt' approx .5 oz *(Premium)*	5 crackers	60	115	2.0
saltine 'Low Salt' approx .5 oz *(Zesta)*	5 crackers	60	95	2.0
saltine, mild cheddar 'Krispy' *(Sunshine)*	5 crackers	60	180	2.0
saltine, 1 7/8-inch square	10 crackers	123	312	3.4
saltine, original, .5 oz *(Premium)*	5 crackers	60	180	2.0

Food Name	Serv. Size	Total Cal.	Sod. MGS	Fat GMS
saltine, 10 pieces (Rokeach)	1 oz	120	na	3.0
saltine, unsalted tops	.5 oz	62	109	1.7
saltine 'Unsalted' (Estee)	4 crackers	60	0	2.0
saltine 'Unsalted Tops' approx .5 oz (Premium)	5 crackers	60	135	2.0
saltine 'Unsalted Tops' approx .5 oz (Zesta)	5 crackers	60	85	2.0
saltine, wheat, approx .5 oz (Zesta)	5 crackers	60	190	2.0
saltine, wheat 'Whole Wheat Premium Plus' .5 oz (Premium)	4 crackers	60	130	2.0
sandwich, peanut-cheese, 6 sandwiches	1 pkt	206	417	10.0
sandwich, peanut-cheese, 4 sandwiches	1 pkt	137	278	6.7
sandwich, w/cheese filling	.5 oz	68	199	3.0
sandwich, w/peanut butter filling	.5 oz	69	134	3.4
'Schooners' 33 pieces (FFV)	.5 oz	60	130	2.0
sesame (Hain)	1 oz	140	210	7.0
sesame, bread wafer, approx .5 oz (Meal Mates)	3 crackers	70	160	3.0
sesame 'Crisp' (FFV)	1 cracker	60	120	2.0
sesame 'Crispbread' (Dar-Vida)	1 cracker	22	40	1.0
sesame 'Distinctive' (Pepperidge Farm)	4 crackers	80	140	4.0
sesame, golden (American Classic)	4 crackers	70	120	3.0
sesame, golden, .5 oz (American Classic)	4 crackers	70	120	3.0
sesame, golden 'Flutters' (Pepperidge Farm)	.75 oz	110	150	5.0
sesame 'No Salt Added' (Hain)	1 oz	140	5	7.0
sesame 'RyKrisp' (Ralston)	.5 oz	50	105	2.0
sesame, savory 'Crispbread' (Wasa)	1 cracker	30	40	1.0
sesame 'Snack Sticks' (Pepperidge Farm)	8 crackers	140	280	5.0
sesame 'Toasteds' approx .5 oz (Keebler)	4 crackers	60	130	3.0
sesame, wafer 'Crisp' approx .5 oz (FFV)	4 crackers	60	140	2.0
sesame and cheese 'Twigs Snack Sticks' .5 oz (Nabisco)	5 crackers	70	140	4.0
sesame chips (Flavor Tree)	1/4 cup	163	380	9.2
sesame wafer (Westbrae)	4.5 crackers	40	60	0.0
sesame wheat (Delicious)	.5 oz	80	170	4.0
sesame wheat 'Crispbread' (Wasa)	1 cracker	50	65	2.0
sesame wheat 'Stoned Wheat' (Health Valley)	13 crackers	130	150	6.0
sesame wheat 'Stoned Wheat No Salt Added' (Health Valley)	13 crackers	130	20	6.0
seven grain 'Stoned Wheat' (Health Valley)	13 crackers	120	125	5.0
seven grain 'Stoned Wheat No Salt Added' (Health Valley)	13 crackers	120	20	5.0
seven-grain vegetable, organic, fat-free (Health Valley)	.5 oz	40	80	0.0

Food Name	Serv. Size	Total Cal.	Sod. MGS	Fa GM
seven-grain vegetable; organic, no salt added				
(Health Valley)	.5 oz	40	80	0.
snack, approx .5 oz (Finast)	12 crackers	70	135	3.
snack, approx .5 oz (Rokeach)	9 crackers	130	(mq)	5.
'Snack N' Cracker' (Delicious)	.5 oz	70	180	3.
'Snackers' (Delicious)	.5 oz	70	90	3.
'Sociables' approx .5 oz (Nabisco)	6 crackers	70	135	4.
soda (Sailor Boy Pilot)	1 cracker	100	125	3.
soda 'Distinctive English Water Biscuit'				
(Pepperidge Farm)	4 crackers	70	100	1.
soda 'English' (North Castles)	1 cracker	10	14	0.
soda, .5 oz (Crown Pilot)	1 cracker	70	70	2
soda, low salt	.5 oz	62	90	1.
soda, 'Lunch' 1 cracker (Royal)	.5 oz	60	125	3.
soda 'Ocean Crisps' (FFV)	1 cracker	60	120	2
soda, unsalted tops	.5 oz	62	109	1
soup, low salt	.5 oz	62	90	1
soup, unsalted tops	.5 oz	62	109	1
sour cream and chive (Hain)	1 oz	130	150	6.
sour cream and chive 'No Salt Added' (Hain)	1 oz	130	25	6.
sour cream and chive flavor (McCrakens)	1 oz	140	170	8
sour cream and onion 'Discos' (Delicious)	.5 oz	79	162	5
sour cream and onion, for weight control (Spicer's)	1 oz	100	150	4
sour cream and onion 'Mr. Phipp's Tater Crisps'				
(Nabisco)	.5 oz	60	150	2
sourdough (Delicious)	.5 oz	70	160	3
sourdough (Hain)	.5 oz	65	100	3
sourdough 'Low Salt' (Hain)	1 oz	130	10	5
sticks 'Snack Sticks' (Pepperidge Farm)	8 crackers	130	400	5
'Tam Tams' (Manischewitz)	10 crackers	147	171	8
'Tam Tams No Salt' (Manischewitz)	10 crackers	138	10	7
tamari wafer (Westbrae)	4.5 crackers	40	60	0
'Uneeda Biscuits Unsalted Tops' approx .5 oz (Nabisco)	2 crackers	60	100	2
vegetable (Hain)	1 oz	130	180	5
vegetable, garden (Delicious)	.5 oz	70	220	3
vegetable 'Garden Crisps' (Nabisco)	.5 oz	60	135	2
vegetable 'No Salt Added' (Hain)	1 oz	130	50	5
'Vegetable Thins' (Nabisco)	7 crackers	70	140	4
wafer, no salt (Westbrae)	4.5 wafers	40	0	0
water (Sailor Boy Pilot)	1 cracker	100	125	3

Food Name	Serv. Size	Total Cal.	Sod. MGS	Fat GMS
water 'Distinctive English Water Biscuit' (Pepperidge Farm)	4 crackers	70	100	1.0
water 'English' (North Castles)	1 cracker	10	14	0.0
water, .5 oz (Crown Pilot)	1 cracker	70	70	2.0
water 'Gourmet' fat-free (Frookie)	4 crackers	35	60	0.0
water, 'Lunch' 1 cracker (Royal)	.5 oz	60	125	3.0
water 'Ocean Crisps' (FFV)	1 cracker	60	120	2.0
water 'Table Water, Bite Size' (Carr's)	2 crackers	25	15	1.0
'Waverly Crackers' approx .5 oz (Nabisco)	4 crackers	70	160	3.0
'Waverly Crackers Low Salt' approx .5 oz (Nabisco)	4 crackers	70	80	3.0
'Waverly Wafer' approx .5 oz (Nabisco)	4 crackers	70	160	3.0
wheat (Delicious)	.5 oz	70	85	3.0
wheat, approx .5 oz (Sociables)	6 crackers	70	135	3.0
wheat 'Bits' approx .5 oz (Triscuit)	8 crackers	60	75	2.0
wheat 'Crispy Wafer' approx .5 oz (FFV)	6 crackers	70	80	3.0
wheat, low salt	.5 oz	67	40	2.9
wheat 'Low Salt' approx .5 oz (Triscuit)	3 crackers	60	35	2.0
'Wheat On' (Delicious)	.5 oz	68	86	3.0
wheat 'Original Snackbread' (Ryvita)	1 cracker	20	20	<1.0
wheat 'Original Wheat Thins' approx .5 oz (Nabisco)	8 crackers	70	120	3.0
wheat, regular	.5 oz	67	113	2.9
wheat, sandwich, w/cheese filling	.5 oz	70	129	3.5
wheat, sandwich, w/peanut butter filling	.5 oz	70	114	3.8
wheat 'Snack Wells' (Nabisco)	.5 oz	50	160	0.0
wheat 'Snacks' approx .5 oz (Finast)	7 crackers	70	85	3.0
wheat 'Stone Ground' approx .5 oz (Wheatsworth)	4 crackers	70	135	3.0
wheat 'Stoned Wheat' (Health Valley)	13 crackers	120	85	6.0
wheat 'Stoned Wheat No Salt Added' (Health Valley)	13 crackers	120	10	6.0
wheat 'Stoned Wheat Wafer' approx .5 oz (FFV)	4 crackers	60	170	2.0
wheat 'Stoned Wheat Wafers Salt Free' (Hickory Farms)	8 crackers	100	0	2.0
wheat toasted (McCrakens)	1 oz	140	170	8.0
wheat, toasted 'Distinctive' (Pepperidge Farm)	4 crackers	80	140	3.0
wheat, toasted 'Flutters' (Pepperidge Farm)	.75 oz	110	170	5.0
wheat 'Wheat Krisp' (Ralston)	.5 oz	50	220	1.0
wheat 'Wheat Mill Wafers Salt Free' (Hickory Farms)	4 crackers	50	na	1.0
wheat 'Wheat Tams' (Manischewitz)	10 crackers	150	180	8.0
wheat 'Wheat Thins' (Nabisco)	8 crackers	70	120	3.0
wheat 'Wheat Thins Low Salt' approx .5 oz (Nabisco)	8 crackers	70	60	3.0
wheat 'Wheats' (Sunshine)	8 crackers	70	170	4.0
wheat 'Whole Wheat'N Bran Wafers' (Triscuit)	3 crackers	60	75	2.0
'Wheatine' bits (Barbara's Bakery)	.5 oz	60	132	2.0

Food Name	Serv. Size	Total Cal.	Sod. MGS	Fat GMS
'Wheatines' cracked pepper (Barbara's Bakery)	.5 oz	60	132	2.0
'Wheatines' lightly salted tops (Barbara's Bakery)	.5 oz	60	132	2.0
'Wheatines' sesame (Barbara's Bakery)	.5 oz	60	132	2.0
'Wheatines' unsalted tops (Barbara's Bakery)	.5 oz	60	45	2.0
wheatstone (Delicious)	.5 oz	70	180	3.0
whole grain 'Crispbread' approx .35 oz (Wasa)	1 slice	30	40	1.0
whole grain 'Harvest Wheats' approx .5 oz (Keebler)	4 crackers	60	95	3.0
whole wheat	.5 oz	63	93	2.4
whole wheat (Carr's)	2 crackers	70	15	1.0
whole wheat (Manischewitz)	10 crackers	90	10	1.0
whole wheat, approx .5 oz (Ritz)	5 crackers	70	135	3.0
whole wheat 'Gourmet' fat-free (Frookie)	4 crackers	35	60	0.0
whole wheat, low salt	.5 oz	63	35	2.4
whole wheat, organic, fat-free (Health Valley)	.5 oz	40	80	0.0
whole wheat 'Wheatables' approx .5 oz (Keebler)	12 crackers	70	140	3.0
w/bacon and cheese (Handi-Snacks)	1 pkg	130	410	9.0
zesty Italian, approx 13-16 crackers (Frito-Lay's)	.5 oz	70	115	3.0
zwieback	1 oz	121	66	2.8
'Zwieback Teething Toast' approx .5 oz (Nabisco)	2 crackers	60	20	1.0

CRACKER CRUMBS AND MEAL

Food Name	Serv. Size	Total Cal.	Sod. MGS	Fat GMS
meal	1 cup	440	32	2.0
meal	1 oz	109	8	0.5
(Golden Dipt) meal	1 oz	100	0	0.0
(Manischewitz) matzo 'Farfel'	1 cup	280	2	0.0
(Manischewitz) matzo meal 'Daily'	1 cup	514	3	1.
(Nabisco) meal	1/4 cup	110	10	0.5
(Premium) fat-free	2 tbsp	50	0	0.0

CRANBERRY

Food Name	Serv. Size	Total Cal.	Sod. MGS	Fat GMS
raw (Ocean Spray) approx 2 oz	1/2 cup	25	0	0.0
raw, chopped	1 cup	54	1	0.2
raw, whole	1 cup	47	1	0.
trimmed	1 oz	14	<1	0.
trimmed, chopped	1/2 cup	27	1	0.
trimmed, whole	1/2 cup	23	1	0.
w/stems	1 lb	210	5	0.5

CRANBERRY APPLE COCKTAIL

Food Name	Serv. Size	Total Cal.	Sod. MGS	Fat GMS
(Minute Maid) 'Juices To Go'	6 oz	120	20	0.
(Welch's) frozen, diluted	6 oz	120	0	0.0

CRANBERRY APPLE DRINK

Food Name	Serv. Size	Total Cal.	Sod. MGS	Fat GMS
	6 oz	123	4	0.
(A&P)	6 oz	130	<1	(tr

Food Name	Serv. Size	Total Cal.	Sod. MGS	Fat GMS
(Ocean Spray) 'Cran•Apple'	6 oz	120	15	0.0
(Ocean Spray) 'Cran•Apple Low Calorie'	6 oz	35	15	0.0
(P&Q)	6 oz	130	<1	(tr)
(Pathmark)	6 oz	130	10	0.0
CRANBERRY APPLESAUCE, 'Cran•Fruit' (Ocean Spray)	2 oz	100	10	0.0
CRANBERRY APRICOT DRINK				
	6 oz	118	4	0.0
'Cranicot' (Ocean Spray)	6 oz	120	15	0.0
CRANBERRY BEAN/borlotti/Roman bean/rose coco				
boiled	1 cup	241	2	0.8
boiled	1/2 cup	120	1	0.4
boiled	4 oz	154	1	0.5
raw	1 cup	653	12	2.4
raw	1/2 cup	328	6	1.2
raw	1 oz	95	2	0.3
CRANBERRY BEAN, CANNED				
	1 cup	216	863	0.7
(Progresso)	1/2 cup	110	420	<1.0
w/liquid	1/2 cup	108	431	0.4
w/liquid	4 oz	94	376	0.3
CRANBERRY BLUEBERRY JUICE (Knudsen & Sons)	8 oz	115	na	0.0
CRANBERRY COCKTAIL JUICE				
(J. Hungerford)	9.03 oz	141	0	0.0
(J. Hungerford) 50% juice	9.03 oz	134	7	0.1
(J. Hungerford) 100% juice	9.03 oz	133	19	0.0
CRANBERRY DRINK				
(Ocean Spray) citrus 'Refreshers'	6 oz	100	15	0.0
(Ocean Spray) 'Cran•Blueberry'	6 oz	120	10	0.0
(Ocean Spray) 'Cran•Raspberry'	6 oz	110	15	0.0
(Ocean Spray) 'Cran•Raspberry Low Calorie'	6 oz	40	15	0.0
(Ocean Spray) 'Cran•Strawberry'	6 oz	110	15	0.0
(Tropicana) 'Cranberry Orchard Juice Sparkler'	8 oz	120	20	0.0
CRANBERRY GRAPE COCKTAIL				
frozen, prepared (Welch's)	6 oz	110	0	0.0
CRANBERRY GRAPE DRINK				
(Finast)	6 oz	103	5	0.0
(Ocean Spray) 'Cran•Grape'	6 oz	120	15	0.0
(Pathmark)	6 oz	103	5	0.0
CRANBERRY JUICE				
(Knudsen & Sons) 'Just Cranberry'	8 oz	40	na	0.0
(Knudsen & Sons) 'Yankee'	8 oz	125	na	0.0

Food Name	Serv. Size	Total Cal.	Sod. MGS	Fat GMS
(Lucky Leaf)	6 oz	110	10	0.0
(Ocean Spray) 'Cran•tastic'	6 oz	100	15	0.0
(Santa Cruz Natural) organic 'Sparkling'	8 oz	90	na	<1.0
(Snapple) 'Cranberry Royale'	8 oz	150	25	0.0
CRANBERRY JUICE COCKTAIL				
	1 cup	144	5	0.3
	6 oz	108	4	0.2
(A&P)	6 oz	100	0	<1.0
(Ocean Spray)	6 oz	110	10	0.0
(Ocean Spray) 'Low Calorie'	6 oz	40	15	0.0
(P&Q)	6 oz	100	0	<1.0
(Pathmark)	6 oz	100	10	0.0
(Pathmark) 'No Frills'	6 oz	100	10	0.0
(Sunkist)	6 oz	110	8	0.1
(Sunkist) frozen, prepared	6 oz	110	0	0.1
(Veryfine)	8 oz	160	10	0.0
(Welch's) frozen 'No Sugar Added' prepared	6 oz	40	5	0.0
(Welch's) frozen, prepared	6 oz	100	0	0.0
(Welch's) frozen, w/blueberry, prepared	6 oz	110	0	0.0
(Welch's) frozen, w/raspberry, prepared	6 oz	110	0	0.0
CRANBERRY JUICE DRINK				
citrus 'Refreshers' (Ocean Spray)	6 oz	100	15	0.0
CRANBERRY LEMONADE				
(Knudsen & Sons)	8 oz	115	na	0.0
(Santa Cruz Natural) organic	8 oz	100	na	<1.0
CRANBERRY NECTAR				
(Knudsen & Sons)	8 oz	110	na	0.0
(Santa Cruz Natural) organic	8 oz	110	na	<1.0
CRANBERRY RASPBERRY DRINK				
(Tropicana) w/strawberry 'Twister'	6 oz	110	4	<1.0
(Tropicana) w/strawberry 'Twister Light' w/NutraSweet	6 oz	30	15	<1.0
CRANBERRY RASPBERRY JUICE (Knudsen & Sons)	8 oz	100	na	0.0
CRANBERRY RASPBERRY SAUCE				
'Cran•Fruit' (Ocean Spray)	2 oz	100	10	0.0
CRANBERRY SAUCE				
canned (A&P)	2 oz	100	15	<1.0
canned (Knudsen & Sons)	1 oz	30	na	<1.0
canned, sweetened	1 cup	418	80	0.4
canned, sweetened	4 oz	171	33	0.2
jellied (Finast)	2 oz	90	10	0.0
jellied (Ocean Spray)	2 oz	80	10	0.0

Food Name	Serv. Size	Total Cal.	Sod. MGS	Fat GMS
jellied *(Pathmark)*	2 oz	90	10	0.0
jellied 'Old Fashioned' *(S&W)*	1/2 cup	90	20	0.0
whole berry *(Finast)*	2 oz	90	10	0.0
whole berry *(Ocean Spray)*	2 oz	80	10	0.0
whole berry 'Old Fashioned' *(S&W)*	1/2 cup	90	20	0.0
CRANBERRY STRAWBERRY SAUCE				
crushed, for chicken 'Cran•Fruit' *(Ocean Spray)*	2 oz	90	10	0.0
CRAWFISH ENTRÉE, frozen, étouffée *(Cajun Cookin')*	12 oz	390	1110	10.0
CRAYFISH, MIXED SPECIES				
farmed, moist-heat cooked	100 gm	87	97	1.3
farmed, moist-heat cooked	3 oz	74	82	1.1
farmed, raw	3 oz	61	53	0.8
farmed, raw	8 crayfish	19	17	0.3
wild, moist-heat cooked	100 gm	88	94	1.2
wild, moist-heat cooked	3 oz	75	80	1.0
wild, raw	3 oz	65	49	0.8
wild, raw	8 crayfish	21	16	0.3
CREAM				
half and half	1 cup	315	98	27.8
half and half	1 oz	37	12	3.3
half and half	1 tbsp	20	6	1.7
half and half *(Crowley)*	1 oz	35	10	3.0
half and half *(Darigold)*	8 oz	310	120	27.0
half and half *(Knudsen)*	4 oz	150	60	13.0
half and half *(Rockview)*	2 tbsp	35	15	3.0
heavy, whipping	1 cup	821	89	88.1
heavy, whipping	1 tbsp	52	6	5.6
light, whipping	1 cup	699	82	73.9
light, whipping	1 tbsp	44	5	4.6
light, coffee or table	1 cup	469	95	46.3
light, coffee or table	1 oz	55	11	5.5
light, coffee or table	1 tbsp	29	6	2.9
medium, 25% fat	1 cup	583	88	59.7
medium, 25% fat	1 oz	69	10	7.1
medium, 25% fat	1 tbsp	37	6	3.8
CREAM CHEESE. See CHEESE.				
CREAM NUT. See BRAZIL NUT.				
CREAM OF TARTAR	1 tsp	8	2	0.0
CREAM SODA. See SOFT DRINKS AND MIXERS.				
CREAM TOPPING				
creamy white 'Dolci Frutta Crema Bianca' *(Saco Foods)*	1 box	900	110	50.1

Food Name	Serv. Size	Total Cal.	Sod. MGS	Fat GMS
dark chocolate 'Dolci Frutta Con Cioccolatta'				
(Saco Foods)	1 box	886	107	52.8
frozen, whipped (La Creme)	1 tbsp	16	5	1.0
frozen, whipped 'Real Cream' (Kraft)	1/4 cup	30	5	2.0
pressurized can, whipped	1 cup	154	78	13.3
pressurized can, whipped	1 oz	73	37	6.3
pressurized can, whipped	1 tbsp	8	4	0.7
pressurized can, whipped (Crowley)	1 tbsp	20	10	1.0
whipping, heavy	1 oz	98	11	10.5
whipping, heavy (Crowley)	1 oz	110	10	11.0
whipping, heavy (Darigold)	1 cup	790	90	81.0
whipping, heavy 'Classic' (Darigold)	1 cup	858	77	90.0
whipping, heavy 'UHT' (Darigold)	1 cup	790	90	81.0
whipping, heavy, whipped	2 cups	821	89	90.0
whipping, heavy, whipped	2 tbsp	52	6	5.6
whipping, light	1 oz	83	10	8.8
whipping, light, whipped	2 cups	699	82	5.6
whipping, light, whipped	2 tbsp	44	5	8.8
CREAM TOPPING, NONDAIRY				
frozen	1 cup	239	19	19.0
frozen	1 oz	90	7	7.2
frozen	1 tbsp	13	1	1.0
frozen, chocolate 'Cool Whip' (Birds Eye)	1 tbsp	12	0	1.0
frozen 'Cool Whip' (Birds Eye)	1 tbsp	12	0	1.0
frozen 'Cool Whip Lite' (Birds Eye)	1 tbsp	8	0	<1.0
frozen, extra creamy 'Cool Whip Dairy Recipe'				
(Birds Eye)	1 tbsp	14	0	1.0
frozen, semisolid	1 cup	239	19	19.0
frozen, semisolid	1 tbsp	13	1	1.0
frozen 'Whip' (Pet)	1 tbsp	14	0	1.0
frozen 'Whipped Topping' (Kraft)	1/4 cup	35	10	3.0
mix, dry	1.5 oz	245	52	17.0
mix, prepared (D-Zerta)	1 tbsp	8	5	1.0
mix, prepared (Featherweight)	1 tbsp	4	5	0.0
mix, prepared (Dream Whip)	1 tbsp	10	0	0.0
pressurized can	1 cup	184	43	15.6
pressurized can	1 oz	75	18	6.3
pressurized can	1 tbsp	11	2	0.9
pressurized can 'Richwhip' (Rich's)	.25 oz	20	5	2.0
prewhipped (Estee)	1 tbsp	4	0	<1.0
prewhipped 'Richwhip' (Rich's)	1 tbsp	12	0	1.0

Food Name	Serv. Size	Total Cal.	Sod. MGS	Fat GMS
reduced calorie *(D-Zerta)*	1 tbsp	8	5	1.0
unwhipped 'Richwhip' *(Rich's)*	.25 oz	20	10	2.0
CREAMER, NONDAIRY				
Liquid				
frozen	1/2 cup	164	95	12.0
frozen	1 oz	39	22	2.8
frozen	1 tbsp	20	12	1.5
w/hydrogenated vegetable oil and soy protein	1/2 cup	163	95	12.0
w/hydrogenated vegetable oil and soy protein	1/2 oz	20	12	1.5
w/lauric acid oil and sodium caseinate	1/2 cup	164	95	12.0
w/lauric acid oil and sodium caseinate	1/2 oz	20	12	1.5
(Coffee-Mate)	1 tbsp	16	5	1.0
(Coffee-Mate) 'Amaretto'	1 tbsp	40	5	2.0
(Coffee-Mate) 'Cinnamon Creme'	1 tbsp	40	5	2.0
(Coffee-Mate) fat-free	1 tbsp	10	0	0.0
(Coffee-Mate) 'Hazelnut'	1 tbsp	40	5	2.0
(Coffee-Mate) 'Irish Creme'	1 tbsp	40	5	2.0
(Crowley)	.5 oz	16	5	1.0
(Diehl)	1 tsp	10	0	<1.0
(Finast) frozen	.5 oz	20	10	2.0
(IGA)	1 tsp	10	5	<1.0
(N-Rich)	1 tsp	10	2	0.6
(Pathmark) 'No Frills'	1 tsp	10	5	0.0
(Rich's) frozen 'Coffee Rich'	.5 oz	20	10	2.0
(Rich's) frozen 'Farm Rich'	.5 oz	20	5	2.0
(Rich's) frozen 'Poly Rich'	.5 oz	20	5	1.0
(Saco Foods) 'kwik kream'	1 tbsp	10	0	<1.0
(Westbrae)	1 tbsp	10	10	<1.0
Powder				
	1/2 cup	257	85	25.8
	1 oz	155	51	10.1
	1 tsp	11	4	0.7
(Coffee-Mate)	1 tsp	10	5	<1.0
(Coffee-Mate) 'Amaretto'	2 tsp	60	15	3.0
(Coffee-Mate) 'Hazelnut'	2 tsp	60	15	3.0
(Coffee-Mate) 'Irish Creme'	2 tsp	60	15	3.0
(Coffee-Mate) 'Lite'	1 tsp	8	0	<1.0
(Cremora)	1 tsp	10	5	<1.0
CREME DE MENTHE. See ALCOHOLIC BEVERAGES.				
CRÊPE MIX, 7-inch crêpes *(Krusteaz)*	2 crêpes	80	110	1.0

Food Name	Serv. Size	Total Cal.	Sod. MGS	Fa GM
CRESS, GARDEN				
boiled, drained	4 oz	26	9	0.
boiled, drained	1/2 cup	16	5	0.
raw	1/2 cup	8	4	0.
raw, trimmed	1 oz	9	4	0.
raw, untrimmed	1 lb	103	45	2.
CROAKER, ATLANTIC				
raw	1 lb	474	252	14.
raw	3 oz	88	48	2.
raw	1 oz	29	16	0.
raw, approx 2.8 oz	1 fillet	82	44	2.
CROISSANT				
almond, 3.7 oz (Dunkin' Donuts)	1 croissant	420	280	27.
butter (Awrey's)	3 oz	300	280	17.
butter (Awrey's)	2 oz	200	190	11.
butter (Awrey's)	1 oz	100	90	6.
frozen, butter, 1.5 oz (Sara Lee)	1 croissant	170	250	9.
frozen, butter, petite (Pepperidge Farm)	1 croissant	140	160	7.
frozen, butter, petite 1 oz (Sara Lee)	1 croissant	120	160	6.
margarine (Awrey's)	2.5 oz	250	360	14.
margarine (Awrey's)	1.25 oz	120	180	7.
plain, 2.5 oz (Dunkin' Donuts)	1 croissant	310	240	19.
'Sandwich Quartet' (Pepperidge Farm)	1 croissant	170	250	7.
wheat (Awrey's)	2.5 oz	240	390	14.
CROUTONS				
Caesar salad (Brownberry)	.5 oz	62	165	2.
Caesar salad (Reese)	.5 oz	60	130	2.
cheddar and Romano cheese (Pepperidge Farm)	.5 oz	60	200	2.
cheddar cheese (Brownberry)	.5 oz	63	155	2.
cheese and garlic (Pepperidge Farm)	.5 oz	70	180	3.
onion and garlic (Brownberry)	.5 oz	60	190	2.
onion and garlic (Pepperidge Farm)	.5 oz	70	160	3.
plain	1 cup	122	209	2.
plain	.5 oz	58	99	0.
seasoned	1 cup	186	495	7.
seasoned	.5 oz	66	175	2.
seasoned (Brownberry)	.5 oz	59	155	2.
seasoned (Pepperidge Farm)	.5 oz	70	180	3.
seasoned (Weight Watchers)	1 pouch	30	120	0.
sour cream and chive (Pepperidge Farm)	.5 oz	70	170	3.
toasted (Brownberry)	.5 oz	56	145	1

Food Name	Serv. Size	Total Cal.	Sod. MGS	Fat GMS
CRUMPET				
blueberry, low-fat, cholestrol-free *(Wolferman's)*	1 crumpet	90	250	<1.0
brown sugar cinnamon, low-fat *(Wolferman's)*	1 crumpet	110	220	2.0
raspberry, low-fat, cholestrol-free *(Wolferman's)*	1 crumpet	90	260	1.0
CUCUMBER				
raw, approx 10.9 oz	1 med	39	6	0.4
raw, slices	1/2 cup	7	1	0.1
raw, w/peel, trimmed	1 oz	4	1	<.1
raw, w/peel, untrimmed	1 lb	56	9	0.6
CUMIN SEED				
whole	1 oz	106	48	6.3
whole	1 tbsp	22	10	1.3
whole	1 tsp	8	4	0.5
whole *(Durkee)*	1 tsp	10	0	<0.1
whole *(Laurel Leaf)*	1 tsp	10	0	<0.1
whole *(Spice Islands)*	1 tsp	7	3	0.4
CURRANT, BLACK/European currant				
raw	1 cup	71	2	0.5
trimmed	1 oz	18	1	0.1
untrimmed	1 lb	282	8	1.8
CURRANT, RED				
raw	1 cup	63	1	0.2
trimmed	1 oz	16	<1	0.1
untrimmed	1 lb	249	5	0.9
CURRANT, WHITE				
raw	1 cup	63	1	0.2
trimmed	1/2 cup	31	1	0.1
trimmed	1 oz	16	<1	0.1
untrimmed	1 lb	249	5	0.9
CURRANT, ZANTE				
dried	1 lb	1282	35	1.2
dried	1 cup	408	12	0.4
dried	1 oz	80	2	0.1
dried *(Del Monte)*	1/2 cup	200	10	0.0
CURRY POWDER				
ground	1 oz	92	15	3.9
ground	1 tbsp	20	3	0.9
ground	1 tsp	7	1	0.3
CUSK/torsk/tusk				
dry-heat cooked	3 oz	95	34	0.8
raw	1 lb	396	143	3.1

Food Name	Serv. Size	Total Cal.	Sod. MGS	Fa GM
raw	3 oz	74	26	0.
raw	1 oz	25	9	0.
raw, approx 4.3 oz	1 fillet	106	38	0.

CUSTARD. See PUDDING MIX; PUDDING/PIE FILLING, MIX.

CUSTARD APPLE/bullock's heart/cherimoya

raw	100 gm	101	4	0.
trimmed	1 oz	29	1	0.
untrimmed	1 lb	267	11	1.

CUTTLEFISH, MIXED SPECIES

moist-heat cooked	100 gm	158	744	1.
moist-heat cooked	3 oz	134	632	1
raw	1 lb	359	1686	3
raw	3 oz	67	316	0.
raw	1 oz	22	105	0.

CYMLING. See SQUASH, SCALLOP.

D

Food Name	Serv. Size	Total Cal.	Sod. MGS	F G
DAIKON/mullangi/Oriental radish				
boiled, drained	4 oz	19	15	0.
boiled, drained, sliced	1/2 cup	13	10	0
dried	1/2 cup	157	161	0
dried	1 oz	77	79	0
raw, trimmed	1 oz	5	6	<.
raw, trimmed (Frieda's)	1 lb	86	(mq)	0.
raw, trimmed (Frieda's)	1 oz	5	(mq)	<.
raw, trimmed, sliced	1/2 cup	8	9	<.
raw, untrimmed	1 lb	65	75	0.
DAIQUIRI. See ALCOHOLIC BEVERAGES.				
DANDELION GREENS				
boiled, drained	4 oz	37	50	0.
boiled, drained, chopped	1 cup	35	46	0.
raw, chopped	1 oz	13	22	0.
raw, trimmed	1 lb	204	345	3.
DANISH PASTRY				
APPLE				
(Awrey's)				
filled, 'Miniature' 1.7 oz	1 piece	160	170	8
filled 'Round' 4.5 oz	1 piece	390	390	20.

Food Name	Serv. Size	Total Cal.	Sod. MGS	Fat GMS
filled 'Round' 2.75 oz	1 piece	270	310	14.0
filled 'Square' 3 oz	1 piece	220	230	8.0
(Pepperidge Farm) frozen, 2.25 oz	1 piece	220	130	8.0
(Sara Lee)				
frozen 'Free & Light'	1/8 pkg	130	120	0.0
frozen 'Individual' 1.3 oz	1 piece	120	120	6.0
frozen twist	1/8 pkg	190	200	10.0
CARAMEL (Pillsbury) w/nuts, refrigerated	1 piece	160	240	8.0
CHEESE				
(Awrey's)				
filled, 'Miniature' 1.7 oz	1 piece	170	200	9.0
filled 'Round' 4.5 oz	1 piece	420	530	22.0
filled 'Round' 2.75 oz	1 piece	280	350	15.0
filled 'Square' 2.5 oz	1 piece	210	300	11.0
(Pepperidge Farm) frozen, 2.25 oz	1 piece	240	230	14.0
(Sara Lee) frozen, 'Individual' 1.3 oz	1 piece	130	130	8.0
CINNAMON (Sara Lee) twist, frozen	1/8 pkg	200	270	12.0
CINNAMON-RAISIN				
(Awrey's)				
filled 'Square' 3 oz	1 piece	290	280	12.0
filled 'Miniature' 1.5 oz	1 piece	160	150	8.0
(Pepperidge Farm) frozen, 2.25 oz	1 piece	250	170	11.0
(Pillsbury) w/icing, refrigerated	1 piece	150	230	7.0
(Sara Lee) frozen, 'Individual' 1.3 oz	1 piece	150	140	8.0
CINNAMON-WALNUT (Awrey's) 'Round' 2.75 oz	1 piece	300	290	18.0
LEMON (Entenmann's) twist	1.2 oz	140	140	7.0
ORANGE (Pillsbury) w/icing, refrigerated	1 piece	150	250	7.0
PECAN RING (Entenmann's)	1.5 oz	190	130	12.0
PINEAPPLE (Awrey's) filled, 'Miniature' 1.7 oz	1 piece	157	180	8.0
RASPBERRY				
(Awrey's) filled 'Square' 3 oz	1 piece	260	210	8.0
(Entenmann's) twist	1.2 oz	140	120	7.0
(Pepperidge Farm) frozen, 2.25 oz	1 piece	220	140	9.0
(Sara Lee) twist, frozen	1/8 pkg	200	220	9.0
RING (Entenmann's)	1.5 oz	180	160	10.0
STRAWBERRY				
(Awrey's)				
filled 'Miniature' 1.7 oz	1 piece	160	180	8.0
filled 'Round' 4.5 oz	1 piece	400	410	20.0
filled 'Round' 2.75 oz	1 piece	270	320	14.0
WALNUT RING (Entenmann's)	1.5 oz	190	130	12.0

Food Name	Serv. Size	Total Cal.	Sod. MGS	Fat GMS
DASHEEN				
cooked	4 oz	161	11	0.1
cooked, sliced	1/2 cup	94	10	0.1
raw, sliced	1/2 cup	56	6	0.1
raw, trimmed	1 oz	30	3	0.1
raw, untrimmed	1 lb	419	43	0.8
DASHEEN LEAF				
raw	1/2 cup	6	1	0.1
raw, trimmed	1 oz	12	1	0.2
raw, untrimmed	1 lb	115	8	2.0
steamed	1/2 cup	18	2	0.3
steamed	4 oz	27	2	0.5
DASHEEN SHOOTS				
cooked	4 oz	16	2	0.1
cooked, sliced	1/2 cup	10	1	0.1
raw, sliced	1/2 cup	5	<1	<.1
raw, trimmed	1 oz	3	<1	<.1
raw, untrimmed	1 lb	45	4	0.4
DATE				
Domestic, natural and dry				
chopped	1/2 cup	245	3	0.4
w/pits	1 lb	1123	10	1.8
w/o pits	1 oz	78	1	0.1
w/o pits, 2.9 oz	10 dates	228	2	0.4
w/o pits (Dole)	1/2 cup	280	0	0.0
Imported, pitted				
(Amport Foods) chopped	1.5 oz	135	0	0.0
(Amport Foods) whole	1.5 oz	135	0	0.0
(Bordo)	2 oz	204	5	1.2
(Bordo) diced	2 oz	203	5	1.1
(Dromedary) approx 1 oz	5 dates	100	0	0.0
(Dromedary) chopped	1/4 cup	130	0	0.0
DEER				
raw	1 lb	544	231	11.0
raw	1 oz	34	14	0.7
roasted	3 oz	134	46	2.7
DIET BAR. See also SNACK BAR.				
(Figurines)				
chocolate	1 bar	100	50	5.0
chocolate caramel	1 bar	100	65	6.0
chocolate caramel '100'	1 bar	100	55	6.0

Food Name	Serv. Size	Total Cal.	Sod. MGS	Fat GMS
chocolate peanut butter	1 bar	100	50	6.0
'S'mores'	1 bar	100	55	5.0
vanilla	1 bar	100	55	6.0
(Nestlé)				
chewy chocolate brownie 'Sweet Success'	1 bar	120	35	4.0
chewy chocolate chip 'Sweet Success'	1 bar	120	35	4.0
chewy chocolate peanut butter 'Sweet Success'	1 bar	120	35	4.0
(Ultra Slim Fast) chocolate chip crunch	1 bar	120	30	4.0
DIET DRINK				
(Nestlé)				
chocolate mocha, ready to drink, 'Sweet Success'	10 oz	200	230	3.0
chocolate raspberry truffle, powder, 'Sweet Success'	1.13 oz	90	150	2.0
chocolate raspberry truffle, prepared, 'Sweet Success'	8 oz	180	na	2.0
creamy milk chocolate, canned, 'Sweet Success'	10 oz	200	230	3.0
dark chocolate fudge, canned, 'Sweet Success'	10 oz	200	210	3.0
dark chocolate fudge, powder, 'Sweet Success'	1.13 oz	90	na	2.0
dark chocolate fudge, prepared, 'Sweet Success'	8 oz	180	280	2.0
rich chocolate almond, powder, 'Sweet Success'	1.13 oz	90	150	2.0
rich chocolate almond, prepared, 'Sweet Success'	8 oz	180	280	2.0
(Ultra Slim Fast)				
cafe mocha powder	1 scoop	100	130	<1.0
cafe mocha powder, prepared w/skim milk	8 oz	200	280	1.0
chocolate fantasy 'Plus' powder	1 scoop	120	140	1.0
chocolate fantasy 'Plus' powder, prepared w/skim milk	12 oz	250	330	2.0
French vanilla powder	1 scoop	100	120	<1.0
French vanilla powder, prepared w/skim milk	8 oz	190	250	1.0
'French Vanilla' canned	12 oz	220	240	1.0
piña colada 'Plus' powder	1 scoop	90	120	<1.0
piña colada 'Plus' powder, prepared w/skim milk	8 oz	190	260	<1.0
strawberry jubilee 'Plus' powder	1 scoop	110	140	1.0
strawberry jubilee 'Plus' powder, prepared w/skim milk	12 oz	240	330	2.0
DILL SEASONING, 'Parsley Patch It's a Dilly' *(Schilling)*	1 tsp	11	5	0.4
DILL SEED				
whole	1 oz	86	6	4.1
whole	1 tbsp	20	1	1.0
whole	1 tsp	6	0	0.3
whole *(Durkee)*	1 tsp	9	0	<0.1
whole *(Laurel Leaf)*	1 tsp	9	0	<0.1
whole *(Spice Islands)*	1 tsp	9	<1	0.4
DILL WEED				
dried	1 oz	72	79	1.2

Food Name	Serv. Size	Total Cal.	Sod. MGS	Fat GMS
dried	1 tbsp	8	6	0.1
dried	1 tsp	3	2	0.0
fresh, sprigs	1 cup	4	5	0.1

DIP

Food Name	Serv. Size	Total Cal.	Sod. MGS	Fat GMS
ACAPULCO *(Ortega)*	1 oz	8	0	0.0
AVOCADO *(Kraft)*	2 tbsp	50	210	4.0
BACON AND HORSERADISH				
(Breakstone's)	2 tbsp	70	270	6.0
(Kraft)	2 tbsp	60	200	5.0
(Kraft) 'Premium'	2 tbsp	50	270	5.0
(Sealtest)	2 tbsp	70	270	6.0
BACON AND ONION				
(Breakstone's) 'Gourmet'	2 tbsp	70	210	6.0
(Kraft) 'Premium'	2 tbsp	60	170	5.0
BEAN				
(Chi-Chi's) 'Fiesta'	1 oz	30	126	1.0
(Hain) hot	4 tbsp	70	250	1.0
BLACK BEAN				
(Guiltless Gourmet) barbeque, mild	1 oz	23	100	0.0
(Guiltless Gourmet) barbeque, spicy	1 oz	23	100	0.0
(Guiltless Gourmet) mild	1 oz	23	100	0.0
(Guiltless Gourmet) spicy	1 oz	23	100	0.0
(Tostitos) fat free, medium	2 tbsp	30	210	0.0
BLUE CHEESE				
(Kraft) 'Premium'	2 tbsp	50	210	4.0
(Litehouse) 'Lite' and dressing, refrigerated	1 tbsp	33	86	3.0
(Litehouse) 'Original' and dressing, refrigerated	1 tbsp	77	82	8.0
CAESAR *(Litehouse)* and dressing, refrigerated	1 tbsp	57	84	6.0
CHEDDAR CHEESE				
(Frito-Lay's)	1 oz	45	180	3.0
(Guiltless Gourmet) queso, mild	1 oz	20	150	0.0
(Guiltless Gourmet) queso, spicy	1 oz	20	150	0.0
CHEESE *(Chi-Chi's)* 'Fiesta'	1 oz	41	296	3.0
CHILI *(La Victoria)*	1 tbsp	6	90	<1.0
CLAM				
(Breakstone's)	2 tbsp	50	220	4.0
(Breakstone's) 'Gourmet Chesapeake'	2 tbsp	50	200	4.0
(Kraft)	2 tbsp	60	240	4.0
(Kraft) 'Premium'	2 tbsp	45	210	4.0
(Sealtest)	2 tbsp	50	220	4.0

Food Name	Serv. Size	Total Cal.	Sod. MGS	Fat GMS
COUNTRY BLUE CHEESE				
(Litehouse) and dressing, refrigerated	1 tbsp	76	84	8.0
COUNTRY RANCH (Litehouse) and dressing, refrigerated	1 tbsp	61	75	7.0
CUCUMBER (Kraft) creamy 'Premium'	2 tbsp	50	130	4.0
CUCUMBER AND ONION				
(Breakstone's)	2 tbsp	50	160	4.0
(Sealtest)	2 tbsp	50	160	4.0
DILL (Nasoya) creamy 'Vegi-Dip'	1 oz	60	100	4.0
FRENCH ONION				
(Bison)	1 oz	60	180	5.0
(Breakstone's)	2 tbsp	50	140	5.0
(Frito-Lay's)	1 oz	50	180	3.0
(Heluva Good) real sour cream	2 tbsp	50	160	5.0
(Kraft)	2 tbsp	60	140	4.0
(Kraft) 'Premium'	2 tbsp	45	150	4.0
(Lucerne)	2 tbsp	70	160	6.0
(Nasoya) 'Vegi-Dip'	1 oz	50	100	3.0
(Sealtest)	2 tbsp	50	140	5.0
GARLIC (Life) and dressing, w/tofu 'All Natural'	1 tbsp	70	75	7.1
GARLIC AND HERB (Nasoya) 'Vegi-Dip'	1 oz	50	100	2.0
GUACAMOLE				
(Kraft)	2 tbsp	50	210	4.0
(Lucerne)	2 tbsp	80	170	8.0
HONEY MUSTARD (Litehouse) and dressing, refrigerated	1 tbsp	67	55	7.0
HUMMUS (Fantastic Foods)	2 oz	111	263	6.5
ITALIAN (Litehouse) and dressing, creamy, refrigerated	1 tbsp	60	76	6.0
JALAPEÑO				
(Breakstone's) cheddar 'Gourmet'	2 tbsp	70	90	6.0
(Frito-Lay's)	1 oz	30	115	1.0
(Hain) medium	4 tbsp	70	150	1.0
(Kraft)	2 tbsp	50	160	4.0
(Kraft) cheese 'Premium'	2 tbsp	50	160	4.0
(Litehouse) ranch, and dressing, refrigerated	1 tbsp	60	80	6.0
(Old El Paso)	1 tbsp	14	53	0.0
(Price's) nacho	1 oz	80	(mq)	7.1
(Wise)	2 tbsp	25	100	0.0
MEXICAN BEAN (Hain)	4 tbsp	60	260	1.0
MUSHROOM AND HERB (Breakstone's) 'Gourmet'	2 tbsp	50	150	4.0
NACHO CHEESE				
(Kraft) 'Premium'	2 tbsp	55	200	4.0
(Tio Sancho) 'Microwave Snacks' cheese sauce mix	3.5 oz	247	995	20.0

Food Name	Serv. Size	Total Cal.	Sod. MGS	Fa GMS
ONION				
(Breakstone's) toasted 'Gourmet'	2 tbsp	50	170	5.
(Hain) bean	4 tbsp	70	270	1.
(Kraft) creamy 'Premium'	2 tbsp	45	160	4.0
(Kraft) green	2 tbsp	60	170	4.0
PEPPERCORN (Litehouse) and dressing, refrigerated	1 tbsp	67	66	7.
PICANTE SAUCE				
(Frito-Lay's)	1 oz	10	160	0.0
(Wise)	2 tbsp	12	130	0.0
PINTO BEAN				
(Guiltless Gourmet) barbeque, mild	1 oz	27	100	0.
(Guiltless Gourmet) barbeque, spicy	1 oz	27	100	0.
(Guiltless Gourmet) mild	1 oz	27	100	0.
(Guiltless Gourmet) spicy	1 oz	27	100	0.
POPPYSEED (Litehouse) and dressing, refrigerated	1 tbsp	65	83	6.
RANCH				
(Heluva Good) real sour cream	2 tbsp	60	180	5.
(Litehouse) and dressing, refrigerated	1 tbsp	59	67	6.
(Litehouse) 'Lite' and dressing, refrigerated	1 tbsp	35	80	3.
(Litehouse) 'Vegi-Dip' refrigerated	1 tbsp	60	68	7.
(Lucerne)	2 tbsp	110	160	11.
SALSA				
(Pace) 'Chunky' medium	2 tbsp	4	102	<1.
(Pace) 'Chunky' mild	2 tbsp	4	101	<1.
SOUR CREAM AND CHIVES				
(Litehouse) vinaigrette, and dressing, refrigerated	1 tbsp	63	72	7.
TACO				
(Hain) and sauce	4 tbsp	25	350	1.
(Wise)	2 tbsp	12	115	0.
THOUSAND ISLAND (Litehouse) and dressing, refrigerated	1 tbsp	65	99	7.
VEGETABLE (T. Marzetti) and dressing	1 tbsp	88	120	10.
DOCK				
boiled, drained	4 oz	23	3	0.
boiled, drained	100 gm	20	3	0.
raw, chopped	1/2 cup	15	3	0.
raw, trimmed	1 oz	6	1	0.
raw, untrimmed	1 lb	70	13	2
DOLLARFISH				
raw	1 lb	663	401	36.
raw	1 oz	41	25	2.

DOLPHIN FISH. See MAHI MAHI.

Food Name	Serv. Size	Total Cal.	Sod. MGS	Fat GMS
DONUT				
(Awrey's)				
crunch	1 donut	600	730	34.0
plain	1 donut	490	650	30.0
sugared	1 donut	610	735	35.0
(Break Cake)				
chocolate, 1 oz	1 donut	130	115	8.0
chocolate, gem, .5 oz	1 donut	70	60	4.0
chocolate, gem, .5 oz	6 donuts	400	340	24.0
cinnamon, 1 oz	1 donut	120	130	6.0
cinnamon, gem, .5 oz	1 donut	60	70	3.0
dunkin stix, .5 oz	2 stix	420	320	27.0
powdered, 1 oz	1 donut	120	135	5.0
powdered, gem, .5 oz	1 donut	60	70	3.0
powdered, gem, .5 oz	6 donuts	350	400	16.0
(Dunkin' Donuts)				
apple filled, w/cinnamon sugar, 2.8 oz	1 donut	250	280	11.0
Bavarian filled, w/chocolate frosting, 2.8 oz	1 donut	240	260	11.0
blueberry filled, 2.4 oz	1 donut	210	240	8.0
'Boston Kreme'	1 donut	240	250	11.0
cinnamon, apple filled	1 donut	190	220	9.0
coffee roll, glazed, 2.9 oz	1 donut	280	310	12.0
cruller, French, glazed, 1.3 oz	1 donut	140	130	8.0
cruller, honey dipped	1 donut	260	330	11.0
jelly filled, 2.4 oz	1 donut	220	230	9.0
lemon filled, 2.8 oz	1 donut	260	280	12.0
plain, cake w/handle	1 donut	240	370	14.0
ring, buttermilk, glazed, 2.6 oz	1 donut	290	370	14.0
ring, chocolate, glazed, 2.5 oz	1 donut	324	383	21.0
ring, plain, cake	1 donut	262	330	18.0
ring, plain, cake, 2.2 oz	1 donut	270	330	17.0
ring, powdered, cake	1 donut	270	340	16.0
ring, whole wheat, glazed, 2.9 oz	1 donut	330	380	18.0
ring, yeast, chocolate frosted, 1.9 oz	1 donut	200	190	10.0
ring, yeast, glazed, 1.9 oz	1 donut	200	230	9.0
(Entenmann's)				
crumb topped	1 donut	260	220	12.0
devil's food crumb	1 donut	250	200	12.0
rich, frosted	1 donut	280	210	18.0
(Hostess)				
cinnamon, 'Donette Gems'	1 donut	60	70	3.0

Food Name	Serv. Size	Total Cal.	Sod. MGS	Fat GMS
cinnamon, 'Family Pack'	1 donut	120	140	6.0
crumb	1 donut	160	140	10.0
crumb, 'Donette Gems'	1 donut	80	70	5.0
frosted, 1.5 oz	1 donut	190	180	12.0
frosted, 'Donette Gems'	1 donut	80	70	5.0
glazed, 'Old Fashioned'	1 donut	250	230	12.0
glazed whirl	1 donut	190	230	7.0
honey wheat	1 donut	250	280	12.0
plain, 'Old Fashioned'	1 donut	170	230	9.0
(Little Debbie) stick 1.67 oz	1 stick	230	180	13.0
(Rich's)				
frozen, glazed 'Ever Fresh' 1.2 oz	1 donut	141	(mq)	7.0
frozen, jelly 'Ever Fresh' 2.17 oz	1 donut	213	(mq)	9.5
(Tastykake)				
cinnamon, 'Assorted' 1.6 oz	1 donut	179	211	8.2
cinnamon, mini	1 donut	48	54	2.4
frosted, rich, 2 oz	1 donut	258	196	16.0
frosted, rich, mini	1 donut	61	59	3.2
honey wheat, 2 oz	1 donut	209	190	7.5
honey wheat, mini	1 donut	40	48	1.2
orange glazed, 2 oz	1 donut	219	178	9.1
plain, 'Assorted' 1.6 oz	1 donut	185	171	10.1
powdered sugar, 'Assorted' 1.6 oz	1 donut	188	221	8.6
powdered sugar, mini	1 donut	42	71	1.3

DREAM WHIP. See CREAM TOPPING, NONDAIRY.

DRESSING. See SALAD DRESSING.

DRINKS. See ALCOHOL-FREE BEVERAGES; ALCOHOLIC BEVERAGES; COFFEE; DIET DRINK; MILK; SOFT DRINKS AND MIXERS; SPORTS DRINK; TEA; WATER; and individual listings.

DRINK MIX. See individual drink mix flavors.

DRUM, FRESHWATER

dry-heat cooked	3 oz	130	82	5.4
raw	1 lb	541	340	22.4
raw	3 oz	101	64	4.2
raw	1 oz	34	21	1.4

DUCK, DOMESTICATED

Meat and skin

raw	1 oz	115	18	11.2
roasted	4 oz	382	67	32.1

Meat only

raw	1 oz	37	21	1.7

Food Name	Serv. Size	Total Cal.	Sod. MGS	Fat GMS
roasted	4 oz	228	74	12.7
DUCK, WILD				
Breast meat, raw	1 oz	35	16	1.2
Meat and skin, raw	1 oz	60	16	4.3
DUCK FAT				
	1 cup	1846	0	204.6
	1 oz	255	0	28.3
	1 tbsp	115	0	12.8
DUCK LIVER, domesticated, raw	1 oz	39	(mq)	1.3
DULSE, raw	100 gm	0	2085	3.2

E

Food Name	Serv. Size	Total Cal.	Sod. MGS	Fat GMS
EEL, MIXED SPECIES				
broiled	4 oz	268	74	17.0
dry-heat cooked	3 oz	201	55	12.7
raw	1 lb	834	231	52.9
raw	1 oz	52	14	3.3
EGG, ALTERNATIVE				
Frozen				
(Fleischmann's) 'Egg Beaters' cheese omelet	1/2 cup	110	480	5.0
(Fleischmann's) 'Egg Beaters' vegetable omelet	1/2 cup	50	170	0.0
(Morningstar Farms) 'Scramblers'	1/4 cup	60	(mq)	3.0
(Tofutti) 'Egg Watchers'	2 oz	50	100	2.0
Refrigerated				
(Featherweight)	2 eggs	120	250	8.0
(Fleischmann's) 'Egg Beaters'	1/4 cup	25	80	0.0
Mix				
(Healthy Choice) 'Cholesterol Free Egg Product'	1.9-oz serving	30	90	<1.0
(Tofu Scrambler) prepared w/tofu	1/2 cup	98	252	5.0
EGG, CHICKEN. See also EGG WHITE, CHICKEN; EGG YOLK, CHICKEN.				
Cooked				
fried	1 large	91	162	6.9
hard-boiled	1 oz	44	35	3.0
hard-boiled, chopped	1 cup	211	169	14.4
poached	1 large	74	140	5.0
poached	1 oz	42	79	2.8
scrambled	1 cup	365	616	26.9
scrambled	1 large	100	168	7.3

Food Name	Serv. Size	Total Cal.	Sod. MGS	Fat GMS
Dried				
....	1 oz	168	148	11.9
....	1 tbsp	30	26	2.1
sifted	1 cup	505	443	35.5
stabilized, glucose reduced	1 oz	174	155	12.5
stabilized, glucose reduced	1 tbsp	31	27	2.2
stabilized, glucose reduced, sifted	1 cup	523	466	37.4
Pickled (Penrose)	1 large	80	230	5.0
Raw				
fresh or frozen	1 cup	363	307	24.3
fresh or frozen	1 large	75	63	5.0
fresh or frozen	1 oz	42	36	2.8
EGG, DUCK				
raw	1 large	130	102	9.6
raw	1 oz	52	41	3.9
EGG, GOOSE				
raw	1 large	267	199	19.1
raw	1 oz	52	na	3.8
EGG, QUAIL				
raw	1 oz	45	na	3.1
raw	1 large	14	13	1.0
EGG, TURKEY				
raw	1 large	135	120	9.4
raw	1 oz	48	na	3.4
EGG BREAKFAST, ALTERNATIVE, FROZEN				
vegetarian, w/hash browns and links 'Scramblers'				
(Morningstar Farms)	7 oz	360	660	23.0
vegetarian, w/pancakes and links 'Scramblers'				
(Morningstar Farms)	6.8 oz	380	900	19.0
EGG BREAKFAST, FREEZE-DRIED				
(Mountain House)				
cheese omelet, prepared	1/2 pkg	180	207	9.0
w/bacon, prepared	1/2 pkg	170	165	10.0
w/butter, prepared	1/2 pkg	160	174	8.0
EGG BREAKFAST, SCRAMBLED, FROZEN				
w/bacon and home fried potatoes (Swanson)	5.6 oz	340	690	26.0
w/cheddar cheese and fried potatoes (Aunt Jemima)	5.9 oz	250	910	13.0
w/ham and hash browns (Downyflake)	6.25 oz	360	730	26.0
w/ham and pecan twirl (Downyflake)	6.25 oz	470	670	28.0
w/hash browns and sausage link (Downyflake)	6.25 oz	420	790	34.0

Food Name	Serv. Size	Total Cal.	Sod. MGS	Fat GMS
w/home fried potatoes 'Great Starts' Budget Breakfast				
(Swanson)	4.6 oz	260	380	19.0
w/sausages and hash browns (Aunt Jemima)	5.7 oz	290	810	20.0
w/sausages and hash browns (Swanson)	6.5 oz	430	760	34.0
w/sausages and pancakes (Aunt Jemima)	5.2 oz	270	880	14.0
w/sausages and pecan twirl (Downyflake)	6.25 oz	510	710	33.0
EGG FOO YUNG				
(LaChoy) mix, prepared	8.8 oz	164	1250	7.0
(LaChoy) packaged 'Dinner Classics' prepared	2 patties	170	1390	7.0
EGG NOODLE. See NOODLE, EGG.				
EGG ROLL				
Frozen				
(Chun King)				
chicken	3.6 oz	220	600	8.0
meat and shrimp	3.6 oz	220	680	8.0
pork 'Restaurant Style'	3 oz	180	450	6.0
shrimp	3.6 oz	200	480	6.0
(Jeno's)				
chicken 'Snacks' approx 6 rolls	3 oz	190	350	9.0
meat and shrimp 'Snacks' approx 6 rolls	3 oz	200	420	11.0
shrimp and cheese 'Snacks' approx 6 rolls	3 oz	190	290	8.0
(LaChoy)				
almond chicken	3 oz	120	290	3.0
chicken 'Snack'	1.45 oz	90	140	3.0
lobster 'Snack'	1.45 oz	75	150	2.0
meat and shrimp 'Snack'	1.45 oz	80	115	3.0
pork 'Restaurant Style'	3 oz	150	480	5.0
shrimp 'Restaurant Style'	3 oz	130	260	4.0
shrimp 'Snack'	1.45 oz	75	120	2.0
sweet and sour chicken	3 oz	150	280	4.0
(Worthington) vegetarian roll, frozen	3 oz	160	530	6.0
Refrigerated				
(Chung's)				
chicken, white meat	3 oz	150	560	6.0
pork	3 oz	190	590	10.0
shrimp	3 oz	170	496	7.0
vegetable	3 oz	180	510	8.0
EGG ROLL WRAPPER				
(Azumaya Pasta)	2 pieces	130	200	0.0
(Nasoya)	1 piece	23	19	0.0

Food Name	Serv. Size	Total Cal.	Sod. MGS	Fat GMS
EGG WHITE, CHICKEN				
Dried				
stabilized, glucose reduced, flakes	1 oz	100	328	<.1
stabilized, glucose reduced, powder	1 cup	402	1325	<.1
stabilized, glucose reduced, powder	1 oz	107	351	<.1
Raw				
fresh or frozen	1 cup	122	399	0.0
fresh or frozen	1 large	17	55	0.0
fresh or frozen	1 oz	14	46	0.0
EGG WHITE STABILIZER (Tone's)	1 tsp	12	1	(tr)
EGG YOLK, CHICKEN				
Dried				
sifted	1 cup	460	61	41.1
sifted	1 oz	195	26	17.4
sifted	1 tbsp	27	4	2.5
Raw				
fresh	1 cup	870	104	75.0
fresh	1 oz	101	12	8.8
fresh	1 large	59	7	5.1
frozen, salted	100 gm	278	3932	23.4
frozen, sugared	100 gm	317	56	23.4
frozen, sugared	1 oz	92	16	7.2
EGGNOG, NON-ALCOHOLIC				
Canned (Borden)	1/2 cup	160	80	9.0
Chilled				
(Crowley)	6 oz	270	200	13.0
(Darigold)	8 oz	350	120	17.0
(Darigold) 'Classic'	8 oz	390	170	17.0
(Ensure) liquid nutrition	8 oz	250	na	8.8
EGGNOG MIX				
dry, 2 heaping tsp	1 oz	111	44	0.3
1 oz powder, prepared w/whole milk	1 cup	261	163	8.4
1 oz powder, prepared w/2% milk	1 cup	232	166	5.0
1 oz powder, prepared w/1% milk	1 cup	213	167	2.9
1 oz powder, prepared w/skim milk	1 cup	197	170	0.7
EGGPLANT/aubergine				
boiled, drained	4 oz	32	3	0.3
boiled, drained, 1-inch cubes	1 cup	27	3	0.2
raw, 1-inch pieces	1/2 cup	11	1	0.1
raw, peeled, approx 1 lb	1 eggplant	119	14	0.8
raw, trimmed	1 oz	7	1	<.1

Food Name	Serv. Size	Total Cal.	Sod. MGS	Fat GMS
raw, untrimmed	1 lb	95	13	0.4
EGGPLANT APPETIZER, 'Caponata' (Progresso)	1/2 can	70	260	4.0
EGGPLANT ENTRÉE, FROZEN				
(Celentano)				
parmigiana	10 oz	350	500	19.0
parmigiana	8 oz	280	400	15.0
parmigiana	6.25 oz	260	220	10.0
rollettes	11 oz	320	210	14.0
(Mrs. Paul's) parmigiana	5 oz	240	600	16.0
ELBOW MACARONI. See PASTA.				
ELDERBERRY				
fresh	1 lb	329	na	2.3
fresh	1 oz	21	na	0.1
fresh	1 cup	106	na	0.7
ENCHILADA (Gebhardt)	2 enchiladas	310	460	24.0
ENCHILADA DINNER, FROZEN. See also ENCHILADA ENTRÉE, FROZEN.				
BEEF				
(Banquet)	12 oz	500	1810	15.0
(Banquet) chili and gravy 'Family Entrées'	7 oz	270	(mq)	13.0
(Healthy Choice)	13.4 oz	370	450	5.0
(Old El Paso) 'Festive Dinners'	11 oz	390	1200	8.0
(Patio)	13.25 oz	520	1810	24.0
(Swanson)	13.75 oz	480	1350	21.0
(Van de Kamp's) 'Mexican Dinner'	1/2 pkg	200	740	7.0
CHEESE				
(Banquet)	12 oz	550	2170	19.0
(Patio)	12.25 oz	380	2010	10.0
(Old El Paso) 'Festive Dinners'	11 oz	590	1200	31.0
(Van de Kamp's) 'Mexican Dinner'	1/2 pkg	220	620	9.0
CHICKEN				
(Healthy Choice)	13.4 oz	340	470	5.0
(Healthy Choice)	9.5 oz	310	480	9.0
(Old El Paso) 'Festive Dinners'	11 oz	460	770	18.0
(Weight Watchers) nacho grande 'Mexican Style'	9 oz	280	590	8.0
ENCHILADA DINNER, MIX				
(Old El Paso) prepared	1 enchilada	145	325	8.0
(Tio Sancho) 'Dinner Kit'	1 shell	80	2	3.5
(Tio Sancho) 'Dinner Kit' and sauce mix	3 oz	278	4058	1.5
ENCHILADA ENTRÉE, FROZEN. See also ENCHILADA DINNER, FROZEN.				
BEEF				
(Hormel)	1 enchilada	140	573	5.0

Food Name	Serv. Size	Total Cal.	Sod. MGS	Fa GM
(Old El Paso)	1 pkg	210	720	13.0
(Ultimate 200) Ranchero	9.12 oz	190	500	5.0
(Van de Kamp's) 'Mexican Entrées'	1 pkg	270	1040	12.0
(Van de Kamp's) 'Mexican Entrées Family Pack'	1/4 pkg	150	530	5.0
(Van de Kamp's) shredded, 'Mexican Entrées'	1 pkg	360	1010	14.0
BLACK BEAN-VEGETABLE *(Amy's Kitchen)*	4.75 oz	135	290	4.0
CHEESE				
(Amy's Kitchen) organic	4.75 oz	210	290	9.0
(Hormel)	1 enchilada	151	676	6.0
(Old El Paso)	1 pkg	250	830	12.0
(Stouffer's)	9.75 oz	490	550	29.0
(Van de Kamp's) 'Mexican Entrées'	1 pkg	300	980	15.0
(Van de Kamp's) 'Mexican Entrées Family Pack'	1/4 pkg	200	460	10.0
CHICKEN				
(Le Menu) 'Light Style'	8 oz	280	530	8.0
(Old El Paso)	1 pkg	220	740	12.0
(Old El Paso) w/sour cream sauce	1 pkg	280	520	19.0
(Stouffer's)	10 oz	490	860	31.0
(Van de Kamp's) 'Mexican Entrées'	1 pkg	260	1010	11.0
RANCHERO *(Van de Kamp's)* 'Mexican Entrées'	1/2 pkg	260	630	12.0
SUIZA				
(Van de Kamp's) 'Mexican Entrées'	1 pkg	230	390	10.0
(Weight Watchers)	9 oz	230	530	7.0
VEGETABLE *(Legume)* w/tofu and sauce	11 oz	270	390	8.0
ENCHILADA SEASONING MIX				
(Old El Paso)	1/8 pkg	6	80	0.0
(Lawry's) 'Seasoning Blends'	1 pkg	152	1723	1.2
ENDIVE				
approx 1.3 lb	1 head	87	113	1.0
chopped	1/2 cup	4	6	0.1
trimmed	1 oz	5	6	0.1
untrimmed	1 lb	65	87	0.8
ENGLISH MUFFIN				
(Earth Grains)				
oat bran, 12-oz pkg	1 muffin	120	410	1.0
plain, 12.5-oz pkg	1 muffin	130	410	1.0
plain, 12-oz pkg	1 muffin	120	390	1.0
raisin, 14-oz pkg	1 muffin	160	300	2.0
raisin, 'Sun Maid' 15-oz pkg	1 muffin	160	180	1.0
sourdough, 12.5-oz pkg	1 muffin	130	410	1.0
sourdough, 12-oz pkg	1 muffin	120	390	1.0

Food Name	Serv. Size	Total Cal.	Sod. MGS	Fat GMS
whole wheat, 15-oz pkg	1 muffin	140	450	2.0
whole wheat, 14-oz pkg	1 muffin	130	420	1.0
(Hi Fiber)				
cinnamon raisin	1 muffin	110	275	1.0
multigrain	1 muffin	120	240	1.0
plain	1 muffin	110	280	1.0
(Oatmeal Goodness)				
cinnamon and raisin oatmeal	1 muffin	140	160	2.0
honey and oatmeal	1 muffin	140	160	2.0
(Oroweat)				
extra crisp	1 muffin	130	260	1.0
health nut	1 muffin	170	220	4.0
sourdough	1 muffin	140	370	1.0
(Pepperidge Farm)				
cinnamon apple	1 muffin	140	210	1.0
cinnamon chip	1 muffin	160	180	3.0
cinnamon raisin	1 muffin	150	200	2.0
plain	1 muffin	140	220	1.0
sourdough	1 muffin	135	260	1.0
(Roman Meal)				
honey nut and oat bran, refrigerated	1/2 muffin	81	114	1.3
plain, 'Original'	1 muffin	146	350	1.8
wheatberry, 14-oz pkg	1 muffin	140	470	1.0
(Thomas')				
honey wheat	1 muffin	129	200	1.1
oat bran	1 muffin	116	192	1.2
plain	1 muffin	130	206	1.3
raisin	1 muffin	153	200	1.5
rye	1 muffin	120	210	1.0
(Wonder) plain	1 muffin	130	280	1.0

ENSURE NUTRITION DRINK. See individual flavors.

ENTRÉES. See individual entrées.

EQUAL. See SUGAR SUBSTITUTE.

EUCHALON. See CANDLEFISH.

F

Food Name	Serv. Size	Total Cal.	Sod. MGS	Fat GMS
FAJITA ENTRÉE, refrigerated *(Chicken By George)*	5 oz	170	370	6.0

Food Name	Serv. Size	Total Cal.	Sod. MGS	Fat GMS
FAJITA ENTRÉE, FROZEN				
beef *(Healthy Choice)*	7 oz	210	250	4.0
chicken *(Healthy Choice)*	7 oz	200	310	3.0
FAJITA ENTRÉE KIT				
(Tyson)	4 oz	80	240	2.0
(Tyson) wholesale club item	3.5 oz	160	420	5.0
FAJITA MARINADE *(Old El Paso)*	1/8 jar	14	450	0.0
FAJITA SAUCE. See SAUCE.				
FAJITA SEASONING MIX, 'Seasoning Blends' *(Lawry's)*	1 pkg	63	2118	0.4
FALAFEL				
(Casbah) mix, dry	1 oz	103	na	2.0
(Fantastic Foods) mix 'Falafil' prepared	3 oz	129	188	2.0
(Near East) mix, prepared	3 patties	270	680	15.0
FARINA. See CEREAL, HOT.				
FAT, ALTERNATIVE, 'Neutral Nyafat' *(Rokeach)*	1 tbsp	99	0	11.0
FAVA BEAN/horse bean/jack bean				
boiled, drained	4 oz	64	47	0.6
mature seeds, boiled	1/2 cup	94	4	0.3
mature seeds, raw	1/2 cup	256	10	1.1
raw, trimmed	1/2 cup	40	28	0.4
raw, trimmed	1 oz	20	14	0.2
raw, untrimmed	1 lb	317	220	2.6
Canned				
mature seeds	1/2 cup	91	580	0.3
mature seeds, w/liquid	4 oz	81	514	0.2
Dried				
mature seeds, boiled	4 oz	125	6	0.5
mature seeds, boiled	1/2 cup	93	4	0.3
mature seeds, raw	1/2 cup	256	9	1.2
mature seeds, raw	1 oz	97	4	0.4
FENNEL/finocchio				
(Frieda's)	1 lb	68	408	0.5
(Frieda's)	1 oz	4	26	<.1
raw, bulb	1 bulb	73	122	0.5
raw, leaves	100 gm	28	9	0.4
raw, sliced	1 cup	27	45	0.2
FENNEL SEED				
whole	1 oz	98	25	4.2
whole	1 tbsp	20	5	0.9
whole	1 tsp	7	2	0.3
whole *(Durkee)*	1 tsp	7	0	tr

| | FIG | 289 |

Food Name	Serv. Size	Total Cal.	Sod. MGS	Fat GMS
whole *(Laurel Leaf)*	1 tsp	7	0	tr
whole *(Spice Islands)*	1 tsp	8	2	0.2
FENUGREEK SEED				
whole	1 oz	92	19	1.8
whole	1 tbsp	36	7	0.7
whole	1 tsp	12	2	0.2
FETTUCCINE ENTRÉE, FROZEN				
Alfredo *(Healthy Choice)*	8 oz	240	370	7.0
Alfredo *(Lean Cuisine)*	9 oz	280	570	7.0
Alfredo *(Weight Watchers)*	8 oz	230	550	7.0
Alfredo, 10-oz pkg *(Stouffer's)*	5 oz	245	400	14.0
Alfredo, w/broccoli 'Lowfat' *(Weight Watchers)*	8 oz	230	550	7.0
chicken *(Healthy Choice)*	8.5 oz	240	370	4.0
primavera *(Green Giant)*	1 pkg	230	610	8.0
primavera *(Lean Cuisine)*	10 oz	260	510	8.0
primavera 'Microwave Garden Gourmet' *(Green Giant)*	1 pkg	260	640	13.0
w/broccoli *(Dining Lite)*	9 oz	290	1020	12.0
w/meat sauce *(Budget Gourmet)*	10 oz	290	980	10.0
FETTUCCINE ENTRÉE, MIX				
Alfredo 'Pasta & Cheese' prepared *(Kraft)*	1/2 cup	180	590	9.0
Alfredo 'Pasta & Sauce' *(Hain)*	1/4 pkg	180	420	4.0
FETTUCCINE LUNCH, FROZEN				
Alfredo sauce 'Lunch Express' w/chicken *(Lean Cuisine)*	10.25 oz	240	540	6.0
FIELD PEAS, CANNED				
'Fresh' *(Allens)*	1/2 cup	100	370	<1.0
'Fresh' w/snaps *(Allens)*	1/2 cup	100	370	<1.0
tiny, 'Fresh' w/snaps *(Allens)*	1/2 cup	70	340	<1.0
w/snaps *(Bush's Best)*	1/2 cup	80	550	0.0
FIG				
candied	100 gm	299	34	0.2
raw, w/o stem	1 large	47	1	0.2
raw, w/o stem	1 med	37	1	0.2
trimmed	1 oz	21	<1	0.1
w/stems	1 lb	333	5	1.4
Canned				
in extra heavy syrup	4 oz	121	1	0.1
in extra heavy syrup, solid and liquid	1 cup	279	3	0.3
in extra heavy syrup, w/1.75 tbsp liquid	3 fruits	91	1	0.1
in heavy syrup	4 oz	100	1	0.1
in heavy syrup, solid and liquid	1 cup	228	3	0.3
in heavy syrup, whole *(Del Monte)*	1/2 cup	100	10	0.0

Food Name	Serv. Size	Total Cal.	Sod. MGS	Fat GMS
in heavy syrup, whole, Kadota 'Fancy' *(S&W)*	1/2 cup	100	10	0.0
in heavy syrup, w/1.75 tbsp liquid	3 fruits	75	1	0.1
in light syrup	1/2 cup	87	2	0.1
in light syrup	4 oz	78	1	0.1
in light syrup, solid and liquid	1 cup	174	3	0.3
in light syrup, w/1.75 tbsp liquid	3 fruits	59	1	0.1
in water	1/2 cup	65	2	0.1
in water	4 oz	60	1	0.1
in water, solid and liquid	1 cup	131	2	0.3
in water, w/1.75 tbsp liquid	3 fruits	42	1	0.1
Dried				
cooked	4 oz	122	6	0.6
stewed	1/2 cup	140	7	0.6
uncooked	1 cup	507	22	2.3
uncooked	4 oz	289	15	1.3
uncooked, Calimyrna *(Blue Ribbon)*	1/2 cup	250	10	2.0
uncooked, Calimyrna *(Sun•Maid)*	1/2 cup	250	10	2.0
uncooked, Mission *(Blue Ribbon)*	1/2 cup	210	20	(mq)
uncooked, Mission *(Sun•Maid)*	1/2 cup	210	20	(mq)
uncooked, trimmed	10 fruits	477	21	2.2
FILBERT, SHELLED. See HAZELNUT, SHELLED.				
FILBERT BUTTER, roasted *(Maranatha Natural)*	2 tbsp	180	5	16.0
FILO DOUGH. See PHYLLO DOUGH.				
FINNAN HADDIE, smoked	4 oz	132	865	1.1
FINOCCHIO. See FENNEL.				
FISH CAKE				
fried	1 cake	103	106	4.8
fried, bite size	5 cakes	103	106	4.8
frozen *(Mrs. Paul's)*	2 pieces	190	690	7.0
FISH DINNER, FROZEN				
(Healthy Choice) lemon pepper, 10.7 oz	1 serving	300	370	5.0
(Kid Cuisine) nuggets	7 oz	320	750	15.0
(Morton)	9.75 oz	370	910	13.0
(Swanson) 'n chips	10 oz	500	960	21.0
FISH ENTRÉE				
Canned, Dijon 'Light' *(Mrs. Paul's)*	8.75 oz	200	650	5.0
Frozen				
fillet of, divan *(Lean Cuisine)*	10 3/8 oz	210	490	5.0
fillet of, Florentine *(Lean Cuisine)*	9 5/8 oz	220	590	7.0
fillet of, Florentine 'Light' *(Mrs. Paul's)*	8 oz	220	820	8.0
fish 'n fries 'Home Style Recipe' *(Swanson)*	6.5 oz	340	670	16.0

Food Name	Serv. Size	Total Cal.	Sod. MGS	Fat GMS
gems, fancy style *(Wakefield)*	4 oz	80	(mq)	1.0
gems, salad style *(Wakefield)*	3 oz	70	(mq)	1.0
in herb sauce *(Gorton's)*	1 pkg	190	450	8.0
Mornay 'Light' *(Mrs. Paul's)*	9 oz	230	670	10.0
oven baked, w/vegetable medley *(Ultimate 200)*	6.64 oz	120	390	2.0
'Platters' *(Banquet)*	8.75 oz	450	(mq)	22.0
salmon, Keta *(Libby's)*	3.7 oz	130	450	6.0
sticks 'Looney Tunes Sylvester' *(Tyson)*	7.5 oz	290	510	11.0
FISH FILLET, ALTERNATIVE				
vegetarian, frozen *(Worthington)* 1.5-oz pieces	2 pieces	180	910	9.0
FISH FILLET, FROZEN				
battered *(Mrs. Paul's)*	2 pieces	330	650	17.0
battered *(Van de Kamp's)*	1 piece	170	350	10.0
battered 'Crispy Batter' *(Gorton's)*	2 pieces	290	550	19.0
battered 'Crispy Batter' large *(Gorton's)*	1 piece	320	680	21.0
battered 'Crunchy' *(Gorton's)*	2 pieces	230	420	13.0
battered 'Crunchy' *(Mrs. Paul's)*	2 pieces	280	730	14.0
battered 'Crunchy Microwave' *(Gorton's)*	2 pieces	340	400	26.0
battered 'Crunchy Microwave' large *(Gorton's)*	1 piece	320	500	22.0
battered, minced 'Portions' *(Mrs. Paul's)*	2 pieces	300	540	19.0
battered 'Potato Crisp' *(Gorton's)*	2 pieces	300	360	20.0
battered, tempura 'Light Recipe' *(Gorton's)*	1 piece	200	400	14.0
battered 'Value Pack Portions' *(Gorton's)*	1 piece	180	490	11.0
breaded *(Van de Kamp's)*	2 pieces	280	280	18.0
breaded 'Crisp and Healthy' baked *(Van de Kamp's)*	2 pieces	150	350	3.0
breaded 'Crispy Crunchy' *(Mrs. Paul's)*	2 pieces	220	380	9.0
breaded, crispy 'Microwave' *(Van de Kamp's)*	1 piece	140	210	9.0
breaded, crispy 'Microwave' large *(Van de Kamp's)*	1 piece	290	640	17.0
breaded, 8 fillets *(Healthy Choice)*	2.5 oz	120	250	4.0
breaded, 4 fillets *(Healthy Choice)*	3 oz	140	300	4.0
breaded 'Light Recipe' *(Gorton's)*	1 piece	180	380	8.0
breaded, minced 'Crispy Crunchy Portions' *(Mrs. Paul's)*	2 pieces	230	300	15.0
breaded, reheated, 2 oz	1 piece	155	332	7.0
breaded 'Snack Pack' *(Van de Kamp's)*	2 pieces	220	280	10.0
breaded, 2 fillets *(Healthy Choice)*	3.5 oz	160	350	5.0
coated, ranch 'Specialty Microwave' *(Gorton's)*	1 piece	330	520	21.0
crispy, microwave *(Van de Kamp's)*	1 piece	140	210	9.0
crispy, microwave large *(Van de Kamp's)*	1 piece	290	640	17.0
in butter sauce 'Light' *(Mrs. Paul's)*	1 piece	140	520	6.0
marinated, Cajun style, catfish 'Select' *(Gorton's)*	1 fillet	220	560	13.0
FISH LOAF, cooked	1 loaf	1507	2151	45.0

Food Name	Serv. Size	Total Cal.	Sod. MGS	Fat GMS
FISH NUGGET, FROZEN, battered *(Van de Kamp's)*	4 pieces	130	310	9.0
FISH OIL				
herring	1 cup	1966	0	218.0
herring	1 tbsp	123	0	13.6
menhaden	1 cup	1966	0	218.0
menhaden	1 tbsp	123	0	13.6
menhaden, fully hydrogenated	1 cup	1849	0	205.0
menhaden, fully hydrogenated	1 tbsp	113	0	12.5
salmon	1 cup	1966	0	218.0
salmon	1 tbsp	123	0	13.6
sardine	1 cup	1966	0	218.0
sardine	1 tbsp	123	0	13.6
FISH PASTE CAKE				
Japanese, block, steamed 'Kamoboko'	4 oz	111	1134	1.0
Japanese, stick, grilled 'Chikuwa'	4 oz	143	1134	2.4
FISH SEASONING MIX. See SEAFOOD SEASONING MIX.				
FISH STICKS, FROZEN				
battered *(Mrs. Paul's)*	4 pieces	210	590	12.0
battered *(Van de Kamp's)*	4 pieces	160	350	9.0
battered 'Crispy Batter' *(Gorton's)*	4 pieces	260	480	18.0
battered 'Crunchy' *(Gorton's)*	4 pieces	210	240	13.0
battered, minced *(Mrs. Paul's)*	4 pieces	220	630	13.0
battered 'Potato Crisp' *(Gorton's)*	4 pieces	260	390	16.0
battered 'Value Pack' *(Gorton's)*	4 pieces	190	420	9.0
breaded *(Healthy Choice)*	2.4 oz	120	350	4.0
breaded *(Van de Kamp's)*	4 pieces	200	290	12.0
breaded 'Bunch o' Crunch' approx 2.7 oz *(Frionor)*	4 pieces	210	267	14.0
breaded 'Crisp and Healthy,' baked *(Van de Kamp's)*	4 pieces	120	330	2.0
breaded 'Crispy Crunchy' *(Mrs. Paul's)*	4 pieces	140	340	6.0
breaded, crispy 'Microwave' *(Van de Kamp's)*	3 pieces	130	280	7.0
breaded, minced 'Crispy Crunchy' *(Mrs. Paul's)*	4 pieces	190	560	8.0
breaded 'Snack Pack' *(Van de Kamp's)*	4 pieces	170	270	10.0
breaded 'Value Pack' *(Van de Kamp's)*	4 pieces	170	270	10.0
breaded w/whole wheat 'Microwave' *(Booth)*	2 oz	150	210	8.0
FIVE-SPICE, Oriental spice *(Tone's)*	1 tsp	9	2	0.3
FLAN. See PUDDING MIX.				
FLATFISH. See FLOUNDER; HALIBUT; SOLE.				
FLAX OIL				
(Spectrum Naturals) organic 'Veg-Omega 3'	1 tbsp	120	0	14.0
(Spectrum Naturals) organic 'Veg-Omega 3' cinnamon flavored	1 tbsp	120	0	14.0

Food Name	Serv. Size	Total Cal.	Sod. MGS	Fat GMS
FLAXSEED (Arrowhead Mills)	1 oz	140	<1	10.0
FLOUNDER				
dry-heat cooked	3 oz	99	89	1.3
raw	3 oz	77	69	1.0
FLOUNDER, FROZEN				
(Booth) Atlantic	4 oz	90	180	1.0
(Finast)	4 oz	90	150	1.0
(Gorton's) crunch breaded, fillet 'Select'				
approx 2.9 oz	1 fillet	190	420	9.0
(Gorton's) 'Fishmarket Fresh'	5 oz	110	170	1.0
(Mrs. Paul's) battered, fillets 'Crunchy'	2 pieces	220	560	9.0
(Mrs. Paul's) breaded, fillets 'Light'	1 piece	240	450	10.0
(SeaPak)	4 oz	90	120	1.0
(Van de Kamp's) breaded fillets 'Light'	1 piece	260	480	12.0
(Van de Kamp's) fillet 'Light'	1 piece	260	480	12.0
(Van de Kamp's) 'Natural'	4 oz	100	100	2.0
FLOUNDER ENTRÉE, FROZEN				
stuffed 'Microwave Entrees' (Gorton's)	1 pkg	350	850	18.0
FLOUR. See also individual listings.				
all-purpose, 4 oz (Gold Medal)	1 cup	400	0	1.0
all-purpose, 4 oz (Red Band)	1 cup	290	0	1.0
all-purpose, 4 oz (Robin Hood)	1 cup	400	0	1.0
'Better for Bread' 4 oz (Gold Medal)	1 cup	400	0	1.0
'Drifted Snow' 4 oz (Red Band)	1 cup	400	0	1.0
'La Piña' 4 oz (Red Band)	1 cup	400	0	1.0
self-rising, 4 oz (Gold Medal)	1 cup	380	1520	1.0
self-rising, 4 oz (Red Band)	1 cup	380	1520	1.0
self-rising, 4 oz (Robin Hood)	1 cup	380	1520	1.0
'Softasilk' 1 oz (Red Band)	1/4 cup	100	0	0.0
unbleached, 4 oz (Gold Medal)	1 cup	400	0	1.0
unbleached, 4 oz (Robin Hood)	1 cup	400	0	1.0
'Wondra' 4 oz (Red Band)	1 cup	400	0	1.0
FLYING FISH				
raw	1 lb	413	(mq)	0.9
raw	1 oz	26	(mq)	<.1
FONDANT. See CANDY.				
FORMULA, INFANT. See BABY FOOD.				
FRANKFURTER				
beef and pork, 1 oz	1 frank	91	318	8.3
cheesefurter/cheese smokie, 1 oz	1 frank	93	307	8.2
cheesefurter/cheese smokie, approx 1.5 oz	1 frank	141	465	12.5

Food Name	Serv. Size	Total Cal.	Sod. MGS	Fat GM
chicken, 1 oz	1 frank	73	388	5.5
raw, beef and pork, 2 oz	1 frank	182	638	16.6
raw, w/nonfat dry milk and cereal, 2 oz	1 frank	156	627	12.4
turkey, 1 oz	1 frank	64	404	5.
(Ball Park)				
beef 'Lite'	1 frank	140	na	12.8
beef, pork and chicken 'Lite'	1 frank	140	na	12.8
(Boar's Head)				
beef, 1 oz	1 frank	80	(mq)	7.
pork and beef, 1 oz	1 frank	80	250	7.
(Butterball) turkey	1 frank	140	610	11.
(Eckrich)				
beef 'Jumbo'	1 frank	190	520	17.6
beef '1-lb pkg'	1 frank	150	400	14.
'Bunsize'	1 frank	190	500	17.
cheesefurter/cheese smokie	1 frank	180	530	16.
'Jumbo Lean Supreme'	1 frank	140	490	12.
'1-lb pkg'	1 frank	160	420	14.
(Health Valley)				
chicken 'Weiners'	1 frank	96	90	8.
turkey 'Weiners'	1 frank	96	112	8.
(Healthy Choice) turkey, pork, and beef 'Jumbo' lowfat	1 frank	70	570	2.
(Healthy Favorites) w/turkey, 2 oz	1 frank	57	572	1
(Hebrew National) beef, 1.7 oz	1 frank	149	497	14
(Hillshire Farm)				
beef 'Bun Size Wieners' 2 oz	1 frank	180	560	16
beef 'Hot Links' 2 oz	1 frank	190	560	17
cheesefurter/cheese smokie 'Bun Size Wieners' 2 oz	1 frank	180	530	16.
'Hot Links' 2 oz	1 frank	190	530	16.
natural casing 'Wieners' 2 oz	1 frank	180	470	17.
(Hormel)				
batter-wrapped, frozen 'Corn Dogs'	1 frank	220	656	12
batter-wrapped, frozen 'Tater Dogs'	1 frank	210	170	14
beef '1-lb pkg'	1 frank	140	463	13
beef '12-oz pkg'	1 frank	100	362	10
chili 'Frank 'n Stuff'	1 frank	165	517	15
'Light & Lean 97' 1.6 oz	1 frank	45	390	1.
Mexicali Dogs' 5 oz	1 frank	400	952	21
'1-lb pkg'	1 frank	140	486	13
smoked, beef 'Wranglers'	1 frank	170	619	15
smoked 'Range Brand Wranglers'	1 frank	170	600	16

Food Name	Serv. Size	Total Cal.	Sod. MGS	Fat GMS
smoked, w/cheese 'Wranglers'	1 frank	180	546	16.0
'12-oz pkg'	1 frank	110	378	10.0
(Hygrade) chicken 'Grillmaster'	1 frank	130	na	11.0
(JM)				
beef, 1.2 oz	1 frank	100	350	9.0
beef 'Jumbo' 2 oz	1 frank	180	600	16.0
beef '10 per lb pkg' 1.6 oz	1 frank	140	480	13.0
cheesefurter/cheese smokie 'Cheese Franks' 1.6 oz	1 frank	140	540	13.0
'German Brand' 2 oz	1 frank	160	620	14.0
1.2 oz	1 frank	110	370	10.0
'10 per lb' 1.6 oz	1 frank	140	490	13.0
w/cheese 'German Brand' 2 oz	1 frank	160	620	14.0
(Kahn's)				
beef	1 frank	140	500	13.0
beef 'Bun Size Franks'	1 frank	190	560	17.0
beef 'Jumbo'	1 frank	190	560	18.0
beef w/cheddar 'Beef 'n Cheddar'	1 frank	180	640	16.0
cheesefurter/cheese smokie 'Cheese Wiener'	1 frank	150	490	13.0
smoked, beef 'Bun Size Beef Smokey'	1 frank	190	530	17.0
smoked 'Big Red Smokey'	1 frank	170	550	14.0
smoked 'Bun Size Smokey'	1 frank	180	550	15.0
'Wieners'	1 frank	140	500	13.0
(King Kold) beef, 2 oz	1 frank	173	815	16.3
(Longacre)				
chicken	1 frank	63	230	5.0
turkey	1 frank	66	260	6.0
(Louis Rich)				
turkey 'Bun Length' 2 oz	1 frank	128	640	10.4
turkey, cheese, 1.6 oz	1 frank	109	523	8.9
turkey, 1.6 oz	1 frank	101	505	8.2
(Mr. Turkey)				
turkey, 1.6 oz	1 frank	106	440	8.9
turkey, cheese, 1.6 oz	1 frank	109	526	9.1
(OHSE)				
beef, 1 oz	1 frank	85	280	8.0
chicken, beef, and pork, 1 oz	1 frank	85	260	8.0
'Wieners' 1 oz	1 frank	90	300	8.0
(Oscar Mayer)				
bacon and cheddar cheese 'Hot Dogs' 1.6 oz	1 frank	137	501	12.0
beef 'Bun-Length Franks' 2 oz	1 frank	182	568	16.8
beef, deli 'Big & Juicy' 2.7 oz	1 frank	249	677	23.5

Food Name	Serv. Size	Total Cal.	Sod. MGS	Fat GMS
beef 'Franks' 2 oz	1 frank	181	583	16.7
beef, garlic 'Big & Juicy' 2.7 oz	1 frank	239	652	22.5
beef 'Light Franks' 2 oz	1 frank	131	594	11.1
beef, quarter lb, bun length 'Big & Juicy' 4 oz	1 frank	359	1146	33.5
beef w/cheddar 'Franks' 2 oz	1 frank	163	655	14.3
'Bun-Length Wieners' 2 oz	1 frank	184	571	16.9
cheesefurter/cheese smokie 'Hot Dogs' 1.6 oz	1 frank	143	480	12.9
cocktail 'Little Wieners' .3 oz	1 frank	28	92	2.6
hot and spicy 'Big & Juicy' 2.7 oz	1 frank	224	773	20.4
'Hot Dogs' 1.6 oz	1 frank	137	501	12.0
'Light Wieners' 2 oz	1 frank	127	623	10.8
97% fat free, turkey, beef 'Healthy Favorites'	1 frank	60	570	1.5
original 'Big & Juicy' 2.7 oz	1 frank	244	690	23.2
'Wieners' 2 oz	1 frank	181	576	16.9
(Pilgrim's Pride)				
'1-lb pkg' 2-oz frank	1 frank	118	456	8.8
'12-oz pkg' 1.5-oz frank	1 frank	88	342	6.6
(Quick Meal) w/chili, and cheese, 4.5 oz	1 frank	340	540	20.0
(State Fair) beef, batter-wrapped, on stick 'Corn Dogs' 2.67 oz	1 frank	210	na	10.0
(Tyson)				
chicken	1 frank	115	700	10.0
chicken, batter-wrapped 'Corn Dogs' 3.5 oz	1 frank	280	70	14.0
w/cheese	1 frank	145	680	11.0
FRANKFURTER, ALTERNATIVE				
(Smart Dog) 'Lightlife' fat-free, 1.5 oz	1 frank	40	290	0.0
(White Wave Soyfood) 'Healthy' 1.5 oz	1 frank	120	340	8.0
(Worthington)				
canned 'Super-Links' 1.7 oz	1 frank	100	440	7.0
canned 'Veja-Links'	2 franks	140	330	10.0
frozen 'Leanies' 1.4 oz	1 frank	100	440	6.0
frozen, on a stick 'Dixie Dogs' 2.5 oz	1 frank	200	640	10.0
FRENCH ARTICHOKE. See ARTICHOKES, FRENCH.				
FRENCH BEAN				
boiled	4 oz	146	7	0.9
dried, boiled	1/2 cup	111	5	0.7
raw	1/2 cup	316	17	1.9
raw, dried	1 oz	97	5	0.6
FRENCH TOAST, FROZEN				
(Aunt Jemima) cinnamon swirl	3 oz	171	516	4.3
(Aunt Jemima) 'Original'	3 oz	166	554	4.4
(Aunt Jemima) sticks, and syrup 'Homestyle'	5.2 oz	400	640	20.0

~~od~~ Name	Serv. Size	Total Cal.	Sod. MGS	Fat GMS
(Aunt Jemima) wedges, and sausages 'Homestyle'	5.3 oz	360	780	17.0
(Downyflake)	2 slices	270	380	12.0
(Downyflake) 'Extra Thick'	1 slice	150	340	9.0
(Downyflake) Texas style, and sausage	4.25 oz	400	550	24.0
(Krusteaz) cinnamon swirl	2 slices	270	370	5.0
(Krusteaz) regular	2 slices	250	380	6.0
(Morningstar Farms) vegetarian, cinnamon swirl, w/patties	6.5 oz	380	1220	15.0
(Swanson) cinnamon swirl, w/sausages 'Great Starts'	5.5 oz	390	530	21.0
(Swanson) mini, w/sausage 'Great Starts'	2.5 oz	190	320	9.0
(Swanson) oatmeal, w/lite links 'Great Starts'	4.65 oz	310	500	13.0
(Swanson) w/sausages 'Great Starts'	5.5 oz	380	550	21.0
~~F~~RENCH TOAST, STICKS				
apple cinnamon *(Farm Rich)*	3 oz	310	300	15.0
blueberry *(Farm Rich)*	3 oz	310	280	14.0
original *(Farm Rich)*	3 oz	300	280	15.0
~~F~~RENCH FRY SEASONING *(Tone's)*	1 tsp	5	1551	0.1
~~F~~ROG'S LEGS				
raw	100 gm	73	58	0.3
raw	1 oz	21	(mq)	<1.0
~~F~~ROSTING MIX				
(Betty Crocker)				
cherry 'Creamy' prepared w/margarine	1/12 pkg	180	100	6.0
chocolate fudge 'Creamy' dry	1/12 pkg	140	25	2.0
chocolate fudge 'Creamy' prepared w/butter	1/12 pkg	180	70	6.0
chocolate fudge 'Creamy' prepared w/margarine	1/12 pkg	180	70	6.0
coconut pecan 'Creamy' dry	1/12 pkg	110	5	4.0
coconut pecan 'Creamy' prepared w/butter, 2% milk	1/12 pkg	150	50	8.0
coconut pecan 'Creamy' prepared w/margarine, skim milk	1/12 pkg	150	50	8.0
milk chocolate 'Creamy' prepared w/margarine	1/12 pkg	170	40	5.0
rainbow chip 'Creamy' prepared w/margarine	1/12 pkg	190	50	7.0
sour cream, chocolate fudge 'Creamy' prepared w/margarine	1/12 pkg	180	75	6.0
sour cream, white 'Creamy' prepared w/margarine	1/12 pkg	170	100	5.0
vanilla 'Creamy' dry	1/12 pkg	150	5	2.0
vanilla 'Creamy' prepared w/butter	1/12 pkg	170	50	5.0
vanilla 'Creamy' prepared w/margarine	1/12 pkg	170	50	5.0
white 'Fluffy'	1/12 pkg	70	40	0.0
(Estee)	1 tbsp	65	28	1.5
~~F~~ROSTING, READY-TO-SPREAD				
(Betty Crocker)				
amaretto almond 'Creamy Deluxe'	1/12 tub	160	50	6.0

Food Name	Serv. Size	Total Cal.	Sod. MGS	Fa GM
butter pecan 'Creamy Deluxe'	1/12 tub	170	50	7.
cherry 'Creamy Deluxe'	1/12 tub	160	50	6.
chocolate 'Creamy Deluxe'	1/12 tub	160	60	7.
chocolate 'Creamy Deluxe Light'	1/12 tub	130	60	2.
chocolate chip 'Creamy Deluxe'	1/12 tub	170	30	7.
chocolate chip, coated 'Creamy Deluxe Party'	1/12 tub	160	60	7.
chocolate chip, double 'Creamy Deluxe'	1/12 tub	170	60	8.
chocolate coconut almond 'Creamy Deluxe'	1/12 tub	160	55	8.
chocolate w/dinosaurs 'Creamy Deluxe Party'	1/12 tub	160	60	7
chocolate w/red gel 'Creamy Deluxe Party'	1/12 tub	160	50	7.
chocolate w/turbo racers 'Creamy Deluxe Party'	1/12 tub	160	50	7.
coconut pecan 'Creamy Deluxe'	1/12 tub	160	60	9.
cream cheese 'Creamy Deluxe'	1/12 tub	170	70	7.
dark Dutch fudge 'Creamy Deluxe'	1/12 tub	160	70	7.
lemon 'Creamy Deluxe'	1/12 tub	170	70	6.
milk chocolate 'Creamy Deluxe'	1/12 tub	160	55	6.
milk chocolate 'Creamy Deluxe Light'	1/12 tub	140	60	2
rainbow chip 'Creamy Deluxe'	1/12 tub	170	30	7.
rocky road 'Creamy Deluxe'	1/12 tub	150	50	8
sour cream chocolate 'Creamy Deluxe'	1/12 tub	160	100	7:
sour cream white 'Creamy Deluxe'	1/12 tub	160	50	6
vanilla 'Creamy Deluxe'	1/12 tub	160	25	6.
vanilla 'Creamy Deluxe Light'	1/12 tub	140	30	2.
vanilla w/blue gel 'Creamy Deluxe Party'	1/12 tub	160	30	6.
vanilla w/teddy bears 'Creamy Deluxe Party'	1/12 tub	160	25	6
(Duncan Hines)				
chocolate	1/12 tub	160	90	7.
cream cheese	1/12 tub	160	120	8
cream cheese 'Homestyle'	1/12 tub	160	75	6
dark chocolate 'Homestyle'	1/12 tub	160	75	6
Dutch fudge	1/12 tub	160	95	7.
lemon	1/12 tub	120	60	6.
milk chocolate	1/12 tub	160	85	7
milk chocolate 'Homestyle'	1/12 tub	160	75	6
vanilla	1/12 tub	160	80	7.
vanilla 'Homestyle'	1/12 tub	160	75	6
(Finast) milk chocolate	1/12 tub	160	105	6
(Lovin' Lites)				
chocolate fudge	1/12 tub	130	95	2.
milk chocolate	1/12 tub	130	95	2.
vanilla	1/12 tub	130	70	2

Food Name	Serv. Size	Total Cal.	Sod. MGS	Fat GMS
(Pathmark)				
chocolate, creamy	1/12 tub	160	95	6.0
fudge, creamy	1/12 tub	160	100	7.0
white, creamy	1/12 tub	160	95	6.0
(Pillsbury)				
butter fudge 'Frosting Supreme'	1/12 tub	140	50	6.0
caramel pecan 'Frosting Supreme'	1/12 tub	150	70	8.0
chocolate chip 'Frosting Supreme'	1/12 tub	150	70	5.0
chocolate fudge 'Frosting Supreme'	1/12 tub	150	85	6.0
chocolate fudge 'Funfetti'	1/12 tub	140	80	6.0
chocolate, double Dutch 'Frosting Supreme'	1/12 tub	140	45	6.0
coconut almond 'Frosting Supreme'	1/12 tub	150	60	9.0
coconut pecan 'Frosting Supreme'	1/12 tub	160	60	10.0
cream cheese 'Frosting Supreme'	1/12 tub	160	115	6.0
decorator, all flavors except chocolate	1 tbsp	70	na	2.0
decorator, chocolate	1 tbsp	60	na	2.0
double Dutch 'Frosting Supreme'	1/12 tub	140	50	6.0
fudge 'Frosting Supreme'	1/12 tub	150	80	6.0
lemon 'Frosting Supreme'	1/12 tub	160	80	6.0
milk chocolate 'Frosting Supreme'	1/12 tub	150	65	6.0
milk chocolate w/fudge swirl 'Frosting Supreme'	1/12 tub	150	65	6.0
mint 'Frosting Supreme'	1/12 tub	150	80	7.0
mocha 'Frosting Supreme'	1/12 tub	150	60	6.0
sour cream vanilla 'Frosting Supreme'	1/12 tub	160	80	6.0
strawberry 'Frosting Supreme'	1/12 tub	160	75	6.0
vanilla 'Frosting Supreme'	1/12 tub	160	75	6.0
vanilla 'Funfetti'	1/12 tub	150	75	6.0
vanilla 'Funfetti Sunshine'	1/12 tub	150	75	6.0
vanilla, pink and white 'Funfetti'	1/12 tub	150	70	6.0
vanilla w/fudge swirl 'Frosting Supreme'	1/12 tub	150	75	6.0
white, fluffy	1/12 tub	60	65	0.0
FRUCTOSE				
(Estee)	1 tsp	16	0	0.0
(Estee) packet	1 pkt	12	0	0.0
(Featherweight)	1 tsp	12	0	0.0
FRUIT. See individual listings.				
FRUIT, MIXED				
Canned				
(A&P) in light syrup	1/2 cup	75	10	<1.0
(Del Monte) chunky	1/2 cup	80	10	0.0
(Del Monte) chunky 'Lite'	1/2 cup	50	10	0.0

Food Name	Serv. Size	Total Cal.	Sod. MGS	Fat GMS
(Del Monte) 'Fruit Cup'	5 oz	100	10	0.0
(Del Monte) tropical	1/2 cup	90	10	0.0
(Dole) pineapple and Mandarin orange segments	1/2 cup	80	5	<1.0
(Dole) tropical fruit salad	1/2 cup	70	10	0.0
(Finast) in heavy syrup, chunky	1/2 cup	70	10	0.0
(Kraft) salad 'Pure'	1/2 cup	80	10	0.0
(Libby's) in juice, chunky 'Lite'	1/2 cup	50	5	0.0
(Pathmark) in juice, chunky	1/2 cup	50	15	0.0
(Pathmark) in light syrup 'No Frills'	1 cup	150	20	0.0
(S&W) in juice, chunky, sweetened, clarified	1/2 cup	90	5	0.0
(S&W Nutradiet) chunky	1/2 cup	40	5	0.0
(Sun Fresh) jar, chilled, in light syrup 'Tropical Salad'	3.5 oz	88	39	0.9
Dried				
(Del Monte)	2 oz	130	10	0.0
(SunSweet)	2 oz	150	20	0.0
(SunSweet) bits	2 oz	150	50	<1.0
(Sun•Maid)	2 oz	150	20	0.0
(Sun•Maid) bits	2 oz	150	50	<1.0
Frozen (Birds Eye) in syrup 'Quick Thaw pouch'	5 oz	120	5	0.0
FRUIT AND NUT MIX				
(Estee)	14 pieces	70	15	5.0
(Estee)	4 pieces	35	0	2.0
(Planters) 'Caribbean Crunch'	1 oz	150	130	10.0
(Planters) 'Fruit 'n Nut'	1 oz	150	90	9.0
FRUIT BAR, FROZEN. See also ICE BARS AND DESSERTS; SHERBET; SORBET.				
all flavors 'Fruit Juicee' (Minute Maid)	1 bar	60	0	0.0
blueberry and cream 'Fruit & Cream' (Dole)	1 bar	90	20	1.4
cherry 'Fresh Lites' (Dole)	1 bar	25	6	<1.0
cherry and yogurt 'Fruit & Yogurt' (Dole)	1 bar	80	22	<1.0
chocolate/banana and cream 'Fruit & Cream' (Dole)	1 bar	175	20	9.0
chocolate/strawberry and cream 'Fruit & Cream' (Dole)	1 bar	140	20	8.0
coconut (Sunkist)	1 bar	170	70	10.0
grape 'SunTops' (Dole)	1 bar	40	5	<1.0
lemon 'Fresh Lites' (Dole)	1 bar	25	16	<1.0
lemonade (Sunkist)	1 bar	90	5	0.0
lemonade 'SunTops' (Dole)	1 bar	40	5	<1.0
orange 'Juice Bar' (Sunkist)	1 bar	100	0	0.0
orange, tropical 'SunTops' (Dole)	1 bar	40	5	<1.0
peach and cream 'Fruit & Cream' (Dole)	1 bar	90	19	1.4
pineapple 'Fruit 'n Juice' (Dole)	1 bar	70	4	<.1
pineapple-orange 'Fresh Lites' (Dole)	1 bar	25	7	<1.0

d Name	Serv. Size	Total Cal.	Sod. MGS	Fat GMS
piña colada 'Fruit 'n Juice' *(Dole)*	1 bar	90	2	3.0
punch 'SunTops' *(Dole)*	1 bar	40	5	<1.0
raspberry 'Fresh Lites' *(Dole)*	1 bar	25	6	<1.0
raspberry 'Fruit 'n Juice' *(Dole)*	1 bar	70	14	<.1
raspberry and cream 'Fruit & Cream' *(Dole)*	1 bar	90	23	1.4
strawberry and cream *(Sunkist)*	1 bar	90	30	1.0
strawberry and cream 'Fruit & Cream' *(Dole)*	1 bar	90	22	1.4
raspberry and yogurt 'Fruit & Yogurt' *(Dole)*	1 bar	70	18	<1.0
strawberry and yogurt 'Fruit & Yogurt' *(Dole)*	1 bar	70	16	<1.0
strawberry 'Fruit 'n Juice' *(Dole)*	1 bar	70	6	<.1
wildberry *(Sunkist)*	1 bar	140	15	0.0

UIT COCKTAIL, CANNED

(Del Monte)	1/2 cup	80	10	0.0
(Hunt's)	4 oz	90	7	<1.0
fruit for salad *(Del Monte)*	1/2 cup	90	10	0.0
in extra heavy syrup	4 oz	98	7	0.1
in extra heavy syrup, solid and liquid	1/2 cup	114	8	0.1
in extra light syrup	4 oz	51	5	0.1
in extra light syrup, solid and liquid	1/2 cup	55	5	0.1
in heavy syrup	4 oz	83	7	0.1
in heavy syrup *(A&P)*	1/2 cup	90	15	<1.0
in heavy syrup *(Finast)*	1/2 cup	90	9	0.0
in heavy syrup *(Pathmark)*	1 cup	180	35	0.0
in heavy syrup *(S&W)*	1/2 cup	90	15	0.0
in heavy syrup, solid and liquid	1/2 cup	93	8	0.1
in juice	4 oz	52	5	<.1
in juice *(Featherweight)*	1/2 cup	50	10	0.0
in juice *(IGA)*	1/2 cup	60	10	0.0
in juice *(S&W)*	1/2 cup	90	5	0.0
in juice 'Lite' *(Libby's)*	1/2 cup	50	10	0.0
in juice, solid and liquid	1/2 cup	57	5	0.0
in light syrup	4 oz	65	7	0.1
in light syrup, solid and liquid	1/2 cup	72	8	0.1
in pear juice *(A&P)*	1/2 cup	50	15	<1.0
in water	4 oz	36	5	0.1
in water, solid and liquid	1/2 cup	39	5	0.1
Lite' *(Del Monte)*	1/2 cup	50	10	0.0
'No Sugar Added' *(Finast)*	1/2 cup	50	10	0.0
'Regulars Unsweetened' *(S&W Nutradiet)*	1/2 cup	40	5	0.0

UIT DRINK

(Finast)	8 oz	80	15	0.0

Food Name	Serv. Size	Total Cal.	Sod. MGS
(Fruitopia) 'Fruit Integration' real fruit	8 oz	120	25
(Hi-C) 'Bubble Gum' aseptic box or chilled	6 oz	90	20
(Hi-C) 'Double Fruit Cooler'	6 oz	93	18
(Hi-C) 'Double Fruit Cooler' aseptic box	6 oz	90	25
(Hi-C) 'Ecto Cooler'	6 oz	95	17
(Hi-C) 'Ecto Cooler' aseptic box	6 oz	90	20
(Hi-C) 'Hula Cooler'	6 oz	97	17
FRUIT JUICE			
(Juicy Juice) bottled	6 oz	100	10
(Juicy Juice) boxed	8.45 oz	140	10
(McCain) mixed fruit, 100% juice 'Junior'	4.2 oz	60	5
FRUIT JUICE COCKTAIL			
'Orchard Harvest Blend' *(Welch's)*	6 oz	110	20
'Orchard Harvest Blend' 'Cocktails-In-A-Box' *(Welch's)*	8.45 oz	150	20
'Orchard Harvest Blend' frozen, prepared *(Welch's)*	6 oz	110	10
FRUIT JUICE DRINK, mixed 'Fruit Box' *(Tang)*	8.45 oz	140	10
FRUIT JUICE DRINK MIX			
'Mixes w/Fruit Juice' powder *(Ultra Slim Fast)*	1 scoop	90	75
'Mixes w/Fruit Juice' prepared w/orange juice *(Ultra Slim Fast)*	8 oz	200	80
FRUIT JUICE PUNCH DRINK			
concentrate, prepared w/water	1 cup	124	12
concentrate, prepared w/water	1 oz	15	2
concentrate, undiluted	12 oz	739	41
(Veryfine) can, bottle, or box '100% Juice Punch'	8 oz	122	10
FRUIT PUNCH			
(Bright & Early) frozen 'Bright & Early Fruit Punch' prepared	6 oz	90	5
(Juicy Juice) can, bottle, or box	6 oz	100	10
(Minute Maid) aseptic box, canned, or chilled	6 oz	90	20
(Minute Maid) frozen, concentrate, prepared	6 oz	90	0
(Pathmark) can, bottle, or box	6 oz	90	0
(Snapple)	8 oz	120	5
FRUIT PUNCH DRINK			
(All Sport) thirst quencher, caffeine-free	8 oz	80	55
(Bama)	8.45 oz	130	15
(Crowley)	8 oz	130	15
(Gatorade) low sodium, no caffeine	8 oz	50	110
(Hawaiian Punch) island fruit	6 oz	90	30
(Hawaiian Punch) red 'Fruit Juicy'	6 oz	90	20
(Hawaiian Punch) red 'Fruit Juicy Lite'	6 oz	60	30

ood Name	Serv. Size	Total Cal.	Sod. MGS	Fat GMS
(Hawaiian Punch) tropical	6 oz	90	30	0.0
(Hawaiian Punch) tropical, wild fruit	6 oz	90	35	0.0
(Hi-C)	6 oz	96	17	<.1
(Hi-C) aseptic box or chilled	6 oz	90	20	0.0
(Hi-C) 'Hula Punch'	6 oz	87	17	<.1
(Hi-C) 'Hula Punch Drink' aseptic box	6 oz	90	20	0.0
(J. Hungerford) 20% juice	9.03 oz	43	32	0.0
(J. Hungerford) 50% juice	9.03 oz	107	7	0.0
(J. Hungerford) 100% juice	9.03 oz	116	11	0.0
(Mott's)	10 oz	170	4	0.0
(Mott's)	9.5 oz	161	4	0.0
(PowerAde) thirst quencher, high energy	8 oz	70	70	0.0
(10-K)	8 oz	60	55	0.0
(Tropicana)	6 oz	90	15	<1.0
(Tropicana) 'Single Serve'	10 oz	148	3	0.0
(Welch's) 'Orchard Fruit Harvest Punch'	10 oz	180	0	0.0
(Wyler's)	6 oz	84	8	0.1
(Wyler's) tropical	6 oz	157	10	0.0
(Wyler's) tropical 'Fruit Slush'	4 oz	157	10	0.0
RUIT PUNCH DRINK MIX				
frozen concentrate, prepared	12 oz	677	33	0.0
frozen, prepared w/water	1 cup	114	10	0.0
frozen, prepared w/water	1 oz	14	1	0.0
instant 'Thirst Quencher' prepared (Gatorade)	8 oz	60	110	0.0
'No Frills' prepared (Pathmark)	8 oz	90	85	0.0
powder, w/added sodium, dry	2 rounded tbsp	97	30	0.0
powder, w/added sodium, prepared	8 oz	97	37	0.0
powder, w/o added sodium, dry	2 rounded tbsp	97	11	0.0
powder, w/o added sodium, prepared	8 oz	97	10	0.0
sugar-free, prepared (Crystal Light)	8 oz	4	0	0.0
sugar-free, w/NutraSweet, prepared (Crystal Light)	8 oz	4	0	0.0
tropical 'Crystals' prepared (Wyler's)	8 oz	85	18	0.1
RUIT ROLL. See FRUIT SNACK.				
RUIT SALAD, CANNED. See FRUIT COCKTAIL, CANNED.				
RUIT SNACK				
all flavors 'Berry Bears' (Betty Crocker)	1 pouch	100	20	<1.0
all flavors 'Fruit Roll-Ups Peel-Outs' (Betty Crocker)	1 roll	50	40	<1.0
all flavors 'Shark Bites' (Betty Crocker)	1 pouch	100	20	<1.0
apple (Weight Watchers)	1 pouch	50	75	<1.0
apple chips (Weight Watchers)	.75 oz	70	110	0.0
apple roll (Flavor Tree)	1 piece	75	17	0.0

Food Name	Serv. Size	Total Cal.	Sod. MGS	Fc GM
apricot roll (Flavor Tree)	1 piece	76	17	0.
assorted flavors, all shapes 'Fun Fruits' (Sunkist)	1 pouch	100	10	1.
assorted flavors 'Bugs Bunny and Friends' (Betty Crocker)	1 pouch	90	30	1.
assorted flavors 'Chip 'N Dale Rescue Rangers' (Fruit Parade)	1 pouch	100	10	1.
assorted flavors 'Darkwing Duck' (Fruit Parade)	1 pouch	100	10	1.
assorted flavors 'Dinosaurs' (Farley's)	1 oz	90	0	<1.
assorted flavors 'Fruit Circus Fruit Bears' (Flavor Tree)	1.05 oz	117	12	1
assorted flavors 'Tale Spin' (Fruit Parade)	1 pouch	100	10	1
assorted flavors 'Tasmanian Devil' (Betty Crocker)	1 pouch	90	30	1.
assorted flavors 'Teenage Mutant Ninja Turtles' (Farley's)	1 oz	90	0	<1.
assorted flavors 'Trolls' (Farley's)	1 oz	90	0	<1
berry 'Fun Fruits Berry Bunch' (Sunkist)	1 pouch	100	10	1
cherry 'Fruit by the Foot' (Betty Crocker)	1 roll	80	45	2.
cherry 'Fruit Roll-Ups' (Betty Crocker)	.5-oz roll	50	40	<1.
cherry 'Fun Fruits' (Sunkist)	1 pouch	100	10	1
cherry 'Wild Cherry Gushers' w/juicy centers (Betty Crocker)	1 pouch	90	40	1.
cherry roll (Flavor Tree)	1 piece	75	18	0
cinnamon flavor (Weight Watchers)	1 pouch	50	75	<1
compote (Rokeach)	4 oz	120	4	1
crazy colors 'Fruit Roll-Ups' (Betty Crocker)	.5-oz roll	50	40	<1
'Fun Fruits Fantastic Fruit' (Sunkist)	1 pouch	100	10	1
'Garfield and Friends' 'Wild Blue' (Betty Crocker)	1 roll	50	20	<1
grape 'Fruit by the Foot' (Betty Crocker)	1 roll	80	45	2
grape 'Fruit Roll-Ups' (Betty Crocker)	.5-oz roll	50	40	<1.
grape 'Fun Fruits' (Sunkist)	1 pouch	100	10	1
grape 'Gushin Grape Gushers' (Betty Crocker)	1 pouch	90	45	<1
grape roll (Flavor Tree)	1 piece	76	13	0
orange 'Fun Fruits' (Sunkist)	1 pouch	100	10	1
peach (Weight Watchers)	.5 oz	50	75	<1
raspberry 'Fruit Roll-Ups' (Betty Crocker)	.5-oz roll	50	40	<1
raspberry roll (Flavor Tree)	1 piece	75	20	0
strawberry (Weight Watchers)	1 pouch	50	75	<1
strawberry 'Fruit by the Foot' (Betty Crocker)	1 roll	80	45	2
strawberry 'Fruit Roll-Ups' (Betty Crocker)	.5-oz roll	50	40	<1
strawberry 'Fun Fruits' (Sunkist)	1 pouch	100	10	1
strawberry roll (Flavor Tree)	1 piece	74	11	0
strawberry 'Strawberry Splash Gushers' (Betty Crocker)	1 pouch	90	45	1
strawberry, yogurt coated 'Creme Supremes' (Sunkist)	1 pouch	114	19	3

Food Name	Serv. Size	Total Cal.	Sod. MGS	Fat GMS
FRUIT SPREAD				
all flavors 'Homestyle' (Smucker's)	1 tsp	15	0	0.0
all flavors 'Slenderella' (Smucker's)	1 tsp	7	0	0.0
apple, no sugar added (Fifty 50)	1 tsp	2	5	0.0
apricot 'All Fruit Spreadable Fruit' (Polaner)	1 tsp	14	0	0.0
apricot 'Light' w/NutraSweet (Smucker's)	1 tsp	7	0	0.0
apricot, low sugar (Smucker's)	1 tsp	8	10	0.0
apricot 'Simply Fruit' (Smucker's)	1 tsp	16	0	0.0
apricot-pineapple (Knott's Berry Farm)	1 tsp	16	0	0.0
apricot-pineapple 'Light' w/NutraSweet (Knott's Berry Farm)	1 tsp	8	0	0.0
apricot-pineapple, portion pack (Knott's Berry Farm)	.5 oz	35	0	0.0
black cherry 'All Fruit Spreadable Fruit' (Polaner)	1 tsp	14	0	0.0
black raspberry 'Simply Fruit' (Smucker's)	1 tsp	16	0	0.0
blackberry (Knott's Berry Farm)	1 tsp	16	0	0.0
blackberry 'Light' w/NutraSweet (Knott's Berry Farm)	1 tsp	8	0	0.0
blackberry, low sugar (Smucker's)	1 tsp	8	10	0.0
blackberry, portion pack (Knott's Berry Farm)	.5 oz	35	0	0.0
blackberry 'Simply Fruit' (Smucker's)	1 tsp	16	0	0.0
blueberry 'All Fruit Spreadable Fruit' (Polaner)	1 tsp	14	0	0.0
blueberry 'Simply Fruit' (Smucker's)	1 tsp	16	0	0.0
boysenberry (Knott's Berry Farm)	1 tsp	16	0	0.0
boysenberry 'Light' w/NutraSweet (Knott's Berry Farm)	1 tsp	8	0	0.0
boysenberry 'Light' w/NutraSweet (Smucker's)	1 tsp	7	0	0.0
boysenberry, low sugar (Smucker's)	1 tsp	8	10	0.0
boysenberry, portion pack (Knott's Berry Farm)	.5 oz	35	0	0.0
calamansi 'Tropical Rainforest' (Knudsen & Sons)	2 tsp	35	0	0.0
grape (Weight Watchers)	1 tsp	8	0	0.0
grape 'All Fruit Spreadable Fruit' (Polaner)	1 tsp	14	0	0.0
grape, Concord, low sugar (Smucker's)	1 tsp	8	0	0.0
grape 'Imitation' (Smucker's)	1 tsp	2	2	0.0
grape, no sugar added (Fifty 50)	1 tsp	2	5	0.0
grape 'Simply Fruit' (Smucker's)	1 tsp	16	0	0.0
guanabana 'Tropical Rainforest' (Knudsen & Sons)	2 tsp	35	0	0.0
orange 'All Fruit Spreadable Fruit' (Polaner)	1 tsp	14	0	0.0
orange marmalade (Knott's Berry Farm)	1 tsp	16	0	0.0
orange marmalade 'Light' w/NutraSweet (Knott's Berry Farm)	1 tsp	8	0	0.0
orange marmalade 'Light' w/NutraSweet (Smucker's)	1 tsp	7	0	0.0
orange marmalade, low sugar (Smucker's)	1 tsp	8	10	0.0
orange marmalade, no sugar added (Fifty 50)	1 tsp	2	5	0.0

Food Name	Serv. Size	Total Cal.	Sod. MGS	Fat GMS
orange marmalade, portion pack *(Knott's Berry Farm)*	.5 oz	35	0	0.0
orange marmalade 'Simply Fruit' *(Smucker's)*	1 tsp	16	0	0.0
peach 'Simply Fruit' *(Smucker's)*	1 tsp	16	0	0.0
raspberry *(Weight Watchers)*	1 tsp	8	0	0.0
raspberry 'All Fruit Spreadable Fruit' *(Polaner)*	1 tsp	14	0	0.0
raspberry 'All Fruit Spreadable Fruit' seedless *(Polaner)*	1 tsp	14	0	0.0
raspberry, no sugar added *(Fifty 50)*	1 tsp	2	5	0.0
red raspberry *(Knott's Berry Farm)*	1 tsp	16	0	0.0
red raspberry 'Light' w/NutraSweet *(Knott's Berry Farm)*	1 tsp	8	0	0.0
red raspberry 'Light' w/NutraSweet *(Smucker's)*	1 tsp	7	0	0.0
red raspberry, low sugar *(Smucker's)*	1 tsp	8	0	0.0
red raspberry, portion pack *(Knott's Berry Farm)*	.5 oz	35	0	0.0
red raspberry 'Simply Fruit' *(Smucker's)*	1 tsp	16	0	0.0
strawberry *(Weight Watchers)*	1 tsp	8	0	0.0
strawberry 'All Fruit Spreadable Fruit' *(Polaner)*	1 tsp	14	0	0.0
strawberry 'Imitation' *(Smucker's)*	1 tsp	2	2	0.0
strawberry 'Light' w/NutraSweet *(Knott's Berry Farm)*	1 tsp	8	0	0.0
strawberry 'Light' w/NutraSweet *(Smucker's)*	1 tsp	7	0	0.0
strawberry, low sugar *(Smucker's)*	1 tsp	8	0	0.0
strawberry, no sugar added *(Fifty 50)*	1 tsp	2	5	0.0
strawberry 'Simply Fruit' *(Smucker's)*	1 tsp	16	0	0.0
FRUIT SYRUP				
all flavors *(Smucker's)*	2 tbsp	100	0	0.0
'Fruit 'n Maple' *(Knudsen & Sons)*	1 oz	105	na	<1.0
'Fruit 'n Maple' pourable *(Knudsen & Sons)*	1 oz	105	0	0.0
raspberry, pourable *(Knudsen & Sons)*	1 oz	75	0	1.0
strawberry, pourable *(Knudsen & Sons)*	1 oz	75	0	1.0
FUDGE TOPPING				
(Hershey's)	2 tbsp	100	30	4.0
(Kraft) hot	1 tbsp	70	50	2.0
(Mrs. Richardson's) hot	2 tbsp	140	75	7.0
(Mrs. Richardson's) hot, microwavable	2 tbsp	140	75	7.0
(Smucker's)	2 tbsp	130	50	1.0
(Smucker's) hot	2 tbsp	110	55	4.0
(Smucker's) hot 'Light'	2 tbsp	70	35	0.0
(Smucker's) hot 'Special Recipe'	2 tbsp	150	60	5.0
(Smucker's) 'Magic Shell'	2 tbsp	190	50	15.0

G

Food Name	Serv. Size	Total Cal.	Sod. MGS	Fat GMS
GARBANZO BEAN/ceci/chick pea				
boiled	4 oz	186	8	2.9
boiled	1/2 cup	134	6	2.1
raw	1/2 cup	364	24	6.0
raw	1 oz	103	7	1.7
raw *(Arrowhead Mills)*	2 oz	200	9	3.0
Canned				
(A&P)	1/2 cup	100	270	1.0
(Allens)	1/2 cup	110	320	<1.0
(Bush's Best)	1/2 cup	80	350	0.0
(Eden Foods) organic, very low sodium, no salt added	1/2 cup	90	10	1.0
(Eden Foods) organic, w/liquid	1/2 cup	110	15	2.0
(Finast)	8 oz	210	250	3.0
(Green Giant)	1/2 cup	90	320	2.0
(Green Giant) 50% less salt	1/2 cup	90	160	2.0
(Joan of Arc) 50% less salt	1/2 cup	90	160	2.0
(Old El Paso)	1/2 cup	190	250	<1.0
(Progresso)	1/2 cup	110	200	1.0
(S&W) large, 50% less salt 'Lite'	1/2 cup	110	295	1.0
(S&W Nutradiet)	1/2 cup	100	5	1.0
GARBANZO FLOUR/chick pea flour				
(Arrowhead Mills)	2 oz	200	9	3.0
GARDEN SALAD				
(Joan of Arc) canned	1/2 cup	70	500	0.0
(Read) canned	1/2 cup	70	500	0.0
(S&W) refrigerated marinated	1/2 cup	60	670	0.0
(Trader Joe's) refrigerated fresh vegetables, no-oil vinaigrette	1 container	90	770	1.0
(Trader Joe's) refrigerated w/eggless egg salad, no-oil vinaigrette	1 container	140	340	7.0
GARLIC				
trimmed	1 oz	42	5	0.1
untrimmed	1 lb	587	67	2.0
GARLIC BREAD. See BREAD.				
GARLIC BREAD SEASONING				
'Garlic Bread Sprinkle' *(Schilling)*	1/4 tsp	5	25	0.4
GARLIC BREAD SPREAD *(Lawry's)*	1/2 tbsp	47	15	4.6
GARLIC PEPPER, 'Spice Blends' *(Lawry's)*	1 tsp	11	292	<.1

Food Name	Serv. Size	Total Cal.	Sod. MGS	Fat GMS
GARLIC POWDER				
dry	1 oz	94	7	0.2
dry	1 tbsp	28	2	0.1
dry	1 tsp	9	1	0.0
dry *(Durkee)*	1 tsp	10	0	tr
dry *(Laurel Leaf)*	1 tsp	10	0	tr
dry *(Lawry's)* w/parsley	1 tsp	12	5	0.9
dry *(Spice Islands)*	1 tsp	5	<1	tr
GARLIC SALT				
(Lawry's)	1 tsp	4	968	<.1
(Morton)	1 tsp	3	1300	<.1
GARLIC SEASONING				
(Gilroy) crushed	1 tsp	8	4	0.0
(Gilroy) minced	1 tsp	23	4	1.0
(Golden Dipt)	2 grams	8	87	0.0
(Schilling) 'Parsley Patch'	1 tsp	13	1	0.5
(Schilling) 'Season All'	1/4 tsp	2	163	(tr)
GARLIC SPREAD, concentrate *(Lawry's)*	1 tbsp	15	21	1.6
GATORADE. See individual flavors.				
GEFILTE FISH				
Hors d'oeuvres *(Rokeach)*	8 balls	60	(mq)	1.0
In jelled broth				
(Mother's) 'Old Fashioned' 24-oz jar	1 ball	70	(mq)	1.0
(Mother's) 'Old Fashioned' 12-oz jar	1 ball	54	(mq)	0.8
(Mother's) 'Old World'	1 ball	70	(mq)	1.0
(Mother's) 'Unsalted'	1 ball	45	(mq)	1.0
(Rokeach) 'Old Vienna' 31-oz jar	3 oz	81	(mq)	1.0
(Rokeach) 'Old Vienna' 24-oz jar	2.6 oz	70	(mq)	1.0
(Rokeach) 'Old Vienna' 12-oz jar	2 oz	54	(mq)	1.0
(Rokeach) 'Redi-Jelled'	4 oz	92	444	2.0
(Rokeach) 'Redi-Jelled'	3 oz	65	333	1.0
(Rokeach) 'Redi-Jelled'	2 oz	46	222	1.0
In liquid				
(Mother's) 'Old Fashioned' 24- or 31-oz jar	1 ball	70	(mq)	1.0
(Mother's) 'Old Fashioned' 12-oz jar	1 ball	54	(mq)	0.8
In natural broth				
(Rokeach) 24-oz jar	4 oz	60	835	1.0
(Rokeach) 24-oz jar	2.6 oz	50	(mq)	1.0
Sweet *(Mother's)* 'Old World'	1 ball	54	(mq)	0.8

Food Name	Serv. Size	Total Cal.	Sod. MGS	Fat GMS
WHITEFISH				
In jelled broth				
(Mother's) 24- or 31-oz jar	1 ball	60	(mq)	1.0
(Mother's) 12-oz jar	1 ball	46	(mq)	0.8
In liquid				
(Mother's) 24- or 31-oz jar	1 ball	70	(mq)	1.0
(Mother's) 12-oz jar	1 ball	54	(mq)	0.8
WHITEFISH AND PIKE				
In jelled broth				
(Mother's) 24- or 31-oz jar	1 ball	60	(mq)	1.0
(Mother's) 12-oz jar	1 ball	46	(mq)	0.8
(Mother's) 'Old World'	1 ball	54	(mq)	0.8
(Rokeach)	2.6 oz	60	(mq)	1.0
(Rokeach)	2 oz	46	(mq)	1.0
In liquid *(Mother's)*	1 ball	70	(mq)	1.0
GELATIN, JAPANESE				
raw	1 lb	116	40	0.1
raw	1 oz	7	3	tr
GELATIN, UNFLAVORED *(Knox)*	1 pkt	25	10	0.0
GELATIN DESSERT				
PREPARED FROM MIX				
(D-Zerta)				
all flavors	1/2 cup	8	0	0.0
all flavors, low calorie, w/aspartame	1/2 cup	8	0	0.0
(Featherweight)				
all flavors except lemon	1/2 cup	10	5	0.0
lemon	1/2 cup	10	4	0.0
(Jell-O)				
berry blue	1/2 cup	80	50	0.0
black raspberry	1/2 cup	80	35	0.0
cherry	1/2 cup	80	70	0.0
cherry, sugar-free	1/2 cup	8	80	0.0
Concord grape	1/2 cup	80	35	0.0
lemon	1/2 cup	80	75	0.0
lemon, sugar-free	1/2 cup	8	60	0.0
lime	1/2 cup	80	55	0.0
lime, sugar-free	1/2 cup	8	65	0.0
orange, sugar-free	1/2 cup	8	55	0.0
orange-pineapple	1/2 cup	80	65	0.0
raspberry, sugar-free	1/2 cup	8	55	0.0
strawberry, sugar-free	1/2 cup	8	65	0.0

Food Name	Serv. Size	Total Cal.	Sod. MGS	Fat GMS
strawberry banana, sugar-free	1/2 cup	8	55	0.0
watermelon	1/2 cup	80	50	0.0
wild strawberry	1/2 cup	80	75	0.0
(Royal)				
apple	1/2 cup	80	95	0.0
blackberry	1/2 cup	80	95	0.0
cherry	1/2 cup	80	95	0.0
cherry, sugar-free	1/2 cup	8	90	0.0
Concord grape	1/2 cup	80	130	0.0
fruit punch	1/2 cup	80	90	0.0
lemon	1/2 cup	80	125	0.0
lemon-lime	1/2 cup	80	95	0.0
lime	1/2 cup	80	125	0.0
lime, sugar-free	1/2 cup	8	100	0.0
mixed berry	1/2 cup	80	90	0.0
orange	1/2 cup	80	95	0.0
orange, sugar-free	1/2 cup	10	90	0.0
peach	1/2 cup	80	95	0.0
pineapple	1/2 cup	80	95	0.0
raspberry	1/2 cup	80	125	0.0
raspberry, sugar-free	1/2 cup	8	90	0.0
strawberry	1/2 cup	80	105	0.0
strawberry, sugar-free	1/2 cup	8	90	0.0
strawberry banana	1/2 cup	80	105	0.0
strawberry banana, sugar-free	1/2 cup	8	85	0.0
strawberry orange	1/2 cup	80	110	0.0
tropical fruit	1/2 cup	80	110	0.0
READY TO SERVE				
(Estee)	1/2 cup	8	0	0.0
(Jell-O) berry blue, six pack	3.5 oz	80	40	0.0
(Jell-O) cherry, six pack	3.5 oz	80	40	0.0
(Jell-O) strawberry, six pack	3.5 oz	80	40	0.0
GELATIN DRINK MIX				
orange flavor	1 oz	108	47	0.3
orange flavor *(Knox)*	1 envelope	39	17	0.1
GERMAN SAUSAGE. See also individual listings.				
(Hickory Farms)	1 oz	100	385	8.0
GHEE/clarified butter	1 oz	249	na	28.4
GIN. See ALCOHOLIC BEVERAGES.				
GINGER				
ground	1 oz	98	9	1.7

Food Name	Serv. Size	Total Cal.	Sod. MGS	Fat GMS
ground	1 tbsp	19	2	0.3
ground	1 tsp	6	1	0.1
ground *(Durkee)*	1 tsp	7	0	tr
ground *(Laurel Leaf)*	1 tsp	7	0	tr
ground *(Spice Islands)*	1 tsp	6	1	0.1
GINGER, PICKLED, Japanese	1 oz	10	105	<.1
GINGER ALE. See SOFT DRINKS AND MIXERS.				
GINGER ROOT				
candied, crystallized	1 lb	1544	272	0.9
candied, crystallized	1 oz	95	17	0.1
raw, slices, 1-inch diam	1/4 cup	17	3	0.2
raw, slices, 1-inch diam	5 slices	8	1	0.1
trimmed	1 oz	20	4	0.2
untrimmed	1 lb	291	53	3.1
GINGER TERIYAKI MARINADE *(Golden Dipt)*	1 oz	120	920	7.0
GINGERBREAD. See BREAD.				
GINKGO NUT				
canned	1 cup	172	476	2.5
canned, approx 9 large, 14 medium, or 22 small	1 oz	32	87	0.5
dried	1 oz	99	4	0.6
dried, in shell	1 lb	1198	46	6.9
raw	1 oz	52	2	0.5
raw, in shell	1 lb	628	24	5.8
GLOBE ARTICHOKE. See ARTHICHOKES, GLOBE.				
GLUTEN. See WHEAT GLUTEN.				
GOA BEAN. See WINGED BEAN.				
GOAT				
raw	1 lb	494	372	10.5
raw	1 oz	31	23	0.7
roasted	4 oz	162	98	3.4
roasted, diced	1 cup	200	120	4.2
GOATFISH				
raw	1 lb	435	(mq)	4.5
raw	1 oz	27	(mq)	0.3
GOBO. See BURDOCK ROOT.				
GOOSE, DOMESTICATED				
meat and skin, raw	1 oz	105	21	9.5
meat and skin, roasted	4 oz	346	79	24.9
meat only, raw	1 oz	46	25	2.0
meat only, roasted	4 oz	270	86	14.4

Food Name	Serv. Size	Total Cal.	Sod. MGS	Fat GMS
GOOSE FAT				
....	1/2 cup	923	0	102.3
....	1 oz	255	0	28.3
....	1 tbsp	115	0	12.8
GOOSE GIBLETS, raw	100 gm	156	70	7.0
GOOSE GIZZARD, raw	100 gm	139	65	5.3
GOOSE LIVER, raw	1 lb	15	15	0.5
GOOSEBERRY				
whole	1 lb	202	4	2.6
whole	1 oz	12	<1	0.2
whole	1 cup	66	2	0.9
GOOSEBERRY, CANNED, in light syrup	4 oz	83	2	0.2
GOOSEFISH. See MONKFISH.				
GOURD, BOTTLE/calabash gourd/white-flowered gourd				
boiled, drained	4 oz	17	2	<.1
boiled, drained, 1-inch cubes	1/2 cup	11	1	<.1
raw, approx 2.4 lb	1 med	106	19	0.2
raw, 1-inch cubes	1/2 cup	8	1	<.1
raw, trimmed	1 oz	4	1	tr
raw, untrimmed	1 lb	44	8	0.1
GOURD, CALABASH. See GOURD, BOTTLE.				
GOURD, DISHCLOTH/loofah gourd/rag gourd/sponge gourd/towel gourd/vegetable sponge				
boiled, drained	4 oz	64	24	0.4
boiled, drained, 1-inch slices	1/2 cup	50	19	0.3
raw, approx 8.6 oz	1 med	36	5	0.4
raw, 1-inch slices	1 cup	19	3	0.2
raw, trimmed	1 oz	6	1	0.1
raw, untrimmed	1 lb	67	11	0.7
GOURD, RAG. See GOURD, DISHCLOTH.				
GOURD, SPONGE. See GOURD, DISHCLOTH.				
GOURD, WAX				
boiled, drained	4 oz	15	121	0.2
boiled, drained, cubes	1/2 cup	11	93	0.2
raw, cubes	1 cup	17	147	0.3
raw, trimmed	1 oz	4	31	0.1
raw, untrimmed	1 lb	42	358	0.6
GOURD, WHITE/tunka				
boiled, drained	4 oz	15	121	0.2
boiled, drained, cubes	1/2 cup	11	93	0.2
raw, cubes	1 cup	17	147	0.3
raw, trimmed	1 oz	4	31	0.1

Food Name	Serv. Size	Total Cal.	Sod. MGS	Fat GMS
raw, untrimmed	1 lb	42	358	0.6
GOURD, WHITE-FLOWERED. See GOURD, BOTTLE.				
GOVERNOR PLUM, trimmed	1 oz	31	na	0.0
GRANADILLA. See PASSION FRUIT.				
GRANOLA. See CEREAL, READY-TO-SERVE.				
GRANOLA AND CEREAL BAR. See also GRANOLA SNACKS.				
(Barbara's Bakery)				
cinnamon and oats, 2 oz	1 bar	281	na	15.0
coconut almond, 2 oz	1 bar	306	na	20.0
peanut butter, 2 oz	1 bar	275	na	15.0
(Bear Valley)				
carob-cocoa, food bar 'Pemmican' 3.75 oz	1 bar	440	80	12.0
coconut almond, food bar 'Meal Pack' 3.75 oz	1 bar	400	80	12.0
sesame lemon, food bar 'Meal Pack' 3.75 oz	1 bar	410	85	13.0
fruit 'n nut, food bar 'Pemmican' 3.75 oz	1 bar	420	90	13.0
(Glenny's)				
apple, 'Original Fruit Bar'	1 bar	100	15	3.0
'Bee Pollen Sunrise' 1.5 oz	1 bar	190	na	8.0
carob mint w/oat bran 'Brown Rice Treats'	1 bar	180	20	2.0
cinnamon and raisin 'Brown Rice Treats' 1.75 oz ...	1 bar	170	30	1.0
coconut amandine 'Moist and Chewy' 1.5 oz	1 bar	190	20	10.0
'Ginseng Sunrise' 1.5 oz	1 bar	160	na	7.0
oatmeal raisin 'Moist and Chewy' 1.5 oz	1 bar	160	25	3.0
peanut and raisin 'Brown Rice Treats' 2 oz	1 bar	210	29	5.0
peanut snack 'Moist and Chewy' 1.5 oz	1 bar	180	20	7.0
plain and fancy 'Brown Rice Treats' 1.25 oz	1 bar	120	29	1.0
raisin bran 'Brown Rice Treats' 1.75 oz	1 bar	170	17	1.0
'Spirulina Sunrise' 1.5 oz	1 bar	140	na	5.0
sunflower 'Moist and Chewy' 1.5 oz	1 bar	180	15	7.0
toasted almond w/oat bran 'Brown Rice Treats'	1 bar	200	20	5.0
(Golden Temple)				
cashew almond 'Wha Guru Chew Bar'	1 bar	164	63	11.0
peanut cashew 'Wha Guru Chew Bar'	1 bar	167	62	11.0
sesame almond 'Wha Guru Chew Bar'	1 bar	160	61	10.0
(Health Valley)				
blueberry apple, fat-free	1 bar	140	10	0.0
date almond flavor, fat-free	1 bar	140	10	0.0
raspberry, fat-free	1 bar	140	10	0.0
(Hershey's)				
chocolate chip, chocolate coated, 1.2 oz	1 bar	170	50	8.0
cocoa creme, chocolate coated, 1.2 oz	1 bar	180	50	9.0

Food Name	Serv. Size	Total Cal.	Sod. MGS	Fat GMS
cookies and creme, chocolate coated, 1.2 oz	1 bar	170	50	8.0
peanut butter, chocolate coated, 1.2 oz	1 bar	180	65	10.0
raspberry filled 'Common Sense Smart Start'	1 bar	170	160	6.0
(Kudo's)				
chocolate chip	1 bar	180	60	9.0
chocolate chunk 'Simply Kudos'	1 bar	100	50	4.0
fudge, nutty	1 bar	190	60	11.0
honey nut 'Simply Kudos'	1 bar	100	55	4.0
oatmeal raisin 'Simply Kudos'	1 bar	90	55	4.0
peanut butter, chocolate coated, 1.3 oz	1 bar	190	70	12.0
(Natural Nectar)				
almond, 'Treat Yourself Right'	1 bar	150	40	5.0
apple-oatmeal spice, 'Fi-Bar A.M.'	1 bar	150	25	3.0
banana nut, 'Fi-Bar A.M.'	1 bar	150	20	4.0
cocoa almond, 'Fi-Bar Chewy & Nutty'	1 bar	130	20	4.0
cocoa almond crunch, 'Canadian Chewy & Nutty'	1 bar	130	20	4.0
cocoa peanut, 'Fi-Bar Chewy & Nutty'	1 bar	130	20	1.0
cocoa peanut butter crunch, 'Chewy & Nutty'	1 bar	130	20	4.0
coconut	1 bar	120	30	4.0
cranberry, w/wild berries 'Original Fruit Bar'	1 bar	120	15	2.0
lemon 'Original Fruit Bar'	1 bar	100	15	3.0
Mandarin orange 'Original Fruit Bar'	1 bar	100	15	3.0
peanut butter	1 bar	130	30	4.0
peanut butter 'Treat Yourself Right'	1 bar	150	55	5.0
raisin nut bran, 'Fi-Bar A.M.'	1 bar	150	30	4.0
raspberry 'Canadian'	1 bar	120	15	3.0
raspberry 'Original Fruit Bar'	1 bar	120	15	2.0
strawberry 'Canadian'	1 bar	120	15	3.0
strawberry 'Original Fruit Bar'	1 bar	120	15	2.0
strawberry-oatmeal w/almonds, 'Fi-Bar A.M.'	1 bar	150	30	4.0
vanilla almond, 'Fi-Bar Chewy & Nutty'	1 bar	130	20	4.0
vanilla almond crunch, 'Canadian Chewy & Nutty'	1 bar	130	20	4.0
vanilla peanut, 'Fi-Bar Chewy & Nutty'	1 bar	130	20	4.0
wild cranberry 'Canadian'	1 bar	120	15	3.0
(Nature Valley)				
cinnamon, .8 oz	1 bar	120	70	5.0
oat bran-honey graham, .8 oz	1 bar	110	90	4.0
oats and honey, .8 oz	1 bar	120	65	5.0
peanut butter, .8 oz	1 bar	120	70	6.0
(Nature's Choice)				
carob chip, .75 oz	1 bar	90	15	3.0

Food Name	Serv. Size	Total Cal.	Sod. MGS	Fat GMS
cinnamon-raisin, .75 oz	1 bar	90	10	3.0
oats 'n honey, .75 oz	1 bar	90	15	3.0
peanut butter, .75 oz	1 bar	90	25	3.0
(Nutri Grain)				
blueberry 'Smart Start' 1.5 oz	1 bar	180	170	8.0
corn flakes, mixed berry-filled 'Smart Start'	1 bar	170	160	7.0
raisin bran 'Smart Start' 1.5 oz	1 bar	160	170	5.0
rice krispies w/almonds 'Smart Start' 1 oz	1 bar	130	65	6.0
strawberry 'Smart Start' 1.5 oz	1 bar	180	170	8.0
(Quaker)				
apple berry 'Chewy'	1 bar	120	95	4.0
caramel nut 'Granola Dipps' 1 oz	1 bar	148	81	6.4
chocolate chip 'Chewy'	1 bar	128	90	4.7
chocolate chip 'Granola Dipps' 1 oz	1 bar	139	78	6.3
chocolate fudge 'Granola Dipps' 1 oz	1 bar	160	74	7.9
chunky nut and raisin 'Chewy' 1 oz	1 bar	131	86	5.8
honey and oats 'Chewy' 1 oz	1 bar	125	95	4.4
peanut butter 'Chewy' 1 oz	1 bar	128	116	4.9
peanut butter, chocolate chip 'Chewy' 1 oz	1 bar	131	112	5.7
peanut butter, chocolate chip 'Granola Dipps'	1 bar	174	102	10.0
peanut butter 'Granola Dipps' 1 oz	1 bar	170	74	9.1
raisin and cinnamon 'Chewy' 1 oz	1 bar	128	92	5.0
S'mores 'Chewy' 1 oz	1 bar	126	108	4.4
trail mix 'Chewy' 1 oz	1 bar	130	105	5.0
(Sunbelt)				
apple bar, baked, 1.31 oz	1 bar	130	130	2.0
chocolate chip, chewy, 1.25 oz	1 bar	150	75	7.0
chocolate chip, fudge dipped, chewy, 1.63 oz	1 bar	220	60	11.0
chocolate chip, fudge dipped, chewy, 1.5 oz	1 bar	210	55	10.0
oats and honey, chewy, 1 oz	1 bar	130	35	5.0
oats and honey, fudge dipped, chewy, 1.38 oz	1 bar	190	55	10.0
w/almonds, chewy, 1 oz	1 bar	120	65	6.0
w/chocolate chips, chewy, 1.75 oz	1 bar	220	105	9.0
w/peanuts, fudge dipped, chewy, 2.25 oz	1 bar	300	90	18.0
w/peanuts, fudge dipped, chewy, 1.38 oz	1 bar	190	55	10.0
w/raisins, chewy, 1.25 oz	1 bar	150	65	6.0
w/raisins, fudge dipped, chewy, 1.5 oz	1 bar	200	60	12.0

GRANOLA SNACKS. See also GRANOLA AND CEREAL BAR.

Food Name	Serv. Size	Total Cal.	Sod. MGS	Fat GMS
(Natural Nectar)				
almond butter crunch 'Nectar Nuggets'	1 cup	120	30	7.0
almond cappuccino crunch 'Nectar Nuggets'	1 cup	110	30	5.0

Food Name	Serv. Size	Total Cal.	Sod. MGS	Fat GMS
coconut almond crunch 'Nectar Nuggets'	1 cup	110	20	5.0
peanut butter crunch 'Nectar Nuggets'	1 cup	120	30	7.0
(Nature Valley)				
apple-cinnamon 'Granola Bites'	1 pkg	170	100	7.0
honey nut 'Granola Bites'	1 pkg	170	120	8.0
variety pack 'Granola Bites'	1 pkg	170	120	8.0
(Nature's Choice)				
chocolate chip 'Grrr-Nola Treats'	.75 oz	80	5	2.0
cinnamon toast 'Grrr-Nola Treats'	.75 oz	80	5	2.0
peanut butter and jelly 'Grrr-Nola Treats'	.75 oz	80	5	3.0
tutti-frutti 'Grrr-Nola Treats'	.75 oz	75	5	2.0
GRAPE				
AMERICAN *(Concord, Delaware, Niagara)*				
(Dole)	1.5 cup	85	3	0.0
Slipskin				
peeled and seeded	1 oz	18	<1	0.1
trimmed	10 fruits	15	0	0.1
untrimmed	1 lb	165	4	0.9
untrimmed	1 cup	58	2	0.3
EUROPEAN *(Muskat, Tokay, Thompson)*				
Adherent skin				
trimmed	10 fruits	35	1	0.3
untrimmed	1 lb	287	7	2.3
untrimmed	1 cup	114	3	0.9
untrimmed w/o seeds	1 lb	309	7	2.5
w/seeds	1/2 cup	57	2	0.5
w/seeds	1 oz	20	1	0.2
w/o seeds	1/2 cup	57	2	0.5
w/o seeds	1 oz	20	1	0.2
w/o seeds, approx 1.75 oz	10 grapes	36	1	0.3
GRAPE, CANNED				
THOMPSON, seedless				
in heavy syrup	1 cup	187	13	0.3
in heavy syrup	4 oz	83	6	0.1
in heavy syrup *(S&W)*	1/2 cup	100	5	0.0
in water	1 cup	98	15	0.3
in water	4 oz	45	7	0.1
GRAPE APPLE DRINK, bottle *(Mott's)*	10 oz	167	<1	0.0
GRAPE DRINK				
Can, bottle, or box				
(A&P)	6 oz	100	0	<1.0

Food Name	Serv. Size	Total Cal.	Sod. MGS	Fat GMS
(All Sport) thirst quencher, caffeine-free	8 oz	70	55	0.0
(Bama)	8.45 oz	120	25	0.0
(Bright & Early) frozen, diluted	6 oz	100	0	0.0
(Crowley)	8 oz	130	15	0.0
(Fruitopia) 'The Grape Beyond' real fruit	8 oz	130	25	0.0
(Gatorade) low sodium, no caffeine	8 oz	50	110	0.0
(Hi-C) aseptic box	6 oz	90	25	0.0
(J. Hungerford)	9.03 oz	41	31	0.0
(Kool-Aid) 'Koolers'	8.45 oz	140	10	0.0
(Pathmark)	6 oz	90	0	0.0
(Squeezit) 'Grumpy Grape'	6.75 oz	120	5	0.0
(10-K) 'Clear'	8 oz	60	55	0.0
(Tropicana)	6 oz	90	10	<1.0
(Veryfine)	8 oz	130	10	0.0
(Wyler's) 'Fruit Slush'	4 oz	157	10	0.0
Prepared from mix				
(Finast)	8 oz	80	15	0.0
(Gatorade) instant 'Thirst Quencher'	8 oz	60	110	0.0
(Kool-Aid) sugar-sweetened	8 oz	80	25	0.0
(Kool-Aid) unsweetened, prepared w/sugar	8 oz	100	0	0.0
(Kool-Aid) unsweetened, prepared w/o sugar	8 oz	2	0	0.0
(Kool-Aid) w/NutraSweet	8 oz	4	0	0.0
(Pathmark) 'No Frills'	8 oz	90	20	0.0
(Pathmark) 'No Frills Sodium Free'	6 oz	80	0	0.0
GRAPE JUICE				
Can, bottle, or box				
(IGA) 'Unsweetened'	6 oz	120	5	0.0
(J. Hungerford)	9.03 oz	160	0	0.0
(J. Hungerford) 100% juice	9.03 oz	155	11	0.0
(J. Hungerford) 50% juice	9.03 oz	135	0	0.0
(J. Hungerford) 20% juice	9.03 oz	41	31	0.0
(Juicy Juice) blend	6 oz	100	5	0.0
(Juicy Juice) bottled	6 oz	90	5	0.0
(Juicy Juice) boxed	8.45 oz	130	10	0.0
(Knudsen & Sons)	8 oz	130	na	0.0
(Knudsen & Sons) Concord	8 oz	130	na	0.0
(Kraft) 'Pure 100% Unsweetened'	6 oz	104	0	0.0
(Pathmark) 'No Frills'	6 oz	113	10	0.0
(Lucky Leaf)	6 oz	130	0	0.0
(Minute Maid) aseptic box	6 oz	100	20	1.0
(Pathmark) 'Unsweetened'	6 oz	120	10	0.0

Food Name	Serv. Size	Total Cal.	Sod. MGS	Fat GMS
(S&W) Concord 'Unsweetened'	6 oz	100	9	0.0
(Sippin' Pak)	8.45 oz	130	25	0.0
(Squeezit 100) 'Caped Grape' 100% natural fruit juice	6.75 oz	100	20	0.0
(Veryfine) '100%'	8 oz	153	20	0.0
(Welch's) purple	6 oz	120	10	0.0
(Welch's) red	8.45 oz	170	20	0.0
(Welch's) red	6 oz	120	15	0.0
(Welch's) sparkling red	6 oz	128	30	0.0
(Welch's) sparkling white	6 oz	120	30	0.0
(Welch's) 'USDA'	6 oz	120	10	0.0
(Welch's) white	8.45 oz	160	20	0.0
(Welch's) white	6 oz	120	15	0.0
Frozen, diluted as directed				
(Minute Maid)	6 oz	90	0	0.0
(Sunkist)	6 oz	69	3	0.1
(Welch's) 'No Sugar Added'	6 oz	40	5	0.0
(Welch's) 'Orchard'	10 oz	170	10	0.0
(Welch's) 'Orchard'	6 oz	110	20	0.0
(Welch's) 'Orchard Cocktails-In-A-Box'	8.45 oz	150	20	0.0
(Welch's) purple	6 oz	100	0	0.0
(Welch's) white	6 oz	100	0	0.0
GRAPE JUICE DRINK				
(Hi-C)	8.45 oz	136	24	0.1
(Hi-C)	6 oz	96	17	0.1
(Sunkist) frozen, diluted	6 oz	69	3	0.1
(Tang) 'Fruit Box'	8.45 oz	130	10	0.0
GRAPE PUNCH				
(Minute Maid) chilled	6 oz	90	20	0.0
(Minute Maid) frozen concentrate	6 oz	90	0	0.0
GRAPEFRUIT				
PINK AND RED				
Arizona/California				
fresh, 3.75-inch diam	1/2 fruit	46	1	0.1
sections w/juice	1 cup	85	2	0.2
trimmed	1 oz	11	<1	<.1
untrimmed	1 lb	86	1	0.2
Florida				
fresh (Ocean Spray)	1/2 med	50	0	0.0
fresh, 3.75-inch diam	1/2 fruit	37	0	0.1
sections w/juice	1 cup	69	0	0.2
trimmed	1 oz	9	tr	<.1

Food Name	Serv. Size	Total Cal.	Sod. MGS	Fat GMS
untrimmed	1 lb	69	1	0.2
WHITE				
California				
fresh, 3.75-inch diam	1/2 fruit	44	0	0.1
sections w/juice	1 cup	85	0	0.2
trimmed	1 oz	10	tr	<.1
untrimmed	1 lb	81	1	0.2
Florida				
fresh (Ocean Spray)	1/2 med	45	0	0.0
fresh, 3.75-inch diam	1/2 fruit	38	0	0.1
sections w/juice	1 cup	74	0	0.2
trimmed	1 oz	9	tr	<.1
GRAPEFRUIT, CANNED				
(Featherweight) in juice	1/2 cup	40	10	0.0
(Finast) in light syrup	1/2 cup	80	10	<.1
(Kraft) chilled 'Pure'	1/2 cup	50	0	0.0
(S&W) in light syrup	1/2 cup	80	0	0.0
(S&W) 'Unsweetened'	1/2 cup	40	10	0.0
(S&W Nutradiet)	1/2 cup	40	0	0.0
(Stokely) in light syrup	1/2 cup	90	5	1.0
GRAPEFRUIT JUICE				
Can, bottle, or box				
(Del Monte)	6 oz	70	10	0.0
(J. Hungerford) regular	9.03 oz	120	0	0.0
(J. Hungerford) 100% juice	9.03 oz	98	6	0.0
(J. Hungerford) 50% juice	9.03 oz	109	0	0.0
(Knudsen & Sons)	8 oz	70	na	0.0
(Knudsen & Sons) pink	8 oz	80	na	0.0
(Kraft) '100% pure'	6 oz	70	0	0.0
(Libby's)	6 oz	70	na	0.0
(Minute Maid)	6 oz	70	20	0.0
(Minute Maid) 'Juices to Go'	6 oz	70	20	0.0
(Mott's)	9.5 oz	118	5	0.0
(Mott's)	10 oz	124	5	0.0
(Ocean Spray)	6 oz	70	10	0.0
(Ocean Spray) 100%	6 oz	60	15	0.0
(Ocean Spray) pink 'Pink Premium'	6 oz	60	10	0.0
(Ocean Spray) 'Ruby Red'	6 oz	100	15	0.0
(S&W)	6 oz	80	10	0.0
(Snapple)	8 oz	110	45	0.0
(Stokely)	6 oz	76	5	1.0

Food Name	Serv. Size	Total Cal.	Sod. MGS	Fat GMS
(Sunkist) 'Fresh Squeezed'	8 oz	96	3	0.2
(Tree Top)	6 oz	80	0	0.0
(TreeSweet) pink	6 oz	72	15	0.0
(TreeSweet) regular	6 oz	72	15	0.0
(Tropicana) 100% pure	6 oz	70	20	<1.0
(Tropicana) 'Ruby Red' 100% pure	6 oz	70	20	<1.0
(Veryfine) '100%'	8 oz	101	10	0.0
Fresh				
juice from one 3.75-inch diam fruit	6 oz	76	2	0.2
pink	1 cup	96	2	0.3
white	1 cup	96	2	0.3
Frozen, diluted as directed				
(A&P)	6 oz	80	0	<1.0
(Minute Maid)	6 oz	80	0	0.0
(Minute Maid) pink	6 oz	80	0	0.0
(Sunkist)	6 oz	56	1	0.2
(TreeSweet)	6 oz	78	15	0.0
GRAPEFRUIT JUICE COCKTAIL				
(IGA)	6 oz	80	15	0.0
(Minute Maid) 'Juices To Go'	6 oz	80	20	0.0
(Ocean Spray)	6 oz	80	15	0.0
(Pathmark)	6 oz	80	15	0.0
(TreeSweet) 'Lite'	6 oz	40	15	0.0
(Tropicana) 'Twister'	8 oz	110	1	0.0
(Tropicana) 'Twister Light' w/NutraSweet	6 oz	30	20	<1.0
(Veryfine)	8 oz	120	15	0.0
GRAPEFRUIT JUICE DRINK				
(Citrus Hill) 'Plus Calcium'	6 oz	70	10	<1.0
(Tropicana) 'Juice Sparkler'	8 oz	110	50	0.0
(Wyler's) 'Fruit Slush'	4 oz	157	10	0.0
GRAPESEED OIL				
	1 cup	1927	0	218.0
	1 oz	251	0	28.4
	1 tbsp	120	0	13.6
GRAVY. See also SAUCE.				
AU JUS				
Canned or in jars				
(Franco-American)	2 oz	10	330	0.0
(Heinz) 'HomeStyle'	1/4 cup	18	350	1.0
Prepared from mix				
(French's)	1/4 cup	10	260	0.0

Food Name	Serv. Size	Total Cal.	Sod. MGS	Fat GMS
(Lawry's)	1 cup	84	3454	1.6
(McCormick/Schilling)	1/4 cup	20	786	0.3
BEEF				
Canned				
(Franco-American)	2 oz	25	340	1.0
(Hormel) w/chunky beef 'Great Beginnings'	5 oz	136	904	7.0
BROWN				
Canned or in jars				
(Heinz) 'HomeStyle'	1/4 cup	25	320	1.0
(Heinz) 'HomeStyle' w/onions	1/4 cup	25	330	1.0
(LaChoy)	1/2 tsp	15	15	<1.0
Prepared from mix				
(French's)	1/4 cup	20	250	1.0
(Lawry's)	1 cup	94	1500	1.4
(McCormick/Schilling)	1/3 cup	30	417	1.0
(McCormick/Schilling)	1/4 cup	23	313	0.8
(McCormick/Schilling) 'Lite'	1/4 cup	10	450	1.0
(Pillsbury)	1/4 cup	15	300	0.0
(Weight Watchers)	1/4 cup	10	360	0.0
(Weight Watchers) w/mushrooms	1/4 cup	10	270	0.0
(Weight Watchers) w/onions	1/4 cup	10	310	0.0
CHICKEN				
Canned or in jars				
(Franco-American)	2 oz	45	240	4.0
(Franco-American) giblet	2 oz	30	310	2.0
(Heinz) 'HomeStyle'	1/4 cup	35	350	2.0
(Heinz) 'Homestyle' w/mushrooms and onions	1/4 cup	35	330	2.0
(Hormel) 'Great Beginnings' w/chunky chicken	5 oz	147	567	8.0
(Weight Watchers)	1/4 cup	10	410	0.0
Prepared from mix				
(French's)	1/4 cup	25	270	1.0
(Lawry's)	1 cup	99	980	2.8
(McCormick/Schilling)	1/4 cup	22	300	0.4
(Pillsbury)	1/4 cup	25	230	1.0
COUNTRY				
(Heinz) 'Homestyle' jar	2 oz	25	210	1.0
CREAM (Franco-American) canned	2 oz	35	220	2.0
HERB (McCormick/Schilling) mix, prepared	1/4 cup	20	312	0.5
MUSHROOM				
Canned or in jars				
(Franco-American)	2 oz	25	290	1.0

Food Name	Serv. Size	Total Cal.	Sod. MGS	Fat GMS
(Heinz) 'HomeStyle'	1/4 cup	25	340	1.0
Prepared from mix				
(French's)	1/4 cup	20	250	1.0
(McCormick/Schilling)	1/4 cup	19	270	0.5
ONION				
(French's) mix, prepared	1/4 cup	25	270	1.0
(McCormick/Schilling) mix, prepared	1/4 cup	22	na	0.6
PORK				
Canned or in jars				
(Franco-American)	1/4 cup	40	330	3.0
(Heinz) 'HomeStyle'	1/4 cup	25	310	1.0
(Hormel) 'Great Beginnings' w/chunky pork	5 oz	140	567	8.0
Prepared from mix				
(French's)	1/4 cup	20	250	1.0
(McCormick/Schilling)	1/4 cup	20	297	0.6
TURKEY				
Canned or in jars				
(Franco-American)	2 oz	30	290	2.0
(Heinz) 'HomeStyle'	1/4 cup	25	370	1.0
(Hormel) 'Great Beginnings' w/chunky turkey	5 oz	138	585	8.0
Prepared from mix				
(Lawry's)	1 cup	102	1400	4.1
(McCormick/Schilling)	1/4 cup	22	353	0.5
GREAT NORTHERN BEAN				
boiled	4 oz	134	2	0.5
boiled, mature seeds	1/2 cup	104	2	0.4
raw	1/2 cup	308	13	1.0
raw	1 oz	96	4	0.3
Canned				
(A&P)	1 cup	210	0	1.0
(Allens)	1/2 cup	105	440	<1.0
(Allens) w/pork	1/2 cup	100	320	1.0
(Bush's Best)	1/2 cup	70	380	0.0
(Eden Foods) organically grown, w/liquid	1/2 cup	110	15	<1.0
(Green Giant)	1/2 cup	80	290	1.0
(Joan of Arc)	1/2 cup	80	290	1.0
(Luck's) w/pork	7.25 oz	220	645	5.0
GREEK SALAD, w/feta cheese and pitted Kalamata olives, refrigerated *(Trader Joe's)*	1 salad	310	530	28.0
GREEN BEAN/string bean				
boiled, drained	4 oz	40	3	0.3

Food Name	Serv. Size	Total Cal.	Sod. MGS	Fat GMS
boiled, drained	1/2 cup	22	2	0.2
raw, trimmed	1/2 cup	17	3	0.1
raw, trimmed	1 oz	9	2	<.1
raw, untrimmed	1 lb	123	23	0.5

GREEN BEAN, CANNED
Cut

Food Name	Serv. Size	Total Cal.	Sod. MGS	Fat GMS
(A&P)	1/2 cup	20	350	<1.0
(A&P) 'No Salt Added'	1/2 cup	20	10	<1.0
(Allens)	1/2 cup	20	350	<1.0
(Bush's Best)	1/2 cup	20	360	0.0
(Del Monte) w/liquid	1/2 cup	20	355	0.0
(Del Monte) w/liquid 'No Salt Added'	1/2 cup	20	10	0.0
(Bush's Best) 'Blue Lake'	1/2 cup	20	360	0.0
(Bush's Best) w/Shelly beans	1/2 cup	35	290	0.0
(Featherweight)	1/2 cup	25	10	0.0
(Finast)	1/2 cup	20	400	0.0
(Finast) 'No Salt Added'	1/2 cup	20	10	0.0
(Finast) 'Veri-Green'	1/2 cup	20	320	0.0
(Freshlike)	1/2 cup	20	340	0.0
(Freshlike) no salt added	1/2 cup	20	5	0.0
(Freshlike) no sugar or salt, in water	1/2 cup	20	5	0.0
(Freshlike) wax, water packed, w/o salt	1/2 cup	18	5	0.0
(Freshlike) wax, water packed, w/o sugar or salt	1/2 cup	18	5	0.0
(Green Giant)	1/2 cup	16	300	0.0
(Green Giant) 50% less salt	1/2 cup	16	195	0.0
(Green Giant) kitchen sliced	1/2 cup	16	390	0.0
(Green Giant) 'Pantry Express'	1/2 cup	12	20	0.0
(IGA)	1/2 cup	20	10	0.0
(Pathmark)	1/2 cup	20	430	0.0
(Pathmark) 'Blue Lake'	1/2 cup	20	430	0.0
(Pathmark) 'No Frills'	1 cup	35	640	0.0
(Pathmark) 'No Salt Added'	1/2 cup	20	10	0.0
(Quincy's)	4.3 oz	40	500	1.0
(S&W) 'Premium Blue Lake'	1/2 cup	20	385	0.0
(S&W) 'Premium Gold'	1/2 cup	20	385	0.0
(S&W) stringless, w/liquid	1/2 cup	20	3850	0.0
(S&W Nutradiet)	1/2 cup	20	5	0.0
(Stokely)	1/2 cup	20	360	0.0
(Stokely) 'No Salt or Sugar'	1/2 cup	20	5	0.0
(Veg•All)	1/2 cup	20	340	0.0

Food Name	Serv. Size	Total Cal.	Sod. MGS	Fat GMS
French style				
(A&P)	1/2 cup	20	350	<1.0
(A&P) 'No Salt Added'	1/2 cup	20	10	<1.0
(Allens)	1/2 cup	20	350	<1.0
(Bush's Best)	1/2 cup	20	360	0.0
(Del Monte) seasoned, w/liquid	1/2 cup	20	355	0.0
(Finast)	1/2 cup	20	400	0.0
(Freshlike)	1/2 cup	20	340	0.0
(Freshlike) in water, w/o salt	1/2 cup	20	5	0.0
(Green Giant)	1/2 cup	16	390	0.0
(Pathmark) 'Blue Lake'	1/2 cup	20	430	0.0
(Pathmark) 'No Frills'	1 cup	35	640	0.0
(Pathmark) 'No Salt Added'	1/2 cup	20	10	0.0
(S&W) 'Premium Blue Lake'	1/2 cup	20	385	0.0
(S&W) stringless, w/liquid	1/2 cup	20	3850	0.0
(Veg•All)	1/2 cup	20	340	0.0
Italian				
(Allens)	1/2 cup	18	260	<1.0
(Del Monte) cut	1/2 cup	25	355	0.0
Whole				
(A&P)	1/2 cup	20	350	<1.0
(Allens) Shelly beans	1/2 cup	35	395	<1.0
(Bush's Best)	1/2 cup	20	360	0.0
(Del Monte) w/liquid	1/2 cup	20	355	0.0
(Finast)	1/2 cup	25	400	0.0
(Freshlike)	1/2 cup	20	340	0.0
(Green Giant) amandine	1/2 cup	45	300	3.0
(IGA)	1 cup	45	640	0.0
(Pathmark)	1/2 cup	20	430	0.0
(S&W) dilled	1/2 cup	60	3850	0.0
(S&W) stringless, w/liquid	1/2 cup	20	3850	0.0
(S&W) 'Vertical Pak'	1/2 cup	20	385	0.0

GREEN BEAN, FREEZE-DRIED

| (Mountain House) diluted as directed | 1/2 cup | 35 | tr | 0.0 |

GREEN BEAN, FROZEN

Cut				
(A&P)	3 oz	25	140	<1.0
(Birds Eye)	3 oz	25	0	0.0
(Birds Eye) 'Portion Pack'	3 oz	25	0	0.0
(Finast)	3 oz	25	5	0.0
(Freshlike)	3 oz	25	5	0.0

Food Name	Serv. Size	Total Cal.	Sod. MGS	Fat GMS
(Frosty Acres)	3 oz	25	3	0.0
(Green Giant) 'Harvest Fresh'	1/2 cup	16	95	0.0
(Green Giant) in butter sauce	1/2 cup	30	230	1.0
(Seabrook)	3 oz	25	3	0.0
(Stokely) 'Singles'	3 oz	30	5	1.0
French style				
(A&P)	3 oz	25	0	<1.0
(Birds Eye)	3 oz	25	0	0.0
(Bird's Eye) w/almonds 'Combination Vegetables'	3 oz	50	340	2.0
(Finast)	3 oz	25	5	0.0
(Freshlike)	3 oz	25	5	0.0
(Frosty Acres)	3 oz	25	3	0.0
(Seabrook)	3 oz	25	3	0.0
(Southern)	3.5 oz	34	20	0.1
(Veg•All)	3 oz	25	5	0.0
Italian				
(Birds Eye)	3 oz	30	0	0.0
(Finast) cut	3 oz	30	5	0.0
(Freshlike)	3 oz	30	5	0.0
(Frosty Acres)	3 oz	30	3	0.0
(Seabrook)	3 oz	30	3	0.0
(Veg•All)	3 oz	30	5	0.0
Whole				
(Bird's Eye) Bavarian style, w/spaetzle	3.3 oz	100	350	5.0
(Birds Eye) 'Deluxe'	3 oz	25	0	0.0
(Bird's Eye) 'Farm Fresh Whole Vegetables'	4 oz	30	0	0.0
(Bird's Eye) petite 'Deluxe'	2.6 oz	20	0	0.0
(Freshlike)	3 oz	25	5	0.0
(Green Giant)	1/2 cup	14	10	0.0
(Green Giant) and creamy mushroom 'Garden Gourmet'	1 pkg	220	860	11.0
(Green Giant) in butter sauce 'One Serving'	5.5 oz	60	370	2.0
(Green Giant) 'Plain Polybag'	1/2 cup	14	10	0.0
(Seabrook)	3 oz	25	1	0.0
(Southern)	3.5 oz	33	20	0.1
(Stouffer's) mushroom casserole	4.75 oz	160	680	11.0
(Veg•All)	3 oz	25	5	0.0

GREEN ONION. See ONION, GREEN.

GRENADINE. See ALCOHOLIC BEVERAGES.

GRITS

Dry

white (Arrowhead Mills)	2 oz	200	1	1.0

Food Name	Serv. Size	Total Cal.	Sod. MGS	Fat GMS
white, enriched	1 cup	579	2	1.9
white, enriched	1 tbsp	36	0	0.1
white, enriched 'Regular/Quick' (Aunt Jemima)	3 tbsp	101	1	0.2
white, unenriched	1 cup	579	2	1.9
white, unenriched	1 tbsp	36	0	0.1
yellow (Arrowhead Mills)	2 oz	200	1	1.0
yelllow, enriched	1 cup	579	2	1.9
yellow, enriched	1 tbsp	36	0	0.1
yellow, enriched (Quick)	3 tbsp	101	1	0.2
yellow, unenriched	1 cup	579	2	1.9
yellow, unenriched	1 tbsp	36	0	0.1
Prepared				
white, enriched, cooked w/water	1 cup	145	0	0.5
white, unenriched, cooked w/water	1 cup	145	0	0.5
yellow, enriched, cooked w/water	1 cup	145	0	0.5
yellow, unenriched, cooked w/water	1 cup	145	0	0.5
GRITS, CANNED				
golden (Allens)	1/2 cup	80	370	<1.0
golden (Bush's Best)	1/2 cup	45	390	0.0
golden (Van Camp's)	1 cup	128	701	0.6
golden, w/red and green peppers (Van Camp's)	1 cup	129	685	0.5
Mexican (Allens)	1/2 cup	80	330	<1.0
white	1 cup	115	336	1.4
white	4 oz	82	238	1.0
white (Allens)	1/2 cup	70	430	<1.0
white (Bush's Best)	1/2 cup	45	450	0.0
white (Van Camp's)	1 cup	138	708	0.7
yellow	1 cup	115	336	1.4
yellow	4 oz	82	238	1.0
GRITS, INSTANT				
white, hominy product, dry, one packet (Quaker)	.8 oz	79	440	0.1
w/imitation bacon bits, dry, one packet (Quaker)	1 oz	101	590	0.4
w/imitation ham bits, dry, one packet (Quaker)	1 oz	99	800	0.3
w/real cheddar cheese flavor, dry, one packet (Quaker)	1 oz	104	497	1.0
GRITS, QUICK-COOKING				
Dry				
white, enriched	1 cup	579	2	1.9
white, enriched	1 tbsp	36	0	0.1
white, unenriched	1 cup	579	2	1.9
white, unenriched	1 tbsp	36	0	0.1
yellow, enriched	1 cup	579	2	1.9

Food Name	Serv. Size	Total Cal.	Sod. MGS	Fat GMS
yellow, enriched	1 tbsp	36	0	0.1
yellow, enriched 'Quick' *(Quaker)*	3 tbsp	101	1	0.2
yellow, unenriched	1 cup	579	2	1.9
yellow, unenriched	1 tbsp	36	0	0.1
Prepared				
white, enriched, cooked w/water	1 cup	145	0	0.5
white, unenriched, cooked w/water	1 cup	145	0	0.5
yellow, enriched, cooked w/water	1 cup	145	0	0.5
yellow, unenriched, cooked w/water	1 cup	145	0	0.5
GROUND CHERRY. See CAPE GOOSEBERRY.				
GROUND HUSK TOMATO. See TOMATILLO.				
GROUPER, MIXED SPECIES				
broiled	4 oz	134	60	1.5
dry-heat cooked	4 oz	134	60	1.5
dry-heat cooked	3 oz	100	45	1.1
microwaved	4 oz	134	60	1.5
raw	1 lb	417	239	4.6
raw	3 oz	78	45	0.9
raw	1 oz	26	15	0.3
GUACAMOLE. See DIP, AVOCADO.				
GUACAMOLE SEASONING				
(Lawry's) 'Seasoning Blend' dry mix	1 pkg	60	1495	0.4
(Old El Paso) dry mix	1/7 pkg	7	240	0.0
GUANABANA NECTAR *(Libby's)*	6 oz	110	15	0.0
GUANABANA PUNCH, 'Rain Forest' *(Knudsen & Sons)*	8 oz	125	na	0.0
GUAVA				
trimmed	1 cup	84	5	1.0
trimmed	1 fruit	46	3	0.5
trimmed	1 oz	15	1	0.2
untrimmed	1 lb	183	9	2.2
w/edible seeds *(Sunfresh)*	3.5 oz	70	15	0.0
GUAVA, STRAWBERRY				
trimmed	1 cup	168	90	1.5
trimmed	1 oz	20	11	0.2
trimmed	1 fruit	4	2	0.0
untrimmed	1 lb	268	141	2.3
GUAVA CRANBERRY JUICE				
organic 'Cruz' *(Santa Cruz Natural)*	8 oz	130	na	<1.0
GUAVA FRUIT DRINK				
Hawaiian 'Mauna La'i' *(Ocean Spray)*	6 oz	100	15	0.0

Food Name	Serv. Size	Total Cal.	Sod. MGS	Fat GMS
GUAVA JUICE				
'Orchard Tropicals' bottled, diluted *(Welch's)*	6 oz	100	20	0.0
'Orchard Tropicals' frozen, diluted *(Welch's)*	6 oz	100	20	0.0
GUAVA NECTAR				
(Kern's)	6 oz	110	0	0.0
(Libby's)	6 oz	110	15	0.0
GUAVA PASSION DRINK				
Hawaiian 'Hawaii' *(Pathmark)*	6 oz	100	10	0.0
Hawaiian 'Mauna La'i' *(Ocean Spray)*	6 oz	100	10	0.0
GUAVA STRAWBERRY DRINK 'Refresher' *(Veryfine)*	8 oz	120	25	0.0
GUINEA HEN				
giblets, raw	100 gm	157	70	7.0
meat and skin, raw	1 lb	567	241	23.2
meat only, raw	1 oz	31	(mq)	0.7
GUMBO. See OKRA.				
GUMBO FILE POWDER *(Tone's)*	1 tsp	8	<1	0.2

H

Food Name	Serv. Size	Total Cal.	Sod. MGS	Fat GMS
HADDOCK				
baked	4 oz	127	99	1.1
broiled	4 oz	127	99	1.1
dry-heat cooked	3 oz	95	74	0.8
microwaved	4 oz	127	99	1.1
raw	1 lb	396	310	3.3
raw	3 oz	74	58	0.6
smoked	3 oz	99	649	0.8
HADDOCK FILLET, FROZEN				
(SeaPak)	4 oz	90	120	1.0
battered *(Van de Kamp's)*	2 pieces	250	580	15.0
battered, 'Crunchy' *(Mrs. Paul's)*	2 pieces	190	580	5.0
breaded *(Van de Kamp's)*	2 pieces	270	290	16.0
breaded, in lemon butter, 'Microwave' *(Gorton's)*	1 pkg	360	730	21.0
breaded, 'Light' *(Mrs. Paul's)*	1 piece	220	350	9.0
breaded, 'Light' *(Van de Kamp's)*	1 piece	240	380	11.0
'Fishmarket Fresh' *(Gorton's)*	5 oz	110	120	1.0
natural *(Van de Kamp's)*	4 oz	90	125	1.0

od Name	Serv. Size	Total Cal.	Sod. MGS	Fat GMS

ALIBUT

TLANTIC

	Serv. Size	Total Cal.	Sod. MGS	Fat GMS
broiled	4 oz	159	78	3.3
dry-heat cooked	4 oz	159	78	3.3
dry-heat cooked	3 oz	119	59	2.5
microwaved	4 oz	159	78	3.3
raw	1 lb	497	245	10.4
raw	3 oz	94	46	2.0
raw	1 oz	31	15	0.6

REENLAND

	Serv. Size	Total Cal.	Sod. MGS	Fat GMS
dry-heat cooked	3 oz	203	88	15.1
raw	1 lb	845	363	62.8
raw	3 oz	158	68	11.8
raw	1 oz	53	23	3.9

ACIFIC

	Serv. Size	Total Cal.	Sod. MGS	Fat GMS
broiled	4 oz	159	78	3.3
dry-heat cooked	4 oz	159	78	3.3
dry-heat cooked	3 oz	119	59	2.5
microwaved	4 oz	159	78	3.3
raw	1 lb	497	245	10.4
raw	3 oz	94	46	2.0
raw	1 oz	31	15	0.6
raw, fillet portions, skinless (Peter Pan Seafoods)	3.5 oz	110	54	2.3

ALIBUT, FROZEN

	Serv. Size	Total Cal.	Sod. MGS	Fat GMS
fillet, battered (Van de Kamp's)	2 pieces	150	400	6.0
steaks, w/o seasoning mix (SeaPak)	6-oz pkg	160	120	1.0

AM. See HAM, ALTERNATIVE; HAM, CANNED; HAM, CURED; HAM, FRESH; HAM, MINCED; HAM PATTY.

AM, ALTERNATIVE

	Serv. Size	Total Cal.	Sod. MGS	Fat GMS
(Worthington) frozen, roll 'Wham' approx .9-oz slices	3 slices	120	940	7.0

AM, CANNED

	Serv. Size	Total Cal.	Sod. MGS	Fat GMS
chopped	1 oz	68	387	5.3
chopped	.75-oz slice	50	287	4.0
cured, extra lean, approx 4% fat, baked	3 oz	116	965	4.2
cured, extra lean, approx 4% fat, unheated	1 oz	34	356	1.3
cured, extra lean and regular, baked	3 oz	142	908	7.2
cured, extra lean and regular, unheated	1 oz	41	362	2.1
cured, regular, approx 13% fat, baked	3 oz	192	800	12.9
cured, regular, approx 13% fat, unheated	1 oz	54	352	3.7
Armour) chopped	3 oz	190	1260	14.0

Food Name	Serv. Size	Total Cal.	Sod. MGS	F G
(Black Label)				
'5-lb can'	4 oz	140	1245	7
'3-lb can'	4 oz	140	1315	7
'1 1/2-lb can'	4 oz	150	1324	7
(Chi-Chi's) 'Black Label'	1 oz	37	303	1
(EXL) 'Deli Ham' 10-lb can	4 oz	130	1368	6
(Holiday Glaze) '3-lb can'	4 oz	130	(mq)	4
(Hormel)				
'Bone-In'	4 oz	210	(mq)	15
chopped, '8-lb can'	3 oz	240	1062	21
chopped, '12-oz can'	2 oz	120	703	9
chunk	6.75 oz	310	2241	20
chunk	2.5 oz	110	780	7
'Cure/81'	4 oz	160	1322	8
'Cure/81'	1 oz	31	291	2
'Curemaster'	4 oz	140	1361	5
'Curemaster'	2 oz	60	627	2
'Light and Lean 97'	2 oz	60	450	2
roll	4 oz	170	1338	10
spiced	3 oz	240	1093	21
(JM) '95% Fat-free'	2 oz	60	680	2
(Light & Lean) 'Boneless'	2 oz	60	574	2
(Oscar Mayer) 'Jubilee'	1 oz	29	287	0
(Rath) hickory smoked, 'Black Hawk'	2 oz	60	720	2
HAM, CURED				
(NOTE: TRIMMED = Lean; separable fat removed. UNTRIMMED = Separable fat not remov				
BONELESS				
center slice, country-style, trimmed, unheated	1 oz	55	764	2
center slice, untrimmed, unheated	1 oz	58	393	3
extra lean, approx 5% fat, baked	3 oz	123	1023	4
extra lean, approx 5% fat, unheated	1 oz	37	405	1
extra lean and regular, baked	3 oz	140	1177	6
extra lean and regular, unheated	1 oz	46	362	2
extra lean and regular, unheated, 4 x 6 1/4 inch slice	1 slice	46	362	2
mini *(JM)*	3 oz	90	40	3
regular, approx 11% fat, baked	3 oz	151	1275	7
regular, approx 11% fat, unheated	1 oz	52	373	3
steak, 'Jubilee' *(Oscar Mayer)*	2 oz	57	754	1
steak, unheated	2 oz	69	720	2
w/natural juices, 'EZ Cut' *(JM)*	2 oz	70	660	3

Food Name	Serv. Size	Total Cal.	Sod. MGS	Fat GMS
WHOLE				
trimmed, fully cooked, baked	3 oz	133	1128	4.7
trimmed, fully cooked, unheated	1 oz	42	430	1.6
trimmed *(JM)*	3 oz	140	40	8.0
untrimmed, fully cooked, baked	3 oz	207	1009	14.2
untrimmed, fully cooked, unheated	1 oz	70	364	5.3

HAM, FRESH. See also PORK.

(NOTE: TRIMMED = Lean; separable fat removed. UNTRIMMED = Separable fat not removed.)

Food Name	Serv. Size	Total Cal.	Sod. MGS	Fat GMS
LEG, RUMP HALF				
Trimmed				
raw	1 lb	621	313	23.5
raw	1 oz	39	20	1.5
roasted	3 oz	175	55	6.9
roasted, diced	1 cup	278	88	11.0
Untrimmed				
raw	1 lb	1007	277	71.2
raw	1 oz	63	17	4.4
roasted	3 oz	214	53	12.1
roasted	1.5 oz	117	26	7.6
roasted, diced	1 cup	340	84	19.3
LEG, SHANK HALF				
Trimmed				
raw	1 lb	631	304	25.5
raw	1 oz	39	19	1.6
roasted	3 oz	183	54	8.9
roasted, diced	1 cup	290	86	14.2
Untrimmed				
raw	1 lb	1193	249	95.4
raw	1 oz	75	16	6.0
roasted	3 oz	246	50	17.0
roasted	1.5 oz	129	25	9.4
roasted, diced	1 cup	390	80	27.1
LEG, WHOLE				
Trimmed				
raw	1 lb	617	249	24.5
raw	1 oz	39	16	1.5
roasted	3 oz	179	54	8.0
roasted	1.5 oz	94	27	4.7
roasted	1 cup	285	86	12.7
Untrimmed				
raw	1 lb	1111	213	85.6

Food Name	Serv. Size	Total Cal.	Sod. MGS	Fo GM
raw	1 oz	69	13	5.
roasted	3 oz	232	51	15.
roasted	1.5 oz	125	25	8.
roasted, diced	1 cup	369	81	23.
HAM, MINCED	1 oz	75	353	5.
HAM ENTRÉE, FROZEN				
and asparagus bake (Stouffer's)	9.5 oz	520	1100	35.
and cheese casserole, 'Microwave Classic' (Pillsbury)	1 pkg	470	1300	29.
dinner (Morton)	10 oz	290	1400	4.
'Platters' (Banquet)	10 oz	400	1180	17.
steak (Le Menu)	10 oz	300	1500	11.
steak 'Classics' (Armour)	10.75 oz	270	1320	7.
w/scalloped potatoes 'Homestyle Recipe' (Swanson)	9 oz	300	1080	13.
HAM LUNCHEON MEAT. See LUNCHEON MEAT.				
HAM PATTY				
canned (Hormel)	1 patty	180	456	16.
canned, w/cheese (Hormel)	1 patty	190	468	18.
cured, boneless steak, extra lean, unheated	2-oz slice	69	720	2.
cured, unheated	1 oz	89	308	8.
grilled	4 oz	388	1205	35.
'Premium Brown 'N Serve' (Swift)	1 patty	130	260	13.
HAM SPREAD				
deviled	1 cup	790	2776	72.
deviled	4.5-oz can	449	1580	41.
deviled (Hormel)	1 oz	76	214	6.
deviled (Hormel)	1 tbsp	35	108	3.
deviled (Underwood)	2 1/8 oz	220	430	19.
deviled (Underwood) 'Light'	2 1/8 oz	120	250	8.
deviled (Underwood) 'Smoked'	2 1/8 oz	190	260	18.
ham and cheese	1 oz	69	339	5.
ham and cheese	1 tbsp	37	179	2.
ham salad	1 oz	61	259	4.
ham salad	1 tbsp	32	137	2.
ham salad 'Spreadables' (Libby's)	1.9 oz	70	380	3.
HAM TACO, refrigerated, 'Border Breakfasts' (Owens)	2.17 oz	90	430	6.
HAMBURG PARSLEY. See PARSLEY ROOT.				
HAMBURGER. See BEEF, GROUND.				
HAMBURGER BUN. See BUN, HAMBURGER.				
HAMBURGER ENTRÉE MIX				
(Betty Crocker) 'Hamburger Helper'				
beef noodle, dry	1/5 pkg	140	1000	2.

d Name	Serv. Size	Total Cal.	Sod. MGS	Fat GMS
beef noodle, prepared	1 cup	320	1050	15.0
beef Romanoff, dry	1/5 pkg	180	1030	3.0
beef Romanoff, prepared	1 cup	350	1070	16.0
beef taco, dry	1/5 pkg	160	930	1.0
beef taco, prepared	1 cup	330	970	14.0
beef teriyaki, dry	1/5 pkg	180	1110	1.0
beef teriyaki, prepared	1 cup	360	1160	14.0
cheddar and bacon, dry	1/5 pkg	190	950	6.0
cheddar and bacon, prepared	1 cup	400	1020	20.0
cheeseburger macaroni, dry	1/5 pkg	190	980	6.0
cheeseburger macaroni, prepared	1 cup	370	1030	19.0
cheesy Italian, dry	1/5 pkg	160	970	3.0
cheesy Italian, prepared w/2% milk	1 cup	360	1040	17.0
chili macaroni, dry	1/5 pkg	150	920	1.0
chili macaroni, prepared	1 cup	330	960	14.0
chili tomato, dry	1/5 pkg	150	1360	1.0
chili tomato, prepared	1 cup	330	1410	14.0
chili w/beans, dry	1/4 pkg	130	1680	1.0
chili w/beans, prepared	1 1/4 cup	350	1740	17.0
creamy Stroganoff, dry	1/5 pkg	190	800	5.0
creamy Stroganoff, prepared w/whole milk	1 cup	390	870	20.0
hamburger hash, dry	1/5 pkg	140	970	2.0
hamburger hash, prepared	1 cup	320	1020	15.0
hamburger stew, dry	1/5 pkg	120	960	1.0
hamburger stew, prepared	1 cup	300	1010	14.0
lasagna, dry	1/5 pkg	160	1000	1.0
lasagna, prepared	1 cup	340	1050	14.0
meat loaf, dry	1/5 pkg	70	620	1.0
meat loaf, prepared	1 cup	360	710	22.0
mushroom and wild rice, dry	1/5 pkg	180	880	3.0
mushroom and wild rice, prepared	1 cup	380	950	16.0
nacho cheese, dry	1/5 pkg	160	980	2.0
nacho cheese, prepared	1 cup	360	1050	15.0
pizza dish, dry	1/5 pkg	180	960	1.0
pizza dish, prepared	1 cup	360	1010	14.0
'Pizzabake' dry	1/6 pkg	150	800	2.0
'Pizzabake' prepared	4.5 oz	320	840	14.0
potato au gratin, dry	1/5 pkg	150	860	2.0
potato au gratin, prepared	1 cup	320	910	15.0
potato Stroganoff, dry	1/5 pkg	140	900	2.0
potato Stroganoff, prepared	1 cup	320	950	15.0

Food Name	Serv. Size	Total Cal.	Sod. MGS	
rice Oriental, dry	1/5 pkg	180	1070	
rice Oriental, prepared	1 cup	340	1120	1
'Sloppy Joe Bake' dry	1/6 pkg	180	1060	
'Sloppy Joe Bake' prepared	5 oz	340	1100	1
spaghetti, dry	1/5 pkg	170	1060	
spaghetti, prepared	1 cup	340	1110	1
'Tacobake' dry	1/6 pkg	170	920	
'Tacobake' prepared	5.75 oz	320	940	1
tamale pie, dry	1/5 pkg	200	890	
tamale pie, prepared	1 cup	380	940	1
three cheese, dry	1/5 pkg	210	910	
three cheese, prepared	1/5 pkg	400	980	2
zesty Italian, dry	1/5 pkg	170	940	
zesty Italian, prepared	1 cup	340	980	1

HAWAIIAN YAM. See YAM, MOUNTAIN.

HAWS/hawthorn tree fruit

scarlet, flesh and skin, raw	100 gm	87	0	

HAZELNUT, SHELLED/cobnut/filbert

blanched	1 oz	191	1	1
dry-roasted, unblanched	1 oz	188	1	1
dry-roasted, unblanched, w/salt	1 oz	188	221	1
oil-roasted, unblanched	1 oz	187	1	1
oil-roasted, unblanched, w/salt	1 oz	187	223	1
unblanched	1 oz	179	1	1
unblanched, chopped	1 cup	727	3	7

HAZELNUT BUTTER, gourmet (Roaster Fresh) | 1 oz | 188 | 1 | 1

HAZELNUT OIL

	1 cup	1927	0	21
	1 oz	251	0	2
	1 tbsp	120	0	1

HAZELNUT SPREAD, Nutella, with milk and cocoa (Ferrero) | 1 tbsp | 80 | 10 |

HERB AND GARLIC MARINADE, w/lemon (Lawry's) | 2 tbsp | 36 | 3688 | <

HERB SEASONING MIX

Italian, 'Bag 'n Season' (Schilling)	1 pkg	94	1367	
mixed, 'Pinch of Herbs' (Lawry's)	1 tsp	9	259	

HERRING

ATLANTIC

broiled	4 oz	230	130	1
dry-heat cooked	4 oz	230	130	1
dry-heat cooked	3 oz	173	98	
kippered	4 oz	246	1041	1

od Name	Serv. Size	Total Cal.	Sod. MGS	Fat GMS
kippered snacks, w/smoke flavoring, drained *(Beach Cliff)*	3.3 oz	220	350	17.0
microwaved	4 oz	230	130	13.1
pickled	4 oz	297	987	20.4
raw	1 lb	718	407	41.0
raw	3 oz	134	77	7.7
raw	1 oz	.45	26	2.6
steaks, in soybean oil, drained *(Beach Cliff)*	3 oz	240	350	20.0
steaks, in water, drained *(Beach Cliff)*	3 oz	230	350	18.0
steaks, w/mustard, drained *(Beach Cliff)*	3 oz	227	350	18.0
steaks, w/tomato, drained *(Beach Cliff)*	3 oz	210	350	17.0
AKE				
raw	1 lb	446	249	8.7
raw	2.8-oz fillet	78	47	1.5
raw	1 oz	28	16	0.5
smoked	4 oz	201	545	13.5
ACIFIC				
dry-heat cooked	3 oz	213	81	15.1
raw	1 lb	885	335	63.0
raw	3 oz	166	63	11.8
raw	1 oz	55	21	3.9
BISCUS COOLER *(Knudsen & Sons)*	8 oz	95	na	0.0
BISCUS CRANBERRY JUICE *(Knudsen & Sons)*	8 oz	110	na	0.0
CKORY NUT				
in shell	1 lb	954	1	93.4
shelled	1 oz	187	0	18.3
OMINY GRITS. See GRITS.				
ONEY				
extracted	1 cup	1031	17	0.0
extracted	1 tbsp	64	1	0.0
strained	1 cup	1031	17	0.0
strained	1 tbsp	64	1	0.0
(Golden Blossom)	1 tbsp	60	na	0.0
(Knott's Berry Farm)	1 oz	90	0	0.0
(Knott's Berry Farm)	1 tbsp	60	0	0.0
(Knott's Berry Farm)	.5 oz	30	0	0.0
(Sioux)	1 tbsp	60	na	0.0
ONEY BUTTER	1 tbsp	50	5	1.0
ONEY ROLL SAUSAGE				
	1 oz	52	375	3.0
4-inch diam	1/8-inch slice	42	304	2.4

Food Name	Serv. Size	Total Cal.	Sod. MGS	
HONEYDEW MELON				
pulp	1 oz	10	3	<
raw, cubed	1 cup	59	17	0
raw, wedge	7 x 2 inches	45	13	0
untrimmed	1 lb	74	21	0
untrimmed *(Dole)*	7 x 2 inches	50	50	0
HORSE BEAN. See FAVA BEAN.				
HORSERADISH				
Prepared				
	1 tbsp	6	14	0
	1 tsp	2	5	0
(Crowley)	1 oz	10	25	<1
(Kraft)	1 tbsp	10	140	●
(Kraft) cream style	1 tbsp	12	85	0
(Gold's) hot	1 tsp	4	60	<1
(Gold's) red	1 tsp	4	75	●
(Gold's) white	1 tsp	4	55	<1
(Silver Spring) cream style	1 tsp	0	10	●
Raw	1 lb	288	27	1
HORSERADISH, JAPANESE. See WASABI.				
HORSERADISH TREE				
Leafy tips				
boiled, drained	4 oz	68	10	<
boiled, drained, chopped	1 cup	25	4	●
raw, chopped	1 cup	13	2	●
raw, trimmed	1 oz	18	3	●
raw, untrimmed	1 lb	181	26	2
Pods				
boiled, drained	4 oz	41	49	●
boiled, drained, sliced	1 cup	42	51	●
boiled, drained, sliced	1/2 cup	21	25	●
raw, sliced	1 cup	37	42	●
raw, trimmed	1 oz	10	12	●
raw, untrimmed	1 lb	88	99	●
raw, whole, approx 15 1/3 inches long	1 pod	4	5	●
HOT CHOCOLATE. See COCOA MIX.				
HOT DOG. See FRANKFURTER.				
HUBBARD SQUASH. See SQUASH, HUBBARD.				
HUMMUS				
mix, dry *(Casbah)*	1 oz	110	na	5
prepared	1/2 cup	210	300	1●

Food Name	Serv. Size	Total Cal.	Sod. MGS	Fat GMS
prepared	1 oz	48	69	2.4
HUSHPUPPY, FROZEN, 'Regular' (SeaPak)	4 oz	330	690	9.0
HUSHPUPPY MIX				
deluxe, dry (Golden Dipt)	1.25 oz	120	520	0.0
jalapeño, dry (Golden Dipt)	1.25 oz	120	570	0.0
w/onion, dry (Golden Dipt)	1.25 oz	120	520	0.0
HYACINTH BEAN				
boiled, drained	4 oz	57	2	0.3
immature, boiled, drained	1/2 cup	22	1	0.1
immature, raw	1/2 cup	18	1	0.1
mature, boiled	1/2 cup	113	7	0.6
mature, raw	1/2 cup	361	22	1.8
raw, trimmed	1 oz	13	<1	0.1
raw, untrimmed	1 lb	196	8	0.8
HYACINTH BEAN, DRIED				
mature, boiled	1/2 cup	114	7	0.6
mature, boiled	4 oz	133	8	0.7
mature, raw	1/2 cup	362	22	1.8
mature, raw	1 oz	98	6	0.5

I

Food Name	Serv. Size	Total Cal.	Sod. MGS	Fat GMS
ICE BARS AND DESSERTS. See also FRUIT BAR, FROZEN; SHERBET; SORBET.				
BAR				
'All Natural' all flavors (Popsicle)	1 bar	60	0	0.0
'Ice Stripes' 1.5 oz, all flavors (Good Humor)	1 bar	35	0	0.0
'Twin Pop' all flavors (Gold Bond)	1 bar	60	0	0.0
'Water Ice' all flavors except cherry and wildberry (Popsicle)	1 bar	50	10	0.0
Cherry				
'Calippo' 4.5 oz (Good Humor)	1 bar	138	5	0.1
'Jumbo Jet Star' 4.5 oz (Good Humor)	1 bar	85	0	0.7
'Water Ice' (Popsicle)	1 bar	70	15	0.0
Fruit				
and juice, 3 oz	1 bar	75	4	0.1
and water, aspartame-sweetened	1 bar	12	3	0.1
Lemon				
'Calippo' 4.5 oz (Good Humor)	1 bar	112	0	0.1
'Great White Shark' 3 oz (Good Humor)	1 bar	68	7	0.1

Food Name	Serv. Size	Total Cal.	Sod. MGS	Fat GMS
Orange				
'Calippo' 4.5 oz *(Good Humor)* .... 1 bar		111	0	0.2
Wildberry, 'Water Ice' *(Popsicle)* .... 1 bar		40	10	0.0
DESSERT				
cherry, Italian *(Good Humor)* .... 6 oz		138	0	0.1
daiquiri *(Baskin-Robbins)* .... 1 scoop		140	15	0.0
lime .... 4 oz		75	21	0.0
pineapple-coconut .... 4 oz		108	34	2.5
ICE CREAM. See also ICE CREAM, ALTERNATIVE; ICE CREAM BAR; ICE CREAM BAR, ALTERNATIVE; ICE CREAM CAKE; ICE CREAM CONE; ICE CREAM MIX; ICE CREAM SNACKS AND SANDWICHES; ICE MILK; ICE MILK BAR.				
ALMOND FUDGE *(Baskin-Robbins)* 'Jamoca' .... 1 scoop		270	115	14.0
BANANA				
(Baskin-Robbins) sugar-free 'Chunky Banana' .... 4 oz		100	50	1.0
(Ben & Jerry's) 'Chunky Monkey' .... 1/2 cup		280	50	19.0
BORDEAUX CHERRY *(Healthy Choice)* 'Dairy Dessert' .... 4 oz		120	50	2.0
BORDEAUX CHERRY CHOCOLATE CHIP				
(Healthy Choice) 'Dairy Dessert' .... 4 oz		120	50	2.0
BOYSENBERRY *(Good Humor)* 'King Cone' .... 5 oz		340	151	13.1
BROWNIES 'N CREME *(Weight Watchers)* 'ONE-ders' .... 4 oz		130	115	4.0
BUTTER ALMOND *(Breyers)* .... 4 oz		170	125	10.0
BUTTER CRUNCH *(Sealtest)* .... 4 oz		150	90	7.0
BUTTER PECAN				
(Ben & Jerry's) .... 1/2 cup		310	160	26.0
(Breyers) .... 4 oz		180	125	12.0
(Frusen Glädjé) .... 4 oz		280	160	21.0
(Häagen-Dazs) .... 4 oz		390	100	24.0
(Lady Borden) .... 4 oz		180	65	12.0
(Sealtest) .... 4 oz		160	125	9.0
BUTTER PECAN CRUNCH *(Healthy Choice)* 'Dairy Dessert' .... 4 oz		140	80	2.0
CHERRY				
(Ben & Jerry's) 'Cherry Garcia' .... 1/2 cup		240	60	16.0
(Breyers) vanilla .... 4 oz		150	45	7.0
CHOCOLATE				
(Baskin-Robbins) .... 1 scoop		270	160	14.0
(Baskin-Robbins) 'World Class' .... 1 scoop		280	145	14.0
(Ben & Jerry's) deep dark chocolate .... 1/2 cup		260	55	15.0
(Breyers) .... 4 oz		160	30	8.0
(Darigold) .... 4 oz		140	70	7.0
(Darigold) 'Alpine' .... 4 oz		140	70	7.0
(Darigold) 'Classic' .... 4 oz		180	30	13.0

Food Name	Serv. Size	Total Cal.	Sod. MGS	Fat GMS
(Frusen Glädjé)	4 oz	240	65	17.0
(Häagen-Dazs)	4 oz	270	50	17.0
(Häagen-Dazs) deep	4 oz	290	70	14.0
(Healthy Choice) 'Dairy Dessert'	4 oz	130	70	2.0
(Sealtest)	4 oz	140	50	6.0
CHOCOLATE, DUTCH (Borden) 'Olde Fashioned Recipe'	4 oz	130	65	6.0
CHOCOLATE CARAMEL NUT (Baskin-Robbins) light	4 oz	130	8	5.0
CHOCOLATE CHIP				
(Baskin-Robbins)	1 scoop	260	110	15.0
(Breyers)	4 oz	170	45	10.0
(Dreyer's)	4 oz	150	40	9.0
(Eskimo Pie) cone 'Cookie Dough'	1 cone	280	103	14.0
(Healthy Choice) 'Dairy Dessert'	4 oz	130	70	2.0
(Sealtest)	4 oz	150	50	8.0
(Weight Watchers) 'ONE-ders'	4 oz	120	80	4.0
CHOCOLATE CHIP CHOCOLATE (Häagen-Dazs)	4 oz	290	40	20.0
CHOCOLATE CHIP COOKIE DOUGH (Ben & Jerry's)	1/2 cup	270	92	17.0
CHOCOLATE CHOCOLATE CHIP (Frusen Glädjé)	4 oz	270	60	18.0
CHOCOLATE CHUNK				
(Ben & Jerry's) 'New York Super Fudge Chunk'	1/2 cup	290	55	20.0
CHOCOLATE FUDGE				
(Ben & Jerry's) 'Chocolate Fudge Brownie'	1/2 cup	250	100	14.0
(Ben & Jerry's) double chocolate fudge	1/2 cup	280	60	16.0
(Häagen-Dazs) deep	4 oz	290	70	14.0
CHOCOLATE MINT (Häagen-Dazs)	4 oz	300	50	20.0
CHOCOLATE PEANUT BUTTER COOKIE DOUGH				
(Ben & Jerry's)	1/2 cup	300	85	20.0
CHOCOLATE RASPBERRY TRUFFLE				
(Baskin-Robbins) 'International Creams'	1 scoop	310	115	17.0
CHOCOLATE SWIRL (Borden)	4 oz	130	65	6.0
CHOCOLATE TRIPLE STRIPES (Sealtest)	4 oz	140	50	7.0
CHOCOLATE-PEANUT BUTTER (Häagen-Dazs) deep	4 oz	330	90	19.0
COCONUT ALMOND FUDGE CHIP (Ben & Jerry's)	1/2 cup	320	82	28.0
COFFEE				
(Baskin-Robbins) light 'Espresso and Cream'	4 oz	120	0	5.0
(Ben & Jerry's) Aztec harvest coffee	1/2 cup	230	55	16.0
(Breyers)	4 oz	150	50	8.0
(Häagen-Dazs)	4 oz	270	120	17.0
(Sealtest)	4 oz	140	50	7.0
COFFEE ALMOND FUDGE (Ben & Jerry's)	1/2 cup	290	85	20.0

Food Name	Serv. Size	Total Cal.	Sod. MGS	Fat GMS
COFFEE TOFFEE				
(Ben & Jerry's) 'Coffee Toffee Crunch'	1/2 cup	280	120	19.0
(Healthy Choice) 'Dairy Dessert'	4 oz	130	80	2.0
COOKIE DOUGH DYNAMO (Häagen-Dazs)	4 oz	300	110	18.0
COOKIES 'N CREAM				
(Breyers)	4 oz	170	60	9.0
(Dreyer's)	4 oz	160	80	9.0
(Healthy Choice) 'Dairy Dessert'	4 oz	130	80	2.0
FUDGE, MARBLE (Dreyer's)	4 oz	150	50	8.0
FUDGE BROWNIE (Healthy Choice) 'Dairy Dessert'	4 oz	130	70	2.0
FUDGE ROYALE (Sealtest)	4 oz	140	55	7.0
FUDGE SWIRL, DOUBLE (Healthy Choice) 'Dairy Dessert'	4 oz	130	70	2.0
HEAVENLY HASH				
(Sealtest)	4 oz	150	50	7.0
(Weight Watchers) 'ONE-ders'	4 oz	130	90	3.0
MACADAMIA BRITTLE (Häagen-Dazs)	4 oz	280	60	18.0
MAPLE WALNUT (Sealtest)	4 oz	160	40	9.0
MINT CHOCOLATE (Breyers)	4 oz	170	45	10.0
MINT CHOCOLATE CHIP (Healthy Choice) 'Dairy Dessert'	4 oz	140	80	2.0
MINT WITH CHOCOLATE COOKIE (Ben & Jerry's)	1/2 cup	260	120	17.0
MOCHA ALMOND FUDGE (Breyers)	4 oz	190	60	10.0
MOCHA FUDGE (Ben & Jerry's)	1/2 cup	270	65	18.0
NEAPOLITAN (Healthy Choice) 'Dairy Dessert'	4 oz	120	60	2.0
PEACH				
(Baskin-Robbins) fat-free 'Just Peachy'	4 oz	100	60	0.0
(Breyers) natural	4 oz	130	35	6.0
PEANUT BUTTER CUP (Ben & Jerry's)	1/2 cup	370	140	26.0
PRALINE				
(Baskin-Robbins) light 'Praline Dream'	4 oz	130	85	6.0
(Baskin-Robbins) pralines 'n cream	1 scoop	280	180	14.0
(Healthy Choice) and caramel 'Dairy Dessert'	4 oz	130	70	2.0
(Weight Watchers) pralines 'n cream 'ONE-ders'	4 oz	120	110	4.0
RASPBERRY SWIRL (Healthy Choice) 'Dairy Dessert'	4 oz	120	60	2.0
ROCKY ROAD				
(Baskin-Robbins)	1 scoop	300	135	14.0
(Dreyer's)	4 oz	170	30	10.0
(Healthy Choice) 'Dairy Dessert'	4 oz	160	70	2.0
RUM RAISIN (Häagen-Dazs)	4 oz	250	45	17.0
STRAWBERRY				
(Baskin-Robbins) light 'Strawberry Royale'	4 oz	110	120	3.0
(Baskin-Robbins) 'Very Berry'	1 scoop	220	95	10.0

Food Name	Serv. Size	Total Cal.	Sod. MGS	Fat GMS
(Borden)	4 oz	130	55	6.0
(Borden) cream 'Olde Fashioned Recipe'	4 oz	130	55	5.0
(Breyers)	4 oz	130	40	6.0
(Frusen Glädjé)	4 oz	230	60	15.0
(Häagen-Dazs)	4 oz	250	40	15.0
(Healthy Choice) 'Dairy Dessert'	4 oz	120	50	2.0
(Sealtest)	4 oz	130	40	5.0
SUNDAE				
(Häagen-Dazs) caramel nut	4 oz	310	100	21.0
(Sealtest) chocolate-marshmallow	4 oz	150	40	6.0
(Sealtest) peanut fudge	4 oz	140	50	7.0
(Weight Watchers) hot caramel fudge	4.5 oz	160	140	4.0
(Weight Watchers) hot chocolate fudge	4.5 oz	160	115	4.0
(Weight Watchers) hot mocha fudge	4.5 oz	160	120	5.0
SWISS CHOCOLATE CANDY ALMOND (Frusen Glädjé)	4 oz	270	60	19.0
TOFFEE (Ben & Jerry's) 'English Toffee Crunch'	1/2 cup	310	130	21.0
VANILLA				
regular, 10% fat, hardened	1 oz	57	25	3.1
rich, 16% fat, hardened	1 oz	67	21	4.5
(Baskin-Robbins)	1 scoop	240	115	14.0
(Ben & Jerry's)	1/2 cup	230	55	17.0
(Ben & Jerry's) vanilla bean	1/2 cup	230	55	17.0
(Borden) 'Olde Fashioned Recipe'	4 oz	130	55	7.0
(Breyers)	4 oz	150	50	8.0
(Darigold)	4 oz	130	50	7.0
(Darigold) 'Alpine'	4 oz	130	50	7.0
(Darigold) 'Classic'	4 oz	180	40	12.0
(Dreyer's)	4 oz	160	30	10.0
(Eagle Brand) 'Homestyle'	4 oz	150	55	9.0
(Frusen Glädjé)	4 oz	230	70	17.0
(Good Humor) 'Cup'	3 oz	98	35	5.1
(Häagen-Dazs)	4 oz	260	55	17.0
(Healthy Choice) 'Dairy Dessert'	4 oz	120	60	2.0
(Sealtest)	4 oz	140	50	7.0
VANILLA, FRENCH				
(Baskin-Robbins)	1 scoop	280	90	18.0
(Sealtest)	4 oz	140	50	7.0
VANILLA CARAMEL FUDGE (Ben & Jerry's)	1/2 cup	280	75	17.0
VANILLA CRUNCH				
(Ben & Jerry's) 'Rainforest Crunch'	1/2 cup	300	140	23.0
(Ben & Jerry's) 'Wavy Gravy'	1/2 cup	330	95	24.0

Food Name	Serv. Size	Total Cal.	Sod. MGS	Fat GMS
VANILLA FUDGE *(Häagen-Dazs)*	4 oz	270	100	17.0
VANILLA FUDGE TWIRL *(Breyers)*	4 oz	160	55	8.0
VANILLA HONEY *(Häagen-Dazs)*	4 oz	250	55	16.0
VANILLA SWISS ALMOND				
(Frusen Glädjé)	4 oz	270	65	19.0
(Häagen-Dazs)	4 oz	290	55	19.0
VANILLA TOFFEE CHUNK *(Frusen Glädjé)*	4 oz	270	160	17.0
VANILLA-CHOCOLATE				
(Baskin-Robbins) fat-free 'Just Chocolate Vanilla'	4 oz	100	60	0.0
(Breyers)	4 oz	160	40	8.0
(Good Humor) cup 'Combo'	6 oz	201	80	9.2
VANILLA-CHOCOLATE-STRAWBERRY				
(Breyers)	4 oz	150	40	8.0
(Sealtest)	4 oz	140	50	6.0
(Sealtest) 'Cubic Scoops'	4 oz	130	50	6.0
VANILLA-PEANUT BUTTER SWIRL *(Häagen-Dazs)*	4 oz	280	120	21.0
WHITE RUSSIAN *(Ben & Jerry's)*	1/2 cup	240	55	16.0
ICE CREAM, ALTERNATIVE				
ALL FLAVORS *(Lite Lite Tofutti)*	4 oz	90	80	<1.0
BLACK CHERRY *(Sealtest)* 'Free'	4 oz	100	45	0.0
CAPPUCCINO				
(Rice Dream)	4 oz	130	80	5.0
(Tofutti) 'Love Drops'	4 oz	230	120	12.0
CAROB *(Rice Dream)*	4 oz	130	80	5.0
CAROB ALMOND *(Rice Dream)*	4 oz	140	80	6.0
CAROB CHIP *(Rice Dream)*	4 oz	140	80	6.0
CHOCOLATE				
(Lite Lite Tofutti) soft-serve	4 oz	90	80	<1.0
(Rice Dream) 'Dream Pie'	1 pie	380	225	19.0
(Sealtest) 'Free'	4 oz	100	50	0.0
(Simple Pleasures)	4 oz	140	15	<1.0
(Tofutti) 'Love Drops'	4 oz	230	100	13.0
(Tofutti) supreme	4 oz	210	130	13.0
(Weight Watchers)	4 oz	80	75	0.0
CHOCOLATE CHIP *(Low, Lite 'n Luscious)*	4 oz	100	80	2.0
CHOCOLATE SWIRL *(Weight Watchers)*	4 oz	90	75	0.0
COCOA MARBLE FUDGE *(Rice Dream)*	4 oz	140	80	6.0
COFFEE *(Simple Pleasures)*	4 oz	120	15	<1.0
COOKIES N' DREAM *(Rice Dream)*	4 oz	130	80	5.0
JAMOCA SWISS ALMOND *(Low, Lite 'n Luscious)*	4 oz	90	100	2.0
LEMON *(Rice Dream)*	4 oz	130	80	5.0

Food Name	Serv. Size	Total Cal.	Sod. MGS	Fat GMS
MINT *(Rice Dream)* 'Dream Pie'	1 pie	380	225	19.0
MINT CAROB CHIP *(Rice Dream)*	4 oz	140	80	6.0
MOCHA *(Rice Dream)* 'Dream Pie'	1 pie	380	225	19.0
NEAPOLITAN				
(Rice Dream)	4 oz	130	80	5.0
(Weight Watchers)	4 oz	80	75	0.0
PEACH				
(Sealtest) 'Free'	4 oz	100	45	0.0
(Simple Pleasures)	4 oz	135	5	<1.0
PEANUT BUTTER FUDGE *(Rice Dream)*	4 oz	160	100	7.0
PINEAPPLE COCONUT *(Low, Lite 'n Luscious)*	4 oz	90	70	1.0
RUM RAISIN *(Simple Pleasures)*	4 oz	130	10	<1.0
STRAWBERRY				
(Low, Lite 'n Luscious)	4 oz	80	70	1.0
(Rice Dream)	4 oz	130	80	5.0
(Sealtest) 'Free'	4 oz	100	40	0.0
(Simple Pleasures)	4 oz	120	55	<1.0
VANILLA				
(Lite Lite Tofutti) soft-serve	4 oz	90	80	<1.0
(Rice Dream)	4 oz	130	80	5.0
(Rice Dream) 'Dream Pie'	1 pie	380	225	19.0
(Sealtest) 'Free'	4 oz	100	45	0.0
(Tofutti)	4 oz	200	90	11.0
(Tofutti) 'Love Drops'	4 oz	220	100	12.0
(Weight Watchers)	4 oz	80	75	0.0
VANILLA ALMOND BARK *(Tofutti)*	4 oz	230	950	14.0
VANILLA CHOCOLATE *(Tofutti)* dipped 'O's	1 piece	40	20	2.0
VANILLA SWISS ALMOND *(Rice Dream)*	4 oz	140	80	6.0
VANILLA-CHOCOLATE-STRAWBERRY *(Sealtest)* 'Free'	4 oz	100	40	0.0
VANILLA-FUDGE *(Rice Dream)*	4 oz	140	80	6.0
VANILLA-FUDGE ROYALE *(Sealtest)* 'Free'	4 oz	100	50	0.0
VANILLA-STRAWBERRY ROYALE *(Sealtest)* 'Free'	4 oz	100	35	0.0
WILDBERRY				
(Rice Dream)	4 oz	130	80	5.0
(Tofutti)	4 oz	210	100	12.0
ICE CREAM BAR				
ALMOND *(Good Humor)* toasted, 3 oz	1 bar	212	34	11.8
CARAMEL ALMOND *(Häagen-Dazs)* 'Crunch Bar'	1 bar	240	65	18.0
CHIP CANDY CRUNCH *(Good Humor)* 3 oz	1 bar	255	40	17.9
CHOCOLATE				
(Häagen-Dazs) w/dark chocolate coating	1 bar	390	60	27.0

Food Name	Serv. Size	Total Cal.	Sod. MGS	Fat GMS
(Klondike) 5 oz	1 bar	270	60	19.0
(Nestlé) w/milk chocolate coating 'Quik' 3 oz	1 bar	210	40	14.0
(Weight Watchers) 'Treat Bars' 2.75 oz	1 bar	100	75	1.0
CHOCOLATE DIP (Weight Watchers) 1.7 oz	1 bar	110	35	7.0
CHOCOLATE ECLAIR (Good Humor) 3 oz	1 bar	188	54	9.9
CHOCOLATE FUDGE				
(Baker's) sundae, crunchy 'Fudgetastic' 4 oz	1 bar	230	40	14.0
(Baker's) sundae 'Fudgetastic' 4 oz	1 bar	220	45	15.0
(Good Humor) cake, 6.3 oz	1 bar	214	50	15.0
(Weight Watchers) double, 1.75 oz	1.75 oz	60	50	1.0
CHOCOLATE MOUSSE				
(Weight Watchers) sugar-free, 1.75 oz	1 bar	35	30	<1.0
MILK CHOCOLATE				
(Nestlé) w/almonds, milk chocolate coating, 3.7 oz	3.7 oz	350	45	23.0
ORANGE-VANILLA				
(Weight Watchers) 'Sugar-free Treat Bars'	1 bar	30	40	<1.0
PEANUT BUTTER (Häagen-Dazs) 'Crunch Bar'	4 oz	270	55	21.0
STRAWBERRY SHORTCAKE (Good Humor) 3 oz	1 bar	176	88	8.2
VANILLA				
(Eskimo Pie) w/dark chocolate coating	1 bar	180	35	12.0
(Eskimo Pie) w/dark chocolate coating 'Sugar-freedom'	1 bar	140	30	11.0
(Eskimo Pie) w/milk chocolate coating	1 bar	190	16	12.0
(Eskimo Pie) w/milk chocolate coating and almonds 'Sugar-freedom'	1 bar	140	35	13.0
(Eskimo Pie) w/milk chocolate coating and crisp rice 'Sugar-freedom'	1 bar	150	40	11.0
(Good Humor) w/chocolate flavor coating, 3 oz	1 bar	198	44	13.7
(Häagen-Dazs) 'Crunch Bar' 4 oz	1 bar	220	55	16.0
(Häagen-Dazs) w/dark chocolate coating, 4 oz	1 bar	390	60	27.0
(Häagen-Dazs) w/milk chocolate coating, 4 oz	1 bar	360	55	27.0
(Häagen-Dazs) w/milk chocolate-almond coating, 4 oz	1 bar	370	55	27.0
(Häagen-Dazs) w/milk chocolate-brittle coating, 4 oz	1 bar	370	160	25.0
(Klondike) w/chocolate flavor coating 'Lite'	1 bar	110	50	6.0
(Nestlé) w/chocolate coating and crisp rice 'Crunch' 3 oz	1 bar	180	(mq)	13.0
(Nestlé) w/chocolate coating and crisp rice 'Crunch Lite'	1 bar	120	50	5.0
(Nestlé) w/white chocolate coating 'Alpine Premium' 3.7 oz	1 bar	350	5	25.0
(Oh Henry!) w/caramel peanut, milk chocolate coating, 3 oz	1 bar	320	75	20.0
ICE CREAM BAR, ALTERNATIVE				
(Rice Dream) chocolate	1 bar	270	115	16.0
(Rice Dream) chocolate nutty bar	1 bar	330	110	23.0

Food Name	Serv. Size	Total Cal.	Sod. MGS	Fat GMS
(Rice Dream) strawberry	1 bar	260	110	14.8
(Rice Dream) vanilla	1 bar	275	120	15.8
(Rice Dream) vanilla nutty bar	1 bar	330	100	23.0
ICE CREAM CAKE (Breyers) 'Viennetta'	1 slice	190	40	12.0
ICE CREAM CONE				
Cup style, wafer				
(Bozo) cake	1 cone	16	13	0.0
(Keebler)	1 cone	15	20	1.0
(Keebler) assorted colors	1 cone	15	20	1.0
(Little Debbie)	1 cone	15	15	0.1
(Nabisco) 'Comet'	1 cone	18	5	<1.0
Sugar				
(Baskin-Robbins)	1 cone	60	45	1.0
(Bozo)	1 cone	53	29	1.0
(Keebler)	1 cone	45	35	1.0
(Nabisco)	1 cone	50	40	<1.0
(Nabisco) 'Comet'	1 cone	50	40	<1.0
Waffle, Baskin-Robbins	1 cone	140	5	2.0
ICE CREAM MIX				
Dutch chocolate, prepared (Salada)	8 oz	310	75	19.0
peach, prepared (Salada)	8 oz	310	60	18.0
vanilla, prepared (Salada)	8 oz	310	60	18.0
wild strawberry, prepared (Salada)	8 oz	310	60	18.0
ICE CREAM SNACKS AND SANDWICHES				
Nuggets				
vanilla, dark chocolate coated 'Bon Bons' (Carnation)	5 pieces	170	50	11.0
vanilla, milk chocolate coated 'Bon Bons' (Carnation)	5 pieces	165	50	11.0
Round novelties				
mocha, 4 oz (Natural Nectar)	1 bar	300	135	14.0
nectar, 4 oz (Natural Nectar)	1 bar	300	120	15.0
Sandwich				
chocolate chip cookie, 4 oz (Good Humor)	1 sandwich	246	181	10.5
chocolate chip cookie, 2.7 oz (Good Humor)	1 sandwich	204	166	8.3
vanilla (Weight Watchers)	1 sandwich	150	170	3.0
vanilla, 5 oz (Klondike)	1 sandwich	230	220	9.0
vanilla 'Lite' (Klondike)	1 sandwich	100	110	2.0
vanilla, 1.5-oz snacks (Weight Watchers)	1 sandwich	90	120	2.0
vanilla, 3 oz (Good Humor)	1 sandwich	191	155	5.7
vanilla, 2.5 oz (Good Humor)	1 sandwich	165	134	4.9
vanilla 'Sugar-freedom' (Eskimo Pie)	1 sandwich	170	142	6.0

Food Name	Serv. Size	Total Cal.	Sod. MGS	Fat GMS
Stick novelties				
banana cream *(Natural Nectar)*	1 bar	170	70	8.0
cocoa-fudge 'n' cream *(Natural Nectar)*	1 bar	170	70	8.0
strawberries 'n' cream *(Natural Nectar)*	1 bar	120	40	5.0
wildberry cream *(Natural Nectar)*	1 bar	120	50	3.0
ICE CREAM TOPPING. See individual toppings.				
ICE MILK				
CARAMEL NUT *(Light n' Lively)*	4 oz	120	85	4.
CHOCOLATE				
(Breyers) 'Light'	4 oz	120	55	4.0
(Borden)	4 oz	100	80	2.
(Darigold) 'Lite'	4 oz	110	65	3.
(Weight Watchers) 'Grand Collection'	4 oz	110	75	3.
CHOCOLATE CHIP				
(Light n' Lively)	4 oz	120	35	4.
(Weight Watchers) 'Grand Collection'	4 oz	120	75	4.
CHOCOLATE CHOCOLATE CHIP *(Breyers)* 'Light'	4 oz	140	55	5.
CHOCOLATE FUDGE TWIRL *(Breyers)* 'Light'	4 oz	130	60	4.
CHOCOLATE SWIRL *(Weight Watchers)* 'Grand Collection'	4 oz	120	75	3.
COFFEE *(Light n' Lively)*	4 oz	100	40	3.
COOKIES N' CREAM *(Light n' Lively)*	4 oz	110	65	3.
HEAVENLY HASH				
(Breyers) 'Light'	4 oz	150	55	5.
(Light n' Lively)	4 oz	120	35	4.
NEAPOLITAN *(Weight Watchers)* 'Grand Collection'	4 oz	110	75	3.
PECAN PRALINES 'N CREME				
(Weight Watchers) 'Grand Collection'	4 oz	120	80	4.
PRALINE ALMOND *(Breyers)* 'Light'	4 oz	130	70	5.
STRAWBERRY				
(Borden)	4 oz	90	65	2.
(Breyers) 'Light'	4 oz	110	50	3.
SWISS ALMOND FUDGE TWIRL *(Breyers)*	4 oz	150	65	6.
TOFFEE FUDGE PARFAIT *(Breyers)* 'Light'	4 oz	140	90	5.
VANILLA				
(Borden)	4 oz	90	60	2
(Breyers) 'Light'	4 oz	120	60	4.
(Darigold)	4 oz	110	66	3.
(Light n' Lively)	4 oz	100	40	3.
(Light n' Lively) w/chocolate covered almonds	4 oz	120	45	4.
(Weight Watchers) 'Grand Collection'	4 oz	100	75	3.

Food Name	Serv. Size	Total Cal.	Sod. MGS	Fat GMS
VANILLA-CHOCOLATE-STRAWBERRY				
(Breyers) 'Light'	4 oz	120	55	4.0
(Light n' Lively)	4 oz	100	35	3.0
VANILLA-FUDGE TWIRL (Light n' Lively)	4 oz	110	45	3.0
VANILLA-RASPBERRY				
(Breyers) parfait 'Light'	4 oz	130	50	3.0
(Light n' Lively) swirl	4 oz	110	35	3.0
ICE MILK BAR				
Chocolate Almond Crunch (Weight Watchers)	1 bar	120	45	7.0
CHOCOLATE FUDGE, DOUBLE (Light n' Lively) nonfat	1 bar	50	45	0.0
CHOCOLATE MOUSSE (Light n' Lively) nonfat	1 bar	50	45	0.0
CHOCOLATE W/FUDGE SWIRL (Sealtest) nonfat 'Free'	1 bar	80	55	0.0
ORANGE VANILLA (Light n' Lively) nonfat	1 bar	40	15	0.0
PRALINE (Weight Watchers) 'Crispy Praline 'N Creme'	1 bar	120	45	6.0
STRAWBERRY (Light n' Lively) nonfat	1 bar	80	25	0.0
TOFFEE (Weight Watchers) 'English Toffee Crunch'	1 bar	120	60	8.0
VANILLA				
(Light n' Lively) chocolate dipped	1 bar	110	35	6.0
(Sealtest) w/fudge swirl, nonfat 'Free'	1 bar	80	55	0.0
(Sealtest) w/strawberry swirl, nonfat 'Free'	1 bar	70	60	0.0
ICED TEA. See TEA, ICED.				
IMBU. See JOBO.				
INDIAN DATE. See TAMARIND.				
INDIAN FRY BREAD. See BREAD.				
INFANT FORMULA. See BABY FOOD.				
IRISH MOSS. See SEAWEED.				
ITALIAN SEASONING (Schilling) 'Spice Blends'	1/4 tsp	1	<1	na

Food Name	Serv. Size	Total Cal.	Sod. MGS	Fat GMS
JALAPEÑO. See PEPPER, JALAPEÑO.				
JAM. See also FRUIT SPREAD; JELLY; PRESERVES.				
(Bama) all flavors	2 tsp	30	5	0.0
(Estee) all flavors	1 tsp	2	10	0.0
(Featherweight) all flavors	1 tsp	4	0	0.0
(Kraft) all flavors	1 tsp	17	0	0.0
(S&W Nutradiet) all flavors	1 tsp	4	0	0.0
APRICOT				
(Finast)	2 tsp	35	1	0.0

Food Name	Serv. Size	Total Cal.	Sod. MGS	Fat GMS
(Smucker's) natural ingredients	1 tsp	18	0	0.0
APRICOT-PINEAPPLE (Smucker's) natural ingredients	1 tsp	18	0	0.
BLACK RASPBERRY (Smucker's) natural ingredients	1 tsp	18	0	0.
BLACKBERRY				
(Finast)	2 tsp	16	5	0.0
(Smucker's) natural ingredients	1 tsp	18	0	0.
BLUEBERRY				
(Finast)	2 tsp	16	5	0.
(Smucker's) natural ingredients	1 tsp	18	0	0.
BOYSENBERRY (Smucker's) natural ingredients	1 tsp	18	0	0.
CHERRY				
(Finast)	2 tsp	25	5	0.
(Smucker's) natural ingredients	1 tsp	18	0	0.
GRAPE				
(Finast) Concord or regular	2 tsp	35	5	0.
(Polaner)	2 tsp	35	5	0.
(Smucker's) Concord, natural ingredients	1 tsp	18	0	0.
(Welch's)	2 tsp	35	5	0.
ORANGE MARMALADE (Polaner)	2 tsp	35	5	0.
PEACH				
(Finast)	2 tsp	35	1	0.
(Smucker's) natural ingredients	1 tsp	18	0	0.
PINEAPPLE				
(Finast)	2 tsp	35	1	0.
(Smucker's) natural ingredients	1 tsp	18	0	0.
PLUM (Smucker's) natural ingredients	1 tsp	18	0	0.
RASPBERRY				
(Finast)	2 tsp	35	3	0.
(Smucker's) natural ingredients, seedless	1 tsp	18	0	0.
RASPBERRY-APPLE (Welch's)	2 tsp	35	5	0.
STRAWBERRY				
(Finast)	2 tsp	35	3	0.
(Kraft) 'Reduced Calorie'	1 tsp	6	5	0.
(Piedmont)	2 tsp	35	10	0.
(Smucker's) natural ingredients, seedless	1 tsp	18	0	0.
(Welch's)	2 tsp	35	5	0.
TOMATO (Smucker's) natural ingredients	1 tsp	18	0	0.
JAMBERRY, fresh (Frieda's)	3.5 oz	25	na	

JAPANESE MEDLAR. See LOQUAT.

JAPANESE WHITE RADISH. See RADISH, ORIENTAL.

Food Name	Serv. Size	Total Cal.	Sod. MGS	Fat GMS
JAVA PLUM/jambolan				
raw	1 cup	81	19	0.3
raw	3 fruits	5	1	0.0
w/seeds	1 lb	222	50	0.9
w/o seeds	1 oz	17	4	0.1
JELLY. See also JAM; FRUIT SPREAD; PRESERVES.				
(Bama) and peanut butter, spread, all flavors	2 tbsp	150	75	7.0
(Estee) all flavors	1 tsp	2	10	0.0
(Featherweight) all flavors, except grape	1 tsp	4	0	0.0
(Kraft) all flavors	1 tsp	17	0	0.0
(Smucker's) 'Slenderella' all flavors	1 tsp	7	0	0.0
APPLE				
(Bama)	2 tsp	30	5	0.0
(Finast)	2 tsp	35	2	0.0
(Lucky Leaf)	1 oz	80	5	0.0
(Musselman's)	1 oz	80	5	0.0
(Polaner)	2 tsp	35	5	0.0
(Smucker's) cinnamon-flavored, natural ingredients	1 tsp	18	0	0.0
(Smucker's) mint-flavored, natural ingredients	1 tsp	18	0	0.0
(Smucker's) natural ingredients	1 tsp	18	0	0.0
APPLE-BLACKBERRY *(Musselman's)*	1 oz	80	0	0.0
APPLE-CHERRY *(Musselman's)*	1 oz	80	5	0.0
APPLE-GRAPE				
(Musselman's)	1 oz	80	5	0.0
(Welch's)	2 tsp	35	5	0.0
APPLE-RASPBERRY *(Musselman's)*	1 oz	80	0	0.0
APPLE-STRAWBERRY *(Musselman's)*	1 oz	80	5	0.0
APRICOT-PINEAPPLE				
(Knott's Berry Farm) 'Light' w/NutraSweet	1 tsp	8	0	0.0
BLACK RASPBERRY *(Smucker's)* natural ingredients	1 tsp	18	0	0.0
BLACKBERRY				
(Bama)	2 tsp	30	5	0.0
(Knott's Berry Farm) 'Light' w/NutraSweet	1 tsp	8	0	0.0
(Smucker's) natural ingredients	1 tsp	18	0	0.0
BOYSENBERRY *(Knott's Berry Farm)* 'Light' w/NutraSweet	1 tsp	8	0	0.0
CHERRY *(Smucker's)* natural ingredients	1 tsp	18	0	0.0
CRABAPPLE *(Smucker's)* natural ingredients	1 tsp	18	0	0.0
CURRANT				
(Finast)	2 tsp	35	2	0.0
(Polaner)	2 tsp	35	5	0.0
(Smucker's) natural ingredients	1 tsp	18	0	0.0

Food Name	Serv. Size	Total Cal.	Sod. MGS	Fat GMS
ELDERBERRY *(Smucker's)* natural ingredients	1 tsp	18	0	0.0
GRAPE				
(Bama)	2 tsp	30	5	0.0
(Featherweight)	1 tsp	4	5	0.0
(Finast)	2 tsp	35	5	0.0
(Kraft) 'Reduced Calorie'	1 tsp	6	5	0.0
(Musselman's)	1 oz	80	0	0.0
(Polaner)	2 tsp	35	5	0.0
(Smucker's) Concord, natural ingredients	1 tsp	18	0	0.0
(Welch's)	2 tsp	35	5	0.0
GREEN PEPPER *(Great Impressions)*	1 tbsp	50	<1	0.0
GUAVA *(Smucker's)* natural ingredients	1 tsp	18	0	0.0
JALAPEÑO				
(Great Impressions)	1 tbsp	58	51	0.0
(Knott's Berry Farm)	1 oz	70	0	0.0
(Knott's Berry Farm)	1 tsp	18	0	0.0
MINT				
(Finast)	2 tsp	35	2	0.0
(Polaner)	2 tsp	35	5	0.0
MIXED FRUIT *(Smucker's)* natural ingredients	1 tsp	18	0	0.0
PLUM *(Smucker's)* natural ingredients	1 tsp	18	0	0.0
QUINCE *(Smucker's)* natural ingredients	1 tsp	18	0	0.0
RASPBERRY				
(Knott's Berry Farm) 'Light' w/NutraSweet	1 tsp	8	0	0.0
(Polaner)	2 tsp	35	5	0.0
(Smucker's) natural ingredients	1 tsp	18	0	0.0
RED PEPPER *(Great Impressions)*	1 tbsp	50	9	0.0
STRAWBERRY				
(Finast)	2 tsp	35	2	0.0
(Knott's Berry Farm) 'Light' w/NutraSweet	1 tsp	8	0	0.0
(Polaner)	2 tsp	35	5	0.0
(Smucker's) natural ingredients	1 tsp	18	0	0.0
STRAWBERRY-APPLE *(Polaner)*	2 tsp	35	5	0.0
JERKY. See BEEF JERKY.				
JICAMA/Chinese yam/fon goot yam/Mexican potato/sicama/yambean tuber				
boiled, drained	4 oz	52	7	0.1
raw, trimmed	1 oz	12	2	0.1
raw, trimmed, sliced	1/2 cup	25	4	0.1
raw, untrimmed	1 lb	170	26	0.3
JUICE. See individual listings.				

Food Name	Serv. Size	Total Cal.	Sod. MGS	Fat GMS
JUJUBE, CHINESE				
dried	100 gm	287	9	1.1
dried	1 oz	81	3	0.3
raw	100 gm	79	3	0.2
raw	1 oz	22	1	0.1
raw, w/seeds	1 lb	331	11	0.8
JUNKET MIX				
CHOCOLATE				
mix only, dry	2-oz pkg	207	40	1.9
mix only, dry	1 tbsp	33	6	0.3
prepared (Junket)	1/2 cup	120	65	4.0
prepared w/2% milk	1/2 cup	110	71	2.9
prepared w/whole milk	1/2 cup	125	69	4.5
STRAWBERRY OR RASPBERRY				
mix only, dry	1.5-oz pkg	165	3	0.0
mix only, dry	1 tbsp	38	1	0.0
prepared (Junket)	1/2 cup	120	60	4.0
prepared w/whole milk	1 cup	238	115	9.0
VANILLA				
mix only, dry	1.5-oz pkg	165	3	0.0
mix only, dry	1 tbsp	41	1	0.0
prepared (Junket)	1/2 cup	120	60	4.0
prepared w/2% milk	1/2 cup	101	61	2.4
prepared w/whole milk	1/2 cup	116	61	4.1
JUTE POTHERB				
boiled, drained	4 oz	42	12	0.2
raw, trimmed	1 oz	10	2	0.1
raw, untrimmed	1 lb	96	23	0.7

K

Food Name	Serv. Size	Total Cal.	Sod. MGS	Fat GMS
KALE /borecole/cole/colewort				
boiled, drained	4 oz	36	26	0.5
boiled, drained, chopped	1 cup	42	30	0.5
chopped (Dole)	1/2 cup	17	15	0.5
raw, chopped	1 cup	33	29	0.5
raw, trimmed	1 oz	14	12	0.2
raw, untrimmed	1 lb	137	119	1.9
Canned, chopped (Allen's)	1/2 cup	25	15	<1.0

Food Name	Serv. Size	Total Cal.	Sod. MGS	Fa GM
Frozen				
boiled, drained	4 oz	34	17	0.
boiled, drained, chopped	1 cup	39	20	0.
chopped *(Frosty Acres)*	3.3 oz	25	15	0.
chopped *(Seabrook)*	3.3 oz	25	14	0.0
chopped *(Southern)*	3.5 oz	30	30	0.
unprepared, 10-oz pkg	3.3 oz	26	14	0.
KALE, SCOTCH				
boiled, drained	4 oz	32	51	0.
boiled, drained, chopped	1 cup	36	58	0.
raw, chopped	1 cup	28	47	0.
raw, trimmed	1 oz	12	20	0.
raw, untrimmed	1 lb	115	194	1.
KASHA. See BUCKWHEAT GROATS.				
KATSUO. See TUNA, SKIPJACK.				
KATURAY/sesbania flower				
raw, approx .1 oz	1 flower	1	tr	
raw, trimmed	1 cup	5	3	<.
raw, trimmed	1 oz	8	4	<.
raw, untrimmed	1 lb	106	59	0.
steamed	4 oz	25	12	0.
KAUAI PUNCH, organic *(Santa Cruz Natural)*	8 oz	120	na	1.
KEFIR, CULTURED				
black cherry *(Alta•Dena)*	1 cup	200	120	9.
boysenberry *(Alta•Dena)*	1 cup	200	120	9.
peach *(Alta•Dena)*	1 cup	200	120	9.
red raspberry *(Alta•Dena)*	1 cup	200	120	9.
KELP. See SEAWEED.				
KETCHUP. See CATSUP.				
KIDNEY BEAN				
California red, mature				
boiled	4 oz	141	5	0.
boiled	1/2 cup	109	4	0.
raw	1/2 cup	304	10	0.
raw	1 oz	94	3	0.
Red, mature				
boiled	1/2 cup	112	2	0.
boiled	4 oz	144	2	0.
boiled *(A&P)*	1 cup	230	5	1.
raw	1/2 cup	310	11	1.
raw	1 oz	96	3	0.

Food Name	Serv. Size	Total Cal.	Sod. MGS	Fat GMS
raw (Arrowhead Mills)	2 oz	190	3	1.0
Royal red, mature				
boiled	4 oz	139	6	0.2
boiled	1/2 cup	108	4	0.2
raw	1/2 cup	303	12	0.4
raw	1 oz	93	4	0.1
Sprouted, mature				
boiled, drained	4 oz	37	(mq)	0.7
raw	1 lb	132	(mq)	2.3
raw	1 cup	53	11	0.9
raw	1 oz	8	(mq)	0.1
KIDNEY BEAN, CANNED				
Dark red				
(Allens)	1/2 cup	105	290	<1.0
(Bush's Best)	1/2 cup	70	300	0.0
(Finast)	1/2 cup	110	350	2.0
(Green Giant)	1/2 cup	90	330	<1.0
(Green Giant) 50% less salt	1/2 cup	90	165	<1.0
(Joan of Arc)	1/2 cup	90	330	<1.0
(Joan of Arc) 50% less salt	1/2 cup	90	165	<1.0
(Pathmark)	1/2 cup	110	370	0.0
(S&W) 50% less salt 'Lite'	1/2 cup	120	355	1.0
(S&W) 'Premium'	1/2 cup	120	596	1.0
(Stokely)	1/2 cup	110	360	1.0
(Van Camp's)	1 cup	182	830	0.5
Light red				
(Allens)	1/2 cup	105	290	<1.0
(Bush's Best)	1/2 cup	70	300	0.0
(Finast)	1/2 cup	110	350	2.0
(Green Giant)	1/2 cup	90	330	<1.0
(Green Giant) 50% less salt	1/2 cup	90	165	<1.0
(Joan of Arc)	1/2 cup	90	330	<1.0
(Joan of Arc) 50% less salt	1/2 cup	90	165	<1.0
(Stokely)	1/2 cup	110	360	1.0
(Van Camp's)	1 cup	184	650	0.5
Red				
(A&P)	1/2 cup	110	440	<1.0
(B&M) baked	8 oz	250	640	7.0
(Eden Foods) organic, very low sodium, no salt added	1/2 cup	60	20	<1.0
(Friends) baked	8 oz	340	1060	4.0
(Friends) baked, w/pork	8 oz	270	990	4.0

Food Name	Serv. Size	Total Cal.	Sod. MGS	Fat GMS
(Green Giant)	1/2 cup	90	250	0.0
(Hunt's)	4 oz	120	400	0.0
(Joan of Arc)	1/2 cup	90	250	0.0
(Pathmark)	1/2 cup	110	370	0.0
(Progresso)	1/2 cup	100	210	<1.0
(S&W) 50% less salt 'Lite'	1/2 cup	120	355	1.0
(S&W) 'Premium'	1/2 cup	120	596	1.0
(S&W Nutradiet)	1/2 cup	90	1	1.0
(Stokely)	1/2 cup	110	360	1.0
(Van Camp's)	1 cup	184	650	0.5
(Van Camp's) 'New Orleans Style'	1 cup	178	940	0.6
KIELBASA/kolbassy				
'Bun Size' *(Hillshire Farm)*	2 oz	180	570	16.0
'Kolbase' *(Hormel)*	3 oz	220	904	19.0
'Lean Supreme Polska' *(Eckrich)*	1 oz	72	224	6.0
'Polska Flavorseal' *(Hillshire Farm)*	2 oz	190	540	17.0
'Polska Flavorseal' beef *(Hillshire Farm)*	2 oz	190	550	17.0
'Polska Flavorseal Lite' *(Hillshire Farm)*	2 oz	160	(mq)	13.0
'Polska Flavorseal' mild *(Hillshire Farm)*	2 oz	190	530	17.0
'Polska Links' *(Hillshire Farm)*	2 oz	190	530	17.0
'Polska' skinless *(Eckrich)*	1 link	180	420	16.0
skinless *(Hormel)*	1/2 link	180	826	14.0
KIWI FRUIT/Chinese gooseberry				
fresh, raw, w/o skin	1 large	56	5	0.4
fresh, raw, w/o skin	1 med	46	4	0.
trimmed	1 oz	17	1	0.
untrimmed *(Dole)*	2 fruit	90	0	1.0
w/skin	1 lb	237	18	1.
KIWI NECTAR *(Knudsen & Sons)*	8 oz	60	na	0.
KNACKWURST				
	4-inch link	209	687	18.9
	1 oz	87	286	7.
beef *(Hebrew National)*	3-oz link	263	877	25.0
'Links' *(Hillshire Farm)*	2 oz	180	460	16.0
KOHLRABI/cabbage turnip				
boiled, drained	4 oz	33	24	0.
boiled, drained, sliced	1/2 cup	24	17	0.
raw, sliced	1/2 cup	19	14	0.
raw, trimmed	1 oz	8	6	<.
raw, untrimmed	1 lb	57	42	0.
KOLBASSY. See KIELBASA.				

od Name	Serv. Size	Total Cal.	Sod. MGS	Fat GMS
OOL-AID. See individual flavors.				
UMQUAT				
raw, trimmed	1 fruit	12	1	0.0
w/seeds	1 lb	266	25	0.4

L

ood Name	Serv. Size	Total Cal.	Sod. MGS	Fat GMS
AMB, DOMESTIC				
NOTE: All USDA choice grade. TRIMMED = Lean; separable fat removed.				
UNTRIMMED = Separable fat not removed.)				
RAINS				
braised	3 oz	123	114	8.6
braised, yield from 1 lb raw	12.25 oz	503	465	35.3
pan-fried	3 oz	232	133	18.9
raw	4 oz	138	127	9.7
OMPOSITE CUTS/LEG AND SHOULDER				
Trimmed				
braised, cubes	3 oz	190	59	7.5
broiled, cubes	3 oz	158	65	6.2
broiled, ground	3 oz	241	69	16.7
raw, cubes	1 lb	608	295	24.0
raw, cubes	1 oz	38	18	1.5
raw, ground	1 lb	1279	268	106.2
raw, ground	1 oz	79	17	6.6
stewed, cubes	4 oz	253	79	10.0
EART				
braised	3 oz	157	54	6.7
raw	4 oz	138	101	6.4
simmered	4 oz	210	71	9.0
IDNEYS				
braised	3 oz	116	128	3.1
raw	4 oz	110	177	3.3
EG/FORESHANK				
Trimmed				
braised	3 oz	159	63	5.1
braised	1 oz	53	21	1.7
braised, diced	1 cup	262	104	8.4
broiled, ground	1 cup	328	94	23.1
broiled, ground	4 oz	321	92	22.3

Food Name	Serv. Size	Total Cal.	Sod. MGS	F G
raw	1 lb	544	358	14
raw	1 oz	34	22	0
raw, ground	1 cup	637	133	52
stewed	4 oz	212	84	6
stewed	1 oz	53	21	1
stewed, diced	1 cup	262	104	8
Untrimmed				
braised	3 oz	207	61	11
braised	1 oz	69	20	3
braised, diced	1 cup	340	101	18
raw	1 lb	912	327	60
raw	1 oz	56	20	3
stewed	1 oz	69	20	3
stewed, diced	1 cup	340	101	18
LEG/SHANK				
Trimmed				
raw	1 lb	567	277	19
raw	1 oz	35	17	1
roasted	3 oz	153	56	5
roasted	1 oz	51	19	1
roasted, diced	1 cup	252	92	9
Untrimmed				
raw	1 lb	912	259	61
raw	1 oz	56	16	3
roasted	3 oz	191	55	10
roasted	1 oz	64	18	3
roasted, diced	1 cup	315	91	17
LEG/SIRLOIN				
Trimmed				
raw	1 lb	608	290	23
raw	1 oz	38	18	1
roasted	3 oz	173	60	7
roasted	1 oz	58	20	2
roasted, diced	1 cup	286	99	12
Untrimmed				
raw	1 lb	1234	254	100
raw	1 oz	76	16	6
roasted	3 oz	248	58	17
roasted	1 oz	83	19	5
roasted, diced	1 cup	409	95	28

Food Name	Serv. Size	Total Cal.	Sod. MGS	Fat GMS
LEG/WHOLE				
Trimmed				
raw	1 lb	581	281	20.5
raw	1 oz	36	17	1.3
roasted	3 oz	162	58	6.6
roasted	1 oz	54	19	2.2
roasted, diced	1 cup	267	95	10.8
Untrimmed				
raw	1 lb	1043	254	77.4
raw	1 oz	64	16	4.8
roasted	3 oz	219	56	14.0
roasted	1 oz	73	19	4.7
roasted, diced	1 cup	361	92	23.0
LIVER				
braised	3 oz	187	48	7.5
pan-fried	3 oz	202	105	10.8
raw	4 oz	158	79	5.7
LOIN				
Trimmed				
broiled	3 oz	184	71	8.3
raw	1 oz	40	19	1.7
roasted	3 oz	172	56	8.3
Untrimmed				
broiled	3 oz	269	65	19.6
roasted	3 oz	263	54	20.0
LUNGS				
braised	3 oz	96	71	2.6
raw	4 oz	108	178	3.0
PANCREAS				
braised	3 oz	199	44	12.8
raw	4 oz	172	85	11.1
RIB				
Trimmed				
broiled	3 oz	200	72	11.0
raw	1 lb	767	327	41.9
raw	1 oz	47	20	2.6
roasted	3 oz	197	69	11.3
Untrimmed				
broiled	3 oz	307	65	25.1
raw	1 lb	1687	254	156.0
raw	1 oz	104	16	9.6

Food Name	Serv. Size	Total Cal.	Sod. MGS	Fat GMS
roasted	3 oz	305	62	25.3
SHOULDER/ARM				
Trimmed				
braised	3 oz	237	65	12.0
broiled	3 oz	170	70	7.7
raw	1 oz	37	19	1.5
roasted	3 oz	163	57	7.9
Untrimmed				
braised	3 oz	294	61	20.4
broiled	3 oz	239	65	16.6
raw	1 oz	73	17	5.8
roasted	3 oz	237	55	17.2
SHOULDER/BLADE				
Trimmed				
braised	1 oz	81	22	4.7
broiled	3 oz	179	75	9.6
raw	3 oz	128	59	6.5
roasted	3 oz	178	58	9.8
Untrimmed				
braised	3 oz	293	64	21.0
broiled	3 oz	236	70	17.0
raw	1 lb	1175	281	94.6
raw	1 oz	73	17	5.8
roasted	3 oz	239	56	17.5
SHOULDER/WHOLE				
Trimmed				
braised	4 oz	321	90	10.0
braised, diced	1 cup	396	111	22.2
broiled	4 oz	238	94	11.9
roasted	4 oz	231	77	12.2
roasted, diced	1 cup	286	95	15.1
stewed	4 oz	321	90	10.0
stewed, diced	1 cup	396	111	22.2
Untrimmed				
braised, diced	1 cup	482	105	34.4
broiled	4 oz	315	88	21.8
broiled, diced	1 cup	389	109	27.0
roasted	4 oz	313	75	22.6
roasted, diced	1 cup	386	92	28.0
stewed	4 oz	390	85	27.8
stewed, diced	1 cup	482	105	34.4

Food Name	Serv. Size	Total Cal.	Sod. MGS	Fat GMS
TONGUE				
braised	3 oz	234	57	17.2
raw	4 oz	252	88	19.5
LAMB, NEW ZEALAND, FROZEN				
COMPOSITE CUTS				
Trimmed				
cooked	4 oz	234	57	10.0
raw	1 oz	36	13	1.3
Untrimmed				
raw	1 oz	182	6	19.2
LEG/FORESHANK				
Trimmed				
braised	3 oz	158	42	5.1
braised, diced	1 cup	260	69	8.5
raw	1 lb	535	227	14.9
raw	1 oz	33	14	0.9
stewed	4 oz	211	56	6.8
stewed, diced	1 cup	260	69	8.5
Untrimmed				
braised	3 oz	219	40	13.5
braised, diced	1 cup	361	66	22.2
raw	1 lb	1012	204	73.3
raw	1 oz	62	13	4.5
stewed	4 oz	293	53	18.0
stewed, diced	1 cup	361	66	22.2
LEG/WHOLE				
Trimmed				
raw	1 lb	558	200	17.2
raw	1 oz	34	12	1.1
roasted	3 oz	154	38	6.0
roasted, diced	1 cup	253	63	9.8
Untrimmed				
raw	1 lb	980	181	69.4
raw	1 oz	60	11	4.3
roasted	3 oz	209	37	13.2
roasted, diced	1 cup	344	60	21.8
LOIN				
Trimmed				
broiled	4 oz	226	62	9.3
raw	1 oz	36	13	1.2
roasted	3 oz	169	47	7.0

Food Name	Serv. Size	Total Cal.	Sod. MGS	Fat GMS
Untrimmed				
broiled	3 oz	268	42	20.3
raw	1 oz	85	10	7.3
RIB				
Trimmed				
raw	1 lb	644	236	27.5
raw	1 oz	40	15	1.7
roasted	3 oz	167	41	8.6
Untrimmed				
raw	1 lb	1569	181	142.0
raw	1 oz	97	11	8.8
roasted	3 oz	289	37	24.4
SHOULDER/WHOLE				
Trimmed				
braised	3 oz	242	48	13.2
braised, diced	1 cup	399	78	21.7
raw	1 lb	612	213	24.6
raw	1 oz	38	13	1.5
stewed	6.5 oz	522	103	28.3
stewed, diced	1 cup	399	78	21.7
Untrimmed				
braised	3 oz	303	43	22.3
braised, diced	1 cup	491	73	35.5
raw	1 lb	1234	186	100.8
stewed	4 oz	398	59	28.8
stewed, diced	1 cup	491	73	35.5
LAMB'S QUARTERS				
boiled, drained	4 oz	36	(mq)	0.8
boiled, drained, chopped	1 cup	58	52	1.2
raw	100 gm	43	43	0.8
raw, trimmed	1 lb	195	(mq)	3.6
raw, trimmed	1 oz	12	(mq)	0.2
LARD				
pork, fresh	1 cup	1849	0	205.0
pork, fresh	1 tbsp	115	0	12.8
pork leaf, fresh	1 oz	243	1	26.7
LASAGNA ENTRÉE, FROZEN				
(Banquet) 'Extra Helping'	16.5 oz	645	1582	23.0
(Celentano)	10 oz	460	870	24.0
(Celentano)	8 oz	370	700	19.0
(Celentano)	6.25 oz	230	600	14.0

Food Name	Serv. Size	Total Cal.	Sod. MGS	Fat GMS
(Chef Boyardee)	5.97 oz	280	900	8.0
(Green Giant) 'Entrées'	12 oz	490	1660	20.0
(Stouffer's) 96-oz tray	9.75 oz	400	940	14.0
(Stouffer's) 21-oz pkg	10.5 oz	360	1020	13.0
(Stouffer's) 10-oz pkg	10 oz	340	840	12.0
(Tyson) 'Gourmet Selection'	11.5 oz	380	840	14.0
(Weight Watchers)	10.25 oz	270	510	6.0
CHEESE				
(Budget Gourmet) three cheese	10 oz	400	760	17.0
(Dining Lite)	9 oz	260	800	6.0
(Lean Cuisine) casserole 'Lunch Express'	9.5 oz	290	560	6.0
(Weight Watchers) Italian	11 oz	290	510	7.0
FLORENTINE *(Smart Ones)* w/spinach cheese	11 oz	220	460	1.0
IN SAUCE *(Buitoni)* 'Family Style'	7.3 oz	370	940	13.0
LOW FAT *(Celentano)* 'Great Choice'	10 oz	260	650	2.0
MEAT *(Buitoni)* 'Single Serving'	9 oz	580	820	19.0
PRIMAVERA *(Celentano)*	11 oz	330	470	14.0
SAUSAGE *(Budget Gourmet)* Italian	10 oz	420	950	20.0
SEAFOOD *(Mrs. Paul's)* seafood 'Light'	9.5 oz	290	750	8.0
TOFU				
(Amy's Kitchen) vegetable, organic	9.5 oz	310	500	10.0
(Legume) and sauce 'Classic'	8 oz	210	410	8.0
TUNA *(Lean Cuisine)* w/spinach noodles	9.75 oz	240	520	7.0
VEGETABLE				
(Amy's Kitchen) organic	9.5 oz	310	470	8.5
(Le Menu) garden 'Light Style'	10.5 oz	260	500	8.0
(Legume) w/tofu and sauce	12 oz	240	520	8.0
(Stouffer's)	10.5 oz	430	820	23.0
(Stouffer's) 96-oz tray	9.5 oz	400	760	20.0
(Weight Watchers) garden 'Lowfat'	11 oz	260	430	7.0
W/MEAT SAUCE				
(Banquet) 'Family Entrees'	7 oz	270	(mq)	10.0
(Dining Lite)	9 oz	240	800	5.0
(Freezer Queen) 'Deluxe Family Suppers'	7 oz	200	730	6.0
(Healthy Choice)	10 oz	260	420	5.0
(Le Menu) 'LightStyle'	10 oz	290	510	8.0
(Lean Cuisine)	10.25 oz	280	560	6.0
(Swanson) 'Homestyle Recipe'	10.5 oz	400	1070	15.0
ZUCCHINI				
(Healthy Choice)	11.5 oz	250	400	3.0
(Lean Cuisine)	11 oz	260	520	6.0

Food Name	Serv. Size	Total Cal.	Sod. MGS	Fat GM
LASAGNA ENTRÉE, MICROWAVE				
(Chef Boyardee)	7.5 oz	230	1080	9.
(Chef Boyardee) hearty 'Main Meals'	10.5 oz	290	na	8.0
(Chef Boyardee) in garden vegetable sauce	7.5 oz	170	940	1.
(Hormel)	7.5 oz	250	949	13.
(Libby's) w/meat sauce 'Diner'	7.75 oz	200	790	5.
(Lunch Bucket) w/meat sauce	7.5 oz	220	870	4.0
LASAGNA ENTRÉE, PACKAGED				
(Dinty Moore) w/meat sauce 'American Classics'	10 oz	320	870	14.
(Top Shelf) Italian	10 oz	350	840	16.
(Top Shelf) vegetable	10.6 oz	275	1024	8.0
(Ultra Slim Fast) vegetable	12 oz	240	730	4.0
(Ultra Slim Fast) w/meat sauce	12 oz	330	980	9.
LASAGNA NOODLE. See PASTA.				
LAVER. See SEAWEED.				
LEEK				
boiled, drained	4 oz	35	11	0.
boiled, drained, chopped	1/4 cup	8	3	0.
raw, chopped	1/2 cup	32	10	0.
raw, trimmed	1 oz	17	6	0.
raw, untrimmed	1 lb	122	40	0.0
LEEK, FREEZE-DRIED				
bulb-lower leaf portion	1 oz	91	10	0.
bulb-lower leaf portion	1/4 cup	3	0	0.0
bulb-lower leaf portion	1 tbsp	1	0	0.0
LEMON				
w/peel, approx 3.9 oz	1 med	22	3	0.
w/peel, whole	1 lb	89	13	1.
w/o peel, approx 3.9 oz	1 med	17	1	0.
w/o peel, approx 5.6 oz	1 large	24	2	0.
w/o peel, trimmed	1-oz wedge	5	1	0.
LEMON AND HERB SEASONING				
(Schilling) 'Spice Blends'	1/4 tsp	1	154	0.
LEMON DILL SEASONING MIX				
(Schilling) 'Bag 'n Season'	1 pkg	161	2035	11.
LEMON DRINK. See also LEMONADE.				
(Crowley) chilled	8 oz	130	15	0.0
(Gatorade) 'Thirst Quencher'	8 oz	50	110	0.
(Pathmark) 'No Frills' mix, prepared	8 oz	90	55	0.
LEMON GINGER JUICE				
(Santa Cruz Natural) organic 'Cruz'	8 oz	125	na	<1.0

od Name	Serv. Size	Total Cal.	Sod. MGS	Fat GMS
EMON HERB MARINADE (Golden Dipt)	1 oz	130	210	14.0
EMON JUICE				
	1 cup	61	2	0.0
	1 oz	8	<1	0.0
	1 tbsp	4	0	0.0
Canned or bottled				
(A&P) reconstituted, natural strength	1 oz	6	0	<1.0
(Lucky Leaf)	6 oz	30	35	0.0
(ReaLemon) reconstituted, natural strength, refrigerated	1 oz	6	10	0.0
(ReaLemon) reconstituted, '100%'	1 oz	6	5	0.0
Frozen				
single strength	1/2 cup	27	1	0.4
single strength	1 tbsp	3	tr	0.1
(Minute Maid) concentrate	6 oz	8	0	0.0
(Sunkist)	1 oz	7	<1	0.1
EMON PEEL				
candied	1 oz	88	0	0.1
raw	1 tbsp	na	0	0.0
raw	1 tsp	na	0	0.0
EMON PEPPER				
Dry seasoning				
(Lawry's)	1 tsp	6	340	0.1
(Schilling) 'Parsley Patch'	1 tsp	13	2	0.6
(Schilling) 'Spice Blends'	1 tsp	7	618	0.0
Marinade (Lawry's)	1 oz	20	800	1.1
EMONADE				
Can, bottle, or box				
(Fruitopia) 'Lemonade, Love & Hope' real fruit	8 oz	110	25	0.0
(Fruitopia) 'Pink Lemonade Euphoria' real fruit	8 oz	120	25	0.0
(Hi-C)	8.45 oz	109	73	0.1
(J. Hungerford) pink, 20% plus juice	9.03 oz	41	39	0.0
(Knudsen & Sons) 'Natural'	8 oz	100	na	0.0
(Minute Maid)	6 oz	80	20	0.0
(Minute Maid) country style	6 oz	80	20	0.0
(Minute Maid) cranberry	6 oz	90	20	0.0
(Minute Maid) pink	6 oz	80	20	0.0
(Minute Maid) raspberry	6 oz	90	20	0.0
(Santa Cruz Natural) organic	8 oz	60	na	<1.0
(Santa Cruz Natural) organic 'Sparkling'	8 oz	85	na	<1.0
(Shasta)	12 oz	146	106	0.0
(Sunkist)	8 oz	141	0	0.0

Food Name	Serv. Size	Total Cal.	Sod. MGS	F· G·
(10-K) pink	8 oz	60	55	0
(Tropicana)	6 oz	100	35	<1
(Tropicana) 'Single Serve'	8 oz	120	3	0
(Veryfine)	8 oz	120	25	0
(Wyler's)	6 oz	64	33	0
(Wyler's) pink 'Fruit Slush'	4 oz	157	10	0
LEMONADE DRINK MIX				
Prepared from dry mix				
(Country Time)	8 oz	80	20	0
(Country Time) pink	8 oz	80	20	0
(Country Time) pink, 'Sugar Free'	8 oz	4	0	0
(Country Time) pink, sugar sweetened	8 oz	80	20	0
(Country Time) pink, sugar-free, w/NutraSweet	8 oz	4	0	0
(Country Time) 'Sugar-free'	8 oz	4	0	0
(Crystal Light) 'Sugar-free'	8 oz	4	0	0
(Crystal Light) sugar-free, w/NutraSweet	8 oz	4	0	0
(Finast)	8 oz	80	15	0
(Gatorade) instant 'Thirst Quencher'	8 oz	60	110	0
(Kool-Aid) pink, unsweetened, prepared w/sugar	8 oz	100	0	0
(Kool-Aid) pink, unsweetened, prepared w/o sugar	8 oz	2	0	0
(Kool-Aid) sugar free, w/NutraSweet	8 oz	4	0	0
(Kool-Aid) sugar sweetened	8 oz	80	0	0
(Wyler's) 'Crystals' 32-serving pkg	8 oz	78	39	0
Prepared from frozen concentrate				
(A&P)	8 oz	110	0	<1
(A&P) pink	8 oz	110	0	<1
(Minute Maid)	6 oz	90	0	0
(Minute Maid) country style	6 oz	90	0	0
(Minute Maid) cranberry	6 oz	90	0	0
(Minute Maid) pink	6 oz	90	0	0
(Minute Maid) raspberry	6 oz	90	0	0
(Sunkist)	8 oz	92	1	0
LEMONADE PUNCH MIX (Country Time) sugar sweetened	8 oz	80	15	0
LEMON-LIME DRINK				
Can, bottle, or box				
(All-Sports) thirst quencher, caffeine-free	8 oz	70	55	0
(Gatorade) 'Thirst Quencher'	8 oz	50	110	0
(Gatorade) 'Thirst Quencher Light'	8 oz	25	80	0
(PowerAde) thirst quencher, high energy	8 oz	70	70	0
(10-K)	8 oz	60	55	0
(Veryfine)	8 oz	120	10	0

Food Name	Serv. Size	Total Cal.	Sod. MGS	Fat GMS
Prepared from dry mix				
(Crystal Light) w/NutraSweet	8 oz	4	0	0.0
(GatorAde) instant 'Thirst Quencher'	8 oz	60	110	0.0
(Kool-Aid) unsweetened, prepared w/sugar	8 oz	100	0	0.0
(Kool-Aid) unsweetened, prepared w/o sugar	8 oz	2	0	0.0
LENTIL				
boiled	1/2 cup	115	2	0.4
boiled	4 oz	132	2	0.4
boiled (A&P)	1 cup	210	0	1.0
raw	1/2 cup	324	9	0.9
raw	1 oz	96	3	0.3
raw, green (Arrowhead Mills)	2 oz	190	9	1.0
raw, red (Arrowhead Mills)	2 oz	195	10	1.0
raw, sprouted	1 oz	30	3	0.2
LENTIL DINNER, CANNED				
hearty, w/garden vegetables 'Fast Menu' fat-free				
(Health Valley)	7.5 oz	160	204	4.0
hearty, w/garden vegetables 'Fast Menu' fat-free				
(Health Valley)	5 oz	80	140	0.0
LETTUCE				
BIBB, BOSTON, OR BUTTERHEAD				
raw, approx 7.75 oz, 5-inch diam	1 head	21	8	0.4
trimmed	1 oz	4	1	0.1
untrimmed	1 lb	45	18	0.7
COS				
raw, shredded	1/2 cup	4	2	0.1
trimmed	1 oz	5	2	0.1
untrimmed	1 lb	68	32	0.9
ICEBERG				
raw, 6-inch diam	1 head	70	49	1.0
trimmed	1 oz	4	3	0.1
untrimmed	1 lb	55	39	0.8
LEAF, shredded (Dole)	1.5 cups	12	40	0.0
LOOSELEAF				
raw, shredded	1/2 cup	5	3	0.1
trimmed	1 oz	5	3	0.1
untrimmed	1 lb	52	26	0.9
ROMAINE				
raw, shredded	1/2 cup	4	2	0.1
trimmed	1 oz	5	2	0.1
untrimmed	1 lb	68	32	0.9

Food Name	Serv. Size	Total Cal.	Sod. MGS	Fat GMS
LIMA BEAN /butterbean				
boiled, drained	4 oz	139	19	0.4
raw, trimmed	1 oz	32	2	0.2
raw, untrimmed	1 lb	226	16	1.7
MATURE, DRY				
Baby				
boiled	4 oz	143	3	0.4
boiled (A&P)	1 cup	230	15	1.0
boiled, thin-seeded	1/2 cup	115	3	0.4
raw	1 oz	95	4	0.3
raw, thin-seeded	1/2 cup	338	13	0.9
Large				
boiled	4 oz	130	2	0.4
boiled	1/2 cup	108	2	0.4
boiled (A&P)	1 cup	230	0	1.0
raw	1/2 cup	301	16	0.6
raw	1 oz	96	5	0.2
LIMA BEAN, CANNED				
(A&P)	1/2 cup	110	380	<1.0
(Allens) large	1/2 cup	110	370	<1.0
(Featherweight)	1/2 cup	80	25	0.0
(Freshlike)	1/2 cup	80	320	0.0
(Freshlike) water packed, w/o salt	1/2 cup	80	5	0.0
(Green Giant)	1/2 cup	80	420	0.0
(Joan of Arc)	1/2 cup	80	420	0.0
(S&W)	1/2 cup	100	440	1.0
(Stokely)	1/2 cup	80	390	0.0
(Stokely) 'No Salt or Sugar Added'	1/2 cup	80	5	0.0
(Van Camp's)	1 cup	162	710	0.5
(Veg•All)	1/2 cup	80	320	0.0
FORDHOOK (Stokely)	1/2 cup	80	300	0.0
GREEN				
(A&P)	1/2 cup	80	320	<1.0
(Allens) medium	1/2 cup	90	350	<1.0
(Allens) tiny, small	1/2 cup	90	350	<1.0
(Bush's Best)	1/2 cup	90	400	0.0
(Del Monte) w/liquid	1/2 cup	70	355	0.0
(Luck's) small, w/pork	7.5 oz	220	640	7.0
(S&W) small 'Fancy'	1/2 cup	80	390	0.0
GREEN AND WHITE				
(Allens)	1/2 cup	90	370	<1.0

Food Name	Serv. Size	Total Cal.	Sod. MGS	Fat GMS
(Bush's Best) gem	1/2 cup	80	300	0.0
W/HAM (Dennison's)	7.5 oz	250	935	7.0
W/PORK (Luck's)	7.5 oz	230	720	7.0
LIMA BEAN, FROZEN				
(Green Giant)	1/2 cup	100	30	0.0
(Green Giant) 'Harvest Fresh'	1/2 cup	80	170	0.0
(Green Giant) in butter sauce	1/2 cup	100	310	2.0
(Health Valley)	1/2 cup	94	26	0.0
BABY				
boiled, drained	10-oz pkg	376	147	1.3
boiled, drained	4 oz	119	33	0.3
boiled, drained, immature seeds	10-oz pkg	327	90	0.9
boiled, drained, immature seeds	1/2 cup	94	26	0.3
unprepared, immature seeds	10-oz pkg	375	148	1.3
unprepared, immature seeds	1/2 cup	108	43	0.4
(A&P) green	3.3 oz	130	130	<1.0
(Birds Eye)	3.3 oz	130	115	0.0
(Freshlike)	3.3 oz	130	100	1.0
(Frosty Acres)	3.3 oz	130	125	0.0
(Seabrook)	3.3 oz	130	125	0.0
(Seabrook) butter	3.3 oz	140	213	1.0
(Southern)	3.5 oz	135	125	0.5
(Stokely) in butter sauce 'Singles'	4 oz	140	450	2.0
(Veg•All)	3.3 oz	130	100	1.0
FORDHOOK				
boiled, drained	10-oz pkg	301	166	1.0
boiled, drained	4 oz	113	60	0.4
boiled, drained, immature seeds	10-oz pkg	311	165	1.1
boiled, drained, immature seeds	1/2 cup	85	45	0.3
unprepared, immature seeds	1/2 cup	85	46	0.3
(A&P)	3.3 oz	100	70	<1.0
(Birds Eye)	3.3 oz	100	100	0.0
(Frosty Acres)	3.3 oz	100	71	0.0
(Seabrook)	3.3 oz	100	71	0.0
(Southern)	3.5 oz	105	100	0.3
SPECKLED				
(Seabrook)	3.3 oz	120	19	0.0
(Southern)	3.5 oz	135	30	0.4
TINY (Seabrook)	3.3 oz	110	144	1.0
LIME				
peeled and seeded	1 oz	9	1	0.1

Food Name	Serv. Size	Total Cal.	Sod. MGS	Fat GMS
raw, 2-inch diam	1 med	20	1	0.1
untrimmed	1 lb	115	8	0.8
LIME JUICE				
fresh	1 cup	66	2	0.3
fresh	1 oz	8	<1	<.1
fresh	1 tbsp	4	0	0.0
Canned or bottled				
	1/2 cup	26	20	0.3
	1 tbsp	3	2	<.1
unsweetened	1 cup	52	39	0.6
unsweetened	1 tbsp	3	2	0.0
(ReaLime) reconstituted, natural strength	1 oz	6	10	0.0
(Roses)	1 oz	48	6	0.0
(Santa Cruz Natural) organic, 'Cruz'	8 oz	120	na	<1.0
LIMEADE				
(Minute Maid) frozen concentrate, diluted	6 oz	70	0	0.0
(Santa Cruz Natural) organic, 'Sparkling'	8 oz	60	na	<1.0
LINGCOD				
dry-heat cooked	3 oz	93	65	1.2
raw	1 lb	385	266	4.8
raw	3 oz	72	50	0.9
raw	1 oz	24	17	0.3
LINGUINE ENTRÉE				
Frozen				
(Banquet) w/meat sauce 'Healthy Balance'	11.5 oz	290	560	6.0
(Budget Gourmet) w/shrimp	10 oz	330	1250	15.0
(Healthy Choice) w/shrimp	9.5 oz	230	420	2.0
(Lean Cuisine) w/clam sauce	9 5/8 oz	280	560	8.0
Packaged (Top Shelf) w/clam sauce	1 serving	330	1420	18.0
Refrigerated				
(Contadina) egg, angel hair 'Fresh'	3 oz	260	30	3.0
(DiGiorno) herb, approx 1 1/3 cups cooked	3 oz	250	135	3.0
LINGUINE NOODLE. See PASTA.				
LINSEED OIL				
edible	1/2 cup	964	0	109.0
edible	1 oz	251	0	28.4
edible	1 tbsp	120	0	13.6
LIQUEUR. See ALCOHOLIC BEVERAGES.				
LIQUOR. See ALCOHOLIC BEVERAGES.				

Food Name	Serv. Size	Total Cal.	Sod. MGS	Fat GMS
LITCHI / lychee				
Dried				
.... 100 gm		277	3	1.2
.... 1 oz		79	1	0.3
Raw				
approx .6 oz .... 1 med		6	tr	<.1
shelled and seeded .... 1/2 cup		63	1	0.4
shelled and seeded .... 1 oz		19	<1	0.1
untrimmed .... 1 lb		179	2	1.2
LIVER. See individual animal listings.				
LIVERWURST. See LUNCHEON MEATS.				
LIVERWURST SPREAD				
(Hormel) canned .... .5 oz		35	(mq)	3.0
(Underwood) canned .... 2 1/8 oz		180	470	15.0
LOBSTER, NORTHERN				
boiled .... 1 cup		142	551	0.9
boiled .... 4 oz		111	431	0.7
moist-heat cooked .... 1 cup		142	551	0.9
moist-heat cooked .... 3 oz		83	323	0.5
poached .... 1 cup		142	551	0.9
poached .... 4 oz		111	431	0.7
raw .... 1 lb		410	(mq)	4.1
raw .... 3 oz		77	252	0.8
raw .... 1 oz		26	(mq)	0.3
steamed .... 1 cup		142	551	0.9
steamed .... 4 oz		111	431	0.7
LOBSTER, SPINY, MIXED SPECIES				
moist-heat cooked .... 3 oz		122	193	1.6
raw .... 1 lb		506	803	6.9
raw .... 3 oz		95	150	1.3
raw .... 1 oz		32	50	0.4
LOBSTER PASTE, canned .... 1 tsp		13	10	0.7
LONGAN				
raw, approx .2 oz .... 1 med		2	tr	tr
raw, shelled and seeded .... 1 oz		17	tr	<.1
raw, untrimmed .... 1 lb		144	1	0.2
LONGAN, DRIED				
.... 100 gm		286	48	0.4
.... 1 oz		81	14	0.1
LOGANBERRY				
fresh, trimmed .... 1 lb		281	5	2.7

Food Name	Serv. Size	Total Cal.	Sod. MGS	Fat GMS
fresh, trimmed	1 cup	89	1	0.9
fresh, untrimmed	1 lb	267	4	2.6
frozen	1 cup	81	1	0.5
frozen	4 oz	62	1	0.4
LONGBEAN				
boiled, drained	4 oz	53	5	0.1
boiled, drained, sliced	1/2 cup	25	2	0.1
boiled, drained, 13 1/4 inches long x 1/4 inch diam	1 pod	7	1	<.1
raw, sliced	1/2 cup	22	2	0.2
raw, 13 1/4 inches long x 1/4 inch diam	1 pod	6	tr	0.1
raw, trimmed	1 oz	13	1	0.1
raw, untrimmed	1 lb	203	17	1.7
LONGBEAN, DRIED				
boiled	1/2 cup	102	4	0.4
boiled	4 oz	134	6	0.5
raw	1/2 cup	292	14	1.1
raw	1 oz	98	5	0.4
LOOFAH GOURD. See GOURD, DISHCLOTH.				
LOQUAT/Japanese medlar				
peeled and seeded	1 oz	13	<1	0.1
trimmed, .6 oz	1 med	5	0	0.0
untrimmed	1 lb	132	3	0.6
LOTTE. See MONKFISH.				
LOTUS ROOT				
boiled, drained	4 oz	75	51	0.1
boiled, drained, 2.5-inch diam	10 slices	59	40	0.1
raw, 2.5-inch diam	10 slices	45	32	0.1
raw, 9.5 inches long	1 root	64	46	0.1
raw, trimmed	1 oz	16	11	<.1
raw, untrimmed	1 lb	201	145	0.4
LOTUS SEED				
dried	1 cup	106	2	0.6
dried, approx 42 medium seeds	1 oz	94	1	0.6
raw	1 oz	25	0	0.2
raw, in shell	1 lb	214	3	1.3
LOX. See SALMON, CHINOOK.				
LUNCHEON MEAT				
BARBECUE LOAF (Oscar Mayer)	1 oz	46	333	2.3
BOLOGNA				
(Eckrich)	1 oz	100	240	9.0
(Eckrich) 'German Brand'	1 oz	80	300	7.0

Food Name	Serv. Size	Total Cal.	Sod. MGS	Fat GMS
(Eckrich) 'Lean Supreme'	1 oz	70	240	6.0
(Eckrich) 'Sandwich'	1 oz	100	240	9.0
(Eckrich) 'Smorgas Pac'	1 oz	100	240	9.0
(Eckrich) 'Thick Sliced, 1-lb pkg'	1.8 oz	170	430	15.0
(Hillshire Farm) 'Large'	1 oz	90	(mq)	8.0
(Hillshire Farm) 'Ring'	1 oz	89	(mq)	8.0
(Hormel) 'Fine Ground, 1-lb'	2 oz	170	596	16.0
(Hormel) 'Perma-Fresh'	2 slices	180	599	16.0
(JM)	1 oz	90	350	8.0
(JM) 'German Brand'	1 oz	70	270	6.0
(Kahn's)	1 slice	90	330	8.0
(Kahn's) 'Deluxe Club'	1 slice	90	290	8.0
(Kahn's) 'Deluxe Club Family Pack'	1 slice	70	220	6.0
(Kahn's) 'Giant Deluxe'	1 slice	90	290	8.0
(Kahn's) 'Giant Thick Deluxe'	1 slice	110	330	10.0
(Kahn's) 'Thick Deluxe'	1 slice	140	450	13.0
(Kahn's) 'Thin Sliced Deluxe'	1 slice	60	190	5.0
(Light & Lean)	2 slices	140	(mq)	12.0
(Light & Lean) 'Thin Sliced'	2 slices	70	(mq)	6.0
(OHSE)	1 oz	75	280	6.0
(Oscar Mayer)	1.6 oz	144	500	13.3
(Oscar Mayer)	1 oz	90	311	8.3
(Oscar Mayer)	.53 oz	48	167	4.4
(Oscar Mayer) 'Light'	1 oz	64	310	5.4
(Oscar Mayer) Wisconsin made, ring	1 oz	90	230	8.0
(Oscar Mayer) w/cheese	.8 oz	74	232	6.8
(Pilgrim's Pride)	1 oz	59	228	4.4
Beef				
(Boar's Head)	1 oz	74	270	7.0
(Boar's Head) 'Premium' low cholesterol	1 oz	70	270	7.0
(Eckrich)	1 oz	90	230	8.0
(Eckrich) 'Thick Sliced'	1.5 oz	130	340	12.0
(Hebrew National) 'Original Deli Style'	1 oz	90	330	3.0
(Hormel) 'Coarse Ground, 1 lb'	2 oz	160	576	14.0
(Hormel) 'Perma-Fresh'	2 slices	170	592	16.0
(JM)	1 oz	90	350	8.0
(Kahn's)	1 slice	90	300	8.0
(Kahn's) 'Family Pack'	1 slice	70	230	6.0
(Kahn's) 'Giant'	1 slice	90	300	8.0
(Kahn's) 'Pounder'	1 slice	90	300	8.0
(OHSE)	1 oz	85	310	8.0

Food Name	Serv. Size	Total Cal.	Sod. MGS	Fat GMS
(Oscar Mayer)	1.6 oz	143	489	13.3
(Oscar Mayer)	1 oz	89	304	8.2
(Oscar Mayer)	.53 oz	48	163	4.4
(Oscar Mayer) 'Light'	1 oz	64	316	5.3
Beef and cheddar *(Kahn's)*	1 slice	90	320	8.0
Beef and pork				
(Boar's Head)	1 oz	80	250	7.0
(Boar's Head) 'Premium' low cholesterol	1 oz	80	250	7.0
(Healthy Deli)	1 oz	41	200	2.0
Chicken				
(Health Valley)	1 slice	85	329	8.0
(OHSE) '15% Chicken'	1 oz	90	320	8.0
(Tyson)	1 slice	44	185	0.5
Garlic				
(Eckrich)	1 oz	90	230	9.0
(Eckrich) w/cheese	1 oz	90	250	9.0
(JM)	1 oz	90	350	8.0
(Kahn's)	1 slice	90	290	8.0
Ham				
(Boar's Head)	1 oz	40	(mq)	2.0
(Oscar Mayer)	1 oz	90	301	8.3
Lebanon *(Oscar Mayer)*	.8 oz	46	302	2.9
Turkey				
(Butterball) 'Cold Cuts'	1 oz	70	370	6.0
(Butterball) 'Deli/Slice 'n Serve'	1 oz	70	370	6.0
(Butterball) 'Turkey Variety Pak'	.75 oz	50	280	4.0
(Healthy Choice) beef and pork	.75-oz slice	25	240	1.0
(Longacre) sliced	1 oz	61	270	5.0
(Louis Rich)	1 oz	61	244	5.0
(Louis Rich) mild	1 oz	59	298	4.5
(Norbest) 'Blue Label' 2-2.5 lb	1 oz	68	331	5.6
(Norbest) 'Blue Label' 5-lb	1 oz	57	339	4.4
(OHSE)	1 oz	70	300	6.0
CHICKEN				
Breast				
(Healthy Choice) deli-thin, 97% fat-free	1 slice	10	90	<1.0
(Healthy Choice) oven roasted, 97% fat-free	1 slice	30	300	<1.0
(Healthy Favorites) oven roasted	.4-oz slice	12	110	<1.0
(Hillshire Farm) smoked 'Deli Select'	1 oz	31	290	0.2
(Longacre) 'Premium'	1 oz	45	280	3.0
(Louis Rich) hickory smoked	1 oz	30	356	0.8

Food Name	Serv. Size	Total Cal.	Sod. MGS	Fat GMS
(Louis Rich) oven roasted 'Deluxe'	1 oz	30	332	0.8
(Louis Rich) oven roasted 'Thin Sliced'	.4-oz slice	12	130	0.3
(Louis Rich) oven roasted, white meat	1-oz slice	35	301	1.7
(Mr. Turkey)	1 oz	32	242	1.1
(Oscar Mayer) oven roasted	1 oz	29	414	0.7
(Oscar Mayer) smoked	1 oz	25	397	0.4
(Oscar Mayer) 'Thin Sliced'	.4-oz slice	13	151	0.4
(Tyson) hickory smoked	1 slice	25	195	1.0
(Tyson) honey flavored	1 slice	25	na	1.0
(Tyson) mesquite, oven roasted	1 slice	25	na	1.0
(Tyson) oven roasted	1 slice	25	185	0.5
Roll				
(Longacre)	1 oz	60	210	5.0
(Pilgrim's Pride)	1-oz slice	35	260	1.2
(Tyson)	1 slice	26	153	0.5
CHICKEN HAM				
(Healthy Favorites) smoked, w/natural juices	.4-oz slice	13	116	0.4
(Pilgrim's Pride)	1-oz slice	35	430	1.8
CORNED BEEF LOAF, jellied	1 oz	43	270	1.7
DUTCH BRAND LOAF				
	1-oz slice	68	354	5.1
(Eckrich)	1-oz slice	70	300	6.0
(Eckrich) 'Lean Supreme'	1-oz slice	60	250	4.0
(Eckrich) 'Smorgas Pac'	1-oz slice	70	300	6.0
(Kahn's)	1 slice	80	280	7.0
HAM				
(Boar's Head) boiled 'Deluxe'	1 oz	28	275	<1.0
(Boar's Head) deluxe 'Deli-trition' low cholesterol	1 oz	30	280	1.0
(Boar's Head) 'Lower Salt'	1 oz	28	250	<1.0
(Healthy Deli)	1 oz	33	120	0.8
(Healthy Deli) 'Deluxe'	1 oz	31	245	0.9
(Healthy Deli) 'Lessalt'	1 oz	32	190	0.9
(Healthy Deli) 'Light AM'	1 oz	27	200	0.6
(Healthy Deli) 'Taverne'	1 oz	31	210	0.8
(Healthy Favorites) boiled	.4-oz slice	12	115	<1.0
(Hormel)	1 oz	29	344	1.0
(JM)	1 oz	30	360	1.0
(JM) 'Slice 'n Eat' 93% fat-free	2 oz	70	630	3.0
(JM) 'Slice 'n Eat' 95% fat-free, presliced	2 slices	60	620	2.0
(Jones Dairy Farm) 'Farm'	1 slice	50	381	1.1
(Jones Dairy Farm) 'Four Family Ham'	1 oz	35	298	1.2

Food Name	Serv. Size	Total Cal.	Sod. MGS	Fat GMS
(Kahn's)	1 slice	30	360	1.0
(Kahn's) 'Low Salt'	1 slice	30	290	1.0
(Light & Lean)	2 slices	50	(mq)	2.0
(OHSE)	1 oz	30	260	1.0
(Oscar Mayer) boiled	.75-oz slice	23	275	0.7
(Oscar Mayer) boiled 'Thin Sliced'	.4 oz	13	157	0.4
(Oscar Mayer) 'Breakfast Ham'	1.5-oz slice	47	582	1.5
(Oscar Mayer) 'Jubilee'	1 oz	43	365	2.4
(Oscar Mayer) 'Lower Salt'	.7 oz	23	174	0.7
(Swift) 'Premium Hostess'	1 oz	30	330	1.0
(Swift) 'Premium Sugar Plum'	1 oz	30	280	1.0
Baked				
(Healthy Deli) Virginia	1 oz	34	245	0.9
(Healthy Deli) Virginia 'Lessalt'	1 oz	32	19	0.9
(Louis Rich) 'Carving Board' cooked w/natural juices	22 grams	22	248	0.4
(Oscar Mayer)	.75-oz slice	21	238	0.5
Barbecue (Light & Lean)	2 slices	50	(mq)	2.0
Black Forest (Healthy Deli)	1 oz	32	220	0.6
Cajun (Hillshire Farm) 'Deli Select'	1 oz	31	350	0.9
Capocollo (Hormel)	1 oz	80	273	6.0
Chopped				
(Eckrich)	1-oz slice	45	350	2.0
(Eckrich) 'Lean Supreme'	1-oz slice	35	350	2.0
(Hormel) 'Black Label'	1 oz	70	326	6.0
(Hormel) 'Perma-Fresh'	2 slices	88	685	5.0
(JM)	1-oz slice	80	370	7.0
(Kahn's)	1 slice	50	360	3.0
(Light & Lean)	2 slices	70	(mq)	4.0
(OHSE)	1 oz	65	260	5.0
(Oscar Mayer)	1-oz slice	41	303	2.3
Glazed (Light & Lean)	2 slices	50	(mq)	2.0
Honey				
(Boar's Head) 'Premium' low cholesterol	1 oz	35	310	1.0
(Carl Buddig) 'Lean' smoked, chopped	1 oz	50	na	3.0
(Healthy Choice) 'Deli-Thin'	1 slice	10	90	<1.0
(Healthy Deli) 'Honey Valley'	1 oz	31	26	0.8
(Healthy Favorites)	1 slice	14	115	<1.0
(Healthy Favorites) 'Breakfast' water added	1 oz	30	346	0.9
(Hillshire Farm) 'Deli Select'	1 oz	31	270	0.9
(Louis Rich) 'Carving Board' w/natural juices	2.1 oz	68	761	1.9
(Oscar Mayer)	.75-oz slice	23	268	0.6

Food Name	Serv. Size	Total Cal.	Sod. MGS	Fat GMS
(Oscar Mayer) 'Thin Sliced'	.4-oz slice	13	153	0.4
Jalapeño (Healthy Deli)	1 oz	25	260	0.6
Peppered				
(Light & Lean) black pepper	2 slices	50	(mq)	2.0
(Light & Lean) red pepper	2 slices	50	(mq)	2.0
(Oscar Mayer) cracked black pepper	.75-oz slice	22	284	0.8
Prosciutto (Hormel)	1 oz	90	502	7.0
Smoked				
(Carl Buddig) 'Lean' chopped	1 oz	50	na	3.0
(Eckrich) 'Slender Sliced'	1 oz	40	360	2.0
(Healthy Favorites)	.4-oz slice	14	115	<1.0
(Hillshire Farm) 'Deli Select'	1 oz	31	300	0.9
(JM) golden	2 oz	80	630	5.0
(JM) golden, water added	2 oz	70	810	2.0
(Light & Lean)	2 slices	50	(mq)	2.0
(Louis Rich) 'Carving Board' w/natural juices	10 grams	11	124	0.4
(OHSE) '95% Fat-Free'	1 oz	30	310	1.0
(Oscar Mayer)	.75-oz slice	22	266	0.7
HAM AND CHEESE LOAF				
(Eckrich)	1-oz slice	50	300	4.0
(Hormel) '8 lb' canned	3 oz	260	1135	22.0
(Hormel) 'Perma-Fresh'	2 slices	110	668	7.0
(Kahn's)	1 slice	70	310	6.0
(Light & Lean)	2 slices	90	(mq)	6.0
(OHSE)	1 oz	65	190	5.0
(Oscar Mayer)	1-oz slice	66	358	5.0
HEAD CHEESE (Oscar Mayer)	1-oz slice	55	347	4.0
HONEY LOAF				
(Eckrich)	1-oz slice	35	280	1.0
(Eckrich) 'Smorgas Pac'	1-oz slice	35	280	1.0
(Hormel) 'Perma-Fresh'	2 slices	90	584	5.0
(Kahn's)	1 slice	40	320	2.0
(Oscar Mayer)	1-oz slice	34	378	1.0
IOWA BRAND LOAF (Hormel) 'Perma-Fresh'	2 slices	90	607	6.0
JALAPEÑO LOAF (Kahn's)	1 slice	70	340	6.0
LIVER CHEESE				
(JM)	1-oz slice	70	(mq)	6.0
(Oscar Mayer)	1.34-oz slice	116	418	10.0
LIVER LOAF				
(Hormel) 'Perma-Fresh'	2 slices	160	704	13.0
(Kahn's)	1 slice	170	370	15.0

Food Name	Serv. Size	Total Cal.	Sod. MGS	Fat GMS
LIVERWURST/liver sausage				
(Hickory Farms)	1 oz	97	249	9.0
(Jones Dairy Farm) 'Farm Club'	1 oz	80	254	6.3
(Jones Dairy Farm) 'Farm Slices'	1 slice	75	186	6.6
LOAF				
(Hormel) spiced, canned	3 oz	280	1110	26.0
(JM) 'P&B'	1-oz slice	70	330	5.0
(Kahn's) 'P&B'	1 slice	40	270	2.0
(OHSE)	1 oz	75	320	6.0
MACARONI AND CHEESE LOAF				
(Eckrich)	1-oz slice	75	320	6.0
(OHSE)	1 oz	60	310	3.0
OLD-FASHIONED LOAF (Oscar Mayer)	1-oz slice	62	337	4.0
OLIVE LOAF				
(Eckrich)	1-oz slice	80	320	6.0
(Hormel) 'Perma-Fresh'	2 slices	110	810	7.0
(Oscar Mayer)	1-oz slice	63	392	4.3
PASTRAMI. See also TURKEY PASTRAMI.				
(Boar's Head) 'Round'	1 oz	40	270	1.5
(Carl Buddig) 'Lean' smoked, chopped, sliced	1 oz	40	na	2.0
(Healthy Deli) 'Deli Round'	1 oz	34	195	1.1
(Hillshire Farm) 'Deli Select'	1 oz	31	290	0.4
(Oscar Mayer)	.6-oz slice	16	217	0.3
PEPPERED BEEF				
(Carl Buddig) 'Lean' smoked, chopped, sliced	1 oz	40	na	2.0
(Eckrich)	1-oz slice	35	340	1.0
(Kahn's)	1 slice	40	340	2.0
(Oscar Mayer)	1-oz slice	39	367	1.5
PICKLE LOAF				
(Eckrich)	1-oz slice	80	270	6.0
(Eckrich) 'Smorgas-Pac'	1-oz slice	80	270	6.0
(Hormel) 'Perma-Fresh'	2 slices	102	752	7.0
(Kahn's)	1 slice	80	280	7.0
(Kahn's) 'Family-Pack'	1 slice	70	220	6.0
(Light & Lean)	2 slices	100	(mq)	6.0
(OHSE)	1 oz	60	330	4.0
PICKLE-PIMIENTO LOAF (Oscar Mayer)	1-oz slice	66	370	4.1
PORK LOAF (Eckrich) 'Slender Sliced'	1 oz	45	320	2.0
ROAST BEEF				
(Healthy Deli)	1 oz	30	130	0.4
(Healthy Deli) Italian	1 oz	31	140	0.6

Food Name	Serv. Size	Total Cal.	Sod. MGS	Fat GMS
(Hillshire Farm) 'Deli Select' oven roasted, cured, w/o added ingredients	1 oz	31	270	0.5
(Oscar Mayer) 'Thin Sliced'	.4-oz slice	14	55	0.4
SALAMI. See also TURKEY SALAMI.				
Beef				
(Boar's Head)	1 oz	60	288	4.0
(Hebrew National) 'Original Deli-Style'	1 oz	80	230	7.0
(Hormel) 'Party'	1 oz	90	399	8.0
(Hormel) 'Perma-Fresh'	2 slices	50	219	5.0
(Kahn's)	1 slice	70	250	6.0
(Kahn's) 'Family-Pack'	1 slice	60	190	5.0
(Oscar Mayer) 'Machiaeh Brand'	.8-oz slice	60	265	5.0
Beer				
(Eckrich)	1-oz slice	70	330	6.0
(Oscar Mayer) 'Salami for Beer'	.8-oz slice	50	286	4.0
(Oscar Mayer) 'Salami for Beer' beef	.8-oz slice	63	280	5.6
Cooked				
(Kahn's)	1 slice	60	300	4.0
(OHSE)	1 oz	65	330	5.0
Cotto				
(Eckrich)	1-oz slice	70	380	6.0
(Eckrich) beef	1.3 oz	100	460	8.0
(Hormel) 'Club'	1 oz	100	385	5.0
(Hormel) 'Perma-Fresh'	2 slices	105	750	7.0
(JM)	1-oz slice	80	270	6.0
(Kahn's) 'Family Pack'	1 slice	45	230	3.0
(Light & Lean)	2 slices	80	(mq)	6.0
(Oscar Mayer) beef	.8-oz slice	45	296	3.4
(Oscar Mayer) beef	.5-oz slice	29	193	2.2
Dry or hard				
(Hickory Farms)	1 oz	120	535	10.0
(Hormel)	1 oz	110	468	10.0
(Hormel) 'Homeland'	1 oz	117	448	10.0
(Hormel) 'National Brand'	1 oz	120	463	11.0
(Hormel) 'Perma-Fresh'	2 slices	80	339	7.0
(Hormel) 'Sliced'	1 oz	110	483	10.0
(JM)	1-oz slice	110	580	9.0
(Oscar Mayer)	.8-oz slice	52	287	4.2
(Oscar Mayer) 'Hard'	.3-oz slice	33	169	2.8
Genoa				
(Hickory Farms)	1 oz	110	540	10.0

Food Name	Serv. Size	Total Cal.	Sod. MGS	Fat GMS
(Hormel)	1 oz	110	456	10.0
(Hormel) 'DiLusso'	1 oz	100	443	8.0
(Hormel) 'Gran Valore'	1 oz	110	453	10.0
(Hormel) 'San Remo Brand'	1 oz	118	541	10.0
(JM)	1-oz slice	100	540	8.0
(Oscar Mayer)	.3-oz slice	34	162	2.8
Piccolo (Hormel) 'Stick'	1 oz	120	512	11.0
SOUSE LOAF (Kahn's)	1 slice	90	190	7.0
SPICE LOAF				
(Hormel) canned	3 oz	280	1110	26.0
(Hormel) 'Perma-Fresh'	2 slices	118	702	9.0
(JM)	1-oz slice	70	370	6.0
(Kahn's) 'Family Pack'	1 slice	70	180	6.0
(Kahn's) 'Family Pack' beef	1 slice	60	200	5.0
(Kahn's) 'Luncheon Loaf'	1 slice	80	240	7.0
TURKEY. See also TURKEY LOAF/ROLL.				
(Boar's Head) 'Premium' skin on, low cholesterol	1 oz	35	200	1.0
(Butterball) 'Cold Cuts'	1 oz	30	230	1.0
(Butterball) 'Deli No Salt Added'	1 oz	45	15	2.0
(Healthy Choice) 97% fat-free	1 slice	30	240	1.0
(Healthy Deli) 'Gourmet'	1 oz	28	170	0.6
(Healthy Deli) 'Lessalt'	1 oz	25	140	0.5
(Hormel) 'Perma-Fresh'	2 slices	60	484	2.0
(Light & Lean)	2 slices	60	(mq)	2.0
(Longacre) 'Catering'	1 oz	35	280	1.0
(Norbest) white meat, diced	1 oz	31	318	0.9
(Tyson)	1 slice	20	136	0.4
Honey roasted (Healthy Deli)	1 oz	28	170	0.5
Honey roasted and smoked				
(Healthy Choice)	1-oz slice	35	230	1.0
(Healthy Choice) deli thin	1 slice	10	70	<1.0
Oven roasted				
(Healthy Choice) deli thin	1 slice	10	85	<1.0
(Healthy Choice) 97% fat-free	1-oz slice	30	290	1.0
(Healthy Deli)	1 oz	26	180	0.2
(Healthy Favorites)	.4-oz slice	12	100	<1.0
(Hillshire Farm) 'Deli Select'	1 oz	31	340	0.2
(Longacre)	1 oz	30	280	1.0
(Louis Rich)	1 oz	31	323	0.8
(Louis Rich) 'Thin Sliced'	.4-oz slice	12	127	0.3
(Oscar Mayer)	.75-oz slice	23	290	0.5

ood Name	Serv. Size	Total Cal.	Sod. MGS	Fat GMS
(Oscar Mayer) 'Thin Sliced'	.4-oz slice	12	151	0.2
Smoked				
(Butterball) 'Cold Cuts'	1 oz	35	190	1.0
(Butterball) 'Turkey Variety Pak'	.75 oz	25	160	1.0
(Carl Buttig) 'Lean' chopped, sliced	1 oz	50	na	3.0
(Healthy Choice) deli thin	1 slice	10	70	<1.0
(Healthy Deli) '3 lb'	1 oz	29	180	0.5
(Healthy Favorites)	1 slice	12	80	<1.0
(Hillshire Farm) 'Deli Select'	1 oz	31	290	0.2
(Longacre)	1 oz	26	260	<1.0
(Louis Rich)	.74-oz slice	21	211	0.3
(Louis Rich) 'Thin Sliced'	.4-oz slice	11	111	0.1
(Mr. Turkey)	1 oz	31	332	0.7
(Oscar Mayer)	.75-oz slice	20	300	0.2
URKEY HAM				
(Butterball) 'Cold Cuts'	1 oz	35	390	1.0
(Butterball) 'Deli Thin'	1 oz	35	390	1.0
(Butterball) 'Slice 'n Serve'	1 oz	35	340	2.0
(Longacre)	1 oz	33	310	1.0
(Longacre) lean lite 'Deli'	1 oz	37	150	2.0
(Louis Rich) cured	1 oz	25	217	0.7
Chopped				
(Louis Rich)	1 oz	46	289	2.8
(Louis Rich) 92% fat-free, water added	1 oz	45	285	2.0
(Mr. Turkey)	1 oz	37	301	1.6
Chunk (Longacre)	1 oz	37	360	2.0
Honey cured				
(Butterball) 'Cold Cuts'	1 oz	35	380	1.0
(Butterball) 'Cold Cuts' chopped	1 oz	35	290	1.0
(Butterball) 'Slice 'n Serve'	1 oz	40	370	2.0
(Louis Rich) 96% fat-free	1 oz	25	215	<1.0
(Mr. Turkey)	1 oz	32	286	1.0
(Mr. Turkey) breakfast	1 oz	33	306	1.3
(Mr. Turkey) buffet style	1 oz	32	340	1.3
(Mr. Turkey) 'Chub'	1 oz	32	340	1.3
Smoked				
(Louis Rich) 'Deli Thin' 96% fat-free	1 slice	15	110	<1.0
(Louis Rich) 94% fat-free, water added	1 oz	35	300	2.0
(Louis Rich) 'Round'	1 oz	34	300	1.2
(Louis Rich) 'Round' 95% fat-free, water added	1-oz slice	30	325	1.0
(Louis Rich) 'Square'	.75-oz slice	24	213	0.7

Food Name	Serv. Size	Total Cal.	Sod. MGS	Fa GMS
(Louis Rich) 'Square' 96% fat free	1-oz slice	25	215	<1.0
(Louis Rich) 'Thin Sliced'	.4-oz slice	12	111	0.4
(Louis Rich) 'Water Added'	1 oz	33	294	1.4
(Norbest) roll	1 oz	31	346	1.1
(Norbest) thigh meat, Canadian style	1 oz	35	331	1.4
(Norbest) thigh meat 'Gold Label'	1 oz	27	297	0.7
(Norbest) thigh meat 'Tavern' 5-6 lb, whole	1 oz	27	311	0.8
(Norbest) thigh meat 'Tavern' 2-2.5 lb, half	1 oz	29	312	0.9
(OHSE)	1 oz	30	370	1.0
TURKEY LOAF/ROLL				
(Louis Rich)	1 oz	45	270	2.8
(Louis Rich) 89% fat-free	1 oz	45	270	3.0
(Mr. Turkey) spiced	1 oz	51	292	3.6
TURKEY PASTRAMI				
(Butterball) 'Cold Cuts'	1 oz	30	290	1.0
(Butterball) 'Slice 'n Serve'	1 oz	35	320	1.0
(Longacre)	1 oz	32	260	1.0
(Louis Rich) 'Deli Thin' 96% fat-free	1 oz	10	125	<1.0
(Louis Rich) 'Round'	1 oz	32	288	1.1
(Louis Rich) 'Round' 96% fat-free	1 oz	35	290	1.0
(Louis Rich) 'Square'	1 oz	24	262	0.7
(Louis Rich) 'Square' 96% fat-free	1 oz	25	260	<1.0
(Louis Rich) Thin Sliced	1 oz	11	125	0.4
(Mr. Turkey)	1 oz	28	383	0.9
(Norbest) '5-6 lb Slab'	1 oz	29	305	0.6
(Norbest) '3 lb'	1 oz	29	302	0.8
TURKEY SALAMI				
(Butterball) 'Cold Cuts'	1 oz	50	350	4.0
(Butterball) 'Deli/Slice 'n Serve'	1 oz	50	350	4.0
(Butterball) 'Turkey Variety Pak'	.75 oz	40	260	3.0
(Longacre)	1 oz	52	290	4.0
(Louis Rich)	1 oz	54	263	4.0
(Louis Rich) cotto	1 oz	53	271	3.8
(Louis Rich) cotto, 85% fat-free	1-oz slice	55	275	4.0
(Louis Rich) 85% fat-free	1-oz slice	55	265	4.0
(Mr. Turkey) cotto	1 oz	45	369	2.9
(Norbest) 'Blue Label' 5 lb	1 oz	46	270	2.9
(Norbest) 'Blue Label' 2-2.5 lb	1 oz	45	314	2.6
(OHSE)	1 oz	50	260	3.0
LUNCHEON MEAT, ALTERNATIVE				
(Worthington) canned 'Numete' 1/2-inch slice	2.4 oz	160	570	11.0

Food Name	Serv. Size	Total Cal.	Sod. MGS	Fat GMS
(Worthington) canned 'Protose' 1/2-inch slice	2.7 oz	180	470	8.0
BOLOGNA TYPE				
(Worthington) frozen 'Bolono' approx .65-oz slices	2 slices	60	390	2.0
SALAMI TYPE				
(Worthington) frozen, roll, approx 1.5-oz slices	2 slices	90	760	5.0
(Worthington) frozen, sliced, approx 1.3-oz slices	2 slices	80	675	4.0
LUNCHEON MEAT, CANNED. See also POTTED MEAT SPREAD; SANDWICH SPREAD.				
(Armour) 'Treet'	2 oz	200	840	17.0
(Armour) 'Treet' low salt	2 oz	190	610	16.0
(Spam)	1 oz	86	376	8.0
(Spam) less salt	2 oz	176	550	15.0
(Spam) lite	2 oz	140	560	12.0
(Spam) smoke flavored	2 oz	170	774	15.0
(Spam) w/cheese chunks	2 oz	170	811	16.0
LUNCHEON MEAT COMBINATIONS, PACKAGED				
(Eckrich) 'Lunch Makers'				
ham/Swiss cheese/crackers	1 pc each	40	170	2.0
turkey/cheddar cheese/crackers	1 pc each	40	160	2.0
(Hillshire Farms) 'Lunch 'n Munch'				
bologna/American cheese/crackers/Snickers	4.25 oz	490	1110	34.0
bologna/American cheese/crackers/Snickers/6-oz drink ...	4.25 oz	590	1130	34.0
chicken/Monterey jack cheese/crackers/Snickers	4.25 oz	400	1080	23.0
ham/cheddar cheese/crackers/Snickers	4.25 oz	400	1010	23.0
ham/cheddar cheese/crackers/Snickers/6-oz drink	4.25 oz	500	1030	23.0
ham/Swiss cheese/crackers/Oreo	4.1 oz	370	1160	21.0
turkey/cheddar cheese/crackers/brownie	4.5 oz	400	1240	22.0
(Louis Rich) 'Lunch Breaks'				
turkey/cheddar cheese	1 pkg	410	1715	26.0
turkey/Monterey jack cheese	1 pkg	400	1665	25.0
turkey ham/Swiss cheese	1 pkg	380	1875	22.0
turkey salami/cheddar cheese	1 pkg	430	1595	29.0
(Oscar Mayer) 'Lunchables'				
bologna/American cheese/crackers	4.5 oz	480	1520	38.0
chicken/Monterey jack cheese/crackers/pudding	6.2 oz	380	1200	21.0
ham/American cheese/crackers/pudding	6.2 oz	410	1380	23.0
ham/cheddar cheese/crackers	4.5 oz	370	1680	25.0
ham/Swiss cheese/crackers	4.5 oz	340	1660	21.0
ham/Swiss cheese/crackers/cookie	4.2 oz	380	1370	23.0
turkey/cheddar cheese/crackers	4.5 oz	360	1600	22.0
turkey/cheddar cheese/crackers/trail mix	5 oz	460	1230	26.0
turkey/ham, deluxe variety pak	5.1 oz	370	1760	20.0

Food Name	Serv. Size	Total Cal.	Sod. MGS	Fat GMS
turkey/Monterey jack cheese/wheat crackers	4.5 oz	360	1600	22.0

M

Food Name	Serv. Size	Total Cal.	Sod. MGS	Fat GMS
MACADAMIA NUT/bushnut				
in shell	1 lb	987	6	103.7
shelled	1 cup	941	7	98.8
shelled	1 oz	199	1	20.9
shelled, oil roasted, chopped	1 cup	790	8	84.2
shelled, oil roasted, kernels, 10-12	1 oz	204	2	21.7
shelled, oil roasted, whole or halves	1 cup	962	9	102.5
shelled, w/salt *(Maunu Loa)*	1 oz	210	75	21.0
MACADAMIA NUT BUTTER, roasted *(Maranatha Natural)*	2 tbsp	200	5	19.0
MACARONI. See PASTA.				
MACARONI ENTRÉE, CANNED				
(Chef Boyardee) shells	7.5 oz	150	930	1.0
(Heinz)	7.5 oz	190	1105	8.0
W/BEEF, IN TOMATO SAUCE				
(Heinz)	7.5 oz	200	850	8.0
(Pathmark) 'No Frills'	7.5 oz	200	880	8.0
W/CHEESE				
(Chef Boyardee)	7.5 oz	170	970	2.0
(Franco-American)	7 3/8 oz	170	870	6.0
Shells w/cheddar *(Lipton)* 'Hearty Ones'	11 oz	367	1406	7.4
MACARONI ENTRÉE, FROZEN				
W/BEEF				
(Swanson)	12 oz	370	930	15.0
(Weight Watchers)	9 oz	220	510	4.0
In tomato sauce *(Lean Cuisine)*	10 oz	250	540	6.0
W/tomatoes *(Stouffer's)*	11.5-oz pkg	340	1440	12.0
W/CHEESE				
(Banquet)	10 oz	420	450	20.0
(Banquet) 'Casserole'	8 oz	350	930	17.0
(Banquet) 'Family Entrees'	8 oz	290	(mq)	13.0
(Budget Gourmet) 'Side Dish'	5.3 oz	210	370	8.0
(Freezer Queen) 'Family Side Dish'	4 oz	110	420	2.0
(Green Giant)	5.7 oz	220	480	8.0
(Green Giant) 'One Serving'	5.7 oz	230	590	9.0
(Healthy Choice)	9 oz	280	520	6.0

Food Name	Serv. Size	Total Cal.	Sod. MGS	Fat GMS
(Healthy Choice)	8.5 oz	260	490	5.0
(Kid Cuisine) 'Mega Meal'	12.45 oz	470	1270	13.0
(Lean Cuisine)	9 oz	290	550	9.0
(Myers)	3.5 oz	168	516	9.0
(Stouffer's) 76-oz pkg	9.5 oz	440	1150	24.0
(Stouffer's) 12-oz pkg	6 oz	250	640	13.0
(Swanson)	12.25 oz	370	1070	15.0
(Swanson) 'Homestyle Recipe'	10 oz	390	1150	19.0
Casserole (Morton)	6.5 oz	290	760	14.0
Organic (Amy's Kitchen)	9 oz	452	434	18.0
Pot pie (Swanson)	7 oz	200	740	8.0
W/broccoli (Lean Cuisine) 'Lunch Express'	9.75 oz	240	560	7.0
W/cheddar and parmesan cheese (Budget Gourmet) 'Light & Healthy'	10.5 oz	330	760	8.0
W/mini franks (Kid Cuisine)	9 oz	380	1000	14.0
W/soy cheese, organic (Amy's Kitchen)	9 oz	380	500	14.0
W/three cheeses (Weight Watchers)	9 oz	280	550	6.0
MACARONI ENTRÉE, MICROWAVE				
W/BEEF				
(Chef Boyardee) 'Beefaroni'	7.5 oz	220	1145	7.0
(Chef Boyardee) elbows in sauce	7.5 oz	210	1000	7.0
(Kid's Kitchen) microwave cup	7.5 oz	200	780	6.0
(Nalley's)	7.5 oz	180	900	3.0
W/CHEESE				
(Chef Boyardee)	7.5 oz	180	970	5.0
(Hormel) micro cup	7.5 oz	189	874	6.0
(Kid's Kitchen) microwave cup	7.5 oz	260	650	11.0
(Libby's) 'Diner' microwave cup	7.5 oz	360	1020	22.0
(Lunch Bucket) microwave cup	7.5 oz	210	990	9.0
MACARONI ENTRÉE, PACKAGED				
(Ultra Slim Fast) w/cheese sauce, prepared	1 cup	230	700	3.0
MACARONI ENTRÉE MIX				
(Kraft) 'Dinner' spirals, prepared	3/4 cup	340	600	18.0
MEXICAN STYLE				
(Velveeta) 'Touch of Mexico' shells, prepared	1/2 cup	210	630	8.0
W/CHEDDAR				
(Fantastic Foods) 'Traditional' prepared	1/2 cup	112	205	2.0
(Golden Grain) dry mix	1.81 oz	190	466	2.1
(Golden Grain) prepared	1 serving	310	620	15.0
W/CHEESE				
(Kraft) 'Deluxe Dinner' prepared	3/4 cup	260	590	8.0

Food Name	Serv. Size	Total Cal.	Sod. MGS	Fat GMS
(Kraft) 'Dinner' prepared	3/4 cup	290	530	13.0
(Kraft) 'Dinomac Dinner' prepared	3/4 cup	310	560	14.0
(Kraft) 'Family Size Dinner' prepared	3/4 cup	290	490	13.0
(Kraft) 'Teddy Bears Dinner' prepared	3/4 cup	310	560	14.0
(Kraft) 'Wild Wheels Dinner' prepared	3/4 cup	310	560	14.0
(Velveeta) 'Bits of Bacon' shells, w/bacon, prepared	1/2 cup	240	690	10.0
(Velveeta) shells, prepared	1/2 cup	210	570	8.0
W/CURRY				
(Tofu Classics) 'Shells 'n Curry' prepared w/tofu	1/2 cup	103	275	3.0
(Tofu Classics) 'Shells 'n Curry' prepared w/tofu and salted butter	1/2 cup	143	330	7.0
W/PARMESAN AND HERBS				
(Fantastic Foods) prepared w/whole milk	1/2 cup	109	264	2.0
MACE				
ground	1 oz	135	23	9.2
ground	1 tbsp	25	4	1.7
ground	1 tsp	8	1	0.6
ground *(Durkee)*	1 tsp	10	0	<0.1
ground *(Laurel Leaf)*	1 tsp	10	0	<0.1
ground *(Spice Islands)*	1 tsp	10	1	0.7
MACKEREL				
ATLANTIC				
baked	4 oz	297	94	20.2
broiled	4 oz	297	94	20.2
dry-heat cooked	3 oz	223	71	15.1
microwaved	4 oz	297	94	20.2
raw	1 lb	929	408	63.0
raw	3 oz	174	77	11.8
raw	1 oz	58	26	3.9
JACK, mixed species				
canned, drained	1 cup	296	720	12.0
canned, drained	4 oz	177	430	7.1
dry-heat cooked	3 oz	171	94	8.6
raw	1 lb	712	391	35.8
raw	3 oz	134	73	6.7
raw	1 oz	45	24	2.2
KING				
dry-heat cooked	3 oz	114	173	2.2
raw	1 lb	475	717	9.1
raw	3 oz	89	134	1.7
raw	1 oz	30	45	0.6

ood Name	Serv. Size	Total Cal.	Sod. MGS	Fat GMS
PACIFIC, mixed species				
dry-heat cooked	3 oz	171	94	8.6
raw	1 lb	712	391	35.8
raw	3 oz	134	73	6.7
raw	1 oz	45	24	2.2
SPANISH				
baked	5.1-oz fillet	230	96	9.2
baked	4 oz	179	75	7.2
broiled	5.1-oz fillet	230	96	9.2
broiled	4 oz	179	75	7.2
dry-heat cooked	3 oz	134	56	5.4
microwaved	5.1-oz fillet	230	96	9.2
microwaved	4 oz	179	75	7.2
raw	1 lb	631	266	28.6
raw	3 oz	118	50	5.3
raw	1 oz	39	17	1.8
MAHI MAHI/dolphin fish				
dry-heat cooked	3 oz	93	96	0.8
raw	1 lb	387	397	3.2
raw	3 oz	72	75	0.6
raw	1 oz	24	25	0.2
Fillet portions *(Peter Pan Seafoods)* raw	3.5 oz	85	88	0.7
MALT, DRY	1 oz	103	22	0.5
MALT EXTRACT, DRIED	1 oz	103	22	0.0
MALT LIQUOR. See ALCOHOLIC BEVERAGES.				
MALT SYRUP				
	1 cup	1221	134	0.0
	1 tbsp	76	8	0.0
MALTED MILK DRINK MIX. See also BREAKFAST DRINK MIX, INSTANT.				
CHOCOLATE FLAVOR				
	1 oz	106	71	1.1
w/added nutrients	1 oz	101	168	1.0
w/added nutrients	4-5 heap tsp	75	125	0.7
(Carnation)	3 heap tsp	80	55	0.8
(Kraft) 'Instant'	3 tsp	90	45	1.0
NATURAL FLAVOR				
	1 oz	117	140	2.2
w/added nutrients	1 oz	109	115	0.8
w/added nutrients	4-5 heap tsp	80	85	0.6
w/o added nutrients	3/4 cup	87	104	1.7
(Carnation) 'Original'	3 heap tsp	90	100	1.8

Food Name	Serv. Size	Total Cal.	Sod. MGS	Fat GMS
(Kraft) 'Instant'	3 tsp	90	100	2.0
MAMMY APPLE				
peeled, w/o seeds	1 oz	14	4	0.1
raw	3 1/2 oz	51	15	0.5
raw, trimmed, approx 3.1 lb	1 med	431	127	4.2
raw, untrimmed	1 lb	139	41	1.4
MANDARIN ORANGE				
fresh, whole, approx 2 3/8-inch diam, 4.1 oz	1 med	37	1	0.2
peeled, w/o seeds	1 oz	12	<1	0.1
sections, w/o membrane	1/2 cup	43	2	0.2
untrimmed	1 lb	144	4	0.6
MANDARIN ORANGE, CANNED *(Dole)* sections	1/2 cup	70	10	<1.0
MANDARIN ORANGE DRINK				
w/papaya *(Tropicana)* 'Twister'	6 oz	90	30	<1.0
MANGO				
peeled, w/o seed	1 oz	18	1	0.1
raw, sliced	1 cup	107	3	0.5
raw, trimmed, approx 10.6 oz	1 med	135	4	0.6
raw, untrimmed	1 lb	204	6	0.9
sliced, chilled, in jar *(Sun Fresh)*	3.5 oz	89	11	0.3
MANGO DRINK				
(Arizona) 'Mucho Mango Cowboy Cocktail'	8 oz	100	20	0.0
(Kern's) nectar, canned or bottled	6 oz	100	0	0.0
(Libby's) nectar, canned or bottled	6 oz	110	0	0.0
MANGO FLAVOR DRINK MIX *(Tang)* prepared	6 oz	80	0	0.0
MANGO-PEACH JUICE *(Knudsen & Sons)*	8 oz	110	na	0.0
MANHATTAN. See ALCOHOLIC BEVERAGES.				
MANICOTTI ENTRÉE, FROZEN				
(Budget Gourmet) cheese, w/meat sauce	10 oz	450	920	26.0
(Buitoni) 'Single Serving'	9 oz	470	830	14.0
(Celentano)	8 oz	300	690	11.0
(Celentano) cheese, w/sauce	10 oz	380	860	14.0
(Celentano) cheese, w/sauce	7 oz	360	580	16.0
(Celentano) low-fat, 'Great Choice'	10 oz	250	675	3.0
(Healthy Choice) cheese	9.25 oz	220	310	3.0
(Le Menu) three cheese	11.75 oz	390	870	15.0
(Legume) cheese, w/spinach, tofu, and sauce	11 oz	260	650	7.0
(Legume) cheese, w/tofu and sauce, 'Classic'	8 oz	220	370	11.0
(Weight Watchers) cheese	9.25 oz	260	510	8.0
MANICOTTI NOODLE. See PASTA.				
MANIOC. See CASSAVA.				

Food Name	Serv. Size	Total Cal.	Sod. MGS	Fat GMS
MAPLE SYRUP. See also PANCAKE SYRUP.				
....	1 cup	825	28	0.6
....	1 tbsp	52	2	0.0
(Knudsen & Sons) 'Fruit 'N Maple'	1 oz	105	na	<1.0
(Maple House) 100% pure	1 oz	100	4	0.0
MARGARINE				
hydrogenated and regular corn oil	1 stick	815	1070	91.3
hydrogenated and regular corn oil	1 tsp	34	44	3.8
hydrogenated and regular soybean oil	1 stick	815	1070	91.3
hydrogenated and regular soybean oil	1 tsp	34	44	3.8
hydrogenated safflower and soybean oil	1 stick	815	1070	91.3
hydrogenated safflower and soybean oil	1 tsp	34	44	3.8
hydrogenated soybean and cottonseed oil	1 stick	815	1070	91.3
hydrogenated soybean and cottonseed oil	1 tsp	34	44	3.8
(A&P)				
'Corn Oil Quarters'	1 tbsp	100	105	11.0
'Premium'	1 tbsp	100	110	11.0
(Ann Page) 'Quarters'	1 tbsp	100	110	11.0
(Blue Bonnet) stick	1 tbsp	100	95	11.0
(Canoleo) 100% canola oil, all natural, dairy-free	1 tbsp	100	120	11.0
(Fleischmann's)				
reduced calorie, 'Diet'	1 tbsp	50	50	6.0
stick	1 tbsp	100	95	11.0
unsalted, stick	1 tbsp	100	0	11.0
(Hain)				
safflower oil	1 tbsp	100	170	11.0
safflower oil, unsalted	1 tbsp	100	5	11.0
(Hollywood)				
safflower oil	1 tbsp	100	130	11.0
safflower oil, unsalted	1 tbsp	100	2	11.0
(Imperial) reduced calorie, 'Diet'	1 tbsp	50	140	6.0
(Land O'Lakes)				
premium, corn oil, stick	1 tsp	35	35	4.0
regular, soy oil, stick	1 tsp	35	35	4.0
tub	1 tsp	35	35	4.0
(Mazola)				
reduced calorie, 'Diet'	1 tbsp	50	130	6.0
regular	1 tbsp	100	100	11.0
unsalted	1 tbsp	100	0	11.0
(Nucoa)	1 tbsp	100	160	11.0
(Parkay)	1 tbsp	100	105	11.0

Food Name	Serv. Size	Total Cal.	Sod. MGS	F GM
(Quincy's)	1 oz	204	268	22
(Spectrum Naturals) non-hydrogenated canola oil, 100% dairy-free	1 tbsp	94	84	11.
MARGARINE, ALTERNATIVE				
hydrogenated and regular corn oil	1 cup	801	2226	90
hydrogenated and regular corn oil	1 tsp	17	46	1
hydrogenated soybean and cottonseed oil	1 cup	801	2226	90
hydrogenated soybean and cottonseed oil	1 tsp	17	46	1.
hydrogenated soybean oil	1 cup	801	2226	90
hydrogenated soybean oil	1 tsp	17	46	1
MARGARINE, SOFT				
(A&P) bowl	1 tbsp	100	105	11
(Blue Bonnet)	1 tbsp	100	95	11.
(Chiffon)				
cup	1 tbsp	90	95	10
stick	1 tbsp	100	105	11.
unsalted	1 tbsp	90	0	10
(Fleischmann's)				
lightly salted	1 tbsp	100	95	11
unsalted	1 tbsp	100	0	11
(Imperial)	1 tbsp	100	95	11
(Nucoa)	1 tbsp	90	150	10
(Parkay)				
reduced calorie, 'Diet'	1 tbsp	50	110	6
regular	1 tbsp	100	105	11
'Squeezable'	1 tbsp	90	110	10
MARGARINE, WHIPPED				
(Blue Bonnet) stick	1 tbsp	70	70	7
(Chiffon)	1 tbsp	70	80	8
(Fleischmann's)				
lightly salted	1 tbsp	70	60	7
unsalted	1 tbsp	70	0	7
(Miracle Brand)				
cup	1 tbsp	60	70	7
stick	1 tbsp	70	65	7
(Parkay)				
cup	1 tbsp	70	70	7
stick	1 tbsp	70	65	7
MARGARINE SPREAD				
hydrogenated soybean and cottonseed oil, tub	1 cup	1236	2276	139
hydrogenated soybean and cottonseed oil, tub	1 tsp	26	48	2

Food Name	Serv. Size	Total Cal.	Sod. MGS	Fat GMS
hydrogenated soybean and hydrogenated and regular palm oils	1 tsp	26	48	2.9
hydrogenated soybean and hydrogenated and regular palm oils, tub	1 cup	1236	2276	139.2
hydrogenated soybean and palm oil, stick	1 cup	1236	2276	139.2
hydrogenated soybean and palm oil, stick	1 tsp	26	48	2.9
60% corn oil margarine, 40% butter	1 stick	811	1014	91.2
60% corn oil margarine, 40% butter	1 tsp	36	45	4.0
(Blue Bonnet)				
48% vegetable oil	1 tbsp	60	115	6.0
75% vegetable oil	1 tbsp	90	95	11.0
whipped, 60% vegetable oil	1 tbsp	80	100	8.0
(Blue Bonnet) 'Better Blend'				
soft	1 tbsp	90	95	11.0
stick	1 tbsp	90	95	11.0
unsalted	1 tbsp	90	0	11.0
(Country Crock)				
'Churn Style' stick	1 tbsp	80	55	9.0
regular	1 tbsp	60	110	7.0
(Fleischmann's) 'Move Over Butter'	1 tbsp	90	100	10.0
(Hollywood) soft	1 tbsp	90	135	10.0
(Imperial) 'Light'	1 tbsp	60	110	6.0
(Kraft) 'Touch of Butter'				
bowl	1 tbsp	50	110	6.0
stick	1 tbsp	90	110	10.0
(Land O'Lakes) 'Country Morning Blend'				
stick	1 tsp	35	35	4.0
tub	1 tsp	30	25	3.0
unsalted, stick	1 tsp	35	0	4.0
unsalted, tub	1 tsp	30	0	3.0
(Land O'Lakes) 'Country Morning Light'				
stick	1 tsp	20	30	2.0
tub	1 tsp	20	25	2.0
(Land O'Lakes) w/sweet cream				
stick	1 tsp	30	35	4.0
tub	1 tsp	25	25	3.0
unsalted	1 tsp	30	0	4.0
(Mazola) 'Corn Oil Light'	1 tbsp	50	100	6.0
(Nucoa) 'Heart Beat'				
regular	1 tbsp	25	110	3.0
unsalted	1 tbsp	24	0	3.0

Food Name	Serv. Size	Total Cal.	Sod. MGS	Fat GMS
(P&Q) 60% vegetable oil, stick	1 tbsp	80	105	8.0
(Parkay) 50% vegetable oil	1 tbsp	60	110	7.0
(Promise)				
'Extra Light'	1 tbsp	50	50	6.0
regular	1 tbsp	90	90	10.0
'Ultra' fat-free	1 tbsp	5	90	0.0
'Ultra' w/canola oil	1 tbsp	35	50	4.0
(Shedd's Spread) 52% vegetable oil	1 tbsp	60	110	7.0
(Van Den Bergh Foods) 'I Can't Believe It's Not Butter'				
light	1 tbsp	60	110	7.0
regular	1 tbsp	90	0	10.0
(Weight Watchers)				
'Country Cottage Farms' extra light, sweet, unsalted	1 tbsp	50	0	6.0
'Country Cottage Farms' extra light, tub	1 tbsp	45	75	4.0
'Country Cottage Farms' light	1 tbsp	50	130	6.0
light, stick	1 tbsp	60	130	7.0
MARGARITA. See ALCOHOLIC BEVERAGES.				
MARINADE. See individual listings.				
MARJORAM				
dried	1 oz	77	22	2.0
dried	1 tbsp	5	1	0.1
dried	1 tsp	2	0	0.0
dried *(Durkee)*	1 tsp	2	0	tr
dried *(Laurel Leaf)*	1 tsp	2	0	tr
dried *(Spice Islands)*	1 tsp	4	1	0.1
MARMALADE, ORANGE				
(Finast)	2 tsp	35	0	0.0
(Knott's Berry Farm) light, w/NutraSweet	1 tsp	8	0	0.0
(Knudsen & Sons)	2 tsp	35	na	<1.0
(Smucker's)	1 tsp	18	0	0.0
(Smucker's) low-sugar	1 tsp	8	0	0.0
(Smucker's) 'Simply Fruit'	1 tsp	16	0	0.0
(Smucker's) sweet, natural ingredients	1 tsp	18	0	0.0
MARSHMALLOW				
(Campfire) large	2 pieces	40	10	0.0
(FunMallows)	1 piece	30	15	0.0
(FunMallows) miniature	10 pieces	18	5	0.0
(Kraft) 'Jet Puffed'	1 piece	25	5	0.0
(Kraft) miniature	10 pieces	18	5	0.0
MARSHMALLOW CREME TOPPING				
(Finast)	1 oz	95	45	0.0

Food Name	Serv. Size	Total Cal.	Sod. MGS	Fat GMS
(Kraft)	1 oz	90	20	0.0
(Marshmallow Fluff)	1 tsp	59	12	0.0
(Smucker's)	2 tbsp	120	0	0.0
MATZO. See cracker.				
MAYONNAISE				
(Bama)	1 tbsp	100	65	11.0
(Bennett's) 'Real'	1 tbsp	110	65	12.0
(Best Foods)	1 tbsp	100	80	11.0
(Cains)	1 tbsp	100	80	11.0
(Finast)	1 tbsp	100	80	11.0
(Hain) cold processed	1 tbsp	110	70	12.0
(Hellmann's)	1 tbsp	100	80	11.0
(Hollywood)	1 tbsp	110	80	12.0
(Kraft) 'Real'	1 tbsp	100	70	12.0
(Pathmark)	1 tbsp	100	70	11.0
(Pathmark) 'No Frills'	1 tbsp	100	75	11.0
(Rokeach)	1 tbsp	100	70	11.0
(Westbrae)	1 tbsp	100	75	11.0
CANOLA				
(Hain)	1 tbsp	100	100	11.0
(Hollywood)	1 tbsp	100	100	11.0
(Spectrum Naturals)	1 tbsp	100	80	12.0
(Spectrum Naturals) 'Lite Mayo'	1 tbsp	35	60	3.0
(Westbrae)	1 tbsp	100	75	11.0
LOW-SODIUM				
(Hain) 'Real No Salt Added'	1 tbsp	110	0	12.0
(Weight Watchers) 'Low Sodium'	1 tbsp	50	45	5.0
REDUCED CALORIE				
(Best Foods) 'Light'	1 tbsp	50	115	5.0
(Estee)	1 tbsp	50	80	5.0
(Featherweight)	1 tbsp	30	40	2.0
(Finast) 'Lite'	1 tbsp	40	100	4.0
(Hain) 'Light Low Sodium'	1 tbsp	60	95	6.0
(Hellmann's) 'Light'	1 tbsp	50	115	5.0
(Janet Lee) 'Light'	1 tbsp	50	115	5.0
(Kraft) 'Light'	1 tbsp	50	110	5.0
(Pathmark)	1 tbsp	40	100	4.0
(Smart Beat) 'Golden Corn Light'	1 tbsp	40	110	4.0
(Weight Watchers) 'Light'	1 tbsp	50	100	5.0
SAFFLOWER				
(Hain)	1 tbsp	110	70	12.0

Food Name	Serv. Size	Total Cal.	Sod. MGS	Fat GMS
(Hollywood)	1 tbsp	100	75	12.0
SAFFLOWER AND SOYBEAN	1 tbsp	99	78	11.0
SOYBEAN				
	1 tbsp	99	78	11.0
(Featherweight) 'Soyamaise'	1 tbsp	100	3	11.0
MAYONNAISE, ALTERNATIVE				
(Best Foods) 'Cholesterol Free'	1 tbsp	50	80	5.0
(Hain) 'Eggless No Salt Added'	1 tbsp	110	5	12.0
(Hellman's) 'Cholesterol Free'	1 tbsp	50	80	5.0
(Kraft) 'Free'	1 tbsp	8	125	0.0
(Nucoa) 'Heart Beat'	1 tbsp	40	110	4.0
(Weight Watchers) 'Cholesterol Free'	1 tbsp	50	90	5.0
CANOLA *(Hain)* reduced calorie	1 tbsp	60	160	5.0
MILK CREAM	1 tbsp	15	76	0.8
SOYBEAN	1 tbsp	35	75	2.9
SUNFLOWER *(Life)* 'All Natural'	1 tbsp	71	3	8.0
TOFU *(Nasoya)* 'Nayonaise'	1 tbsp	40	50	4.0
MEAT. See individual listings.				
MEAT, ALTERNATIVE. See also individual listings.				
chops *(Worthington)* 'Choplets' canned	2 slices	100	350	2.0
cutlet *(Worthington)* 'Multigrain' canned	2 slices	90	260	1.0
unflavored *(Heartline)* lite	.5 oz	22	135	0.0
MEAT EXTENDER				
soybean	1 cup	275	8	2.6
soybean	1 oz	88	3	0.8
MEAT LOAF ENTRÉE, FROZEN				
(Armour) 'Classics'	11.25 oz	360	1170	17.0
(Banquet)	11 oz	440	770	27.0
(Banquet) 'Cookin' Bags'	4 oz	200	(mq)	14.0
(Freezer Queen)	10 oz	350	910	19.0
(Freezer Queen) 'Family Suppers' w/tomato sauce	7 oz	230	850	13.0
(Healthy Choice) low-fat, low-cholesterol	12 oz	340	560	8.0
(Lean Cuisine) w/macaroni and cheese	9 3/8 oz	280	540	8.0
(Morton)	10 oz	310	1520	17.0
(Stouffer's) homestyle, in gravy, w/whipped potatoes	9 7/8 oz	370	860	20.0
(Swanson)	10.75 oz	360	960	15.0
MEAT LOAF ENTRÉE, PACKAGED				
(Dinty Moore) 'American Classics' w/mashed potatoes and gravy	10 oz	262	na	9.0
(Ultra Slim Fast) w/tomato sauce	10.5 oz	340	780	9.0

Food Name	Serv. Size	Total Cal.	Sod. MGS	Fat GMS
MEAT LOAF MIX				
(Hunt's) 'Meatloaf Fixins'	2.222 oz	23	600	0.4
(Lipton) 'Microeasy' homestyle	1/4 pkg	90	630	1.0
MEAT LOAF MIX, ALTERNATIVE				
(Natural) 'Touch Loaf Mix' vegetarian	4 oz	180	25	7.0
MEAT LOAF SEASONING				
(French's)	1/8 pkg	20	620	0.0
(Lawry's) 'Seasoning Blends'	1 pkg	355	6547	1.2
(Schilling) 'Bag 'n Season'	1 pkg	111	3090	0.7
MEAT MARINADE MIX (French's)	1/8 pkg	10	540	0.0
MEAT STICKS				
smoked	1 oz	156	420	14.1
smoked	1 stick	109	293	9.8
MEAT TENDERIZER				
(Tone's) seasoned	1 tsp	7	1650	0.2
(Tone's) unseasoned	1 tsp	7	1760	0.2
MEATBALL, ALTERNATIVE				
vegetarian (Worthington) 'Non-Meat Balls'	3 pieces	100	220	6.0
MEATBALL ENTRÉE				
Canned, stew				
(Chef Boyardee)	8 oz	350	1315	24.0
(Dinty Moore)	8 oz	240	980	16.0
Frozen, BBQ homestyle (Banquet) 'Healthy Balance'	10.25 oz	270	680	5.0
Microwave (Dinty Moore) microwave cup	7.5 oz	240	980	16.0
MEATBALL SEASONING (French's) dry mix	1/4 pkg	35	830	0.0
MELBA TOAST. See CRACKER.				
MELON. See individual listings.				
MESQUITE MARINADE (Lawry's)	2 tbsp	24	4142	0.4
MESQUITE SEASONING (Tone's)	1 tsp	13	467	<.1
MEXICAN FOODS. See individual listings.				
MEXICAN POTATO. See JICAMA.				
MEXICAN SEASONING (Tone's)	1 tsp	6	4185	0.1
MEXICAN STYLE DINNER, FROZEN. See also individual listings.				
(Banquet)	12 oz	490	2000	18.0
(Banquet) combination	12 oz	520	1980	17.0
(Morton)	10 oz	300	1390	10.0
(Patio)	13.25 oz	540	1940	25.0
(Patio) 'Fiesta'	12.25 oz	470	2040	20.0
(Swanson) combination	14.25 oz	490	1760	18.0
(Swanson) 'Hungry Man'	20.25 oz	820	2080	41.0
(Van de Kamp's)	1/2 pkg	220	640	10.0

Food Name	Serv. Size	Total Cal.	Sod. MGS	Fat GMS
MILK, ALTERNATIVE. See RICE BEVERAGE; SOY BEVERAGE.				
MILK, COW'S, CANNED				
CONDENSED, SWEETENED				
. . . .	1 cup	982	389	26.6
(Borden)	1/3 cup	320	115	8.0
(Carnation)	1/3 cup	320	110	8.0
(Diehl) 'Jerzee'	1/3 cup	320	120	9.0
(Eagle)	1/2 cup	320	120	9.0
EVAPORATED				
. . . .	1/2 cup	169	133	9.5
(Carnation)	1/2 cup	170	135	10.0
(Diehl)	1/2 cup	170	135	10.0
(Finast)	1/2 cup	170	135	10.0
(IGA)	1/2 cup	170	140	10.0
(Pathmark)	1/2 cup	170	140	10.9
(Pet)	1/2 cup	170	140	10.0
Filled (Pet)	1/2 cup	150	140	8.0
Low-fat (Carnation)	1/2 cup	110	140	3.0
Skim				
. . . .	1/2 cup	100	147	0.3
(Carnation) 'Lite'	1/2 cup	100	150	<1.0
(Diehl)	1/2 cup	100	150	<1.0
(Finast)	1/2 cup	100	150	<1.0
(Pathmark)	1/2 cup	100	15	0.0
(Pet) 'Lite'	1/2 cup	100	150	<1.0
MILK, COW'S, DRY				
LOW-FAT				
(Milkman)	1/4 pkg	90	125	1.0
(Milkman) reconstituted	1 quart	380	500	5.0
SKIM				
(Alba) reconstituted	8 oz	80	190	0.0
(Carnation)	1/3 cup	80	125	0.0
(Lucerne)	1/3 cup	80	125	0.0
(Saco Foods)	5 tbsp	80	125	<1.0
(Sanalac) 'Dairy Fresh' reconstituted	8 oz	80	85	0.1
(Sanalac) reconstituted	9.03 oz	80	110	0.1
(Weight Watchers) 'Dairy Creamer'	1 pkt	10	15	0.0
MILK, COW'S, FLUID				
WHOLE				
(A&P)	1 cup	150	120	8.0
(Borden)	1 cup	150	130	8.0

od Name	Serv. Size	Total Cal.	Sod. MGS	Fat GMS
(Borden) 'Hi-Calcium'	1 cup	150	130	8.0
(Carnation)	1 cup	150	120	8.0
(Crowley)	1 cup	150	125	8.0
(Darigold)	1 cup	150	125	8.0
(Knudsen)	1 cup	160	180	8.0
Low-sodium	1 cup	149	6	8.4
3.7% fat	1 cup	157	119	8.9
3.3% fat	1 cup	150	120	8.1
% FAT				
	1 cup	121	122	4.7
Protein-fortified				
	1 cup	137	145	4.9
(A&P)	1 cup	120	120	5.0
(Borden) 'Hi-Protein'	1 cup	140	150	5.0
(Crowley) 'Tone Acidophilus'	1 cup	120	125	5.0
(Darigold) 'Nutrish Acidophilus'	1 cup	120	130	5.0
(Finast)	1 cup	130	130	5.0
(Knudsen) 'Sweet Acidophilus'	1 cup	140	150	5.0
(Viva)	1 cup	120	125	5.0
W/non-fat milk solids added	1 cup	125	128	4.7
% FAT				
	1 cup	102	123	2.6
(Crowley)	1 cup	100	130	2.0
Protein-fortified				
	1 cup	119	143	2.9
(A&P)	1 cup	100	120	3.0
(Borden)	1 cup	100	130	2.0
(Crowley)	1 cup	120	150	2.0
(Crowley) 'Lactaid'	1 cup	100	125	2.0
(Darigold)	1 cup	100	130	2.0
(Knudsen) 'Nice n' Light'	1 cup	130	153	3.0
W/calcium added (Darigold)	1 cup	100	130	2.0
W/non-fat milk solids added	1 cup	104	128	2.4
KIM				
	1 cup	86	126	0.4
Protein-fortified				
(A&P)	1 cup	90	125	<1.0
(Borden)	1 cup	90	130	1.0
(Borden) 'Skim-Line'	1 cup	100	150	1.0
(Crowley)	1 cup	90	130	<1.0
(Darigold) 'Trim'	1 cup	80	130	1.0

Food Name	Serv. Size	Total Cal.	Sod. MGS	Fo GM
(Knudsen)	1 cup	80	130	(mo
(Weight Watchers)	1 cup	90	140	<1.
W/non-fat milk solids added	1 cup	90	130	0.
W/vitamin A added	1 cup	86	126	0.
MILK, GOAT'S				
evaporated (Meyenberg) canned, undiluted	4 oz	143	86	7.
fluid, whole	1 cup	168	122	10.
fluid, whole	1 oz	20	14	1.
MILK, LACTOSE-REDUCED				
2% FAT				
(Lactaid) 70% lactose reduced, w/vitamins A and D	1 cup	130	125	5.
(Lucerne) 70% lactose reduced, w/vitamins A and D	1 cup	120	110	5.
1% FAT				
(First Alternative) lactose free	1 cup	80	180	2.
SKIM				
(Lactaid) 70% lactose reduced, w/calcium and vitamins A and D	1 cup	80	125	0.
(Lactaid) 70% lactose reduced, w/vitamins A and D	1 cup	80	125	0.
(Lactaid 100) lactose free, w/vitamins A and D	1 cup	80	125	0.
(Lucerne) 70% lactose reduced, w/vitamins A and D	1 cup	80	115	0.
MILKFISH. See AWA.				
MILKSHAKE				
chocolate, thick	10.6 oz	356	333	8.
vanilla, thick	11 oz	350	299	9.
(MicroMagic) chocolate, frozen	11.5 oz	340	120	8.
(MicroMagic) chocolate, frozen	7 oz	200	70	4.
(MicroMagic) strawberry, frozen	11.5 oz	340	120	9.
(MicroMagic) vanilla, frozen	11.5 oz	380	150	13.
MILKSHAKE MIX				
(Alba '77) chocolate, 'Fit'N' prepared	6 oz	346	709	2.
(Alba '77) chocolate marshmallow, 'Fit'N' prepared	6 oz	346	690	3.
(Alba '77) double fudge, frosty, 'Fit'N' prepared	6 oz	346	728	3.
(Alba '77) strawberry, 'Fit'N' prepared	6 oz	333	805	1.
(Alba '77) vanilla, 'Fit'N' prepared	6 oz	333	810	1.
(Weight Watchers) chocolate fudge	1 pkt	70	170	1.
(Weight Watchers) orange sherbet	1 pkt	70	210	0.
MILLET				
pearl, cooked	1/2 cup	143	2	1.
pearl, cooked	4 oz	135	2	1.
pearl, raw	1/2 cup	378	5	4.
pearl, raw	1 oz	107	1	1.

Food Name	Serv. Size	Total Cal.	Sod. MGS	Fat GMS
pearl, raw, hulled *(Arrowhead Mills)*	1 oz	90	1	1.0
Proso/hog millet, whole grain	3 1/2 oz	327	1	2.9
MILLET FLOUR, whole grain *(Arrowhead Mills)*	2 oz	185	1	2.0
MINCEMEAT. See PIE FILLING.				
MISO				
	1/2 cup	284	5033	8.4
	1 oz	58	1034	1.7
w/barley malt/mugi-koji	1 oz	56	1191	1.2
w/rice malt, dark yellow/kome-koji	1 oz	53	1446	1.6
w/rice malt, sweet/kome-koji	1 oz	62	680	0.9
w/soybean malt/mame-koji	1 oz	62	1219	3.9
(Eden Foods) barley/mugi, organic	1 tbsp	25	760	<1.0
(Eden Foods) brown rice/genmai, organic	1 tbsp	25	810	1.0
(Eden Foods) rice/shiro, organic	1 tbsp	35	410	1.0
(Eden Foods) soybean and rice/kome, organic	1 tbsp	25	850	1.0
(Eden Foods) soybean/hacho, organic	1 tbsp	35	600	2.0
(Westbrae) barley, pasteurized	1 tsp	12	310	0.0
(Westbrae) brown rice, pasteurized	1 tsp	10	360	0.0
(Westbrae) red, instant	.35 oz	35	750	1.0
(Westbrae) red, pasteurized	1 tsp	10	375	0.0
(Westbrae) soybean, pasteurized	1 tsp	12	265	0.0
(Westbrae) soybean/hacho	1 tsp	14	240	0.0
(Westbrae) white, instant	.35 oz	35	740	1.0
MOLASSES				
	1 cup	872	121	0.3
	1 tbsp	53	7	0.0
Barbados	1 cup	889	49	0.0
Barbados	1 oz	111	6	0.0
1st extraction/light	1 cup	827	49	0.0
1st extraction/light	1 oz	103	6	0.0
2nd extraction/medium	1 cup	761	121	0.0
2nd extraction/medium	1 oz	95	15	0.0
3rd extraction/blackstrap	1 cup	771	180	0.0
3rd extraction/blackstrap	1 tbsp	47	11	0.0
(Br'er Rabbit) dark	1 oz	110	20	0.0
(Br'er Rabbit) light	1 oz	110	15	0.0
(Grandma's) mild flavor, gold	1 tbsp	70	28	0.0
(Grandma's) robust flavor, green	1 tbsp	70	57	0.0
(LaChoy) bead	.7055 oz	52	48	0.0
(LaChoy) bead	1/2 tsp	7	1	0.0

Food Name	Serv. Size	Total Cal.	Sod. MGS	Fat GMS
MONKFISH/angler fish/bellyfish/frogfish/goosefish/lotte/sea devil				
dry-heat cooked	3 oz	82	20	1.7
raw	1 lb	343	84	6.9
raw	3 oz	65	15	1.3
raw	1 oz	22	5	0.4
MONOSODIUM GLUTAMATE/MSG				
flavor enhancer *(Tone's)* 'MSG'	1 tsp	0	638	0.0
MOSTACCIOLI. See PASTA.				
MOSTACCIOLI ENTRÉE				
(Banquet) frozen, w/meat sauce 'Family Entrees'	7 oz	170	(mq)	3.0
MOUNTAIN YAM. See YAM.				
MOUSSE *(Estee)* orange chocolate	1/2 cup	70	50	3.0
MOUSSE, FROZEN				
(Weight Watchers) 'Sweet Celebrations' chocolate	2.5 oz	170	190	6.0
(Weight Watchers) 'Sweet Celebrations' praline pecan	2.75 oz	190	180	7.0
(Weight Watchers) 'Sweet Celebrations' triple chocolate caramel	2.75 oz	170	120	4.0
MOUSSE MIX				
(Jell-O) 'Rich & Luscious' chocolate, dry mix	1 pkg	110	45	3.0
(Jell-O) 'Rich & Luscious' chocolate, prepared	1/2 cup	150	75	6.0
(Jell-O) 'Rich & Luscious' chocolate fudge, dry mix	1 pkg	110	45	4.0
(Jell-O) 'Rich & Luscious' chocolate fudge, prepared	1/2 cup	140	75	6.0
(Weight Watchers) chocolate, prepared w/skim milk	1/2 cup	60	45	3.0
(Weight Watchers) chocolate cheesecake, prepared w/skim milk	1/2 cup	60	75	2.0
(Weight Watchers) chocolate raspberry, prepared w/skim milk	1/2 cup	60	75	3.0
(Weight Watchers) white chocolate almond, prepared w/skim milk	1/2 cup	60	50	3.0
MSG. See MONOSODIUM GLUTAMATE.				
MUFFIN. See also ENGLISH MUFFIN.				
APPLE				
(Awrey's) 1.5-oz muffin	1 muffin	130	210	6.0
(Awrey's) 2.5-oz muffin	1 muffin	220	350	10.0
(Awrey's) w/banana nut 'Grande' 4.2-oz muffin	1 muffin	260	160	16.0
(Hostess) w/banana walnut, mini muffin	5 muffins	160	90	9.0
APPLE SPICE				
(Dunkin' Donuts) 3.5-oz muffin	1 muffin	300	360	8.0
(Health Valley) fat-free	1 muffin	130	110	0.0
APPLE STREUSEL *(Awrey's)* 'Grande' 4.2-oz muffin	1 muffin	340	540	13.0
BANANA *(Health Valley)* fat-free	1 muffin	130	110	0.0

Food Name	Serv. Size	Total Cal.	Sod. MGS	Fat GMS
BANANA NUT				
(Break Cake) .5-oz muffin	1 muffin	60	45	3.0
(Dunkin' Donuts) 3.6-oz muffin	1 muffin	310	410	10.0
BLUEBERRY				
(Awrey's) 1.5-oz muffin	1 muffin	130	180	5.0
(Awrey's) 2.5-oz muffin	1 muffin	210	280	8.0
(Awrey's) 'Grande' 4.2-oz muffin	1 muffin	360	480	14.0
(Break Cake)	1 muffin	60	50	3.0
(Dunkin' Donuts) 3.6-oz muffin	1 muffin	280	340	8.0
(Entenmann's)	1 muffin	200	250	8.0
(Hostess) mini muffin	5 muffins	240	180	13.0
BLUEBERRY-APPLE (Health Valley) fat-free, twin pack	1 muffin	140	100	0.0
BRAN (Dunkin' Donuts) w/raisins, 3.7-oz muffin	1 muffin	310	560	9.0
CARROT (Health Valley) fat-free, twin pack	1 muffin	130	110	0.0
CINNAMON APPLE (Hostess) mini muffin	5 muffins	260	180	16.0
CORN				
(Awrey's) 1.5-oz muffin	1 muffin	130	270	5.0
(Awrey's) 2.5-oz muffin	1 muffin	220	430	8.0
(Dunkin' Donuts) 3.4-oz muffin	1 muffin	340	560	12.0
CRANBERRY (Awrey's) 1.5-oz muffin	1 muffin	120	210	4.0
CRANBERRY NUT (Dunkin' Donuts) 3.5-oz muffin	1 muffin	290	360	9.0
OAT BRAN				
(Awrey's) 2.75-oz muffin	1 muffin	180	330	7.0
(Awrey's) pineapple raisin, 2.75-oz muffin	1 muffin	180	320	6.0
(Dunkin' Donuts) 3.4-oz muffin	1 muffin	330	450	11.0
(Hostess)	1 muffin	160	150	7.0
(Hostess) banana nut	1 muffin	140	160	5.0
(Health Valley) almond and date	1 muffin	180	81	4.0
(Health Valley) blueberry	1 muffin	180	99	4.0
(Health Valley) 'Fancy Fruit Muffins' raisin	1 muffin	180	90	5.0
RAISIN				
(Dunkin' Donuts)	1 muffin	310	560	9.0
(Wonder) 'Raisin Rounds'	1 muffin	140	280	2.0
RAISIN BRAN				
(Awrey's) 1.5-oz muffin	1 muffin	110	170	4.0
(Awrey's) 2.5-oz muffin	1 muffin	190	280	7.0
(Awrey's) 'Grande' 4.2-oz muffin	1 muffin	320	470	12.0
RAISIN SPICE (Health Valley) fat-free	1 muffin	140	100	0.0
RASPBERRY (Health Valley) fat-free, twin pack	1 muffin	130	110	0.0
RICE BRAN-RAISIN (Health Valley)	1 muffin	215	124	7.0
SOURDOUGH (Wonder)	1 muffin	130	250	1.0

Food Name	Serv. Size	Total Cal.	Sod. MGS	Fat GMS
MUFFIN, FROZEN				
APPLE SPICE				
(Healthy Choice) 2.5-oz muffin	1 muffin	190	90	4.0
(Sara Lee) 2.5-oz muffin	1 muffin	220	280	8.0
(Weight Watchers) 'Microwave' 2.5-oz muffin	1 muffin	160	260	5.0
BANANA NUT				
(Healthy Choice) 2.5-oz muffin	1 muffin	180	80	6.0
(Weight Watchers) 'Microwave' 2.5-oz muffin	1 muffin	170	250	5.0
BLUEBERRY				
(Healthy Choice) 2.5-oz muffin	1 muffin	190	110	4.0
(Pepperidge Farm) 'Old Fashioned'	1 muffin	170	250	7.0
(Sara Lee) 2.5-oz muffin	1 muffin	200	290	8.0
(Sara Lee) 'Free & Light'	1 muffin	120	140	0.0
(Weight Watchers) 'Microwave' 2.5-oz muffin	1 muffin	170	220	5.0
CHEESE STREUSEL (Sara Lee) 2.1-oz muffin	1 muffin	220	170	11.0
CHOCOLATE CHUNK (Sara Lee) 2.1-oz muffin	1 muffin	220	210	8.0
CINNAMON SWIRL (Pepperidge Farm) 'Old Fashioned'	1 muffin	190	170	6.0
CORN (Pepperidge Farm) 'Old Fashioned'	1 muffin	180	260	7.0
HONEY BRAN				
(Sara Lee) golden, 2.5-oz muffin	1 muffin	250	310	13.0
(Weight Watchers) 2.5-oz muffin	1 muffin	160	150	4.0
OAT BRAN				
(Pepperidge Farm) apple 'Old Fashioned Cholesterol Free'	1 muffin	190	200	7.0
(Sara Lee) 2.5-oz muffin	1 muffin	210	320	8.0
(Sara Lee) apple, 2.5-oz muffin	1 muffin	210	320	8.0
RAISIN BRAN				
(Pepperidge Farm) 'Old Fashioned Cholesterol Free'	1 muffin	170	280	6.0
(Sara Lee) 2.5-oz muffin	1 muffin	220	400	7.0
MUFFIN MIX				
ALMOND (Krusteaz) w/poppy seed, prepared	1 muffin	160	230	4.0
APPLE CINNAMON				
(Betty Crocker) prepared w/egg, 2% milk	1/12 recipe	120	140	4.0
(Betty Crocker) prepared w/egg white, skim milk	1/12 recipe	110	140	3.0
(General Mills) prepared	1 muffin	100	130	3.0
(General Mills) prepared w/egg, 1/2 cup 2% milk	1 muffin	120	140	4.0
(General Mills) prepared w/egg white, skim milk	1 muffin	110	140	3.0
(Krusteaz) prepared	1 muffin	180	340	3.0
(Martha White) prepared	1/16 recipe	140	250	3.0
(Martha White) prepared w/2% milk	1 muffin	140	250	3.0
APPLE STREUSEL				
(Betty Crocker) Dutch, prepared w/egg, whole milk	1/12 recipe	200	240	7.0

Food Name	Serv. Size	Total Cal.	Sod. MGS	Fat GMS
APPLESAUCE				
(Gold Medal) 'Pouch Mix' prepared w/egg, whole milk	1/6 recipe	160	240	5.0
(Robin Hood) 'Pouch Mix' prepared w/egg, whole milk	1/6 recipe	160	240	5.0
BANANA				
(Gold Medal) 'Pouch Mix' prepared w/egg, whole milk	1/12 recipe	150	240	5.0
(Robin Hood) 'Pouch Mix' prepared w/egg, whole milk	1/12 recipe	150	240	5.0
BANANA NUT				
(Betty Crocker) prepared w/egg, 2% milk	1/12 recipe	120	140	5.0
(Betty Crocker) prepared w/egg white, skim milk	1/12 recipe	110	140	4.0
(General Mills) prepared	1 muffin	110	140	4.0
(General Mills) prepared w/egg, 1/3 cup 2% milk	1 muffin	120	150	4.0
(General Mills) prepared w/egg white, skim milk	1 muffin	120	150	4.0
(Martha White) prepared w/2% milk	1 muffin	180	240	8.0
BLACKBERRY				
(Martha White) prepared	1/6 recipe	140	250	3.0
(Martha White) prepared w/2% milk	1 muffin	140	250	3.0
BLUEBERRY				
(Betty Crocker) streusel 'Bake Shop' prepared	1/12 recipe	210	230	8.0
(Betty Crocker) wild blueberries, prepared w/egg, 2% milk	1/12 recipe	120	150	4.0
(Betty Crocker) wild blueberries, prepared w/egg white, skim milk	1/12 recipe	110	150	3.0
(Duncan Hines) 'Bakery Style' prepared	1 muffin	190	250	6.0
(Duncan Hines) prepared	1 muffin	120	185	3.0
(General Mills) 'Twice the Blueberries' prepared	1 muffin	100	130	3.0
(General Mills) 'Twice the Blueberries' prepared, no cholesterol recipe	1 muffin	110	140	3.0
(General Mills) 'Twice the Blueberries' prepared w/egg, 1/2 cup 2% milk	1 muffin	120	140	4.0
(Gold Medal) 'Pouch Mix' prepared w/egg, whole milk	1/6 recipe	170	240	6.0
(Krusteaz) prepared	1 muffin	150	260	4.0
(Lovin' Lites) dry mix	1/12 pkg	100	150	1.0
(Lovin' Lites) prepared w/egg, water	1/12 recipe	100	160	1.0
(Lovin' Lites) prepared w/2 egg whites, water	1/12 recipe	100	160	1.0
(Martha White) prepared	1/6 recipe	140	260	3.0
(Martha White) prepared w/2% milk	1 muffin	140	260	3.0
(Robin Hood) 'Pouch Mix' prepared w/egg, whole milk	1/6 recipe	170	240	6.0
BRAN				
(Duncan Hines) w/honey 'Bakery Style' prepared	1 muffin	200	220	7.0
(Martha White) prepared	1/6 recipe	150	330	5.0
(Martha White) prepared w/2% milk	1 muffin	150	330	5.0

Food Name	Serv. Size	Total Cal.	Sod. MGS	Fat GMS
CARAMEL				
(Gold Medal) 'Pouch Mix' prepared w/egg, whole milk	1/6 recipe	150	250	5.0
(Robin Hood) 'Pouch Mix' prepared w/egg, whole milk	1/6 recipe	150	250	5.0
CARROT NUT				
(Betty Crocker) prepared w/egg, 2% milk	1/12 recipe	150	160	5.0
(Betty Crocker) prepared w/egg white, skim milk	1/12 recipe	150	160	5.0
CHOCOLATE CHIP				
(Betty Crocker) prepared	1/12 recipe	140	180	5.0
(Betty Crocker) prepared w/egg, 2% milk	1/12 recipe	150	180	6.0
(Krusteaz) prepared	1 muffin	200	340	5.0
CINNAMON				
(Betty Crocker) streusel, prepared w/egg, 2% milk	1/12 recipe	200	240	9.0
(Duncan Hines) swirl 'Bakery Style' prepared	1 muffin	200	245	7.0
(General Mills) streusel, prepared	1 muffin	190	220	8.0
CORN				
(Arrowhead Mills) blue, prepared	1 muffin	110	na	4.0
(Dromedary) dry mix	3 1/2 tbsp	110	250	3.0
(Dromedary) prepared	1 muffin	120	270	4.0
(Flako) prepared	1 muffin	116	351	3.3
(Gold Medal) prepared w/egg, whole milk	1/6 pkg	130	250	2.0
(Krusteaz) prepared	1 muffin	220	450	7.0
(Martha White) yellow, prepared w/water	1 muffin	160	230	3.0
(Robin Hood) prepared w/egg, whole milk	1/6 pkg	130	250	2.0
CRANBERRY-ORANGE NUT				
(Duncan Hines) 'Bakery Style' prepared	1 muffin	200	215	8.0
HONEY BRAN				
(Gold Medal) 'Pouch Mix' prepared w/egg, whole milk	1/6 recipe	170	240	6.0
(Krusteaz) prepared	1 muffin	140	290	4.0
(Martha White) w/poppy seed, prepared w/2% milk	1 muffin	200	260	9.0
(Robin Hood) 'Pouch Mix' prepared w/egg, whole milk	1/6 recipe	170	240	6.0
OAT				
(Gold Medal) 'Pouch Mix' prepared w/egg, 2% milk	1/6 recipe	150	220	5.0
(Robin Hood) 'Pouch Mix' prepared w/egg, 2% milk	1/6 recipe	150	220	5.0
OAT BRAN				
(Arrowhead Mills) apple spice, prepared	1 muffin	120	(mq)	4.0
(General Mills) prepared	1 muffin	170	230	6.0
(Krusteaz) prepared	1 muffin	190	310	5.0
(Hain) apple cinnamon, prepared	1 muffin	140	200	3.0
(Hain) banana nut, prepared	1 muffin	140	190	4.0
(Hain) raspberry spice, prepared	1 muffin	140	190	3.0

Food Name	Serv. Size	Total Cal.	Sod. MGS	Fat GMS
OATMEAL RAISIN				
(Arrowhead Mills) wheat-free, prepared	1 muffin	100	na	5.0
(Betty Crocker) prepared w/egg, 2% milk	1/8 recipe	190	240	8.0
(Betty Crocker) prepared w/egg white, skim milk	1/8 recipe	180	240	7.0
(General Mills) prepared w/egg, 1/2 cup 2% milk	1 muffin	180	250	7.0
(General Mills) prepared w/egg white, skim milk	1 muffin	170	260	6.0
ORANGEBERRY				
(Martha White) prepared	1/6 recipe	140	220	3.0
(Martha White) prepared w/2% milk	1 muffin	140	220	3.0
PECAN CRUNCH *(Duncan Hines)* 'Bakery Style' prepared	1 muffin	220	250	11.0
RASPBERRY				
(Martha White) prepared	1/6 recipe	140	184	3.0
(Martha White) prepared w/2% milk	1 muffin	140	180	3.0
STRAWBERRY				
(Arrowhead Mills) wheat bran, prepared	2 muffins	270	(mq)	7.0
(Betty Crocker) prepared w/egg, 2% milk	1/10 recipe	150	170	5.0
(Betty Crocker) prepared w/egg white, skim milk	1/10 recipe	140	170	4.0
(Martha White) prepared	1/6 recipe	140	270	3.0
(Martha White) prepared w/2% milk	1 muffin	140	270	3.0
WILD BERRY				
(General Mills) 'Light' prepared	1 muffin	90	140	<1.0
(General Mills) 'Light' prepared w/egg	1 muffin	90	140	1.0
(General Mills) prepared	1 muffin	100	140	3.0
(General Mills) prepared w/egg, 1/2 cup 2% milk	1 muffin	120	150	4.0
(General Mills) prepared w/egg white, skim milk	1 muffin	110	150	3.0
MUFFIN/PASTRY, TOASTER				
APPLE				
(Kellogg's) Dutch, 'Frosted Pop-Tarts' 1.8 oz each	1 pastry	210	200	6.0
(Pastry Poppers) fruit juice sweetened, low-sodium, 2 oz each	1 pastry	212	115	5.4
(Pillsbury) 'Toaster Strudel'	1/6 pkg	200	190	9.0
(Toastettes) 'Frosted Tarts' 1.5 oz each	1 pastry	190	170	5.0
(Toastettes) 'Tarts' 1.5 oz each	1 pastry	190	170	5.0
APPLE SPICE *(Toaster)* 'Muffins'	1 muffin	130	100	5.0
APPLE-CINNAMON				
(Pepperidge Farm) 'Croissant Toaster Tarts'	1 pastry	170	120	7.0
BANANA NUT				
(Pastry Poppers) fruit juice sweetened, low-sodium, 2 oz each	1 pastry	212	115	4.5
(Thomas') 'Toast-r-Cakes'	1 muffin	111	192	4.4
(Toaster) 'Muffins'	1 muffin	130	85	6.0

Food Name	Serv. Size	Total Cal.	Sod. MGS	Fat GMS
(Toaster) 'Strudel Breakfast Pastries'	1 pastry	190	190	8.0
BLUEBERRY				
(Kellogg's) 'Frosted Pop-Tarts' 1.8 oz each	1 pastry	210	210	6.0
(Kellogg's) 'Pop-Tarts' 1.8 oz each	1 pastry	210	210	6.0
(Pillsbury) 'Toaster Strudel'	1/6 pkg	190	210	9.0
(Thomas') 'Toast-r-Cakes'	1 muffin	108	158	3.3
(Toaster) 'Strudel Breakfast Pastries'	1 pastry	190	200	8.0
(Toaster) wild, Maine	1 muffin	120	135	3.0
(Toastettes) 'Frosted Tarts' 1.5 oz each	1 pastry	190	200	5.0
(Toastettes) 'Tarts' 1.5 oz each	1 pastry	190	200	5.0
BRAN *(Thomas')* 'Toast-r-Cakes'	1 muffin	103	163	2.9
BROWN SUGAR-CINNAMON				
(Kellogg's) 'Frosted Pop-Tarts'	1 pastry	210	180	7.0
(Toastettes) 'Frosted Tarts' 1.5 oz each	1 pastry	190	180	5.0
(Kellogg's) 'Pop-Tarts' 1.8 oz each	1 pastry	210	210	8.0
CHEESE *(Pepperidge Farm)* 'Croissant Toaster Tarts'	1 pastry	190	180	10.0
CHERRY				
(Kellogg's) 'Frosted Pop-Tarts' 1.8 oz each	1 pastry	200	220	5.0
(Kellogg's) 'Pop-Tarts' 1.8 oz each	1 pastry	210	220	6.0
(Pastry Poppers) fruit juice sweetened, low-sodium, 2 oz each	1 pastry	212	115	4.5
(Toaster) 'Strudel Breakfast Pastries'	1 pastry	190	200	9.0
(Toastettes) 'Frosted Tarts' 1.5 oz each	1 pastry	190	200	5.0
(Toastettes) 'Tarts' 1.5 oz each	1 pastry	190	200	5.0
CHOCOLATE FUDGE				
(Kellogg's) 'Frosted Pop-Tarts' 1.8 oz each	1 pastry	200	220	5.0
CHOCOLATE-VANILLA CREME				
(Kellogg's) 'Frosted Pop-Tarts' 1.8 oz each	1 pastry	200	230	5.0
CINNAMON				
(Pillsbury) 'Toaster Strudel'	1/6 pkg	200	200	10.0
(Toaster) 'Strudel Breakfast Pastries'	1 pastry	190	200	8.0
CORN				
(Thomas') 'Toast-r-Cakes'	1 muffin	120	142	4.0
(Toaster) 'Old Fashioned Muffins'	1 muffin	120	200	5.0
FRUIT PUNCH *(Toastettes)* 'Frosted Tarts' 1.5 oz each	1 pastry	190	200	5.0
FUDGE *(Toastettes)* 'Frosted Tarts' 1.5 oz each	1 pastry	200	280	5.0
GRAPE *(Kellogg's)* 'Frosted Pop-Tarts' 1.8 oz each	1 pastry	200	200	5.0
OAT BRAN *(Awrey's)* 'Toastums' w/raisins	1 muffin	130	310	5.0
PEACH-APRICOT *(Pastry Poppers)* fruit juice sweetened, low-sodium, 2 oz each	1 pastry	212	115	4.5
RAISIN BRAN *(Toaster)* 'Muffins'	1 muffin	120	220	5.0

Food Name	Serv. Size	Total Cal.	Sod. MGS	Fat GMS
RASPBERRY				
(Kellogg's) 'Frosted Pop-Tarts' 1.8 oz each	1 pastry	200	210	5.0
(Pastry Poppers) fruit juice sweetened, low-sodium, 2 oz each	1 pastry	212	115	4.5
(Toaster) 'Strudel Breakfast Pastries'	1 pastry	190	200	8.0
STRAWBERRY				
(Kellogg's) 'Frosted Pop-Tarts' 1.8 oz each	1 pastry	200	190	5.0
(Kellogg's) 'Pop-Tarts' 1.8 oz each	1 pastry	210	200	6.0
(Pastry Poppers) fruit juice sweetened, low-sodium, 2 oz each	1 pastry	212	115	4.5
(Pepperidge Farm) 'Croissant Toaster Tarts'	1 pastry	190	120	7.0
(Pillsbury) 'Toaster Strudel'	1/6 pkg	190	200	9.0
(Toaster) 'Strudel Breakfast Pastries'	1 pastry	190	200	8.0
(Toastettes) 'Frosted Tarts' 1.5 oz each	1 pastry	190	200	5.0
(Toastettes) 'Tarts' 1.5 oz each	1 pastry	190	200	5.0
MULBERRY				
raw	1 lb	197	46	1.8
raw	1 cup	60	14	0.6
raw	1/2 cup	31	7	0.3
raw	1 oz	12	3	0.1
MULLANGI. See DAIKON.				
MULLET, STRIPED				
baked	4 oz	170	81	5.5
broiled	4 oz	170	81	5.5
dry-heat cooked	3 oz	127	60	4.1
microwaved	4 oz	170	81	5.5
raw	1 lb	530	294	17.2
raw	3 oz	99	55	3.2
raw	1 oz	33	18	1.1
MUNG BEAN				
boiled	4 oz	119	2	0.4
boiled	1/2 cup	106	2	0.4
raw	1/2 cup	361	16	1.2
raw	1 oz	98	4	0.3
sprouted, boiled, drained	4 oz	24	11	0.1
sprouted, boiled, drained	1/2 cup	13	6	0.1
sprouted, raw	1 lb	136	26	0.8
sprouted, raw	1/2 cup	16	3	0.1
sprouted, raw	1 oz	9	2	0.1
sprouted, stir-fried	4 oz	57	(mq)	0.2
sprouted, stir-fried	1/2 cup	31	6	0.1

Food Name	Serv. Size	Total Cal.	Sod. MGS	Fat GMS
MUNG BEAN, CANNED				
drained	4 oz	14	(mq)	0.1
sprouted *(LaChoy)*	2 oz	8	20	0.1
sprouted, drained	1/2 cup	7	87	0.0
MUNG BEAN LONG RICE				
dehydrated	1/2 cup	246	7	0.0
dehydrated	1 oz	99	3	tr
MUNGO BEAN				
boiled	1/2 cup	94	6	0.5
raw	1/2 cup	365	27	1.9
MUSHROOM, ENOKI				
raw	1 large	2	0	0.0
raw	1 med	1	0	0.0
MUSHROOM, JAPANESE HONEY/hon shimeji				
trimmed	1 lb	136	(mq)	1.4
trimmed	1 oz	9	(mq)	<.1
MUSHROOM, OYSTER/abalone/hiritake/shimeji/tree mushroom				
(Frieda's)	1 lb	113	18	1.8
(Frieda's)	1 oz	7	1	0.1
MUSHROOM, SHIITAKE				
cooked	4 oz	62	5	0.2
cooked, pieces	1 cup	80	6	0.3
dried	1 lb	1343	60	4.5
dried	1 oz	84	4	0.3
MUSHROOM, STRAW				
(Green Giant) canned	2 oz	12	290	0.0
(Green Giant) canned, whole	1/4 cup	12	290	0.0
MUSHROOM, WHITE				
boiled, drained	4 oz	31	2	0.5
boiled, drained, pieces	1/2 cup	21	2	0.4
raw, pieces	1/2 cup	9	1	0.2
raw, trimmed	1 oz	7	1	0.1
raw, untrimmed	1 lb	111	16	1.9
Canned				
drained	4 oz	27	(mq)	0.3
pieces, drained	1/2 cup	19	331	0.2
(Allens) pieces and stems	1/2 cup	20	450	<1.0
(B In B)	1/4 cup	12	240	0.0
(B In B) w/garlic	1/4 cup	12	200	0.0
(Empress) pieces and stems	2 oz	14	260	na
(Green Giant) in butter sauce	1/2 cup	30	330	1.0

Food Name	Serv. Size	Total Cal.	Sod. MGS	Fat GMS
(Green Giant) whole, pieces, and stems	1/4 cup	12	220	0.0
Frozen				
(Birds Eye) whole 'Deluxe'	2.6 oz	20	0	0.0
(Freshlike)	3.5 oz	30	15	0.0
(Green Giant) creamy 'Right for Lunch'	9.5-oz pkg	220	860	11.0
(Stilwell) battered 'Quick Krisp'	2 oz	140	280	8.0
(Veg•All)	3.5 oz	30	15	0.0
MUSKMELON. See CANTALOUPE.				
MUSSEL, BLUE				
moist-heat cooked	4 oz	195	418	5.1
moist-heat cooked	3 oz	146	314	3.8
raw	1 lb	391	1296	10.2
raw	1 cup	129	429	3.4
raw	3 oz	73	243	1.9
MUSTARD, DRY. See MUSTARD POWDER.				
MUSTARD, PREPARED				
(Featherweight)	1 tsp	5	0	0.0
(French's) 'Medford'	1 tbsp	16	240	1.0
(Grey Poupon) 'Parisian'	1 tsp	6	55	0.0
(Kraft) 'Pure'	1 tbsp	11	160	1.0
(Life) 'English All Natural'	1 tbsp	22	2	2.0
(Westbrae) 'Mt. Fuji'	1 tbsp	16	195	1.0
DIJON				
(French's)	1 tsp	8	140	1.0
(Grey Poupon)	1 tbsp	18	450	1.0
(Grey Poupon) 'Country Style'	1 tsp	6	120	0.0
(Westbrae)	1 tbsp	16	195	1.0
HORSERADISH				
(French's)	1 tbsp	16	265	1.0
(Kraft)	1 tbsp	14	135	1.0
JALAPEÑO *(Great Impressions)*	2 tsp	7	173	0.3
ONION *(French's)*	1 tsp	8	70	0.0
SPICY				
(French's) 'Bold 'n Spicy'	1 tsp	6	50	0.0
(Gulden's) hot, 'Diablo'	.25 oz	8	55	0.0
(Gulden's) 'Spicy Brown'	.25 oz	8	45	0.0
(Heinz) 'Brown'	1 tbsp	14	115	1.0
STONE GROUND				
(Hain)	1 tbsp	14	185	1.0
(Hain) no salt added	1 tbsp	14	10	1.0
(Westbrae)	1 tbsp	16	195	1.0

Food Name	Serv. Size	Total Cal.	Sod. MGS	Fat GMS
(Westbrae) no salt added	1 tbsp	16	195	1.0
YELLOW				
(French's)	1 tbsp	10	180	1.0
(Gulden's) 'Creamy Mild'	.25 oz	6	60	0.0
(Heinz)	1 tsp	3	55	0.2
(Heinz) 'Mild'	1 tbsp	8	175	1.0
(Westbrae)	1 tbsp	16	195	1.0
MUSTARD BLEND *(Best Foods)* 'Dijonnaise'	1 tsp	12	70	1.0
MUSTARD GREENS				
boiled, drained	4 oz	17	18	0.3
boiled, drained, chopped	1/2 cup	10	11	0.2
raw, chopped	1/2 cup	7	7	0.1
raw, untrimmed	1 lb	109	107	0.8
Canned *(Allens)* chopped	1/2 cup	20	35	<1.0
Frozen				
boiled, drained	10-oz pkg	40	53	0.5
boiled, drained	4 oz	22	28	0.3
boiled, drained, chopped	1/2 cup	14	19	0.2
chopped	1/2 cup	15	21	0.2
unprepared	10-oz pkg	57	82	0.8
(Frosty Acres)	3.3 oz	20	20	0.0
(Seabrook) chopped	3.3 oz	20	20	0.0
(Southern) chopped	3.5 oz	25	40	0.3
MUSTARD OIL				
	1 cup	1927	0	218.0
	1 oz	251	0	28.4
	1 tbsp	124	0	14.0
MUSTARD POWDER				
ground *(Durkee)*	1 tsp	19	0	<0.1
ground *(Laurel Leaf)*	1 tsp	19	0	<0.1
ground *(Spice Islands)*	1 tsp	9	<1	0.6
MUSTARD SEED, YELLOW				
whole	1 oz	133	1	8.2
whole	1 tbsp	53	1	3.2
whole	1 tsp	15	0	1.0
MUSTARD SPINACH/tendergreen				
boiled, drained	4 oz	18	(mq)	0.2
boiled, drained, chopped	1/2 cup	14	13	0.2
raw, chopped	1/2 cup	16	16	0.2
raw, trimmed	1 oz	6	(mq)	0.1
raw, untrimmed	1 lb	93	(mq)	1.3

Food Name	Serv. Size	Total Cal.	Sod. MGS	Fat GMS
MUSTARD TALLOW	1 oz	256	0	28.4
MUTTON TALLOW				
	1 cup	1849	0	205.0
	1 tbsp	115	0	12.8

MUTTONFISH. See OCEAN POUT.

N

Food Name	Serv. Size	Total Cal.	Sod. MGS	Fat GMS
NACHO CHIPS. See CORN CHIPS AND SNACKS.				
NACHO SEASONING (Lawry's) 'Seasoning Blends'	1 pkg	141	2168	6.8
NAPA CABBAGE. See CABBAGE, NAPA.				
NATTO. See SOYBEAN, FERMENTED.				
NAVY BEAN				
boiled	4 oz	161	1	0.6
boiled	1/2 cup	129	1	0.5
cooked 'Michigan #1' (A&P)	1 cup	220	15	1.0
raw	1/2 cup	348	15	1.3
raw	1 oz	95	4	0.4
NAVY BEAN, CANNED				
(Allens)	1/2 cup	160	440	<1.0
(Bush's Best)	1/2 cup	60	370	0.0
(Eden Foods) organic, very low sodium	1/2 cup	70	15	<1.0
(Hunt's) w/ham 'Homestyle'	9.03 oz	239	737	2.7
NAVY BEAN, SPROUTED				
boiled, drained	4 oz	88	(mq)	0.9
raw	1 lb	306	(mq)	3.2
raw	1/2 cup	35	7	0.4
raw	1 oz	19	(mq)	0.2
NECTAR. See individual flavors.				
NECTARINE				
pitted	1 oz	14	tr	0.1
sliced	1 cup	68	0	0.6
trimmed, approx 2.5-inch diam	1 med	67	0	0.6
untrimmed (Dole)	1 med	70	0	1.0
whole	1 lb	204	1	1.9
NOODLE. See NOODLE, CHINESE; NOODLE, EGG; NOODLE, JAPANESE; PASTA.				
NOODLE, CHINESE				
cellophane, dehydrated	1 lb	1594	44	0.3
cellophane, dehydrated	2 oz	199	6	<.1

Food Name	Serv. Size	Total Cal.	Sod. MGS	Fat GMS
chow mein	1 cup	237	198	13.8
chow mein	1.5 oz	227	189	13.2
long rice, dehydrated	1 lb	1594	44	0.3
long rice, dehydrated	2 oz	199	6	<.1
NOODLE, EGG				
(NOTE: All of the following egg noodles are dry unless otherwise noted.)				
DUMPLING *(Creamette)* w/pasteurized eggs	2 oz	220	20	3.0
ENRICHED				
	2 oz	217	12	2.4
cooked	1 cup	213	11	2.3
EXTRA WIDE *(American Beauty)* enriched	2 oz	220	15	3.0
FINE				
(American Beauty) enriched	2 oz	220	15	3.0
(Herb's)	2 oz	230	5	2.0
JERUSALEM ARTICHOKE				
(De Boles)	2 oz	210	0	1.0
(De Boles) w/garlic and parsley	2 oz	210	15	1.0
MEDIUM *(American Beauty)* enriched	2 oz	220	15	3.0
PLAIN				
cooked	4 oz	151	8	1.7
(Creamette) enriched	2 oz	221	3	2.5
(Gioia)	2 oz	220	(mq)	3.0
(Golden Grain)	2 oz	210	10	2.2
(Goodman's) 'Country Style'	2 oz	220	15	3.0
(Mrs. Grass)	2 oz	220	200	3.0
(Mueller's)	2 oz	220	10	3.0
(P&R)	2 oz	220	15	3.0
(Prince)	2 oz	210	35	2.0
(San Giorgio)	2 oz	220	15	3.0
SPINACH				
cooked	4 oz	150	14	1.8
enriched	1 cup	145	27	1.7
enriched	2 oz	218	41	2.6
enriched, cooked	1 cup	211	19	2.5
SUBSTITUTE *(No Yolks)* broad	2 oz	200	25	1.0
UNENRICHED				
	2 oz	74	218	0.2
cooked	1 cup	213	11	2.3
VERY LOW SODIUM *(Ronzoni)* 'Egg Pastina'	2 oz	220	15	3.0
WIDE				
(American Beauty) enriched	2 oz	220	15	3.0

Food Name	Serv. Size	Total Cal.	Sod. MGS	Fat GMS
(Creamette) w/pasteurized eggs 'Fancy'	2 oz	220	20	3.0
(Hospitality) enriched 'Valu Pack'	1 1/4 cup	235	5	2.5
(Ronzoni) enriched 'Country Kitchen Style'	2 oz	220	15	3.0
NOODLE, JAPANESE				
GENMAI, dry *(Westbrae)*	2 oz	200	411	1.0
SOBA/BUCKWHEAT				
cooked	1 cup	113	68	0.1
dry	1 lb	1526	3593	3.2
dry	2 oz	192	451	0.4
dry *(Westbrae)*	2 oz	190	5	2.0
SOMEN/WHEAT				
cooked	1 cup	231	283	0.3
cooked	4 oz	149	183	0.2
dry	2 oz	203	1049	0.5
whole wheat, dry *(Westbrae)*	2 oz	200	375	1.0
TRADITIONAL, dry *(Westbrae)*	2 oz	190	198	2.0
UDON/WHEAT				
cooked	4 oz	115	51	0.6
dry	2 oz	159	340	0.7
whole wheat, organic, dry *(Westbrae)*	2 oz	200	375	1.0
NOODLE ENTRÉE/DISH				
(Dinty Moore)				
and chicken 'American Classics'	10 oz	230	1020	7.0
tuna casserole 'American Classics'	10 oz	240	1280	7.0
(LaChoy)				
and beef	9.03 oz	156	1332	3.5
and chicken	8.995 oz	163	859	3.3
and vegetables	9.383 oz	131	1311	1.3
chow mein	2 tbsp	140	209	6.1
chow mein, narrow	1/2 cup	150	230	8.0
chow mein, wide	1/2 cup	150	300	8.0
crispy, wide	2 tbsp	148	258	7.8
rice	1/2 cup	130	420	5.0
rice	2 tbsp	122	362	3.1
(Westbrae)				
brown rice, steamed 'Ramen'	1 oz	100	500	1.0
buckwheat, steamed 'Ramen'	1 oz	100	500	0.0
carrot, steamed 'Ramen'	1 oz	100	460	1.0
curry, steamed 'Ramen'	1 oz	100	420	1.0
five-spice, steamed 'Ramen'	1 oz	100	420	1.0
miso, steamed 'Ramen'	1 oz	100	540	1.0

Food Name	Serv. Size	Total Cal.	Sod. MGS	Fat GMS
mushroom, steamed 'Ramen'	1 oz	100	340	1.0
onion, steamed 'Ramen'	1 oz	100	460	1.0
seaweed, steamed 'Ramen'	1 oz	100	460	1.0
spinach, steamed 'Ramen'	1 oz	100	460	1.0
tofu, steamed 'Ramen'	1 oz	100	460	1.0
whole wheat, steamed 'Ramen'	1 oz	110	480	1.0
NOODLE ENTRÉE/DISH, CANNED				
(Heinz)				
and chicken	7.5 oz	160	930	7.0
w/beef, in sauce	7.5 oz	170	825	8.0
w/tuna	7.5 oz	170	950	5.0
(Nalley's)				
and chicken	7 3/8 oz	150	1000	5.0
and chicken w/vegetables	7 3/8 oz	160	1450	5.0
(Van Camp's) w/franks 'Noodle Weenee'	1 cup	245	1245	8.5
NOODLE ENTRÉE/DISH, FREEZE-DRIED				
(Mountain House) w/chicken, prepared	1 cup	270	201	10.0
NOODLE ENTRÉE/DISH, FROZEN				
(Banquet)				
and beef w/gravy 'Family Entrées'	8 oz	200	(mq)	7.0
and julienne beef w/sauce 'Family Entrées'	7 oz	170	(mq)	3.0
w/chicken	10 oz	350	460	15.0
w/chicken 'Family Favorites'	10 oz	340	455	15.0
(Stouffer's) Romanoff	6 oz	260	1260	14.0
(Swanson) w/chicken	10.5 oz	280	740	8.0
NOODLE ENTRÉE/DISH, MICROWAVE				
(Hormel) and chicken 'Micro-Cup'	7.5 oz	180	1000	8.0
(Kid's Kitchen) rings and chicken	7.5 oz	150	840	4.0
(Minute)				
Alfredo, family size, prepared w/salted butter	1/2 cup	170	670	6.0
Alfredo, single size, prepared w/salted butter	1/2 cup	160	660	5.0
chicken or chicken flavor, family size, prepared	1/2 cup	160	570	5.0
chicken or chicken flavor, single size, prepared	1/2 cup	160	610	4.0
Parmesan, family size, prepared w/salted butter	1/2 cup	170	470	6.0
Parmesan, single size, prepared w/salted butter	1/2 cup	160	460	5.0
w/cheddar cheese, family size, prepared w/salted butter	1/2 cup	160	530	7.0
w/cheddar cheese, single size, prepared w/salted butter	1/2 cup	160	520	6.0
NOODLE ENTRÉE/DISH, MIX				
(Kraft)				
cheese 'Dinner' prepared	3/4 cup	340	670	17.0
chicken flavor 'Dinner' prepared	3/4 cup	240	1050	9.0

Food Name	Serv. Size	Total Cal.	Sod. MGS	Fat GMS
(LaChoy)				
beef flavor 'Ramen' prepared	1 cup	225	865	8.0
chicken flavor 'Ramen' prepared	1 cup	200	740	7.0
(Lipton)				
Alfredo 'Noodles and Sauce' dry mix	1/4 pkg	150	510	4.0
beef 'Noodles and Sauce' dry mix	1/4 pkg	120	640	2.0
broccoli 'Noodles and Sauce' dry mix	1/4 pkg	130	430	2.0
butter 'Noodles and Sauce' dry mix	1/4 pkg	150	450	4.0
butter and herb 'Noodles and Sauce' dry mix	1/4 pkg	140	460	3.0
carbonara Alfredo 'Noodles and Sauce' dry mix	1/4 pkg	140	460	4.0
cheese 'Noodles and Sauce' dry mix	1/4 pkg	140	470	2.0
chicken flavor 'Noodles and Sauce' dry mix	1/4 pkg	130	390	2.0
Parmesan 'Noodles and Sauce' dry mix	1/4 pkg	140	410	4.0
sour cream and chives 'Noodles and Sauce' dry mix	1/4 pkg	150	440	3.0
Stroganoff 'Noodles and Sauce' dry mix	1/4 pkg	130	330	3.0
(Mueller's)				
Alfredo 'Chef's Series' prepared	1/2 cup	190	580	9.0
chicken flavor 'Chef's Series' prepared	1/2 cup	160	550	8.0
garlic and butter 'Chef's Series' prepared	1/2 cup	170	480	7.0
sour cream and chives 'Chef's Series' prepared	1/2 cup	190	470	8.0
Stroganoff 'Chef's Series' prepared	1/2 cup	190	620	9.0
(Noodle Roni)				
angel hair pasta, w/Parmesan cheese, prepared	1/2 cup	210	580	9.0
fettuccini, prepared	1/2 cup	300	560	18.0
garlic, creamy, prepared	1/2 cup	300	630	17.0
herb and butter, prepared	1/2 cup	160	290	7.0
mushroom, prepared	1/2 cup	160	550	4.0
Parmesan, prepared	1/2 cup	240	470	13.0
Parmesano 'Less Fat' prepared	1/2 cup	190	460	8.0
Romanoff, prepared	1/2 cup	240	730	11.0
Stroganoff, prepared	1/2 cup	350	1190	17.0
(Ultra Slim Fast) w/Alfredo sauce, prepared	8 oz	240	1110	4.0

NORI. See SEAWEED.

NORWAY HADDOCK. See OCEAN PERCH, ATLANTIC.

NUT TOPPING

Food Name	Serv. Size	Total Cal.	Sod. MGS	Fat GMS
(Fisher) fancy	1 oz	170	60	15.0
(Fisher) oil-roasted, w/peanuts	1 oz	160	115	14.0
(Planters)	1 oz	180	0	16.0
(Smucker's) pecan, in syrup	2 tbsp	130	0	1.0
(Smucker's) walnut, in syrup	2 tbsp	130	0	1.0

Food Name	Serv. Size	Total Cal.	Sod. MGS	Fat GMS
NUTMEG				
ground	1 oz	149	5	10.3
ground	1 tbsp	37	1	2.5
ground	1 tsp	12	0	0.8
ground (Durkee)	1 tsp	12	0	<0.1
ground (Laurel Leaf)	1 tsp	12	0	<0.1
ground (Spice Islands)	1 tsp	11	<1	0.7
NUTMEG BUTTER OIL				
	1 cup	1927	0	218.0
	1 oz	251	0	28.4
	1 tbsp	120	0	13.6
NUTRASWEET. See SUGAR, ALTERNATIVE.				
NUTS, MIXED				
(Guy's) w/peanuts	1 oz	170	140	14.0
(Planters) 'Select Mix' cashews, almonds, and peanuts	1 oz	170	100	14.0
(Planters) 'Select Mix' cashews, almonds, and pecans	1 oz	180	85	16.0
(Planters) 'Select Mix' cashews, pecans, and peanuts	1 oz	180	80	16.0
Dry-roasted				
(Finast) 'No Frills' w/peanuts, salted	1 oz	180	150	14.0
(Fisher) lightly salted	1 oz	170	na	15.0
(Fisher) salted	1 oz	170	125	15.0
(Pathmark) 'No Frills' w/peanuts, salted	1 oz	180	220	14.0
(Planters)	1 oz	160	250	14.0
✓ (Planters) sesame nut mix	1 oz	160	330	12.0
(Planters) 'Unsalted'	1 oz	170	0	15.0
w/peanuts	1 cup	814	16	70.5
w/peanuts	1 oz	169	3	14.6
w/peanuts, salted	1 cup	814	917	70.5
w/peanuts, salted	1 oz	169	190	14.6
Honey-roasted				
(Fisher) peanuts and cashews	1 oz	150	105	13.0
(Planters)	1 oz	170	140	13.0
(Planters) cashews and peanuts	1 oz	170	170	12.0
Oil-roasted				
(Fisher) lightly salted	1 oz	170	50	16.0
(Fisher) salted	1 oz	170	110	16.0
(Flavor House)	1 oz	180	125	18.0
(Pathmark) 'No Frills' salted	1 oz	180	150	15.0
(Pathmark) 'No Frills' w/peanuts, salted	1 oz	180	150	15.0
(Pathmark) 'No Frills Fancy' salted	1 oz	180	150	15.0
(Planters)	1 oz	180	110	16.0

Food Name	Serv. Size	Total Cal.	Sod. MGS	Fat GMS
(Planters) 'Deluxe'	1 oz	180	110	17.0
(Planters) lightly salted	1 oz	180	80	16.0
(Planters) sesame nut mix	1 oz	160	200	13.0
salted	1 cup	886	1008	80.9
salted	1 oz	175	199	15.9
w/peanuts	1 cup	876	16	80.0
w/peanuts	1 oz	175	3	16.0
w/peanuts, salted	1 cup	876	926	80.0
w/peanuts, salted	1 oz	175	185	16.0

O

Food Name	Serv. Size	Total Cal.	Sod. MGS	Fat GMS
OAT. See also CEREAL, HOT.				
cooked	1 cup	87	2	1.9
cooked	4 oz	45	1	1.0
raw	1 cup	231	4	6.6
raw	1 oz	70	1	2.0
steel-cut *(Arrowhead Mills)*	2 oz	220	1	4.0
whole grain	1 cup	607	3	10.8
whole grain	1 oz	110	1	2.0
OAT BRAN. See CEREAL, HOT.				
OAT FLOUR				
(Arrowhead Mills) whole grain	2 oz	200	1	1.0
(Gold Medal) blend	1 cup	390	0	3.0
OAT GROATS *(Arrowhead Mills)*	2 oz	220	1	4.0
OAT VEGETABLE OIL				
	1 cup	1927	0	218.0
	1 tbsp	120	0	13.6
OATMEAL. See CEREAL, HOT.				
OCEAN CATFISH. See WOLF FISH.				
OCEAN PERCH, ATLANTIC/Norway haddock/red perch/redfish/rosefish/sea perch				
baked	4 oz	137	109	2.4
broiled	4 oz	137	109	2.4
dry-heat cooked	3 oz	103	82	1.8
microwaved	4 oz	137	109	2.4
raw	1 lb	427	339	7.4
raw	1 oz	27	21	0.5
OCEAN PERCH, FROZEN				
(Booth)	4 oz	100	250	1.0

Food Name	Serv. Size	Total Cal.	Sod. MGS	Fat GMS
(Gorton's) 'Fishmarket Fresh'	5 oz	140	100	3.0
(Van de Kamp's) breaded 'Light'	1 piece	280	450	14.0
(Van de Kamp's) 'Natural'	4 oz	130	65	5.0
OCEAN POUT/muttonfish				
dry-heat cooked	3 oz	87	66	1.0
raw	1 lb	360	277	4.1
raw	1 oz	22	17	0.3
OCEANIC BONITO. See TUNA, SKIPJACK.				
OCTOBER BEAN, CANNED, w/pork *(Luck's)*	7.25 oz	230	550	6.0
OCTOPUS				
moist-heat cooked	3 oz	139	391	1.8
raw	1 lb	372	(mq)	4.7
raw	1 oz	23	(mq)	0.3
OIL. See individual listings.				
OKRA/gumbo				
boiled, drained	4 oz	36	6	0.2
boiled, drained, approx 3 inches long	8 pods	27	4	0.1
boiled, drained, sliced	1/2 cup	26	4	0.1
raw, approx 3 inches long	8 pods	36	8	0.1
raw, sliced	1/2 cup	19	4	0.1
raw, trimmed	1 oz	11	2	<.1
raw, untrimmed	1 lb	148	32	0.4
OKRA, FROZEN				
boiled, drained	10 oz	94	8	0.8
boiled, drained, sliced	1/2 cup	34	3	0.3
cut *(Freshlike)*	3.3 oz	25	5	0.0
cut *(Seabrook)*	3.3 oz	25	3	0.0
cut *(Southern)*	3.5 oz	31	20	0.2
cut *(Veg•All)*	3.3 oz	25	5	0.0
whole *(Freshlike)*	3.3 oz	30	5	0.0
whole *(Seabrook)*	3.3 oz	30	2	0.0
whole *(Southern)*	3.5 oz	35	20	0.2
whole *(Veg•All)*	3.3 oz	30	5	0.0
whole, baby *(Frosty Acres)*	3.3 oz	30	2	0.0
OLD FASHIONED. See ALCOHOLIC BEVERAGES.				
OLIVE				
all varieties, all sizes, pickled *(S&W)*	1 oz	46	215	5.1
black, jumbo, canned	1 olive	7	75	0.6
black, large, canned	1 olive	5	38	0.5
black, small, canned	1 olive	4	28	0.3
black, super colossal, canned	1 olive	12	136	1.0

ood Name	Serv. Size	Total Cal.	Sod. MGS	Fat GMS
mixed varieties, chopped, pickled *(Lindsay)*	1 oz	29	249	2.7
mixed varieties, pitted, pickled *(Vlasic)*	1 oz	37	230	3.9
mixed varieties, sliced, pickled *(Lindsay)*	1/2 cup	70	598	6.5
mixed varieties, sliced, pickled *(Lindsay)*	1 oz	29	249	2.7
salad, pickled *(Progresso)*	1/2 cup	120	2400	15.0
OLIVE, ASCOLANO				
all sizes, pitted, pickled	1 oz	23	255	1.9
all sizes, pitted, pickled *(Lindsay)*	1 oz	23	255	1.9
colossal, pitted, pickled *(Lindsay)*	10 olives	90	1010	7.7
jumbo, pitted, pickled	10 olives	67	745	5.7
jumbo, pitted, pickled *(Lindsay)*	10 olives	66	745	5.7
super colossal, pitted, pickled	10 olives	123	1365	10.4
super colossal, pitted, pickled *(Lindsay)*	10 olives	122	1365	10.4
OLIVE, GREEK				
all sizes, pitted, salt-cured, oil-coated, pickled	1 oz	96	932	10.2
extra large, w/pits, salt-cured, oil-coated, pickled	10 olives	89	868	9.5
extra large, w/pits, salt-cured, pickled	10 olives	89	868	9.5
medium, w/pits, salt-cured, oil-coated, pickled	10 olives	65	631	6.9
medium, w/pits, salt-cured, pickled	10 olives	65	631	6.9
OLIVE, GREEN				
all sizes, pitted, pickled	1 oz	33	680	3.6
giant, w/pits, pickled	10 olives	76	1572	8.3
large, w/pits, pickled	10 olives	45	926	4.9
small, select, w/pits, pickled	10 olives	33	686	3.6
small, standard, w/pits, pickled	10 olives	33	686	3.6
OLIVE, MANZANILLA				
all sizes, pitted, pickled	1 oz	33	247	3.0
all sizes, pitted, pickled *(Lindsay)*	1 oz	32	247	3.0
extra large, pitted, pickled *(Lindsay)*	10 olives	63	484	5.9
large, pitted, pickled	10 olives	51	384	4.7
large, pitted, pickled *(Lindsay)*	10 olives	50	388	4.8
medium, pitted, pickled *(Lindsay)*	10 olives	44	336	4.1
small, pitted, pickled	10 olives	37	279	3.4
small, pitted, pickled *(Lindsay)*	10 olives	37	283	3.5
OLIVE, MISSION				
all sizes, pitted, pickled	1 oz	33	247	3.0
all sizes, pitted, pickled *(Lindsay)*	1 oz	32	247	3.0
extra large, pitted, pickled *(Lindsay)*	10 olives	63	484	5.9
large, pitted, pickled	10 olives	51	384	4.7
large, pitted, pickled *(Lindsay)*	10 olives	50	388	4.8
medium, pitted, pickled *(Lindsay)*	10 olives	44	336	4.1

Food Name	Serv. Size	Total Cal.	Sod. MGS	Fa GMs
small, pitted, pickled	10 olives	37	279	3.
small, pitted, pickled *(Lindsay)*	10 olives	37	283	3.
OLIVE, SEVILLANO				
all sizes, pitted, pickled	1 oz	23	255	1.
all sizes, pitted, pickled *(Lindsay)*	1 oz	23	255	1.
colossal, pitted, pickled *(Lindsay)*	10 olives	90	1010	7.
jumbo, pitted, pickled	10 olives	67	745	5.
jumbo, pitted, pickled *(Lindsay)*	10 olives	66	745	5.
super colossal, pitted, pickled	10 olives	123	1365	10.
super colossal, pitted, pickled *(Lindsay)*	10 olives	122	1365	10.
OLIVE APPETIZER				
(Progresso)	1/2 cup	180	1600	21.
(Progresso) 'Condite'	1/2 cup	130	870	14.
OLIVE OIL				
	1/2 cup	955	tr	108.
	1 oz	251	tr	28.
(Amore) 'Extra Virgin'	1 tbsp	130	0	14.
(Amore) 'Pure'	1 tbsp	130	0	14.
(Bertolli)	1 tbsp	120	(tr)	14.
(Filippo Berio)	1 tbsp	120	(tr)	14.
(Hain)	1 tbsp	120	0	14.
(Pope) 100% Italian cold press, no salt	1 tbsp	120	0	14.
(Progresso) all varieties	1 tbsp	119	0	14.
(Spectrum Naturals)	1 tbsp	120	0	14.
(Spectrum Naturals) organic	1 tbsp	120	0	14.
(Wesson)	1 tbsp	120	0	14.
OMELET, FROZEN				
(Healthy Choice) turkey sausage, on English muffin	1 serving	210	470	4.
(Healthy Choice) western style, on English muffin	1 serving	200	480	3.
(Weight Watchers) ham and cheese 'Handy'	4 oz	180	420	5.
ONION				
Mature				
boiled, drained	4 oz	50	3	0.
chopped, boiled, drained	1/2 cup	46	3	0.
chopped, boiled, drained	1 tbsp	7	0	0.
raw *(Dole)*	1 med	60	10	0.
raw, chopped	1/2 cup	30	2	0.
raw, chopped	1 tbsp	4	tr	<.
raw, trimmed	1 oz	11	1	<.
raw, untrimmed	1 lb	154	12	0.

od Name	Serv. Size	Total Cal.	Sod. MGS	Fat GMS
NION, CANNED				
sweet *(Heinz)*	1 oz	40	165	0.0
whole, small *(Pathmark)*	1/2 cup	35	280	0.0
whole, small *(S&W)*	1/2 cup	35	345	0.0
w/liquid	4 oz	22	421	0.1
w/liquid, chopped	1/2 cup	21	416	0.1
NION, COCKTAIL, lightly spiced *(Vlasic)*	1 oz	4	365	0.0
NION, DRIED				
flakes	1 oz	92	6	0.1
flakes	1/4 cup	45	3	0.1
flakes	1 tbsp	16	1	0.0
w/green onion, minced *(Lawry's)*	1 tsp	7	1	0.2
NION, FROZEN				
Chopped				
boiled, drained	1/2 cup	29	13	0.1
boiled, drained	4 oz	32	14	0.1
boiled, drained	1 tbsp	4	2	0.0
unprepared	10 oz	82	34	0.3
(Ore-Ida)	2 oz	20	10	<1.0
(Seabrook)	1 oz	8	2	0.0
Diced				
(Freshlike)	3.3 oz	8	0	0.0
(Veg•All)	3.3 oz	8	0	0.0
Whole				
boiled, drained	4 oz	32	9	0.1
(Birds Eye) small	4 oz	40	10	0.0
(Birds Eye) small, w/cream sauce 'Combination Vegetables'	5 oz	140	400	10.0
(Freshlike)	3.3 oz	35	10	0.0
(Seabrook) small	3.3 oz	35	9	0.0
(Veg•All)	3.3 oz	35	10	0.0
NION, GREEN/scallion/spring onion				
chopped *(Dole)*	1 tbsp	2	0	0.1
trimmed, w/top	1 oz	19	5	<.1
trimmed, w/top, chopped	1/2 cup	16	8	0.1
trimmed, w/top, chopped	1 tbsp	2	1	<.1
untrimmed	1 lb	140	71	0.8
NION, SPRING. See ONION, GREEN.				
NION, WELSH				
trimmed	1 lb	160	na	1.6
trimmed	1 oz	10	na	0.1

Food Name	Serv. Size	Total Cal.	Sod. MGS	
ONION POWDER				
ground	1 tbsp	23	3	
ground	1 tsp	7	1	
ground (Durkee)	1 tsp	8	0	
ground (Laurel Leaf)	1 tsp	8	0	
ground (Spice Islands)	1 tsp	8	1	
ONION RINGS, FROZEN				
breaded, partially fried in vegetable oil, prepared in oven	4 oz	462	425	3
breaded, partially fried in vegetable oil, prepared in oven	2 rings	81	75	
breaded, partially fried in vegetable oil, unprepared	16 oz	1171	1117	6
breaded, partially fried in vegetable oil, unprepared	9 oz	658	627	3
(Farm Rich) battered, precooked 'Batter Dipt'	4 oz	260	580	1
(Farm Rich) crispy 'Onion O's'	5 rings	190	480	
(Mrs. Paul's) crispy	2.5 oz	190	230	1
(Ore-Ida) 'Onion Ringers'	2 oz	140	190	
(Stilwell) battered	3 oz	250	300	1
ONION SALT (Tone's)	1 tsp	1	1599	
ORANGE				
All commercial varieties				
approx 2 5/8-inch diam	1 med	62	0	
peeled and seeded	1 oz	13	0	
sections, w/o membrane	1 cup	85	0	
untrimmed	1 lb	156	0	
California navel				
approx 2 7/8-inch diam	1 med	64	1	
peeled and seeded	1 oz	13	<1	
sections, w/o membrane	1 cup	76	2	
untrimmed	1 lb	142	2	
California Valencia				
approx 2 5/8-inch diam	1 med	59	0	
peeled and seeded	1 oz	14	0	
sections, w/o membrane	1 cup	88	0	
untrimmed	1 lb	167	0	
Florida				
approx 2 5/8 inch diam	1 med	69	0	
peeled and seeded	1 oz	13	tr	
sections, w/o membrane	1 cup	85	0	
untrimmed	1 lb	153	2	
ORANGE APRICOT DRINK (Tropicana) 'Twister'	8 oz	115	2	
ORANGE APRICOT JUICE				
(Musselman's) 'Breakfast Cocktail'	6 oz	90	20	

Food Name	Serv. Size	Total Cal.	Sod. MGS	Fat GMS
ORANGE APRICOT JUICE DRINK	1 oz	16	1	0.0
ORANGE BANANA NECTAR (Kern's)	6 oz	110	0	0.0
ORANGE CRANBERRY JUICE				
(Santa Cruz Natural) organic 'Cruz'	8 oz	125	na	<1.0
ORANGE CRANBERRY JUICE DRINK				
(Ocean Spray) 'Refreshers'	6 oz	100	15	0.0
(Tropicana) 'Single Serve'	10 oz	175	3	0.0
(Tropicana) 'Twister'	8 oz	115	1	0.0
(Tropicana) 'Twister'	6 oz	100	25	<1.0
(Tropicana) 'Twister Light' w/NutraSweet	6 oz	18	27	<1.0
ORANGE DRINK				
Can, bottle, or box				
	8 oz	128	40	tr
(Bama)	8.45 oz	120	60	0.0
(Crowley)	8 oz	130	15	0.0
(Hawaiian Punch)	6 oz	100	20	0.0
(Hi-C)	8.45 oz	134	24	<.1
(Hi-C)	6 oz	95	17	<.1
(Hi-C) aseptic box	6 oz	90	20	0.0
(J. Hungerford) 20% plus juice	9.03 oz	41	23	0.0
(Pathmark) 'No Frills Sodium Free'	6 oz	80	0	0.0
(Squeezit) 'Smarty Arty Orange'	6.75 oz	100	50	0.0
(Sunny Delight) California style	8 oz	130	130	0.0
(Tropicana)	6 oz	90	35	<1.0
(Tropicana) 'Single Serve'	10 oz	132	3	0.0
(Veryfine)	8 oz	130	70	0.0
(Wyler's) 'Fruit Slush'	4 oz	157	10	0.0
Chilled (Hi-C)	6 oz	90	20	0.0
Frozen, w/juice and pulp, diluted	6 oz	85	19	0.0
Mix				
(Finast) breakfast, prepared	8 oz	80	15	0.0
(Kool-Aid) sugar-free, w/NutraSweet, prepared	8 oz	4	0	0.0
(Kool-Aid) sugar-sweetened, prepared	8 oz	80	0	0.0
(Kool-Aid) unsweetened, prepared w/sugar	8 oz	100	0	0.0
(Kool-Aid) unsweetened, prepared w/o sugar	8 oz	2	0	0.0
(Pathmark) breakfast 'No Frills' prepared	4 oz	60	0	0.0
ORANGE FLAVOR DRINK				
Can, bottle, or box	12 oz	729	103	2.2
Chilled (Bright & Early) diluted	6 oz	90	18	0.2
Frozen				
(Bright & Early) diluted	6 oz	90	18	0.2

Food Name	Serv. Size	Total Cal.	Sod. MGS	Fat GMS
w/orange pulp, diluted	1 oz	15	3	tr
Mix				
powder, unprepared	1 oz	109	5	<.1
powder, unprepared	3 rounded tsp	93	4	tr
(Tang) crystals, prepared	6 oz	90	0	0.0
(Tang) crystals 'Sugar-free' prepared	6 oz	6	0	0.0
ORANGE FRUIT JUICE BLEND				
(Mott's)	10 oz	144	6	0.0
(Mott's)	9.5 oz	139	6	0.0
ORANGE GRAPEFRUIT JUICE				
canned	8 oz	106	7	0.3
canned	1 oz	13	1	0.0
(Kraft) chilled 'Pure 100%'	6 oz	80	0	0.0
ORANGE JUICE				
fresh squeezed	8 oz	112	2	0.5
Can, bottle, or box				
	6 oz	78	5	0.3
(Del Monte) 'Unsweetened'	6 oz	80	10	0.0
(J. Hungerford)	9.03 oz	112	1	0.0
(Minute Maid) blend 'Juices to Go'	6 oz	90	20	0.0
(Minute Maid) 'Juices to Go'	6 oz	80	20	0.0
(Ocean Spray)	6 oz	80	15	0.0
(S&W)	6 oz	83	2	0.0
(Sippin' Pak)	8.45 oz	110	25	0.0
(Snapple)	8 oz	130	55	0.0
(Stokely) 'Unsweetened'	6 oz	89	5	1.0
(Sunkist)	6 oz	84	2	0.1
(Tree Top)	6 oz	90	5	0.0
(TreeSweet)	6 oz	78	15	0.0
(Tropicana) '100% Pure'	8 oz	109	3	0.0
(Tropicana) 'Pure Premium' 100% pure	6 oz	80	0	<1.0
(Tropicana) reconstituted, 100% pure	6 oz	80	20	<1.0
(Veryfine) blend '100%'	8 oz	120	35	0.0
(Veryfine) '100%'	8 oz	121	10	0.0
Chilled				
	8 oz	110	2	0.7
(Citrus Hill) 'Plus Calcium'	6 oz	90	10	<1.0
(Citrus Hill) 'Select'	6 oz	90	10	<1.0
(Crowley)	8 oz	110	5	0.0
(Kraft) 'Pure 100% Unsweetened'	6 oz	80	0	0.0
(Minute Maid) calcium fortified	6 oz	80	20	0.0

Food Name	Serv. Size	Total Cal.	Sod. MGS	Fat GMS
(Minute Maid) country style	6 oz	80	20	0.0
(Minute Maid) country style, premium choice	6 oz	90	0	0.0
(Minute Maid) premium choice	6 oz	90	0	0.0
(Minute Maid) regular	6 oz	80	20	0.0
(Sunkist)	6 oz	84	2	0.1
(Sunkist) 'Fresh Squeezed'	6 oz	77	2	0.3
Frozen				
(A&P) diluted	6 oz	80	0	<1.0
(Minute Maid) calcium fortified	6 oz	80	0	0.0
(Minute Maid) country style	6 oz	80	0	0.0
(Minute Maid) reduced acid	6 oz	80	0	0.0
(Minute Maid) regular	6 oz	80	0	0.0
(Sunkist) '8-16 servings per pkg' diluted	6 oz	112	3	0.1
(TreeSweet) diluted	6 oz	84	15	0.0
ORANGE JUICE COCKTAIL				
(Musselman's) w/grapefruit juice 'Breakfast Cocktail'	6 oz	90	20	0.0
(Ocean Spray)	6 oz	100	15	0.0
(Welch's) 'Orchard'	10 oz	150	0	0.0
ORANGE JUICE DRINK				
(Citrus Hill) 'Lite Premium'	6 oz	60	10	<1.0
(Kool-Aid) 'Koolers'	8.45 oz	110	10	0.0
(Tang) 'Fruit Box'	8.45 oz	130	10	0.0
(Tropicana) tropical 'Juice Sparkler'	8 oz	110	50	0.0
ORANGE JUICE FLOAT *(Knudsen & Sons)*	8 oz	120	na	0.0
ORANGE KIWI PASSION JUICE *(Tropicana)* 100% pure	6 oz	80	35	<1.0
ORANGE MANGO DRINK *(Tropicana)* 'Twister'	6 oz	90	45	<1.0
ORANGE MANGO JUICE *(Knudsen & Sons)*	8 oz	110	na	0.0
ORANGE PASSION DRINK				
(Tropicana) 'Twister'	8 oz	90	1	0.0
(Tropicana) 'Twister'	6 oz	80	35	<1.0
ORANGE PEACH DRINK				
(Tropicana) 'Twister'	8 oz	115	2	0.0
(Tropicana) 'Twister'	6 oz	90	35	<1.0
ORANGE PEACH MANGO JUICE *(Tropicana)* 100% pure	6 oz	80	20	<1.0
ORANGE PEEL				
candied	1 oz	88	0	0.1
fresh	1 oz	na	1	0.1
fresh	1 tbsp	na	tr	<.1
fresh	1 tsp	na	tr	tr
ORANGE PINEAPPLE JUICE				
(Kraft) 'Pure 100%'	6 oz	80	0	0.0

Food Name	Serv. Size	Total Cal.	Sod. MGS	Fat GMS
(Musselman's) 'Breakfast Cocktail'	6 oz	90	15	0.0
(Tropicana) 100% pure	6 oz	80	15	<1.0
ORANGE PUNCH *(Minute Maid)* aseptic box	6 oz	80	20	0.0
ORANGE RASPBERRY DRINK				
(Tropicana) 'Twister'	6 oz	80	30	<1.0
(Tropicana) 'Twister Light'	6 oz	30	30	<1.0
ORANGE ROUGHY/slimehead				
dry-heat cooked	3 oz	76	69	0.8
raw	1 lb	571	286	31.8
raw	1 oz	36	18	2.0
ORANGE STRAWBERRY BANANA JUICE				
(Tropicana) 100% pure	6 oz	80	25	<1.0
ORANGE STRAWBERRY DRINK				
(Tropicana) w/banana 'Twister'	6 oz	80	45	<1.0
(Tropicana) w/banana 'Twister Light'	6 oz	25	20	<1.0
(Tropicana) w/guava 'Twister'	6 oz	80	40	<1.0
ORANGEADE				
(Santa Cruz Natural) organic	8 oz	90	na	<1.0
(Santa Cruz Natural) organic 'Sparkling'	8 oz	90	na	<1.0
OREGANO				
dried *(Golden Dipt)*	2 grams	6	88	0.
dried *(Spice Islands)*	1 tsp	6	<1	0.
ground	1 tbsp	14	1	0.5
ground	1 tsp	5	0	0.
ground *(Durkee)*	1 tsp	5	0	t
ground *(Laurel Leaf)*	1 tsp	5	0	t
ORIENTAL SEASONING MIX *(Schilling)* 'Bag 'n Season'	1 pkg	152	1912	8.0
OYSTER, CANNED				
Eastern	1 cup	171	278	6.
Eastern	3 oz	59	95	2.
Eastern, w/liquid	4 oz	78	127	2.8
(Bumble Bee)	1 cup	218	185	5.
(S&W) mole 'Fancy'	2 oz	95	(mq)	3.
OYSTER, EASTERN				
Farmed				
dry-heat cooked	3 oz	67	139	1.
dry-heat cooked	6 med	47	96	1.
raw, approx 3 oz	6 med	50	150	1.
Wild				
dry-heat cooked	3 oz	61	207	1.
dry-heat cooked	6 med	42	144	1.

Food Name	Serv. Size	Total Cal.	Sod. MGS	Fat GMS
moist-heat cooked	4 oz	155	254	5.6
moist-heat cooked	3 oz	116	359	4.2
moist-heat cooked, approx 1.5 oz	6 med	58	177	2.1
raw	1 cup	169	523	6.1
raw	1 oz	20	32	0.7
raw, approx 3 oz	6 med	57	177	2.1
OYSTER, PACIFIC				
moist-heat cooked	3 oz	139	180	3.9
moist-heat cooked	1 med	41	53	1.1
raw	1 lb	370	481	10.4
raw	3 oz	69	90	2.0
raw	1 oz	23	30	0.7
raw, approx 1.75 oz	1 med	41	53	1.1

OYSTER PLANT. See SALSIFY.
OYSTER STEW. See SOUP.

P

Food Name	Serv. Size	Total Cal.	Sod. MGS	Fat GMS
PALM KERNEL OIL /babassu oil				
	1 cup	1927	0	218.0
	1/2 cup	964	0	109.0
	1 oz	251	0	28.4
	1 tbsp	120	0	13.6
PALM OIL				
	1 oz	251	0	28.4
	1 tbsp	120	0	13.6
PANANG CURRY BASE *(A Taste of Thai)*	1 tbsp	25	180	2.0
PANCAKE, FROZEN				
(Aunt Jemima) blueberry	3.5 oz	220	826	3.7
(Aunt Jemima) buttermilk 'Lite Microwave'	3.5 oz	140	660	3.0
(Aunt Jemima) buttermilk 'Microwave'	3.5 oz	210	860	3.0
(Aunt Jemima) 'Original Microwave'	3.5 oz	211	801	3.6
(Downyflake)	3 pancakes	280	920	9.0
(Downyflake) blueberry	3 pancakes	290	920	9.0
(Downyflake) buttermilk	3 pancakes	280	920	9.0
(Krusteaz) blueberry, 4.5 oz	3 pancakes	280	710	5.0
(Krusteaz) buttermilk, 4.75 oz	3 pancakes	290	900	5.0
(Krusteaz) mini, microwave	6 pancakes	120	280	2.0
(Krusteaz) whole wheat honey, 4.75 oz	3 pancakes	250	990	4.0

Food Name	Serv. Size	Total Cal.	Sod. MGS	Fat GMS
(Pillsbury) blueberry 'Microwave'	3 pancakes	250	540	4.0
(Pillsbury) buttermilk 'Microwave'	3 pancakes	260	590	4.0
(Pillsbury) harvest wheat 'Microwave'	3 pancakes	240	420	4.0
(Pillsbury) 'Original Microwave'	3 pancakes	240	550	4.0
(Weight Watchers) buttermilk 'Microwave' approx 2.5 oz	1/2 pkg	140	270	3.0
PANCAKE BATTER, FROZEN				
(Aunt Jemima) blueberry	3.6 oz	204	688	4.0
(Aunt Jemima) buttermilk	3.6 oz	180	778	2.3
(Aunt Jemima) 'Original'	3.6 oz	183	763	2.4
PANCAKE ENTRÉE, FROZEN				
(Aunt Jemima) and sausages 'Homestyle'	6 oz	420	1140	16.0
(Aunt Jemima) lite, w/lite links 'Homestyle'	6 oz	310	970	10.0
(Aunt Jemima) lite, w/lite syrup 'Homestyle'	6 oz	260	860	3.0
(Downyflake) and sausages	5.5 oz	430	1170	23.0
(Swanson) and sausages 'Great Starts'	6 oz	460	920	22.0
(Swanson) silver dollar, and sausage 'Great Starts'	3.75 oz	310	680	14.0
(Swanson) whole wheat, w/lite links 'Great Starts'	5.5 oz	350	600	16.0
(Swanson) w/bacon 'Great Starts'	4.5 oz	400	1000	20.0
PANCAKE MIX. See also PANCAKE/WAFFLE MIX.				
(NOTE: Unless otherwise stated, all pancakes are 4 inches in diameter.)				
(Hungry Jack) dry	1/14 pkg	180	650	3.0
(Hungry Jack) prepared w/water	3 pancakes	180	650	3.0
BLUEBERRY (Krusteaz) imitation, prepared	3 pancakes	205	660	4.0
BLUEBERRY, WILD				
(Hungry Jack) dry	1/5 pkg	170	780	1.0
(Hungry Jack) prepared w/milk/oil/egg	3 pancakes	320	820	14.0
BUCKWHEAT (Krusteaz) prepared	3 pancakes	215	770	3.0
BUTTERMILK				
(Health Valley) 'Biscuit & Pancake'	1 oz	100	170	1.0
(Hungry Jack) 'Complete' dry	1/17 pkg	180	720	1.0
(Hungry Jack) 'Complete' prepared w/water	3 pancakes	180	720	1.0
(Hungry Jack) dry	1/25 pkg	120	530	0.0
(Hungry Jack) prepared w/skim milk/oil/egg whites	3 pancakes	200	570	7.0
(Hungry Jack) prepared w/2% milk/oil/egg	3 pancakes	210	560	9.0
(Krusteaz) prepared	3 pancakes	200	770	3.0
EXTRA LIGHT				
(Hungry Jack) 'Complete' dry	1/17 pkg	180	730	3.0
(Hungry Jack) dry	1/17 pkg	180	730	3.0
(Hungry Jack) dry	1/26 pkg	120	450	0.0
(Hungry Jack) prepared w/skim milk/oil/egg whites	3 pancakes	170	500	4.0
(Hungry Jack) prepared w/2% milk/oil/egg	3 pancakes	190	490	6.0

Food Name	Serv. Size	Total Cal.	Sod. MGS	Fat GMS
OAT BRAN *(Krusteaz)* 'Lite'	3 pancakes	130	370	1.0
WHOLE WHEAT *(Krusteaz)* honey	3 pancakes	215	630	1.0
PANCAKE MIX, MICROWAVE				
(Hungry Jack) blueberry, dry	3/4 pkg	230	550	4.0
(Hungry Jack) buttermilk, dry	3/4 pkg	260	590	4.0
(Hungry Jack) harvest wheat, dry	3/4 pkg	230	560	4.0
(Hungry Jack) oat bran, dry	3/4 pkg	230	580	4.0
(Hungry Jack) original, dry	3/4 pkg	240	570	4.0
PANCAKE SYRUP. See also MAPLE SYRUP.				
15% maple	1 cup	879	328	0.3
15% maple	1 tbsp	56	21	0.0
2% maple	1 cup	762	126	0.6
2% maple	1 tbsp	48	8	0.0
reduced calorie	100 gm	164	200	0.0
(Aunt Jemima)				
'ButterLite'	1 oz	50	65	0.0
'Lite'	1 oz	54	92	0.1
'Original' rich maple taste	1 oz	100	60	0.0
(Br'er Rabbit)				
dark	1 oz	120	0	0.0
light	1 oz	120	0	0.0
(Estee)				
	1 tbsp	4	25	0.0
'Breakfast'	1 tbsp	12	35	0.0
(Featherweight)	1 tbsp	16	25	0.0
(Hungry Jack)				
'Lite'	2 tbsp	50	105	0.0
regular	2 tbsp	100	25	0.0
(Knott's Berry Farm)				
	1 oz	110	0	0.0
'Country'	1 oz	110	0	0.0
'Light' microwavable	1 oz	45	70	0.0
w/30% real maple syrup, microwavable	1 oz	110	90	0.0
(Log Cabin)				
'Country Kitchen'	1 oz	100	20	0.0
'Country Kitchen' butter flavor	1 oz	100	100	0.0
'Country Kitchen Lite'	1 oz	50	85	0.0
'Lite' reduced calorie	1 oz	50	90	0.0
'Pancake and Waffle'	1 oz	100	35	0.0
(Maple Valley)				
maple syrup substitute	2 tbsp	110	50	0.0

Food Name	Serv. Size	Total Cal.	Sod. MGS	Fat GMS
maple syrup substitute, 'Lite'	2 tbsp	60	60	0.0
(Mrs. Butterworth's) thick 'n rich 'Lite'	2 tbsp	60	65	0.
(Mrs. Richardson's)				
'Lite'	1 oz	50	90	0.
original recipe	1 oz	100	60	0.0
(S&W) maple flavor, saccharin sweetened	1 tsp	4	25	0.
(Vermont Maid)	1 tbsp	50	5	0.
(Weight Watchers) 'Reduced Calorie'	1 tbsp	25	40	0.
PANCAKE/WAFFLE MIX. See also PANCAKE MIX.				
(NOTE: Unless otherwise stated, all pancakes are 4 inches in diameter.)				
(Arrowhead Mills) 'Griddle Lite' prepared	1/2 cup	260	(mq)	3.
(Aunt Jemima) 'Original' prepared	3 pancakes	116	609	0.
(Aunt Jemima) 'Original Complete' prepared	3 pancakes	253	1024	3.
(Bisquick) 'Shake 'n Pour' prepared	3 pancakes	260	850	5.
(Estee) prepared, 3 inches each	3 pancakes	100	130	0.
(Featherweight) prepared	3 pancakes	140	90	2.
(Gold Medal) 'Pouch Mix' prepared w/egg	1/8 pouch	100	280	2.
(Hungry Jack) 'Panshakes' prepared	3 pancakes	250	880	6.
(Krusteaz) Belgian waffle, prepared, 4-inch square	1 waffle	170	350	7.
(Martha White) 'FlapStax' 1/4-cup batter per pancake	1 pancake	80	320	1.
(Martha White) 'Light Crust' dry	2 oz	120	290	3.
(Robin Hood) 'Pouch Mix' prepared w/egg	1/8 pouch	100	280	2.
APPLE CINNAMON (Bisquick) 'Shake 'n Pour' prepared	3 pancakes	270	870	5.
BLUE CORN (Arrowhead Mills) prepared	1/2 cup	330	295	5.
BLUEBERRY				
(Bisquick) 'Shake 'n Pour' prepared	3 pancakes	280	860	5.
(Hungry Jack) prepared	3 pancakes	320	820	15.
BUCKWHEAT				
(Arrowhead Mills) prepared	1/2 cup	270	(mq)	2.
(Aunt Jemima) prepared	3 pancakes	143	773	1.
BUTTERMILK				
(Aunt Jemima) 'Complete' prepared	3 pancakes	231	950	2.
(Aunt Jemima) 'Lite Complete' prepared	3 pancakes	130	570	2.
(Aunt Jemima) prepared	3 pancakes	122	698	0.
(Betty Crocker) complete, dry	1/2 cup	210	500	3.
(Betty Crocker) complete, prepared	3 pancakes	210	500	3.
(Betty Crocker) dry	1/2 cup	170	760	1.
(Betty Crocker) prepared w/milk/oil/egg	3 pancakes	280	810	10.
(Bisquick) 'Shake 'n Pour' prepared	3 pancakes	260	860	5.
(Hungry Jack) 'Complete' prepared	3 pancakes	180	710	1.
(Hungry Jack) 'Complete Packets' prepared	3 pancakes	180	680	3.

Food Name	Serv. Size	Total Cal.	Sod. MGS	Fat GMS
(Hungry Jack) prepared	3 pancakes	240	570	11.0
EXTRA LIGHT (Hungry Jack) 'Complete' prepared w/water	3 pancakes	180	730	3.0
MULTIGRAIN (Arrowhead Mills) prepared	1/2 cup	350	(mq)	2.0
OAT BRAN				
(Arrowhead Mills) prepared	1/2 cup	200	230	2.0
(Bisquick) 'Shake 'n Pour' prepared	3 pancakes	240	580	4.0
WHOLE WHEAT (Aunt Jemima) prepared	3 pancakes	161	892	1.0
PAPAYA				
peeled and seeded	1 oz	11	1	<.1
raw (Calavo Growers)	1/2 med	80	15	0.0
raw (Del Monte)	1/3 med	60	5	0.0
raw, approx 3 1/2-inch diam	1 med	119	9	0.4
raw, cubed	1 cup	55	4	0.2
raw, slices in light syrup (Sunfresh)	2/3 cup	80	10	0.0
PAPAYA DRINK (Knudsen & Sons) concentrate	1.5 oz	90	37	0.0
PAPAYA JUICE (Knudsen & Sons) cream	2 oz	25	na	0.0
PAPAYA LIME JUICE (Knudsen & Sons)	8 oz	115	na	0.0
PAPAYA NECTAR				
canned	1 cup	142	13	0.4
canned	1 oz	18	2	0.1
(Kern's)	6 oz	110	5	0.0
(Knudsen & Sons)	8 oz	100	na	0.0
(Knudsen & Sons) concentrate	1.5 oz	90	na	0.0
(Libby's)	6 oz	110	10	0.0
PAPAYA PUNCH (Veryfine)	8 oz	120	10	0.0
PAPRIKA				
ground	1 oz	82	10	3.7
ground	1 tbsp	20	2	0.9
ground	1 tsp	6	1	0.3
ground (Durkee)	1 tsp	8	0	tr
ground (Laurel Leaf)	1 tsp	8	0	tr
ground (Spice Islands)	1 tsp	7	<1	0.2
PARANUT. See BRAZIL NUT.				
PARFAIT				
chocolate (Pearson)	1 oz	120	70	3.0
chocolate (Swiss Miss)	4 oz	170	200	6.0
chocolate vanilla, fat-free (Swiss Miss)	4 oz	104	171	0.3
peanut butter (Pearson)	1 oz	120	70	3.0
vanilla (Swiss Miss)	4 oz	180	150	6.0
vanilla chocolate (Swiss Miss)	4 oz	164	196	6.0
vanilla chocolate 'Light' (Swiss Miss)	4 oz	100	110	1.0

Food Name	Serv. Size	Total Cal.	Sod. MGS	Fat GMS
PARROT FISH/pollyfish				
raw	1 lb	390	(mq)	1.8
raw	1 oz	24	(mq)	0.1
PARSLEY				
dried	1 oz	78	128	1.3
dried	1 tbsp	4	6	0.1
dried	1 tsp	1	1	tr
dried (Durkee)	1 tsp	1	0	tr
dried (Laurel Leaf)	1 tsp	1	0	tr
dried flakes (Spice Islands)	1 tsp	4	6	0.1
freeze-dried	1 oz	77	111	1.5
freeze-dried	1/4 cup	4	5	0.1
freeze-dried	1 tbsp	1	2	tr
raw	10 sprigs	4	6	0.1
raw, chopped	1/2 cup	11	17	0.2
raw, trimmed	1 oz	9	11	0.1
raw, untrimmed	1 lb	140	169	1.3
PARSLEY ROOT/hamburg parsley/turnip-rooted parsley				
fresh	1 lb	50	454	2.7
fresh	1 oz	3	28	0.2
PARSLEY SEASONING				
(Schilling) all-purpose 'Parsley Patch'	1 tsp	6	3	0.0
PARSNIP				
boiled, drained	4 oz	92	11	0.3
boiled, drained, 9 inches long	1 parsnip	130	16	0.5
boiled, drained, slices	1/2 cup	63	8	0.2
raw, slices	1/2 cup	50	7	0.2
raw, trimmed	1 oz	21	3	0.1
raw, untrimmed	1 lb	289	39	1.2
PASSION FRUIT/granadilla				
purple, trimmed	1 oz	27	na	0.2
purple, trimmed, approx 1.2 oz	1 med	17	5	0.1
purple, untrimmed	1 lb	230	na	1.7
PASSION FRUIT BEVERAGES				
COCKTAIL				
fresh, purple	1 cup	126	15	0.1
fresh, purple	1 oz	16	2	0.0
fresh, yellow	1 cup	148	15	0.4
(Welch's) bottled 'Orchard Tropicals' diluted	6 oz	100	20	0.0
(Welch's) frozen 'Orchard Tropicals' diluted	6 oz	100	20	0.0
(Welch's) 'Orchard Tropicals Cocktails-In-A-Box'	8.45 oz	140	20	0.0

Food Name	Serv. Size	Total Cal.	Sod. MGS	Fat GMS
JUICE				
fresh, yellow	1 oz	19	2	0.1
(Knudsen & Sons) raspberry	8 oz	130	na	0.0
(Snapple) passion juice 'Passion Supreme'	8 oz	160	20	0.0
(Veryfine) refresher, w/orange, tropical	8 oz	110	25	0.0

PASTA/macaroni. See also NOODLE, CHINESE; NOODLE, EGG; NOODLE, JAPANESE; TORTELLINI PASTA.

(NOTE: 2 ounces uncooked pasta = approximately 1 cup cooked.)

Food Name	Serv. Size	Total Cal.	Sod. MGS	Fat GMS
ACINI PEPE (Ronzoni) dry	2 oz	210	0	1.0
AGNOLOTTI, refrigerated, 'Fresh' (Contadina)	3 oz	270	230	7.0
ANGEL HAIR				
Dry				
corn (Westbrae)	2 oz	210	10	2.0
Jerusalem artichoke (De Boles)	2 oz	210	0	1.0
Jerusalem artichoke, garlic and parsley (De Boles)	2 oz	210	15	1.0
Jerusalem artichoke, tomato and basil (De Boles)	2 oz	210	10	1.0
100% durum wheat semolina (American Beauty)	2 oz	210	0	1.0
wheat (Creamette)	2 oz	210	0	1.0
wheat (DiGiorno)	3 oz	250	140	3.0
whole wheat (De Boles)	2 oz	210	0	2.0
Refrigerated, fresh				
'Fresh' (Contadina)	3 oz	260	30	3.0
BOW TIE. See FARFELLE.				
CAPELLINI				
100% durum wheat semolina (American Beauty) dry	2 oz	210	0	1.0
CURLY				
100% durum wheat semolina 'Curly-Roni'				
(American Beauty) dry	2 oz	210	0	1.0
ELBOW				
Dry				
corn (Westbrae)	2 oz	210	10	2.0
corn, wheat-free (De Boles)	2 oz	210	0	1.0
Jerusalem artichoke (De Boles)	2 oz	210	0	1.0
100% durum wheat semolina (American Beauty)	2 oz	210	0	1.0
'Primavera' (De Boles)	2 oz	210	0	<1.0
quinoa 'Supergrain Wheat Free' (Ancient Harvest)	2 oz	180	5	2.0
quinoa 'Supergrain Wheat Free' (Quinoa)	2 oz	180	5	2.0
'Valu Pack' (Hospitality)	1/2 cup	240	0	0.5
wheat (Creamette)	2 oz	210	0	1.0
whole wheat	1 cup	365	8	1.5
whole wheat (De Boles)	2 oz	210	0	2.0

Food Name	Serv. Size	Total Cal.	Sod. MGS	Fat GMS
FARFELLE/bow tie				
Dry				
wheat *(De Cecco)*	2 oz	210	0	1.0
wheat *(Ronzoni)*	2 oz	210	0	1.0
FETTUCCINE				
Dry				
basil *(Al Dente)*	2 oz	220	20	2.0
curry *(Al Dente)*	2 oz	220	20	2.0
dill *(Al Dente)*	2 oz	220	20	2.0
egg noodle *(Antoine's)*	2 oz	210	0	1.0
egg noodle, extra long *(Ronzoni)*	2 oz	220	15	3.0
egg noodle 'Home-Style' *(De Cecco)*	2 oz	210	35	3.0
Jerusalem artichoke *(De Boles)*	2 oz	210	0	1.0
spinach *(Al Dente)*	2 oz	220 ·	20	2.0
spinach *(DiGiorno)*	3 oz	250	140	3.0
spinach, Jerusalem artichoke *(De Boles)*	2 oz	210	5	<1.0
spinach and egg 'Florentine' *(American Beauty)*	2 oz	220	35	3.0
tarragon *(Al Dente)*	2 oz	220	20	2.0
wheat *(DiGiorno)*	3 oz	250	140	3.0
wheat, bell pepper/basil, organic *(Herb's)*	2 oz	220	5	2.0
whole wheat *(Al Dente)*	2 oz	210 ·	10	1.0
Refrigerated, fresh				
spinach 'Fresh' *(Contadina)*	3 oz	260	70	4.0
FUSILLI				
Dry				
rainbow *(Antoine's)*	2 oz	210	20	1.0
spinach *(De Cecco)*	2 oz	210	5	1.0
tricolor *(Antoine's)*	2 oz	210	20	1.0
tricolor, vegetable *(Antoine's)*	2 oz	210	25	1.0
vegetable *(Antoine's)*	2 oz	210	20	1.0
wheat *(De Cecco)*	2 oz	210	0	1.0
GEMELLI *(Antoine's)* dry	2 oz	210	0	1.0
LASAGNA				
Dry				
curly edge *(Ronzoni)*	2 oz	210	0	1.0
Jerusalem artichoke *(De Boles)*	2 oz	210	0	1.0
100% durum wheat semolina *(American Beauty)*	2 oz	210	0	1.0
100% semolina *(Creamette)*	2 oz	210	0	1.0
100% semolina *(De Cecco)*	2 oz	210	0	1.0
spinach, whole wheat, no egg *(Westbrae)*	2 oz	210	0	2.0
whole wheat *(De Boles)*	2 oz	210	0	2.0

Food Name	Serv. Size	Total Cal.	Sod. MGS	Fat GMS
whole wheat *(Health Valley)*	2 oz	170	10	1.0
whole wheat, no egg *(Westbrae)*	2 oz	210	0	2.0
whole wheat, spinach *(Health Valley)*	2 oz	170	15	1.0
LINGUINE				
Dry				
Jerusalem artichoke *(De Boles)*	2 oz	210	0	1.0
quinoa 'Supergrain Wheat Free' *(Ancient Harvest)*	2 oz	180	5	2.0
quinoa 'Supergrain Wheat Free' *(Quinoa)*	2 oz	180	5	2.0
wheat *(Creamette)*	2 oz	210	0	1.0
wheat *(De Cecco)*	2 oz	210	0	1.0
wheat *(DiGiorno)*	3 oz	250	135	3.0
wheat *(Ronzoni)*	2 oz	210	0	1.0
Refrigerated, fresh				
(DiGiorno)	3 oz	250	140	3.0
MANICOTTI, extra fancy *(Ronzoni)* dry	2 oz	210	0	1.0
MOSTACCIOLI				
Dry				
100% durum wheat semolina *(American Beauty)*	2 oz	210	0	1.0
wheat *(Creamette)*	2 oz	210	0	1.0
wheat *(Ronzoni)*	2 oz	210	0	1.0
ORZO *(Ronzoni)* dry	2 oz	210	0	3.0
PENNE RIGATI				
Dry				
(Antoine's)	2 oz	210	0	1.0
(De Cecco)	2 oz	210	0	1.0
PENNONI *(De Cecco)* dry	2 oz	210	0	1.0
QUINOA				
Dry				
garden pagodas 'Supergrain Wheat Free'				
(Ancient Harvest)	2 oz	180	5	2.0
veggie curls 'Supergrain Wheat Free' *(Ancient Harvest)*	2 oz	180	5	2.0
veggie curls 'Supergrain Wheat Free' *(Quinoa)*	2 oz	180	5	2.0
RADIATORE				
Dry				
tomato and spinach, tri-color *(Ronzoni)*	2 oz	210	30	1.0
wheat *(Antoine's)*	2 oz	210	0	1.0
RAINBOW 100% durum wheat semolina 'Rainbo Twirl'				
(American Beauty) dry	2 oz	210	30	1.0
RIBBON				
Dry				
spinach *(Creamette)*	2 oz	210	70	1.0

Food Name	Serv. Size	Total Cal.	Sod. MGS	Fat GMS
wheat, mixed vegetable, organic *(Herb's)*	2 oz	220	5	2.0
wheat, paella, w/saffron, organic *(Eden Foods)*	2 oz	228	0	<1.0
wheat, parsley garlic, organic *(Eden Foods)*	2 oz	228	0	<1.0
whole wheat *(De Boles)*	2 oz	210	0	2.0
yolk-free 'Pennsylvania Dutch' *(Creamette)*	2 oz	210	0	1.0
RIGATONI				
Dry				
(Creamette)	2 oz	210	0	1.0
(De Cecco)	2 oz	210	0	1.0
(Ronzoni)	2 oz	210	0	1.0
Refrigerated, fresh				
'Fresh' *(Contadina)*	2.3 oz	200	25	3.0
Jerusalem artichoke *(De Boles)*	2 oz	210	0	1.0
ROTELLE				
Dry				
100% durum wheat semolina *(American Beauty)*	2 oz	210	30	1.0
quinoa 'Supergrain Wheat Free' *(Ancient Harvest)*	2 oz	180	5	2.0
quinoa 'Supergrain Wheat Free' *(Quinoa)*	2 oz	180	5	2.0
wheat *(Creamette)*	2 oz	210	0	1.0
wheat *(De Cecco)*	2 oz	210	0	1.0
wheat *(Ronzoni)*	2 oz	210	0	1.0
ROTINI				
Dry				
garlic and parsley *(De Boles)*	2 oz	210	15	1.0
Jerusalem artichoke *(De Boles)*	2 oz	210	0	1.0
100% durum wheat semolina *(American Beauty)*	2 oz	210	0	1.0
quinoa 'Supergrain' *(Ancient Harvest)*	2 oz	210	11	1.0
vegetable 'Primavera' *(De Boles)*	2 oz	210	0	<1.0
vegetable, tomato, and basil *(De Boles)*	2 oz	210	10	1.0
SALAD PASTA 100% durum wheat semolina 'Salad-Roni' *(American Beauty)* dry	2 oz	210	0	1.0
SEA SHELL durum wheat semolina *(American Beauty)* dry	2 oz	210	0	1.0
SHELL				
Dry				
corn *(Westbrae)*	2 oz	210	10	2.0
corn, wheat-free *(De Boles)*	2 oz	210	0	1.0
extra fancy *(Ronzoni)*	2 oz	210	0	1.0
jumbo *(Ronzoni)*	2 oz	210	0	1.0
medium *(Creamette)*	2 oz	210	0	1.0
medium, 100% durum wheat semolina *(American Beauty)*	2 oz	210	0	1.0

Food Name	Serv. Size	Total Cal.	Sod. MGS	Fat GMS
100% durum wheat semolina 'Shel-Roni'				
(American Beauty) dry	2 oz	210	0	1.0
quinoa 'Supergrain Wheat Free' *(Ancient Harvest)*	2 oz	180	5	2.0
quinoa 'Supergrain Wheat Free' *(Quinoa)*	2 oz	180	5	2.0
'Primavera' *(De Boles)*	2 oz	210	0	<1.0
wheat *(Ronzoni)*	2 oz	210	0	1.0
wheat, vegetable, no eggs, organic *(Eden Foods)*	2 oz	228	0	<1.0
whole wheat *(De Boles)*	2 oz	210	0	2.0
SPAGHETTI				
Dry				
amaranth *(Health Valley)*	2 oz	170	10	1.0
corn *(Westbrae)*	2 oz	210	10	2.0
corn, wheat-free *(De Boles)*	2 oz	210	0	1.0
Jerusalem artichoke *(De Boles)*	2 oz	210	0	1.0
oat bran *(Health Valley)*	2 oz	120	2	1.0
100% durum wheat semolina *(American Beauty)*	2 oz	210	0	1.0
100% semolina *(Hospitality)*	2 oz	210	0	0.5
pepper 'Three Pepper Pasta' *(Al Dente)*	2 oz	220	20	2.0
protein-fortified	2 oz	213	5	1.3
quinoa 'Supergrain' *(Ancient Harvest)*	2 oz	210	11	1.0
quinoa 'Supergrain' *(Quinoa)*	2 oz	210	11	1.0
quinoa 'Supergrain Wheat Free' *(Ancient Harvest)*	2 oz	180	5	2.0
quinoa 'Supergrain Wheat Free' *(Quinoa)*	2 oz	180	5	2.0
spinach	2 oz	212	21	0.9
spinach, Jerusalem artichoke *(De Boles)*	2 oz	210	5	<1.0
spinach, whole wheat, no egg *(Westbrae)*	2 oz	210	0	2.0
thin *(Creamette)*	2 oz	210	0	1.0
thin *(Ronzoni)*	2 oz	210	0	1.0
thin, 100% durum wheat semolina *(American Beauty)*	2 oz	210	0	1.0
unenriched	2 oz	211	4	0.9
wheat *(DiGiorno)*	3 oz	250	140	3.0
wheat *(Rummo)*	2 oz	210	10	1.0
whole wheat	2 oz	198	5	0.8
whole wheat *(De Boles)*	2 oz	210	0	2.0
whole wheat *(Health Valley)*	2 oz	170	10	1.0
whole wheat, no egg *(Westbrae)*	2 oz	210	0	2.0
whole wheat, spinach *(Health Valley)*	2 oz	170	10	1.0
SPAGHETTINI *(De Cecco)* dry	2 oz	210	0	1.0
SPIRAL				
Dry				
spicy *(Antoine's)*	2 oz	210	40	1.0

Food Name	Serv. Size	Total Cal.	Sod. MGS	Fat GMS
vegetable	1 cup	308	36	0.9
wheat, sesame rice, organic *(Eden Foods)*	2 oz	212	0	1.0
wheat, vegetable, no eggs, organic *(Eden Foods)*	2 oz	228	0	<1.0
TRICOLOR				
Dry				
'Primavera' *(De Boles)*	2 oz	200	8	1.0
spirals	1 cup	308	36	0.9
wheat *(Creamette)*	2 oz	210	5	1.0
TRIO ITALIANO rotini, mostaccioli, shells *(American Beauty)* dry	2 oz	210	0	1.0
VERMICELLI				
Dry				
extra thin *(Creamette)*	2 oz	210	0	1.0
100% durum wheat semolina *(American Beauty)*	2 oz	210	0	1.0
wheat *(Ronzoni)*	2 oz	210	0	1.0
ZITI Jerusalem artichoke *(De Boles)* dry	2 oz	210	0	1.0
ZITI RIGATI *(Ronzoni)* dry	2 oz	210	0	1.0
PASTA DINNER, FROZEN				
penne, w/tomato sauce, Italian sausage *(Budget Gourmet)*	10 oz	320	520	9.0
primavera *(Healthy Choice)*	11 oz	280	360	3.0
stuffed, shells, 3-cheese 'LightStyle' *(Le Menu)*	10 oz	280	690	8.0
w/chicken and herb tomato sauce *(Lean Cuisine)*	9.5 oz	270	460	6.0
zesty tomato sauce over ziti 'Classics' *(Healthy Choice)*	12 oz	350	530	5.0
PASTA DINNER MIX				
artichoke elbow 'Mac & Cheese' dry *(De Boles)*	2 oz	210	160	2.0
artichoke elbow 'Mac & Cheese' prepared *(De Boles)*	3/4 cup	220	140	7.0
artichoke shells and cheddar, dry *(De Boles)*	2 oz	210	160	2.0
artichoke shells and cheddar, prepared *(De Boles)*	3/4 cup	220	140	7.0
wheat elbow 'Mac & Cheese' dry *(De Boles)*	2 oz	210	150	3.0
wheat elbow 'Mac & Cheese' prepared *(De Boles)*	3/4 cup	200	120	8.0
w/beef flavored sauce, prepared *(Ultra Slim Fast)*	8 oz	230	1070	3.0
w/chicken flavored sauce, prepared *(Ultra Slim Fast)*	8 oz	220	980	3.0
w/tomato herb sauce, prepared *(Ultra Slim Fast)*	8 oz	220	1090	3.0
w/zesty cheese sauce, prepared *(Ultra Slim Fast)*	8 oz	230	770	4.0
PASTA DISH MIX. See also NOODLE ENTRÉE/DISH MIX; ROTINI ENTRÉE MIX; SPAGHET ENTRÉE MIX.				
Alfredo 'Pasta For One' *(Villa Lorenzo)*	2.3 oz	270	910	8.0
butter and herbs 'Pasta For One' *(Villa Lorenzo)*	2.3 oz	270	800	7.0
cream sauce and mushrooms 'Pasta For One' *(Villa Lorenzo)*	2.3 oz	260	800	6.0
cream sauce and spinach 'Pasta For One' *(Villa Lorenzo)*	2.3 oz	270	900	6.0
pesto and herbs 'Pasta For One' *(Villa Lorenzo)*	2.3 oz	260	850	6.0

Food Name	Serv. Size	Total Cal.	Sod. MGS	Fat GMS
three cheese and broccoli 'Pasta For One' (Villa Lorenzo)	2.3 oz	260	910	5.0
zesty tomato 'Pasta For One' (Villa Lorenzo)	2.3 oz	250	680	3.0

PASTA ENTRÉE, CANNED. See also NOODLE ENTRÉE/DISH, CANNED; RAVIOLI ENTRÉE; SPAGHETTI ENTRÉE, CANNED.

(Chef Boyardee)

Food Name	Serv. Size	Total Cal.	Sod. MGS	Fat GMS
and chicken	7.5 oz	180	850	2.0
in cheese sauce 'ABC's & 123's'	8.6 oz	200	1020	1.0
in cheese sauce 'Dinosaurs'	8.6 oz	200	1060	1.0
in cheese sauce 'Dinosaurs'	7.5 oz	160	790	1.0
in cheese sauce 'Sharks'	7.5 oz	170	780	1.0
in cheese sauce 'Smurfs'	7.5 oz	150	830	1.0
in cheese sauce 'Tic Tac Toes'	8.6 oz	190	1080	1.0
in cheese sauce 'Tic Tac Toes'	7.5 oz	160	870	1.0
in chicken sauce 'Pac Man'	7.5 oz	170	905	7.0
in meat sauce, shells	7.5 oz	190	810	6.0
in pizza sauce, spirals	7.5 oz	180	1080	3.0
in sauce 'ABC's & 123's'	7.5 oz	160	830	1.0
in sauce 'Turtles'	7.5 oz	150	830	1.0
in tomato sauce 'Pac Man'	7.5 oz	150	830	1.0
mini bites	7.5 oz	260	1020	12.0
'Roller Coasters'	7.5 oz	230	1070	10.0
w/meatballs 'ABC's & 123's'	8.6 oz	280	1090	11.0
w/meatballs 'Dinosaurs'	8.6 oz	280	1131	11.0
w/meatballs 'Pac Man'	7.5 oz	230	880	9.0
w/meatballs 'Sharks'	7.5 oz	230	900	8.0
w/meatballs 'Smurfs'	7.5 oz	240	900	9.0
w/meatballs 'Tic Tac Toes'	8.6 oz	290	1045	11.0
w/meatballs 'Tic Tac Toes'	7.5 oz	240	1000	9.0
w/meatballs 'Turtles'	7.5 oz	220	940	8.0
w/meatballs in sauce 'Zooroni'	7.5 oz	240	970	8.0
w/mini meatballs 'ABC's & 123's'	7.5 oz	240	920	9.0
w/mini meatballs 'Dinosaurs'	7.5 oz	230	960	8.0

PASTA ENTRÉE, FROZEN. See also NOODLE ENTRÉE/DISH, FROZEN; RAVIOLI ENTRÉE; ROTINI ENTRÉE, FROZEN; SPAGHETTI ENTRÉE, FROZEN; TORTELLINI PASTA DISH/ENTRÉE, FROZEN; ZITI ENTRÉE, FROZEN.

Food Name	Serv. Size	Total Cal.	Sod. MGS	Fat GMS
angel hair (Smart Ones)	8.55 oz	120	290	<1.0
angel hair pasta (Lean Cuisine)	10 oz	240	410	5.0
baked, and cheese (Celentano)	6 oz	290	350	13.0
broccoli stuffed shells, low fat 'Great Choice' (Celentano)	10 oz	190	520	4.0
creamy cheddar 'Pasta Accents' (Green Giant)	1/2 cup	90	280	3.0
Dijon 'Microwave Garden Gourmet' (Green Giant)	1 pkg	300	560	20.0

Food Name	Serv. Size	Total Cal.	Sod. MGS	Fat GMS
garden herb seasoning 'Pasta Accents' (Green Giant)	1/2 cup	80	290	3.0
garlic seasoning 'Pasta Accents' (Green Giant)	1/2 cup	100	260	4.0
Italiano (Ultimate 200)	8 oz	190	450	4.0
'Looney Tunes Bugs Bunny & Tazmanian Devil' (Tyson)	8 oz	290	420	8.0
'Looney Tunes Daffy Duck' spaghetti & meatballs (Tyson) ..	8.65 oz	340	570	10.0
'Looney Tunes Daffy Duck & Elmer Fudd' (Tyson)	8 oz	270	430	7.0
'Looney Tunes Foghorn Leghorn & Henry Hawk' (Tyson) ...	8 oz	230	320	4.0
'Looney Tunes Sylvester & Tweety' (Tyson)	8 oz	250	380	4.0
'Looney Tunes Tweety' macaroni and cheese (Tyson)	8 oz	340	650	10.0
Parmesan, w/sweet peas 'One Serving' (Green Giant)	5.5 oz	160	420	5.0
Portafino, in wine sauce (Smart Ones)	9.5 oz	160	220	1.0
primavera 'Pasta Accents' (Green Giant)	1/2 cup	110	190	4.0
Romanoff supreme (Weight Watchers)	9 oz	230	540	7.0
shells, cheese, w/tomato sauce (Stouffer's)	9.25 oz	300	820	13.0
shells, stuffed (Celentano)	8 oz	330	680	11.0
shells, stuffed, in tomato sauce 'Classics' (Healthy Choice) ..	12 oz	330	470	3.0
shells, stuffed, low fat 'Great Choice' (Celentano)	10 oz	250	675	2.0
shells, stuffed 'Single Serving' (Buitoni)	9 oz	460	840	13.0
shells, stuffed, w/sauce (Celentano)	10 oz	410	850	14.0
shells, stuffed, w/sauce (Celentano)	6.25 oz	340	420	16.0
shells, stuffed, w/vegetables, tofu, sauce (Legume)	11 oz	240	660	12.0
shells and beef (Budget Gourmet)	10 oz	340	985	14.0
teriyaki pasta, w/chicken 'Classics' (Healthy Choice)	12.6 oz	350	370	3.0
trio 'Gourmet Selection' (Tyson)	11 oz	450	890	17.0
w/shrimp 'Classics' (Healthy Choice)	12.5 oz	270	490	4.0
w/turkey, Dijon sauce 'Lunch Express' (Lean Cuisine)	9 7/8 oz	290	540	7.0

PASTA ENTRÉE, MICROWAVE. See also NOODLE ENTRÉE/DISH, MICROWAVE; RAVIOLI ENTRÉE; SPAGHETTI ENTRÉE, MICROWAVE.

(Chef Boyardee)

Food Name	Serv. Size	Total Cal.	Sod. MGS	Fat GMS
in cheese sauce 'ABC's & 123's'	7.5 oz	180	940	1.0
in cheese sauce 'Dinosaurs'	7.5 oz	180	880	1.0
in cheese sauce 'Tic Tac Toes'	7.5 oz	170	930	1.0
in sauce 'Turtles'	7.5 oz	160	870	1.0
rings and franks	7.5 oz	190	980	5.0
rings and meatballs	7.5 oz	220	990	8.0
shells, in meat sauce	7.5 oz	210	1090	6.0
shells, in mushroom sauce	7.5 oz	170	1080	1.0
w/meatballs 'Dinosaurs'	7.5 oz	240	900	9.0
w/meatballs 'Tic Tac Toes'	7.5 oz	250	1035	10.0
w/meatballs 'Turtles'	7.5 oz	210	990	8.0
w/mini meatballs 'ABC's & 123's'	7.5 oz	260	1005	11.0

Food Name	Serv. Size	Total Cal.	Sod. MGS	Fat GMS
(Lunch Bucket)				
and garden vegetables 'Light 'n Healthy'	7.5 oz	150	630	1.0
elbows, in tomato sauce	7.5 oz	190	860	2.0
in wine sauce, beef 'Light 'n Healthy'	7.5 oz	130	600	3.0
Italian style chicken 'Light 'n Healthy'	7.5 oz	130	630	1.0
'Pasta 'n Chicken'	7.5 oz	180	860	6.0
PASTA SALAD MIX				
Caesar, dry *(Suddenly Salad)*	1/6 pkg	110	450	1.0
Caesar, prepared *(Suddenly Salad)*	1/2 cup	170	450	8.0
creamy macaroni, dry *(Suddenly Salad)*	1/6 pkg	100	210	1.0
creamy macaroni, prepared *(Suddenly Salad)*	1/2 cup	200	280	10.0
garden primavera, dry *(Kraft)*	1/6 box	170	490	7.0
Italian 'Light' dry *(Kraft)*	1/6 box	120	480	1.0
pasta, classic, dry *(Suddenly Salad)*	1/6 pkg	120	530	1.0
pasta, classic, prepared *(Suddenly Salad)*	1/2 cup	160	530	6.0
pasta primavera, dry *(Suddenly Salad)*	1/6 pkg	90	270	1.0
pasta primavera, prepared *(Suddenly Salad)*	1/2 cup	190	340	10.0
ranch and bacon, dry *(Suddenly Salad)*	1/6 pkg	110	250	1.0
ranch and bacon, prepared *(Suddenly Salad)*	1/2 cup	210	320	11.0
tortellini, Italiano, dry *(Suddenly Salad)*	1/5 pkg	120	450	2.0
tortellini, Italiano, prepared *(Suddenly Salad)*	1/2 cup	160	450	7.0
PASTA SAUCE. See SAUCE.				
PASTRAMI. See LUNCHEON MEAT.				
PASTRY. See also BREAD, SWEET; BUN, SWEET; CAKE; DANISH PASTRY; MUFFIN; PIE; ROLL, SWEET; TURNOVER.				
(Charlette Russe) w/lady fingers, whipped cream filling	1 serving	326	49	16.6
(Pillsbury) pocket, refrigerated	1 piece	240	520	13.0
PASTRY, BAVARIAN CREAM				
(Entenmann's)	1.3 oz	80	90	0.0
(Rich's) puff, frozen	1 piece	150	70	8.0
PASTRY, CINNAMON *(Entenmann's)* filbert ring	1.5 oz	190	160	12.0
PASTRY, DATE NUT *(Awrey's)* 1 piece	1.6 oz	230	150	10.0
PASTRY, ÉCLAIR				
(Rich's) frozen, chocolate, 2 oz	1 piece	210	110	10.0
(Weight Watchers) frozen, chocolate 'Sweet Celebrations'	2.1 oz	150	110	4.0
PATÉ, CANNED				
chicken liver	1 oz	57	109	3.7
chicken liver	1 tbsp	26	50	1.7
foie gras, goose liver, smoked	1 oz	131	198	12.4
foie gras, goose liver, smoked	1 tbsp	60	91	5.7
liver *(Sells)*	2 1/8 oz	190	470	16.0

Food Name	Serv. Size	Total Cal.	Sod. MGS	Fat GMS
PATTYPAN SQUASH. See SQUASH, SCALLOP.				
PEACH				
peeled, pitted	1 oz	12	tr	<.1
peeled, sliced	1/2 cup	37	1	0.1
raw, approx 4 oz	1 med	37	0	0.1
raw, slices	1 cup	73	0	0.2
untrimmed	1 lb	148	2	0.3
untrimmed *(Dole)*	2 pieces	70	0	0.0
PEACH, CANNED				
'Fruit Pak' *(Mott's)*	3.75 oz	75	7	0.0
halves *(Hunt's)*	4 oz	90	7	<1.0
slices *(Hunt's)*	4 oz	90	7	<1.0
FREESTONE				
halves *(Del Monte)*	1/2 cup	90	10	0.0
halves *(S&W Nutradiet)*	1/2 cup	30	10	0.0
halves 'Lite' *(Del Monte)*	1/2 cup	60	10	0.0
in heavy syrup, halves *(S&W)*	1/2 cup	100	10	0.0
in heavy syrup, slices *(S&W)*	1/2 cup	100	10	0.0
slices *(Del Monte)*	1/2 cup	90	10	0.0
slices *(S&W Nutradiet)*	1/2 cup	30	10	0.0
slices 'Lite' *(Del Monte)*	1/2 cup	60	10	0.0
YELLOW CLING				
diced 'Fruit Cup' *(Del Monte)*	5 oz	110	10	0.0
halves *(Del Monte)*	1/2 cup	80	10	0.0
halves *(S&W Nutradiet)*	1/2 cup	30	5	0.0
halves 'Lite' *(Del Monte)*	1/2 cup	50	10	0.0
halves 'Lite' *(Finast)*	1/2 cup	50	10	0.0
in heavy syrup, halves *(A&P)*	1/2 cup	100	10	<1.0
in heavy syrup, halves *(S&W)*	1/2 cup	100	10	0.0
in heavy syrup, slices *(A&P)*	1/2 cup	100	10	<1.0
in heavy syrup, slices *(Finast)*	1/2 cup	100	6	0.0
in heavy syrup, slices *(Pathmark)*	1/2 cup	100	10	0.0
in heavy syrup, slices *(S&W)*	1/2 cup	100	10	0.0
in heavy syrup, whole, spiced *(S&W)*	1/2 cup	90	10	0.0
in juice *(A&P)*	1/2 cup	50	10	<1.0
in juice, halves *(A&P)*	1/2 cup	50	10	<1.0
in juice, halves *(Featherweight)*	1/2 cup	50	10	0.0
in juice, halves 'Lite' *(Libby's)*	1/2 cup	50	0	0.0
in juice, slices *(Featherweight)*	1/2 cup	50	10	0.0
in juice, slices *(IGA)*	1/2 cup	50	10	0.0
in juice, slices *(Pathmark)*	1/2 cup	50	10	0.0

Food Name	Serv. Size	Total Cal.	Sod. MGS	Fat GMS
in juice, slices 'Lite' *(Libby's)*	1/2 cup	50	0	0.0
in juice, slices, sweetened *(S&W)*	1/2 cup	90	10	0.0
in light syrup, slices 'No Frills' *(Pathmark)*	1/2 cup	140	15	0.0
slices *(Del Monte)*	1/2 cup	80	10	0.0
slices 'Lite' *(Del Monte)*	1/2 cup	50	10	0.0
slices 'Lite' *(Finast)*	1/2 cup	50	10	0.0
slices, unsweetened *(S&W Nutradiet)*	1/2 cup	30	5	0.0
spiced, w/pits *(Del Monte)*	3.5 oz	80	10	0.0
PEACH, DRIED				
sulfured, cooked, sweetened	4 oz	117	2	0.2
sulfured, cooked, sweetened, halves	1/2 cup	139	3	0.3
sulfured, cooked, unsweetened	4 oz	87	2	0.3
sulfured, cooked, unsweetened, halves	1/2 cup	91	3	0.3
sulfured, uncooked	4 oz	271	8	0.9
sulfured, uncooked, approx 4.6 oz	10 halves	311	9	1.0
sulfured, uncooked, halves	1/2 cup	192	6	0.6
(Del Monte) uncooked	2 oz	140	10	0.0
(Mountain House) freeze-dried, prepared	1/4 cup	50	<1	0.0
(Sun•Maid)	2 oz	140	10	0.0
(SunSweet)	2 oz	140	10	0.0
PEACH, FROZEN				
slices, sweetened	10-oz pkg	267	17	0.4
slices, sweetened	1/2 cup	118	8	0.2
slices, sweetened	4 oz	107	7	0.1
PEACH BUTTER *(Smucker's)*	1 tsp	15	0	0.0
PEACH DRINK				
(Hi-C)	6 oz	101	18	<.1
(Ocean Spray) citrus 'Refreshers'	6 oz	90	15	0.0
PEACH JUICE				
(Dole) orchard blend 'Pure & Light'	6 oz	90	10	0.0
(Smucker's) 'Naturally 100%'	8 oz	120	10	0.0
(Snapple) 'Dixie Peach'	8 oz	160	20	0.0
PEACH NECTAR				
w/added ascorbic acid	1 cup	134	17	0.1
w/added ascorbic acid	1 oz	17	2	0.0
w/o added ascorbic acid	1 cup	134	17	0.1
w/o added ascorbic acid	1 oz	17	2	0.0
(Kern's)	6 oz	110	0	0.0
(Knudsen & Sons)	8 oz	107	na	0.0
(Libby's)	6 oz	100	5	0.0

Food Name	Serv. Size	Total Cal.	Sod. MGS	Fat GMS
PEANUT, SHELLED				
(Beer Nuts)	1 oz	180	60	14.0
(Frito Lay) salted	1 oz	170	170	15.0
(Little Debbie) salted	1.25 oz	230	90	18.0
(Pathmark) 'Sweet and Crunchy'	1 oz	140	30	8.0
(Planters)				
hot spicy 'Heat'	1 oz	170	190	14.0
mild spicy 'Heat'	1 oz	170	130	14.0
'Sweet-N-Crunchy'	1 oz	140	20	8.0
(Weight Watchers)	1 pouch	100	50	7.0
BOILED				
salted	1/2 cup	102	240	7.0
salted	1 oz	90	213	6.2
DRY-ROASTED				
(Finast)				
lightly salted	1 oz	160	15	14.0
salted	1 oz	160	120	14.0
(Flavor House)				
salted	1 oz	180	200	14.0
unsalted	1 oz	180	0	14.0
(Frito Lay) salted	1 1/8 oz	190	300	16.0
(Guy's) salted	1 oz	170	310	14.0
(Pathmark)				
'No Frills' salted	1 oz	170	150	14.0
'No Frills' unsalted	1 oz	180	0	14.0
(Planters)				
lightly salted	1 oz	170	110	15.0
salted	1 oz	160	250	14.0
unsalted	1 oz	170	0	15.0
HONEY-ROASTED				
(Eagle) 'Honey Roast'	1 oz	170	140	13.0
(Fisher)				
lightly salted	1 oz	150	0	13.0
salted	1 oz	150	115	13.0
(Flavor House)	1 oz	160	120	11.0
(Little Debbie)	1.13 oz	190	15	13.0
(Pathmark)	1 oz	170	75	13.0
(Planters)	1 oz	170	180	13.0
(Weight Watchers)	1 pouch	100	50	7.0
OIL-ROASTED				
(Fisher) salted	1 oz	160	130	14.0

Food Name	Serv. Size	Total Cal.	Sod. MGS	Fat GMS
(Flavor House) salted	1 oz	170	125	15.0
(Pathmark) salted	1 oz	180	150	14.0
(Planters)				
cocktail	1 oz	170	160	15.0
cocktail, unsalted	1 oz	170	0	15.0
lightly salted	1 oz	170	80	14.0
redskin	1 oz	170	150	15.0
salted	1 oz	170	160	15.0
unsalted	1 oz	170	0	14.0
PEANUT, SPANISH				
DRY-ROASTED *(Planters)*	1 oz	160	200	14.0
OIL-ROASTED				
salted	1/2 cup	426	319	36.0
salted	1 oz	162	121	13.7
salted *(Flavor House)*	1 oz	170	125	15.0
salted *(Planters)*	1 oz	170	100	15.0
shelled, salted *(Flavor House)*	1 oz	170	125	15.0
shelled, salted *(Guy's)*	1 oz	170	170	14.0
unsalted	1/2 cup	426	4	36.0
unsalted	1 oz	162	2	13.7
RAW				
	1 cup	832	32	72.4
	1 oz	160	6	13.9
(Planters)	1 oz	160	5	14.0
PEANUT, VALENCIA				
oil-roasted	1 cup	848	9	73.8
oil-roasted	1/2 cup	424	4	36.9
oil-roasted	1 oz	165	2	14.4
raw	1/2 cup	417	<1	34.7
raw	1 oz	160	0	13.3
PEANUT, VIRGINIA				
oil-roasted, unsalted	1 cup	827	9	69.5
oil-roasted, unsalted	1 oz	162	2	13.6
raw	1 cup	822	15	71.2
raw	1 oz	158	3	13.6
PEANUT BUTTER				
(Hollywood) 'Unsalted'	1 tbsp	35	0	3.0
(Pathmark) 'Natural'	2 tbsp	200	130	17.0
(Roaster Fresh) gourmet	1 oz	166	2	14.0
(S&W Nutradiet)	1 tbsp	93	10	8.0

Food Name	Serv. Size	Total Cal.	Sod. MGS	Fat GMS
(Smucker's)				
honey sweetened	2 tbsp	200	150	16.0
no salt added 'Natural'	2 tbsp	200	10	16.0
CHUNKY				
(Arrowhead Mills)	2 tbsp	190	<1	16.0
(Bama)	2 tbsp	200	115	17.0
(Estee)	2 tbsp	200	0	18.0
(Featherweight)	1 tbsp	90	5	7.0
(Finast) 'Crunchy'	2 tbsp	195	175	17.0
(Health Valley) 'No Salt Added'	2 tbsp	180	2	14.0
(Hollywood)	1 tbsp	35	25	3.0
(Jif)				
regular	2 tbsp	190	155	16.0
'Simply Jif'	2 tbsp	180	50	16.0
(Maranatha Natural) crunchy	2 tbsp	190	5	15.0
(Pathmark) 'Super Chunky'	2 tbsp	200	140	17.0
(Peter Pan)				
'Extra Crunchy'	2 tbsp	190	122	16.3
regular	2 tbsp	190	120	16.0
'Salt Free'	2 tbsp	190	0	17.0
(Skippy) 'Super Chunk'	2 tbsp	190	130	17.0
(Smucker's) 'Chunky Natural'	2 tbsp	200	120	16.0
(Westbrae)				
'Natural' w/salt	2 tbsp	190	5	16.0
'Natural' w/o salt	2 tbsp	190	0	16.0
SMOOTH				
(Arrowhead Mills)	2 tbsp	190	<1	16.0
(Bama)	2 tbsp	200	140	17.0
(Estee)	1 tbsp	100	2	8.0
(Featherweight)	1 tbsp	90	3	7.0
(Finast)	2 tbsp	195	175	17.0
(Health Valley) 'No Salt Added'	2 tbsp	180	2	14.0
(Hollywood)	1 tbsp	35	25	3.0
(Jif)				
regular	2 tbsp	190	155	16.0
'Simply Jif'	2 tbsp	180	65	16.0
(Pathmark) 'No Frills Creamy'	2 tbsp	200	170	17.0
(Peter Pan)				
'Creamy'	2 tbsp	190	150	16.4
'Creamy Salt Free'	2 tbsp	195	1	17.1
(Skippy) 'Creamy'	2 tbsp	190	150	17.0

Food Name	Serv. Size	Total Cal.	Sod. MGS	Fat GMS
(Smucker's)				
'Natural'	2 tbsp	200	120	16.0
'No Salt Added Natural'	2 tbsp	200	10	17.0
(Westbrae) 'Natural' no salt	2 tbsp	190	0	16.0
(Woodstock) 'Old Fashioned Unsalted'	2 tbsp	200	3	16.0
W/JELLY				
(Bama)	2 tbsp	150	75	7.0
(Smucker's)				
'Goober Grape'	2 tbsp	180	120	10.0
'Goober Strawberry'	2 tbsp	180	120	10.0
PEANUT BUTTER CHIPS *(Hershey's)* 'Reese's'	1.5 oz	230	90	13.0
PEANUT BUTTER TOPPING *(Smucker's)* caramel	2 tbsp	150	120	2.0
PEANUT FLOUR				
defatted	1 cup	196	108	0.3
defatted	1 oz	92	50	0.2
low-fat	1 cup	257	1	13.1
low-fat	1 oz	120	0	6.1
PEANUT OIL				
	1/2 cup	955	0	108.0
	1 oz	251	0	28.4
(Hain)	1 tbsp	120	0	14.0
(Planters)	1 tbsp	120	0	14.0
(Spectrum Naturals)	1 tbsp	120	0	14.0
(Wesson)	1 tbsp	122	0	13.6
PEAR				
Asian, raw	1 fruit	51	0	0.3
raw, slices	1 cup	97	0	0.7
trimmed, w/skin	1 oz	17	tr	0.1
untrimmed	1 lb	247	2	1.7
untrimmed *(Dole)*	1 fruit	100	1	1.0
w/skin, sliced	1/2 cup	49	1	0.3
PEAR, CANNED				
in extra heavy syrup	4 oz	110	6	0.1
in extra heavy syrup, halves	1/2 cup	127	7	0.2
in extra heavy syrup, solid and liquid, halves	1 cup	253	13	0.3
in extra light syrup	4 oz	53	2	0.1
in extra light syrup, halves	1/2 cup	58	3	0.1
in extra light syrup, solid and liquid, halves	1 cup	116	5	0.3
in heavy syrup	4 oz	84	6	0.1
in heavy syrup, halves	1/2 cup	94	7	0.2
in heavy syrup, solid and liquid, halves	1 cup	189	13	0.3

Food Name	Serv. Size	Total Cal.	Sod. MGS	Fat GMS
in juice	4 oz	57	5	0.1
in juice, halves	1/2 cup	62	5	0.1
in juice, solid and liquid, halves	1 cup	124	10	0.2
in light syrup	4 oz	65	6	<.1
in light syrup, halves	1/2 cup	72	7	<.1
in light syrup, solid and liquid, halves	1 cup	143	13	0.1
in water	4 oz	33	2	<.1
in water, halves	1/2 cup	36	3	<.1
in water, solid and liquid, halves	1 cup	71	5	0.1
(A&P)				
in heavy syrup, halves or slices	1/2 cup	95	10	<1.0
in juice, halves or slices	1/2 cup	60	10	<1.0
in light syrup, halves or slices	1/2 cup	70	10	<1.0
(Del Monte)				
Bartlett, halves 'Lite'	1/2 cup	50	10	0.0
Bartlett, halves or slices	1/2 cup	80	10	0.0
Bartlett, slices 'Lite'	1/2 cup	50	10	0.0
(Featherweight) in juice, halves	1/2 cup	60	10	0.0
(Finast)				
Bartlett, halves or slices, in heavy syrup	1/2 cup	100	10	0.0
Bartlett, halves or slices, 'Lite No Sugar Added'	1/2 cup	60	10	0.0
(Hunt's) halves	4 oz	90	6	1.0
(IGA) Bartlett, halves, unsweetened	1/2 cup	60	10	0.0
(Libby's) in juice, halves or slices, 'Lite'	1/2 cup	60	10	0.0
(Pathmark)				
Bartlett, halves, in heavy syrup	1/2 cup	90	10	0.0
Bartlett, halves, in juice	1/2 cup	60	10	0.0
Bartlett, in light syrup 'No Frills'	1 cup	140	10	0.0
Bartlett, slices, in heavy syrup	1 cup	180	20	0.0
(S&W Nutradiet)				
Bartlett, peeled, unsweetened	1/2 cup	35	10	0.0
in heavy syrup, halves	1/2 cup	100	10	0.0
in juice, slices, sweetened 'Natural Style'	1/2 cup	80	10	0.0
peeled, quarters	1/2 cup	35	10	0.0
PEAR, DRIED				
Sulfured				
cooked, sweetened	4 oz	159	3	0.3
cooked, unsweetened	4 oz	144	3	0.4
stewed, w/added sugar, halves	1/2 cup	196	4	0.4
stewed, w/o added sugar, halves	1/2 cup	163	4	0.4
uncooked	10 halves	458	10	1.1

Food Name	Serv. Size	Total Cal.	Sod. MGS	Fat GMS
uncooked	4 oz	297	7	0.7
PEAR JUICE				
(Knudsen & Sons)	8 oz	110	na	0.0
(Santa Cruz Natural) organic 'Cruz'	8 oz	135	na	<1.0
PEAR NECTAR				
(Kern's)	6 oz	120	0	0.0
(Libby's)	6 oz	110	0	0.0
PEAS, CROWDER				
(Allens) canned, 'Fresh'	1/2 cup	80	370	<1.0
(Seabrook) frozen	3 oz	130	na	1.0
PEAS, GREEN				
(NOTE: All peas are shelled unless otherwise noted.)				
boiled, drained	4 oz	95	3	0.2
boiled, drained	1/2 cup	67	2	0.2
boiled, drained, in pod	4 oz	48	5	0.3
boiled, drained, in pod	1/2 cup	34	3	0.2
raw	1/2 cup	58	4	0.3
raw	1 oz	23	1	0.1
raw, in pod	1 lb	140	8	0.7
raw, trimmed	1/2 cup	30	3	0.1
raw, trimmed	1 oz	12	1	0.1
raw, untrimmed	1 lb	180	18	0.9
CANNED				
dietary pack, drained solids	1/2 cup	59	2	0.3
dietary pack, solids and liquid	1/2 cup	61	2	0.4
drained, low-sodium	4 oz	78	2	0.4
regular pack, drained solids	1/2 cup	59	186	0.3
regular pack, solids and liquid	1/2 cup	61	340	0.4
Early/June				
(A&P)	1/2 cup	70	350	<1.0
(Allens) dry	1/2 cup	80	320	<1.0
(Del Monte) small, w/liquid	1/2 cup	50	355	0.0
(Green Giant)	1/2 cup	50	330	0.0
(Green Giant) very young, small	1/2 cup	50	390	0.0
(S&W) 'Petit Pois'	1/2 cup	70	330	0.0
(Stokely)	1/2 cup	60	320	0.0
Mixed sizes				
(A&P)	1/2 cup	60	350	<1.0
(IGA) 'No Salt or Sugar Added'	1/2 cup	50	10	0.0
Sweet				
wrinkled, dietary pack, drained, low-sodium	1 lb	82	14	0.0

Food Name	Serv. Size	Total Cal.	Sod. MGS	Fat GMS
wrinkled, dietary pack, drained, low-sodium	1 oz	5	1	0.0
wrinkled, regular pack, drained	1 lb	100	1071	0.0
wrinkled, regular pack, drained	1 oz	6	66	0.0
(Featherweight)	1/2 cup	70	10	0.0
(Finast)	1/2 cup	70	300	1.0
(Finast) 'No Salt Added'	1/2 cup	60	10	0.0
(Green Giant)	1/2 cup	50	320	0.0
(Green Giant) 50% less salt	1/2 cup	50	195	0.0
(Green Giant) mini	1/2 cup	50	340	0.0
(Green Giant) mini, in brine	1/2 cup	60	240	<1.0
(Green Giant) very young, small	1/2 cup	50	390	0.0
(Green Giant) very young, tender	1/2 cup	50	390	0.0
(IGA) tiny, early/June	1/2 cup	70	340	0.0
(Pathmark) garden, fancy	1/2 cup	70	350	1.0
(Pathmark) large, tender	1/2 cup	70	350	1.0
(Pathmark) 'Little Gem'	1/2 cup	70	350	1.0
(Pathmark) mixed sizes 'No Salt Added'	1/2 cup	50	10	0.0
(Pathmark) 'No Frills'	1 cup	120	640	1.0
(Pathmark) small	1/2 cup	70	350	1.0
(S&W) 'Perfection'	1/2 cup	70	330	0.0
(S&W Nutradiet)	1/2 cup	40	5	0.0
(Stokely)	1/2 cup	60	320	0.0
W/ liquid				
low-sodium	4 oz	56	2	0.3
(Del Monte)	1/2 cup	60	355	0.0
(Del Monte) 'No Salt Added'	1/2 cup	60	10	0.0
FREEZE-DRIED (Mountain House) prepared	1/2 cup	70	21	1.0
FROZEN				
boiled, drained	4 oz	88	99	0.3
boiled, drained	1/2 cup	62	70	0.2
unprepared	1/2 cup	55	81	0.3
(Birds Eye)	3.3 oz	80	130	0.0
(Birds Eye) 'Portion Pack'	3 oz	70	120	0.0
(Freshlike)	3.3 oz	80	75	0.0
(Frosty Acres)	3.3 oz	80	91	0.0
(Health Valley)	1/2 cup	65	70	0.0
(Seabrook)	3.3 oz	80	91	0.0
(Southern)	3.5 oz	79	130	0.5
(Stokely) 'Singles'	3 oz	65	95	1.0
(Veg•All)	3.3 oz	80	75	0.0

Food Name	Serv. Size	Total Cal.	Sod. MGS	Fat GMS
Chinese				
(Chun King)	1.5 oz	20	10	0.0
(Seabrook)	2 oz	20	na	0.0
Combinations				
(Bird's Eye) w/cream sauce 'Combination Vegetables'	5 oz	180	480	11.0
(Bird's Eye) w/pearl onions 'Combination Vegetables'	3.3 oz	70	440	0.0
(Bird's Eye) w/potatoes, cream sauce 'Combination Vegetables'	5 oz	190	490	12.0
(Budget Gourmet) and cauliflower, in cream sauce	5.75 oz	170	280	7.0
(Budget Gourmet) Oriental, and water chestnuts 'Side Dish'	5 oz	120	240	3.0
(Green Giant) 'LeSueur Valley'	1/2 cup	70	400	2.0
(Green Giant) mini, pea pods, water chestnut, butter 'LeSueur Valley'	1/2 cup	80	410	2.0
(Green Giant) w/onions and carrots in butter sauce 'LeSueur Valley'	1/2 cup	80	470	3.0
Early/June				
(Finast) in butter sauce	1/2 cup	80	400	4.0
(Green Giant) 'Harvest Fresh'	1/2 cup	60	140	1.0
(Green Giant) in butter sauce 'One Serving'	4.5 oz	90	500	2.0
(Green Giant) in butter sauce 'Select LeSueur'	1/2 cup	80	440	2.0
(Southern) petite	3.5 oz	64	50	0.4
Sweet				
(Finast)	3.3 oz	80	125	0.0
(Green Giant)	1/2 cup	50	95	0.0
(Green Giant) 'Harvest Fresh'	1/2 cup	50	135	0.0
(Green Giant) in butter sauce	1/2 cup	80	410	2.0
(Stokely) in butter sauce 'Singles'	4 oz	90	335	1.0
Tiny				
(Birds Eye) tender, 'Deluxe'	3.3 oz	60	120	0.0
(Freshlike)	3.3 oz	60	75	0.0
(Frosty Acres)	3.3 oz	60	127	0.0
(Seabrook)	3.3 oz	60	127	0.0
(Veg•All)	3.3 oz	60	75	0.0
PEAS, PIGEON				
immature seeds, boiled, drained	1/2 cup	85	4	1.0
immature seeds, raw	10 seeds	5	0	0.1
raw, in pods	1 lb	296	11	3.6
red gram, mature seeds, boiled	1/2 cup	102	4	0.3
red gram, mature seeds, raw	1/2 cup	350	17	1.5
shelled, boiled, drained	4 oz	126	5	1.5

Food Name	Serv. Size	Total Cal.	Sod. MGS	Fat GMS
shelled, raw	1 oz	39	1	0.5
shelled, raw, approx .1 oz	10 peas	5	tr	0.1
Dried				
shelled, mature, boiled	4 oz	137	6	0.4
shelled, mature, boiled	1/2 cup	102	5	0.3
shelled, mature, raw	1/2 cup	350	17	1.5
shelled, mature, raw	1 oz	97	5	0.4
PEAS, PURPLE HULL				
(Allens) canned 'Fresh'	1/2 cup	100	370	<1.0
(Frosty Acres) frozen	3.3 oz	130	6	0.0
PEAS, SNAP				
(Birds Eye) carrots, water chestnuts	3.2 oz	50	20	0.0
(Birds Eye) 'Deluxe'	2.6 oz	45	5	0.0
(Green Giant) 'Harvest Fresh'	1/2 cup	30	100	0.0
(Green Giant) 'Sugar Snap' frozen	1/2 cup	30	0	0.0
PEAS, SNOW, 'Deluxe' (Birds Eye)	3 oz	35	0	0.0
PEAS, WHITE ACRE, canned (Allens)	1/2 cup	90	440	<1.0
PEAS AND CARROTS, CANNED				
regular pack, solid and liquid	1/2 cup	49	333	0.4
special dietary pack, solid and liquid	1/2 cup	49	5	0.4
w/liquid	4 oz	43	295	0.3
w/liquid, low-sodium	4 oz	43	5	0.3
(A&P) early/June 'No Salt Added'	1/2 cup	60	10	<1.0
(A&P) mixed sizes	1/2 cup	60	10	<1.0
(Del Monte) w/liquid	1/2 cup	50	355	0.0
(Finast)	1/2 cup	55	315	0.0
(Freshlike)	1/2 cup	50	340	0.0
(Freshlike) water pack, w/o salt	1/2 cup	50	30	0.0
(Freshlike) water pack, w/o sugar, salt	1/2 cup	50	30	0.0
(Kohl's)	1/2 cup	50	330	<1.0
(Pathmark)	1/2 cup	60	330	1.0
(S&W)	1/2 cup	50	310	0.0
(S&W Nutradiet)	1/2 cup	35	5	0.0
(Stokely)	1/2 cup	50	320	0.0
(Stokely) 'No Salt or Sugar Added'	1/2 cup	45	20	0.0
(Veg•All)	1/2 cup	50	340	0.0
PEAS AND CARROTS, FROZEN				
boiled, drained	10-oz pkg	133	189	1.2
boiled, drained	4 oz	54	77	0.5
boiled, drained	1/2 cup	38	54	0.3
unprepared	10-oz pkg	151	224	1.3

Food Name	Serv. Size	Total Cal.	Sod. MGS	Fat GMS
unprepared	1/2 cup	37	55	0.3
(A&P)	3.3 oz	60	75	<1.0
(A&P) sweet peas	1/2 cup	80	90	<1.0
(Freshlike)	3.3 oz	60	60	0.0
(Frosty Acres)	3.3 oz	60	75	0.0
(Seabrook)	3.3 oz	60	75	0.0
(Southern)	3.5 oz	64	80	0.0
(Veg•All)	3.3 oz	60	60	0.0
PEAS AND ONIONS, CANNED				
solid and liquid	1/2 cup	31	265	0.2
w/liquid	4 oz	58	501	0.4
(Freshlike) sweet peas, tiny onions	1/2 cup	60	440	0.0
(Green Giant) pearl onions, w/liquid	1/2 cup	50	510	0.0
(S&W) tiny pearl onions, w/liquid	1/2 cup	60	490	1.0
PEAS AND ONIONS, FROZEN				
boiled, drained	4 oz	51	na	0.2
boiled, drained	1/2 cup	41	33	0.2
unprepared	10-oz pkg	199	173	0.9
unprepared	1/2 cup	48	42	0.2
(Birds Eye) pearl onions 'Cheese Sauce Combinations'	5 oz	140	470	5.0
(Birds Eye) pearl onions 'Combination Vegetables'	3.3 oz	70	440	0.0
(Freshlike)	3.3 oz	70	100	0.0
(Frosty Acres) pearl onions	3.3 oz	70	80	0.0
(Seabrook)	3.3 oz	70	na	0.0
(Veg•All)	3.3 oz	70	100	0.0
PECAN, SHELLED				
chopped (Fisher)	1 oz	190	0	19.0
dried, chopped	1 cup	794	1	80.5
dried, ground	1 cup	634	1	64.3
dried, halves	1 cup	721	1	73.1
dried, halves, pieces, or chips (Planters)	1 oz	190	0	20.0
dried, 31 large or 20 medium halves	1 oz	190	tr	19.2
dry-roasted	1 oz	187	0	18.4
ground (Fisher)	1 oz	190	0	19.0
honey-roasted (Planters)	1 oz	200	0	18.0
oil-roasted	1 cup	753	1	78.3
oil-roasted, 15 halves	1 oz	195	0	20.2
raw (Fisher)	1 oz	190	0	19.0
raw, chips (Planters)	1 oz	190	0	20.0
raw, halves (Planters)	1 oz	190	0	20.0
raw, pieces (Planters)	1 oz	190	0	20.0

Food Name	Serv. Size	Total Cal.	Sod. MGS	Fat GMS
PECAN FLOUR	1 oz	93	0	0.4
PECTIN, unsweetened, dry mix	.5 oz	39	24	0.0
PEPITAS				
In shell				
dried	1 lb	1817	59	153.9
roasted, whole	1 cup	285	12	12.4
roasted, whole, approx 85 seeds	1 oz	127	5	5.5
Shelled				
dried	1 cup	747	24	63.3
dried, approx 142 kernels	1 oz	154	5	13.0
roasted	1 cup	1184	40	95.6
roasted	1 oz	148	5	12.0
salted	1 lb	2021	2608	88.0
salted	1 cup	285	368	12.4
salted	1 oz	127	163	5.5
PEPPER, BANANA, hot rings *(Vlasic)*	1 oz	4	465	0.0
PEPPER, BELL. See PEPPER, SWEET.				
PEPPER, CHERRY				
hot *(Progresso)*	1/2 cup	190	130	20.0
hot *(Vlasic)*	1 oz	10	425	0.0
hot, pickled *(Progresso)*	1/2 cup	130	110	12.0
mild *(Vlasic)*	1 oz	8	410	0.0
PEPPER, CHILI				
green, raw, approx 1.6 oz	1 med	18	3	0.1
green, raw, chopped	1/2 cup	30	5	0.2
green, raw, trimmed	1 oz	11	2	0.1
green, raw, untrimmed	1 lb	134	23	0.7
red, raw, approx 1.6 oz	1 med	18	3	0.1
red, raw, chopped	1/2 cup	30	5	0.2
red, raw, trimmed	1 oz	11	2	0.1
red, raw, untrimmed	1 lb	134	23	0.7
Canned				
green, chopped *(Old El Paso)*	2 tbsp	8	70	<1.0
green, diced *(Rosarita)*	1.058 oz	6	85	0.1
green, diced, w/liquid *(Del Monte)*	1/2 cup	20	690	0.0
green, whole *(Old El Paso)*	1 pepper	8	105	<1.0
green, whole *(Rosarita)*	1.235 oz	4	74	0.1
green, whole, diced, sliced, or strips *(Ortega)*	1 oz	10	20	0.0
green, whole, w/liquid *(Del Monte)*	1/2 cup	20	690	0.0
green and red, seeded, chopped, w/liquid	1/2 cup	17	(mq)	0.1
green and red, seeded, w/liquid	4 oz	28	(mq)	0.1

Food Name	Serv. Size	Total Cal.	Sod. MGS	Fat GMS
hot, green, pods, w/o seeds, solid and liquid, chopped	1/2 cup	17	798	0.1
hot, green and red, seeded, w/liquid, approx 2.6 oz	1 med	18	(mq)	0.1

PEPPER, GREEN. See PEPPER, SWEET.

PEPPER, GROUND

Food Name	Serv. Size	Total Cal.	Sod. MGS	Fat GMS
black	1 oz	72	12	0.9
black	1 tbsp	16	3	0.2
black	1 tsp	5	1	0.1
black (Durkee)	1 tsp	8	0	tr
black (Laurel Leaf)	1 tsp	8	0	tr
black (Spice Islands)	1 tsp	9	<1	0.2
cayenne/red	1 oz	90	9	4.9
cayenne/red	1 tbsp	17	2	0.9
cayenne/red	1 tsp	6	1	0.3
cayenne/red (Durkee)	1 tsp	8	0	<0.1
cayenne/red (Laurel Leaf)	1 tsp	8	0	<0.1
cayenne/red (Spice Islands)	1 tsp	9	<1	0.3
chili (Spice Islands)	1 tsp	9	<1	0.3
pizza (Lawry's)	1 tsp	2	11	0.2
seasoned (Lawry's)	1 tsp	9	5	0.1
seasoned 'All Pepper' (Schilling)	1/4 tsp	1	106	0.0
white	1 oz	84	1	0.6
white	1 tbsp	21	0	0.2
white	1 tsp	7	0	0.1
white (Durkee)	1 tsp	9	0	tr
white (Laurel Leaf)	1 tsp	9	0	tr
white (Spice Islands)	1 tsp	9	<1	0.2

PEPPER, JALAPEÑO

Food Name	Serv. Size	Total Cal.	Sod. MGS	Fat GMS
diced (Ortega)	1 oz	10	20	0.0
diced (Rosarita)	1.058 oz	5	121	0.2
for nachos (La Victoria)	14 pieces	5	330	0.0
for nachos (La Victoria)	1 tbsp	2	335	<1.0
hot, diced (Ortega)	1 oz	8	(mq)	0.0
hot 'Mexican' (Vlasic)	1 oz	8	380	0.0
hot, tiny, Mexican (Vlasic)	1 oz	6	430	0.0
hot, whole (Ortega)	1 oz	8	(mq)	0.0
marinated (La Victoria)	1.5 pieces	10	300	0.0
marinated (La Victoria)	1 tbsp	4	251	<1.0
nacho sliced (Rosarita)	1.058 oz	4	448	0.1
sliced, w/liquid (Del Monte)	1/2 cup	30	1690	1.0
whole (Old El Paso)	2 peppers	14	480	1.0
whole (Ortega)	1 oz	10	20	0.0

Food Name	Serv. Size	Total Cal.	Sod. MGS	Fat GMS
whole *(Rosarita)*	1.34 oz	6	568	0.2
whole, w/escabeche *(Rosarita)*	1.164 oz	8	430	0.2
whole, w/liquid *(Del Monte)*	1/2 cup	30	1690	1.0
PEPPER, PEPPERONCINI				
mild, Greek, salad *(Vlasic)*	1 oz	4	450	0.0
Tuscan *(Progresso)*	1/2 cup	20	5	0.0
PEPPER, PICCALILLI *(Progresso)*	1/2 cup	190	220	20.0
PEPPER, SWEET/bell pepper/green pepper/red pepper/yellow pepper				
boiled, drained	4 oz	32	2	0.2
boiled, drained, approx 2.6 oz	1 med	20	1	0.2
boiled, drained, chopped	1/2 cup	19	1	0.1
raw, approx 3.2 oz	1 med	20	1	0.1
raw, chopped	1/2 cup	14	1	0.1
raw *(Dole)*	1 med	25	0	1.0
raw, trimmed	1 oz	8	<1	0.1
raw, untrimmed	1 lb	99	7	0.7
Canned				
roasted *(Progresso)*	1/2 cup	20	2	<1.0
solid and liquid, halves	1/2 cup	13	958	0.2
'Sweet Pepper Mementos' *(Heinz)*	1 oz	6	320	0.0
w/liquid	4 oz	20	1552	0.3
Freeze-dried				
	1 oz	89	55	0.9
	1/4 cup	5	3	0.1
Frozen				
boiled, drained, chopped	4 oz	20	5	0.2
chopped, unprepared	10-oz pkg	57	14	0.6
chopped, unprepared	1 oz	6	1	0.1
green *(Seabrook)*	1 oz	6	1	0.0
red *(Seabrook)*	1 oz	8	na	0.0
PEPPER DILL SEASONING *(Golden Dipt)*	2 grams	8	96	0.0
PEPPER STEAK DINNER				
(Armour) frozen, beef 'Classics Lite'	11.25 oz	220	970	4.0
(Healthy Choice) frozen	11 oz	260	500	5.0
(LaChoy)	3.81 oz	36	942	0.2
(Le Menu) frozen	11.5 oz	370	1020	13.0
PEPPER STEAK DINNER MIX				
(LaChoy) 'Dinner Classics'	1/5 pkg	35	720	<1.0
(LaChoy) 'Dinner Classics' prepared	3/4 cup	180	760	9.0
PEPPER STEAK ENTRÉE				
pork and beef	1 oz	141	578	12.5

Food Name	Serv. Size	Total Cal.	Sod. MGS	Fat GMS
pork and beef, approx .2 oz	1 slice	27	112	2.4
(Budget Gourmet) frozen, w/rice	10 oz	300	800	9.0
(Dining Lite) frozen	9 oz	260	1050	6.0
(Healthy Choice) frozen	9.5 oz	250	560	4.0
(LaChoy) frozen, w/rice & vegetables 'Fresh & Lite'	10 oz	280	1082	8.0
(Stouffer's) frozen, green, w/rice, 1 pkg	10.5 oz	310	700	10.0
(Top Shelf) Oriental, microwave bowl	1 serving	290	1700	10.0
(Tyson) frozen 'Gourmet Selection'	11.25 oz	330	1130	11.0
(Ultra Slim Fast) beef, and parsley rice	12 oz	270	690	4.0
PEPPERONI				
(Hickory Farms)	1 oz	140	578	13.0
(Hormel)				
'Chunk'	1 oz	140	423	12.0
'Leoni Brand'	1 oz	130	508	12.0
'Perma-Fresh'	2 slices	80	281	7.0
'Rosa'	1 oz	140	626	13.0
'Rosa Grande'	1 oz	140	512	13.0
(JM) approx .5 oz	8 slices	70	290	6.0
PEPPERS AND ONIONS (Quincy's)	4 oz	80	11	5.0
PERCH				
frozen (Booth)	4 oz	100	90	1.0
frozen (SeaPak)	4 oz	100	80	2.0
frozen, fillet, battered (Van de Kamp's)	2 pieces	310	500	21.0
mixed species, dry-heat cooked	4 oz	133	90	1.3
mixed species, dry-heat cooked	3 oz	99	67	1.0
mixed species, raw	1 lb	413	280	4.2
mixed species, raw	3 oz	77	53	0.8
mixed species, raw	1 oz	26	18	0.3
PERSIMMON				
Japanese, dried	1 oz	78	1	0.2
Japanese, fresh, trimmed	1 oz	20	<1	0.1
Japanese, fresh, untrimmed	1 lb	268	6	0.7
Japanese, raw, 2.5-inch diam	1 med	118	2	0.3
native, fresh, trimmed	1 oz	36	<1	0.1
native, fresh, untrimmed	1 lb	472	4	1.5
native, raw, trimmed, approx 1.1 oz	1 med	32	0	0.1
PE-TSAI. See CABBAGE, NAPA.				
PHEASANT				
breast meat only, raw	1 oz	38	9	0.9
leg meat only, raw	1 oz	38	13	1.2
meat and skin, raw	1 oz	51	11	2.6

Food Name	Serv. Size	Total Cal.	Sod. MGS	Fat GMS
meat only, raw	1 oz	38	10	1.0
PHYLLO DOUGH				
1 sheet	1 oz	85	137	1.7
1 sheet *(Apollo)*	1 oz	80	200	.4
PICKLES				
BREAD AND BUTTER				
chunks 'Old-Fashion' *(Vlasic)*	1 oz	25	120	0.0
'Deli' *(Vlasic)*	1 oz	25	120	0.0
fresh	2 slices	11	101	0.0
one slice *(Claussen)*	.4 oz	7	61	tr
slices	1 cup	124	1144	0.3
slices *(Claussen)*	1 oz	20	172	0.1
slices, approx 2/3 oz *(Mrs. Fanning's)*	2 slices	16	140	0.0
slices 'Cucumber Slices' *(Heinz)*	1 oz	25	170	0.0
'Sweet Butter Chips' *(Vlasic)*	1 oz	30	160	0.0
'Sweet Butter Stix' *(Vlasic)*	1 oz	18	110	0.0
DILL				
	1 lb	81	5813	0.9
	1 oz	5	363	0.1
baby *(Heinz)*	1 oz	4	285	0.0
baby *(Vlasic)*	1 oz	4	210	0.0
chips *(Heinz)*	1 oz	4	275	0.0
chunks, snack *(Vlasic)*	1 oz	4	220	0.0
chunks, zesty, snacks *(Vlasic)*	1 oz	4	290	0.0
crunchy *(Vlasic)*	1 oz	4	210	0.0
crunchy, half salt *(Vlasic)*	1 oz	4	125	0.0
crunchy, zesty *(Vlasic)*	1 oz	4	250	0.0
gherkins *(Vlasic)*	1 oz	4	210	0.0
halves 'Deli' *(Vlasic)*	1 oz	4	290	0.0
halves 'Deli Style' *(Heinz)*	1 oz	4	280	0.0
hamburger chips, half salt *(Vlasic)*	1 oz	2	175	0.0
hamburger slices *(Heinz)*	1 oz	2	405	0.0
low sodium	1 lb	81	82	0.9
low sodium	1 oz	5	5	0.1
no garlic *(Claussen)*	1 oz	6	313	0.1
no garlic, 1 piece *(Claussen)*	2.9 oz	17	895	0.3
'Original' *(Vlasic)*	1 oz	4	375	0.0
'Polish Snack Chunks' *(Vlasic)*	1 oz	4	300	0.0
spears *(Claussen)*	1 oz	4	330	0.1
spears, half salt *(Vlasic)*	1 oz	4	120	0.0
spears, kosher *(Heinz)*	1 oz	4	295	0.0

od Name	Serv. Size	Total Cal.	Sod. MGS	Fat GMS
spears, kosher (Vlasic)	1 oz	4	175	0.0
spears, no garlic (Vlasic)	1 oz	4	210	0.0
spears, 1 piece (Claussen)	1.1 oz	4	373	0.1
spears, Polish style (Heinz)	1 oz	4	285	0.0
spears, zesty (Vlasic)	1 oz	4	230	0.0
whole (Featherweight)	1 piece	4	5	0.0
whole 'Genuine' (Heinz)	1 oz	2	420	0.0
whole, kosher (Heinz)	1 oz	4	295	0.0
whole, Polish style (Heinz)	1 oz	4	285	0.0
whole, processed (Heinz)	1 oz	2	435	0.0
OT AND SPICY, garden, mixed (Vlasic)	1 oz	4	380	0.0
OSHER. See also DILL.				
chips, 'Old Fashioned' (Heinz)	1 oz	4	270	0.0
halves (Claussen)	1 oz	4	330	0.1
halves 'Old Fashioned Deli Halves' (Heinz)	1 oz	4	275	0.0
halves, 2.3 oz (Claussen)	1 piece	9	769	0.2
slices (Claussen)	1 oz	3	319	0.1
slices, .3 oz (Claussen)	1 piece	1	107	tr
OUR				
	1 lb	48	5477	0.9
	1 oz	3	342	0.1
low sodium	1 lb	48	82	0.9
low sodium	1 oz	3	5	0.1
whole (Claussen)	1 oz	3	332	0.1
whole 'Old Fashioned' (Heinz)	1 oz	4	280	0.0
whole, 1 piece (Claussen)	2.5 oz	9	832	0.2
WEET				
	1 lb	529	4257	1.2
	1 oz	33	266	0.1
cubes, salad (Heinz)	1 oz	30	270	0.0
'Cucumber Stix' (Heinz)	1 oz	25	145	0.0
gherkins (Heinz)	1 oz	35	210	0.0
gherkins, midget (Heinz)	1 oz	35	205	0.0
half salt 'Sweet Butter Chips' (Vlasic)	1 oz	30	80	0.0
low sodium	1 lb	529	82	1.2
low sodium	1 med	41	6	0,1
low sodium	1 oz	33	5	0.1
low sodium	1 slice	7	1	0.0
low sodium, mixed (Heinz)	1 oz	40	200	0.0
low sodium, 3 inches long, approx 1.2 oz	1 large	41	6	0.1
sliced (Featherweight)	3-4 slices	24	5	0.0

Food Name	Serv. Size	Total Cal.	Sod. MGS	
sliced *(Heinz)*	1 oz	35	205	
sliced 'Cucumber Slices' *(Heinz)*	1 oz	20	195	
whole, 3 inches long, approx 1.2 oz	1 large	41	328	
PICKLING SPICE *(Tone's)*	1 tsp	10	1	
PIE				
APPLE				
Fresh				
(Entenmann's) homestyle	2.1 oz	140	150	
(McMillin's)	4 oz	430	340	2
Frozen				
(Amy's Kitchen)	8 oz	282	180	12
(Banquet) 'Family Size' 3 1/3 oz	1/6 pie	250	290	1
(Mrs. Smith's) 'Pie In Minutes' 8-inch pie	1/8 pie	210	250	9
(Pet-Ritz)	1/16 pie	330	385	12
(Sara Lee) apple streusel 'Free & Light'	1/8 pie	170	140	2
(Sara Lee) Dutch apple 'Homestyle' 9-inch pie	1/10 pie	300	310	12
(Sara Lee) 'Homestyle' 9-inch pie	1/10 pie	280	220	1
(Sara Lee) 'Homestyle High' 10-inch pie	1/10 pie	400	450	2
(Weight Watchers) 3.5 oz	1/2 pkg	200	280	5
BANANA CREAM				
Frozen				
(Banquet) 2 1/3 oz	1/6 pie	180	150	1
(Pet-Ritz) 2 1/3 oz	1/6 pie	170	155	9
BERRY, fresh *(McMillin's)*	4 oz	430	410	23
BLACKBERRY, frozen *(Banquet)* 'Family Size' 3 1/3 oz	1/6 pie	270	350	1
BLUEBERRY				
Frozen				
(Banquet) 'Family Size' 3 1/3 oz	1/6 pie	270	350	1
(Mrs. Smith's) 'Pie In Minutes' 8-inch pie	1/8 pie	220	240	9
(Pet-Ritz)	1/6 pie	370	330	12
(Sara Lee) 'Homestyle' 9-inch pie	1/10 pie	300	210	12
BOSTON CREAM, frozen *(Weight Watchers)*	3 oz	160	260	4
CHERRY				
Fresh *(McMillin's)*	4 oz	430	350	24
Frozen				
(Banquet) 'Family Size' 3 1/3 oz	1/6 pie	250	260	1
(Mrs. Smith's) 'Pie In Minutes' 8-inch pie	1/8 pie	220	200	9
(Pet-Ritz)	1/6 pie	300	330	12
(Sara Lee) cherry streusel 'Free & Light'	1/10 pie	160	140	2
(Sara Lee) 'Homestyle' 9-inch pie	1/10 pie	270	270	13

d Name	Serv. Size	Total Cal.	Sod. MGS	Fat GMS
OCOLATE				
resh *(McMillin's)* chocolate pudding	4 oz	420	350	21.0
rozen				
(Banquet) chocolate cream, 2 1/3 oz	1/6 pie	190	110	10.0
(Pet Ritz) chocolate cream, 2 1/3 oz	1/6 pie	190	145	8.0
(Weight Watchers) chocolate mocha 'Sweet				
Celebrations' 2.75 oz	1/2 pkg	160	150	5.0
CONUT				
resh *(McMillin's)* coconut pudding	4 oz	450	420	26.0
rozen				
(Banquet) cream, 2 1/3 oz	1/6 pie	190	120	11.0
(Pet Ritz) cream, 2 1/3 oz	1/6 pie	190	145	8.0
CONUT CUSTARD, fresh *(Entenmann's)*	1.8 oz	140	160	8.0
G CUSTARD, frozen *(Pet-Ritz)*	1/6 pie	200	(mq)	8.0
MON				
resh *(McMillin's)*	4 oz	450	330	25.0
rozen				
(Banquet) cream, 2 1/3 oz	1/6 pie	170	120	9.0
(Mrs. Smith's) meringue, 8-inch pie	1/8 pie	210	130	5.0
(Pet Ritz) cream, 2 1/3 oz	1/6 pie	190	150	9.0
NCE				
rozen				
(Banquet) mincemeat 'Family Size' 3 1/3 oz	1/6 pie	260	370	11.0
(Pet-Ritz)	1/6 pie	280	(mq)	9.0
(Sara Lee) 'Homestyle' 9-inch pie	1/10 pie	300	340	13.0
APOLITAN CREAM, frozen, *(Pet Ritz)* 2 1/3 oz	1/6 pie	180	185	10.0
ACH				
resh *(McMillin's)*	4 oz	430	370	24.0
rozen				
(Banquet) 'Family Size' 3 1/3 oz	1/6 pie	245	280	11.0
(Mrs. Smith's) 'Pie In Minutes' 8-inch pie	1/8 pie	210	190	9.0
(Pet-Ritz)	1/6 pie	320	320	12.0
(Sara Lee) 'Homestyle' 9-inch pie	1/10 pie	280	170	12.0
CAN				
rozen				
(Mrs. Smith's) 'Pie In Minutes' 8-inch pie	1/8 pie	330	200	13.0
(Sara Lee) 'Homestyle' 9-inch pie	1/10 pie	400	290	18.0
MPKIN				
rozen				
(Banquet) 'Family Size' 3 1/3 oz	1/6 pie	200	350	8.0
(Mrs. Smith's) 'Pie In Minutes' 8-inch pie	1/8 pie	190	230	6.0

Food Name	Serv. Size	Total Cal.	Sod. MGS	
(Pet Ritz) pumpkin custard	1/6 pie	250	(mq)	
(Sara Lee) 'Homestyle' 9-inch pie	1/10 pie	240	250	1
RASPBERRY, frozen *(Sara Lee)* 'Homestyle' 9-inch pie	1/10 pie	280	150	1
STRAWBERRY				
Fresh *(McMillin's)*	4 oz	400	370	2
Frozen				
(Banquet) strawberry cream, 2 1/3 oz	1/6 pie	170	120	
(Pet Ritz) strawberry cream, 2 1/3 oz	1/6 pie	170	145	
SWEET POTATO, frozen *(Pet-Ritz)*	1/6 pie	150	110	
PIE, SNACK				
APPLE				
(Break Cake) 'Fried Pie' 4.5 oz	2 pies	430	370	1
(Drake's) approx 2 oz	1 piece	210	135	1
(Hostess)	1 piece	430	390	2
(Hostess) French apple	1 piece	430	390	2
(Little Debbie) Dutch apple, 2.17 oz	1 piece	230	150	
(Little Debbie) Dutch apple, 2.5 oz	1 piece	270	170	
(Tastykake) 4 oz	1 piece	296	339	1
(Tastycake) French apple, 4.2 oz	1 piece	353	225	1
BANANA CREAM *(Tastycake)* 4.2 oz	1 piece	382	428	1
BLACKBERRY *(Hostess)*	1 piece	420	360	1
BLUEBERRY				
(Hostess)	1 piece	420	360	1
(Tastykake) 4 oz	1 piece	308	410	
BLUEBERRY APPLE *(Drake's)* approx 2 oz	1 piece	210	135	1
CHERRY				
(Break Cake) 'Fried Pie' 4.5 oz	2 pies	410	370	1
(Hostess)	1 piece	460	380	2
(Tastykake) 4 oz	1 piece	298	306	
CHERRY APPLE *(Drake's)* approx 2 oz	1 piece	220	135	1
CHOCOLATE PUDDING				
(Hostess) chocolate pudding	1 piece	490	439	1
(Tastycake) chocolate pudding, 4.2 oz	1 piece	443	(mq)	1
COCONUT CREME *(Tastykake)* 4 oz	1 piece	377	416	2
LEMON				
(Break Cake) 'Fried Pie' 4.5 oz	2 pies	490	370	2
(Drake's) approx 2 oz	1 piece	210	115	1
(Hostess)	1 piece	440	370	2
(Tastykake) 4 oz	1 piece	319	375	1
LEMON-LIME *(Tastykake)* 4 oz	1 piece	310	329	

Food Name	Serv. Size	Total Cal.	Sod. MGS	Fat GMS
MARSHMALLOW BANANA				
(Little Debbie) 3 oz	1 piece	360	180	12.0
(Little Debbie) 1.4 oz	1 piece	170	85	6.0
MARSHMALLOW CHOCOLATE				
(Little Debbie) 3 oz	1 piece	370	170	13.0
(Little Debbie) 1.4 oz	1 piece	170	85	6.0
Mississippi mud (Pepperidge Farm) frozen 'American Collection'	1 ramekin	310	60	23.0
OATMEAL CREME				
(Little Debbie) 1.33 oz	1 piece	160	125	6.0
(Little Debbie) 2.75 oz	1 piece	350	260	14.0
PEACH				
(Hostess)	1 piece	420	360	19.0
(Tastykake) 4 oz	1 piece	310	329	8.8
PECAN				
(Little Debbie) 1.83 oz	1 piece	170	200	2.0
(Little Debbie) 3 oz	1 piece	280	340	3.0
PINEAPPLE CHEESE (Tastykake) 4.2 oz	1 piece	343	405	13.2
PUMPKIN (Tastykake) 4 oz	1 piece	324	520	14.2
RAISIN CREME				
(Little Debbie) 2.5 oz	1 piece	290	190	10.0
(Little Debbie) 1.17 oz	1 piece	140	90	6.0
STRAWBERRY				
(Hostess)	1 piece	410	360	19.0
(Tastykake) 4 oz	1 piece	342	303	11.4
PIE CRUST				
Mix				
(Betty Crocker) dry	1/16 pkg	120	140	8.0
(Flako) prepared	1 serving	247	393	15.0
(General Mills) dry	1/16 pkg	120	150	8.0
(Krusteaz) 9-inch pie	1/8 shell	90	120	5.0
(Nabisco) chocolate cookie crumbs 'Oreo' dry	2 tbsp	80	140	3.0
(Nabisco) graham crumbs 'Honey Maid' dry	2 1/2 tbsp	70	90	2.0
(Nabisco) wafer crumbs 'Nilla' dry	2 tbsp	70	55	2.0
(Pillsbury) dry	1/8 pkg	200	300	13.0
Shell				
(Mrs. Smith's) 8-inch pie	1/8 shell	80	105	5.0
(Mrs. Smith's) '9-inch pie'	1/8 shell	90	125	5.0
(Mrs. Smith's) '9 5/8-inch pie'	1/8 shell	120	160	7.0
(Oronoque) deep dish, 9-inch pie	1/6 shell	130	130	9.0
(Oronoque) regular, 9-inch pie	1/6 shell	120	115	8.0

Food Name	Serv. Size	Total Cal.	Sod. MGS	Fo GM
(Pet-Ritz)	1/6 shell	110	110	7.
(Pet-Ritz) all vegetable shortening	1/6 shell	110	60	8.
(Pet-Ritz) deep dish, 1 oz	1/6 shell	130	120	8.
(Pet-Ritz) deep dish, whole-grain	1/6 shell	130	125	8.
(Pet-Ritz) graham cracker	1/6 shell	110	80	6.
(Pet-Ritz) 9 5/8-inch pie	1/6 shell	170	180	11.
(Pet-Ritz) tart	3-inch shell	150	150	10.
(Pet-Ritz) vegetable shortening, deep dish	1/6 shell	140	75	9.
(Pillsbury) 'All Ready' 2-crust pie	1/8 shell	240	210	15.
Stick (Betty Crocker)	1/8 stick	120	140	8.

PIE FILLING. See also PUDDING/PIE FILLING MIX.

(NOTE: All pie fillings are canned unless otherwise noted.)

APPLE

Food Name	Serv. Size	Total Cal.	Sod. MGS	Fo GM
(Comstock)	3.5 oz	120	15	0.
(Comstock) 'Lite'	3.5 oz	80	10	0.
(Lucky Leaf)	4 oz	120	60	0.
(Lucky Leaf) apple turnover, diced	4 oz	120	60	0.
(Lucky Leaf) 'Deluxe'	4 oz	120	40	0.
(Lucky Leaf) 'Plus'	4 oz	121	24	0.
(Musselman's)	4 oz	120	60	0.
(Musselman's) apple turnover, diced	4 oz	120	60	0.
(Musselman's) 'Deluxe'	4 oz	120	40	0.
(Musselman's) 'Plus'	4 oz	121	24	0.
(Pathmark) 'No Frills'	4 oz	130	60	0.
(White House)	3.5 oz	121	44	1.

APRICOT

Food Name	Serv. Size	Total Cal.	Sod. MGS	Fo GM
(Comstock)	3.5 oz	110	100	0.
(Lucky Leaf)	4 oz	150	90	0.
(Musselman's)	4 oz	150	90	0.

BANANA *(Comstock)* | 3.5 oz | 110 | 300 | 2.

BLACKBERRY

Food Name	Serv. Size	Total Cal.	Sod. MGS	Fo GM
(Lucky Leaf)	4 oz	120	140	0.
(Lucky Leaf) 'Plus'	4 oz	121	20	0.
(Musselman's)	4 oz	120	140	0.
(Musselman's) 'Plus'	4 oz	121	20	0.

BLUEBERRY

Food Name	Serv. Size	Total Cal.	Sod. MGS	Fo GM
(Comstock)	3.5 oz	110	15	0.
(Comstock) 'Lite'	3.5 oz	75	15	0.
(Lucky Leaf) cultivated	4 oz	120	150	0.
(Lucky Leaf) 'Plus'	4 oz	145	17	0.
(Musselman's) cultivated	4 oz	120	150	0.

od Name	Serv. Size	Total Cal.	Sod. MGS	Fat GMS
(Musselman's) 'Plus'	4 oz	145	17	0.0
(White House)	3.5 oz	118	48	1.0
OYSENBERRY				
(Lucky Leaf)	4 oz	120	140	0.0
(Musselman's)	4 oz	120	140	0.0
HERRY				
(Comstock)	3.5 oz	110	15	0.0
(Comstock) 'Lite'	3.5 oz	75	15	0.0
(Lucky Leaf)	4 oz	120	50	0.0
(Musselman's)	4 oz	120	50	0.0
(Musselman's) 'Plus'	4 oz	108	10	0.2
(Pathmark) 'No Frills'	4 oz	130	60	0.0
(White House)	3.5 oz	141	54	1.0
HOCOLATE (Comstock)	3.5 oz	130	240	3.0
OCONUT (Comstock)	3.5 oz	120	290	3.0
OOSEBERRY				
(Lucky Leaf)	4 oz	180	30	0.0
(Musselman's)	4 oz	180	30	0.0
EMON				
(Comstock)	3.5 oz	140	110	1.0
(Lucky Leaf)	4 oz	200	235	2.0
(Lucky Leaf) 'French'	4 oz	180	140	1.0
(Musselman's)	4 oz	200	235	2.0
(Musselman's) 'French'	4 oz	180	140	1.0
INCEMEAT				
(Comstock)	3.5 oz	150	180	1.0
(Lucky Leaf)	4 oz	190	145	1.0
(Musselman's)	4 oz	190	145	1.0
(None Such)	1/3 cup	200	280	1.0
(None Such) condensed	1/4 pkg	220	310	2.0
(None Such) w/brandy and rum	1/3 cup	220	260	2.0
(S&W) w/brandy, 'Old Fashioned'	4 oz	234	234	2.3
EACH				
(Comstock)	3.5 oz	110	20	0.0
(Lucky Leaf)	4 oz	150	65	0.0
(Lucky Leaf) 'Plus'	4 oz	113	16	0.0
(Musselman's)	4 oz	150	65	0.0
(Musselman's) 'Plus'	4 oz	113	16	0.0
(White House)	3.5 oz	117	30	1.0
INEAPPLE				
(Comstock)	3.5 oz	100	65	0.0

Food Name	Serv. Size	Total Cal.	Sod. MGS	Fa GM
(Lucky Leaf)	4 oz	110	65	0.(
(Musselman's)	4 oz	110	65	0.(
PUMPKIN				
(Comstock)	3.5 oz	100	180	0.0
(Libby's)	1 cup	260	0	0.3
(Lucky Leaf)	4 oz	170	200	4.(
(Musselman's)	4 oz	170	200	4.(
(Stokely)	1/2 cup	170	420	0.(
RAISIN				
(Comstock)	3.5 oz	120	80	0.(
(Lucky Leaf)	4 oz	130	120	1.(
(Musselman's)	4 oz	130	120	1.(
RASPBERRY, BLACK				
(Lucky Leaf)	4 oz	190	50	0.(
(Musselman's)	4 oz	190	50	0.(
RASPBERRY, RED				
(Lucky Leaf)	4 oz	190	80	0.(
(Musselman's)	4 oz	190	80	0.(
STRAWBERRY				
(Comstock)	3.5 oz	100	20	0.0
(Lucky Leaf)	4 oz	120	75	0.0
(Lucky Leaf) 'Plus'	4 oz	138	17	0.(
(Musselman's)	4 oz	120	75	0.(
(Musselman's) 'Plus'	4 oz	138	17	0.(
STRAWBERRY-RHUBARB				
(Lucky Leaf) strawberry-rhubarb	4 oz	120	95	0.(
(Musselman's) strawberry-rhubarb	4 oz	120	95	0.(
PIE MIX				
BANANA CREAM				
(Jell-O) 'No Bake' dry	1 pkg	140	190	5.(
(Jell-O) 'No Bake' prepared	1/8 pie	240	300	14.(
BOSTON CREAM				
(Betty Crocker) 'Classic' dry	1/8 pkg	230	370	4.0
(Betty Crocker) 'Classic' prepared w/egg and 2% milk	1/8 pkg	270	390	6.0
(Jell-O) mousse 'No Bake' dry	1 pkg	160	320	7.0
(Jell-O) mousse 'No Bake' prepared	1/8 pie	260	430	17.(
CHOCOLATE				
(Royal) chocolate mint 'No-Bake' prepared	1/8 pie	260	280	15.0
(Royal) mousse 'No Bake' prepared	1/8 pie	230	260	12.(
COCONUT CREAM				
(Jell-O) 'No Bake' dry	1 pkg	160	200	7.0

Food Name	Serv. Size	Total Cal.	Sod. MGS	Fat GMS
(Jell-O) 'No Bake' prepared	1/8 pie	260	300	16.0
KEY LIME *(Royal)* dry	1 serving	50	120	0.0
LEMON				
(Royal) dry	1 serving	50	120	0.0
(Royal) lemon meringue 'No Bake' prepared	1/8 pie	310	250	11.0
PUMPKIN				
(Jell-O) 'No Bake' dry	1 pkg	140	330	3.0
(Jell-O) 'No Bake' prepared	1/8 pie	250	450	13.0
(Libby's) prepared	1/6 pie	390	70	17.0
VANILLA CREME				
(Lucky Leaf) prepared	4 oz	150	145	3.0
(Musselman's) prepared	4 oz	150	145	3.0
PIGNOLIA. See PINE NUT.				
PIG'S EAR				
frozen, raw	1 oz	66	54	4.3
frozen, simmered	4 oz	188	189	12.2
PIG'S FEET				
pickled *(Penrose)*	6 oz	220	2890	15.0
pickled, cured	1 lb	921	4187	73.2
pickled, cured	1 oz	58	262	4.6
raw	1 oz	75	18	5.3
simmered	5 oz	275	43	17.6
PIG'S KNUCKLES, pickled *(Penrose)*	6 oz	290	2380	21.0
PIG'S TONGUE				
braised	3 oz	230	93	15.8
cured, '8-lb can' *(Hormel)*	3 oz	190	966	13.0
raw	1 oz	64	31	4.9
PIKE, NORTHERN				
dry-heat cooked	3 oz	96	42	0.8
raw	1 lb	401	177	3.1
raw	3 oz	75	33	0.6
raw	1 oz	25	11	0.2
PIKE, WALLEYE				
dry-heat cooked	3 oz	101	55	1.3
raw	1 lb	420	230	5.5
raw	3 oz	79	43	1.0
raw	1 oz	26	14	0.3
PILAF DINNER, CANNED				
oat bran, w/garden vegetables 'Fast Menu' *(Health Valley)*	7.5 oz	210	445	7.0
PILAF MIX				
lentil, approx 1/2 cup cooked or 1 oz dry *(Casbah)*	1 serving	100	(mq)	0.0

Food Name	Serv. Size	Total Cal.	Sod. MGS	Fat GMS
three-grain, w/herbs, prepared w/salted butter (Quick Pilaf)	1/2 cup	142	324	4.0
three-grain, w/herbs, prepared w/o butter (Quick Pilaf)	1/2 cup	110	278	0.6
PIMIENTO, CAN OR JAR				
	2 oz	13	8	0.2
	1 tbsp	3	2	<.1
all varieties, drained (Dromedary)	1 oz	10	5	0.0
PIMIENTO SPREAD (Price's)	1 oz	80	na	6.0
PIÑA COLADA. See ALCOHOLIC BEVERAGES.				
PINE NUT/Colorado pinyon pine nut/Italian stone pine nut/pignolia/pinocchio/piñon				
whole	1 oz	161	20	17.3
whole	1 tbsp	52	0	5.1
whole	10 kernels	6	1	0.6
PINEAPPLE				
candied, approx 1/2 cup	4-oz pkg	357	7	0.5
raw, diced pieces	1 cup	76	2	0.7
raw, 3 1/2-inch diam	1 slice	41	1	0.4
raw, 3 1/2-inch diam, 3/4 inch thick (Del Monte)	2 slices	90	5	0.0
trimmed	1 oz	14	<1	0.1
untrimmed	1 lb	117	2	1.0
untrimmed (Dole)	2 slices	90	10	1.0
PINEAPPLE, CANNED				
chunks	1/2 cup	75	2	0.1
chunks (A&P)	1/2 cup	70	10	<1.0
chunks, unsweetened 'Hawaiian' (Pathmark)	1/2 cup	70	10	0.0
crushed (A&P)	1/2 cup	70	10	<1.0
crushed (Empress)	1/2 cup	70	10	0.0
crushed, unsweetened 'Hawaiian' (Pathmark)	1/2 cup	70	10	0.0
'Fruit Pak' (Mott's)	3.75 oz	86	2	0.0
in extra heavy syrup	4 oz	94	1	0.1
in extra heavy syrup, chunks	1/2 cup	109	2	0.1
in extra heavy syrup, chunks, w/liquid	1 cup	216	3	0.3
in extra heavy syrup, crushed	1/2 cup	109	2	0.1
in extra heavy syrup, w/1.25 tbsp liquid	1 slice	48	1	0.1
in heavy syrup	4 oz	88	1	0.1
in heavy syrup, chunks (A&P)	1/2 cup	90	10	<1.0
in heavy syrup, chunks 'Hawaiian' (Pathmark)	1/2 cup	90	10	0.0
in heavy syrup, chunks, tidbits, or crushed	1/2 cup	100	2	0.1
in heavy syrup, chunks or crushed, w/liquid	1 cup	199	3	0.3
in heavy syrup, crushed (A&P)	1/2 cup	90	10	<1.0
in heavy syrup, slices (A&P)	2 slices	90	10	<1.0

Food Name	Serv. Size	Total Cal.	Sod. MGS	Fat GMS
in heavy syrup, slices 'Hawaiian' (Pathmark)	1/2 cup	90	10	0.0
in heavy syrup, slices '100% Hawaiian' (S&W)	2 slices	90	0	0.0
in heavy syrup, w/1.25 tbsp liquid	1 slice	45	1	0.1
in juice	4 oz	68	1	0.1
in juice, all cuts (Dole)	1/2 cup	70	1	0.5
in juice, chunks (Del Monte)	1/2 cup	70	10	0.0
in juice, chunks or tidbits, w/liquid	1 cup	150	3	0.2
in juice, crushed (Del Monte)	1/2 cup	70	10	0.0
in juice, slices (A&P)	2 slices	70	10	<1.0
in juice, slices (Del Monte)	1/2 cup	70	10	0.0
in juice, slices (Featherweight)	1/2 cup	70	10	0.0
in juice, slices '100% Hawaiian' (S&W)	1/2 cup	70	10	0.0
in juice, tidbits (Del Monte)	1/2 cup	70	10	0.0
in juice, w/1.25 tbsp liquid	1 slice	35	1	0.1
in light syrup	1/2 cup	66	2	0.1
in light syrup	4 oz	59	1	0.1
in light syrup, w/liquid	1 cup	131	3	0.3
in light syrup, w/1.75 tbsp liquid	1 slice	30	1	0.1
in pineapple juice (Dole)	1/2 cup	70	10	<1.0
in pineapple syrup (Dole)	1/2 cup	90	10	0.0
in syrup, all cuts (Del Monte)	1/2 cup	90	10	0.0
in syrup, all cuts (Dole)	1/2 cup	95	2	0.2
in water	4 oz	36	1	0.1
in water, tidbits	1/2 cup	40	2	0.1
in water, tidbits, w/liquid	1 cup	79	2	0.2
in water, w/1.25 tbsp liquid	1 slice	19	1	0.1
spears, approx 3.1 oz (Del Monte)	2 spears	50	10	0.0
spears or slices, unsweetened 'Hawaiian' (Pathmark)	1/2 cup	70	10	0.0
tidbits	1/2 cup	75	2	0.1
unsweetened, slices (S&W Nutradiet)	1/2 cup	60	10	0.0
PINEAPPLE, FROZEN				
sweetened, chunks	1/2 cup	104	2	0.1
sweetened, chunks	4 oz	96	2	0.1
PINEAPPLE CITRUS DRINK				
'Thirst Quencher Light' (Gatorade)	8 oz	25	80	0.0
PINEAPPLE COCKTAIL JUICE				
w/banana 'Orchard Tropicals' (Welch's) bottled	6 oz	100	20	0.0
w/banana 'Orchard Tropicals' (Welch's) boxed	8.45 oz	140	20	0.0
w/banana 'Orchard Tropicals' (Welch's) frozen	6 oz	100	20	0.0
w/grapefruit juice (Ocean Spray)	6 oz	110	5	0.0
PINEAPPLE COCONUT JUICE (Knudsen & Sons)	8 oz	110	na	0.0

Food Name	Serv. Size	Total Cal.	Sod. MGS	Fat GMS
PINEAPPLE DRINK				
frozen 'Bright & Early Pineapple' prepared *(Bright & Early)*	6 oz	90	0	0.0
w/grapefruit juice	6 oz	90	24	0.2
w/grapefruit juice *(Del Monte)*	6 oz	90	50	0.0
w/grapefruit juice *(Pathmark)*	6 oz	80	0	0.0
w/grapefruit juice *(Tropicana)*	6 oz	100	10	<1.0
w/grapefruit juice 'Single Serve' *(Tropicana)*	10 oz	159	3	0.0
w/grapefruit juice 'Twister' *(Tropicana)*	8 oz	125	2	0.0
w/pink grapefruit juice *(Del Monte)*	6 oz	90	50	0.0
PINEAPPLE GRAPEFRUIT JUICE				
canned	1 cup	117	35	0.3
canned	1 oz	15	4	0.0
PINEAPPLE JUICE				
Can, bottle, or box				
	6 oz	104	2	0.2
(Dole)	6 oz	103	2	0.2
(Knudsen & Sons)	8 oz	110	na	0.0
(Minute Maid)	6 oz	90	20	0.0
(Mott's)	9.5 oz	169	0	0.0
50% juice *(J. Hungerford)*	9.03 oz	123	0	0.0
float *(Knudsen & Sons)*	8 oz	130	na	0.0
'Hawaiian' *(Pathmark)*	6 oz	100	10	0.0
'No Frills Unsweetened' *(Pathmark)*	6 oz	100	0	0.0
'100%' *(Veryfine)*	8 oz	125	10	0.0
100% juice *(J. Hungerford)*	9.03 oz	124	9	0.0
regular *(J. Hungerford)*	9.03 oz	114	0	0.0
'Unsweetened' *(Del Monte)*	6 oz	100	10	0.0
'Unsweetened' *(IGA)*	6 oz	100	10	0.0
'Unsweetened' *(S&W)*	6 oz	100	0	0.0
unsweetened, w/added ascorbic acid	1 cup	140	3	0.2
unsweetened, w/added ascorbic acid	1 oz	18	0	0.0
unsweetened, w/o added ascorbic acid	1 cup	140	3	0.2
unsweetened, w/o added ascorbic acid	1 oz	18	0	0.0
Frozen or chilled				
(Dole)	6 oz	90	5	0.0
(Minute Maid)	6 oz	90	0	0.0
concentrate *(Dole)* diluted	6 oz	100	7	na
unsweetened concentrate, diluted	1 cup	130	3	0.1
unsweetened concentrate, diluted	1 oz	16	0	0.0
unsweetened concentrate, undiluted	6 oz	387	6	0.2
w/grapefruit juice *(Dole)*	6 oz	90	8	na

Food Name	Serv. Size	Total Cal.	Sod. MGS	Fat GMS
w/grapefruit juice '100% Pure' (Tropicana)	8 oz	120	3	0.0
w/pink grapefruit juice (Dole)	6 oz	101	tr	0.1
PINEAPPLE NECTAR (Libby's)	6 oz	110	na	0.0
PINEAPPLE ORANGE DRINK				
	6 oz	96	6	0.0
(Del Monte)	6 oz	90	20	0.0
(Veryfine)	8 oz	130	10	0.0
PINEAPPLE ORANGE JUICE				
(Dole)	6 oz	100	8	na
chilled, carton (Dole)	6 oz	90	10	0.0
chilled, w/banana, carton (Dole)	6 oz	100	10	0.0
chilled, w/guava, carton (Dole)	6 oz	100	10	0.0
frozen, can (Dole)	6 oz	90	10	0.0
frozen, w/banana, can (Dole)	6 oz	90	5	0.0
frozen, w/guava, can (Dole)	6 oz	100	10	0.0
frozen or chilled (Minute Maid)	6 oz	90	0	0.0
w/banana (Dole)	6 oz	90	5	0.1
PINEAPPLE PASSION JUICE				
frozen, can, w/banana (Dole)	6 oz	100	10	0.0
frozen, carton, w/banana (Dole)	6 oz	100	10	0.0
PINEAPPLE TOPPING				
	1 cup	860	214	0.3
	2 tbsp	106	26	0.0
(Kraft)	1 tbsp	50	0	0.0
(Smucker's)	2 tbsp	130	0	0.0
PINK BEAN				
boiled	4 oz	169	2	0.6
mature seeds, boiled	1/2 cup	125	2	0.4
mature seeds, raw	1/2 cup	360	8	1.2
raw	1 oz	97	2	0.3
PINOCCHIO. See PINE NUT.				
PIÑON. See PINE NUT.				
PINTO BEAN				
(Allens)	1/2 cup	105	480	<1.0
boiled	4 oz	155	2	0.6
boiled (A&P)	1 cup	230	5	1.0
mature seeds, boiled	1/2 cup	116	2	0.4
mature seeds, raw	1/2 cup	326	10	1.1
raw	1 oz	96	3	0.3
raw (Arrowhead Mills)	2 oz	200	3	1.0
raw, dry (Evans)	1 cup	660	19	2.0

Food Name	Serv. Size	Total Cal.	Sod. MGS	Fat GMS
sprouted, mature seeds, boiled, drained	4 oz	25	58	0.4
sprouted, mature seeds, raw	1 lb	280	694	4.1
sprouted, mature seeds, raw	1 oz	18	43	0.3
Canned				
(Bush's Best)	1/2 cup	60	350	0.0
(Gebhardt)	4 oz	197	608	0.5
(Green Giant)	1/2 cup	90	280	1.0
(Joan of Arc)	1/2 cup	90	280	1.0
(Old El Paso)	1/2 cup	100	320	0.0
(Progresso)	1/2 cup	110	410	<1.0
baked style, and Great Northern, w/pork (Luck's)	7.25 oz	200	822	5.0
baked style, w/pork, 15-oz can (Luck's)	7.5 oz	220	787	6.0
baked style, w/pork, 29-oz can (Luck's)	7.25 oz	220	520	6.0
mature seeds	1/2 cup	94	499	0.4
organic, very low sodium, no salt added (Eden Foods)	1/2 cup	70	15	<1.0
organic, w/liquid (Eden Foods)	1/2 cup	110	20	<1.0
picante style (Green Giant)	1/2 cup	100	580	1.0
picante style (Joan of Arc)	1/2 cup	100	580	1.0
w/liquid	4 oz	88	472	0.4
Frozen				
	10-oz pkg	484	na	1.4
(Seabrook)	3.2 oz	160	na	0.0
boiled, drained	4 oz	184	na	0.5
immature seeds, boiled, drained, 10-oz pkg	1/3 pkg	152	78	0.5
immature seeds, unprepared, 10-oz pkg	1/3 pkg	160	86	0.5
PIROGIES, FROZEN				
pasta pocket, potato and American cheese filled (Mrs. T's)	1 pocket	70	180	2.0
pasta pocket, potato and cheddar cheese filled (Mrs. T's)	1 pocket	60	170	<1.0
pasta pocket, potato and onion filled (Mrs. T's)	1 pocket	50	140	<1.0
pasta pocket, sauerkraut filled (Mrs. T's)	1 pocket	50	220	<1.0
PISTACHIO BUTTER, roasted (Maranatha Natural)	2 tbsp	170	5	13.0
PISTACHIO NUT				
In shell				
dried	1 lb	1309	13	109.7
dried (Dole)	1 oz	90	250	7.0
dried (Fisher)	1 oz	170	85	14.0
dried (Fisher) red tint	1 oz	170	85	14.0
dry-roasted	1 lb	1429	14	124.5
dry-roasted, salted	1 lb	1429	1840	124.5
Shelled				
dried	1 cup	739	8	61.9

Food Name	Serv. Size	Total Cal.	Sod. MGS	Fat GMS
dried, approx 47 kernels	1 oz	164	2	13.7
dry-roasted	1 cup	776	8	67.6
dry-roasted	1 oz	172	2	15.0
dry-roasted *(Dole)*	1 oz	163	2	14.0
dry-roasted *(Planters)*	1 oz	170	250	15.0
dry-roasted, natural *(Planters)*	1 oz	170	250	14.0
dry-roasted, red tint *(Planters)*	1 oz	170	250	14.0
PITA BREAD. See BREAD.				
PITANGA /Surinam cherry				
raw	1 cup	57	5	0.7
raw, trimmed	1/2 cup	29	3	0.3
raw, trimmed	1 oz	9	1	0.1
raw, trimmed, approx .3 oz	1 med	2	0	0.0
raw, untrimmed	1 lb	132	11	1.6
PIZZA, FRENCH BREAD, FROZEN				
Canadian style bacon, 1 pkg *(Stouffer's)*	5.5 oz	370	1070	15.0
cheese *(Healthy Choice)*	5.6 oz	300	500	3.0
cheese *(Lean Cuisine)*	5 1/8 oz	300	310	9.0
cheese *(Pappalo's)*	1 piece	360	830	15.0
cheese, microwave *(Oven Lovin')*	1 serving	350	700	14.0
cheese 'Microwave' *(Pillsbury)*	1 piece	370	680	15.0
cheese, 1 pkg *(Stouffer's)*	5 1/8 oz	350	630	14.0
cheese 'Zap' *(Banquet)*	4.5 oz	310	800	10.0
combination *(Pappalo's)*	1 piece	430	1120	21.0
combination, microwave *(Oven Lovin')*	1 serving	420	910	21.0
deluxe *(Healthy Choice)*	6.25 oz	330	490	8.0
deluxe *(Lean Cuisine)*	6 1/8 oz	350	580	11.0
deluxe, 1 pkg *(Stouffer's)*	6 1/8 oz	420	950	19.0
deluxe 'Zap' *(Banquet)*	4.8 oz	330	890	13.0
double cheese, 1 pkg *(Stouffer's)*	5 7/8 oz	420	850	18.0
hamburger, 1 pkg *(Stouffer's)*	6 oz	410	650	18.0
Italian turkey sausage *(Healthy Choice)*	6.45 oz	320	440	7.0
pepperoni *(Healthy Choice)*	6.25 oz	320	490	8.0
pepperoni *(Lean Cuisine)*	5 1/4 oz	340	580	11.0
pepperoni *(Pappalo's)*	1 piece	410	1130	20.0
pepperoni, microwave *(Oven Lovin')*	1 serving	410	980	21.0
pepperoni 'Microwave' *(Pillsbury)*	1 piece	430	940	19.0
pepperoni, 1 pkg *(Stouffer's)*	5 3/4 oz	400	880	19.0
pepperoni 'Zap' *(Banquet)*	4.5 oz	350	1060	16.0
pepperoni and mushroom *(Stouffer's)*	6 oz	410	920	19.0
sausage *(Lean Cuisine)*	6 oz	350	600	10.0

Food Name	Serv. Size	Total Cal.	Sod. MGS	Fat GMS
sausage *(Pappalo's)*	1 piece	410	1000	18.0
sausage *(Stouffer's)*	6 oz	430	840	21.0
sausage, microwave *(Oven Lovin')*	1 serving	400	830	20.0
sausage 'Microwave' *(Pillsbury)*	1 piece	410	860	16.0
sausage and pepperoni *(Stouffer's)*	6.25 oz	460	920	23.0
sausage combo, and pepperoni 'Microwave' *(Pillsbury)*	1 piece	450	950	21.0
three cheese *(Lean Cuisine)*	5.5 oz	330	350	10.0
vegetable deluxe *(Stouffer's)*	6.5 oz	420	830	20.0

PIZZA, FROZEN

(Banquet)

Food Name	Serv. Size	Total Cal.	Sod. MGS	Fat GMS
pepperoni 'Pizza Pie'	6-oz pie	470	970	27.0
sausage 'Pizza Pie'	6-oz pie	500	860	29.0
sausage and pepperoni 'Pizza Pie'	6-oz pie	470	930	27.0

(Celeste)

Food Name	Serv. Size	Total Cal.	Sod. MGS	Fat GMS
cheese	1/4 pie	315	690	17.0
cheese 'Pizza for One'	1 pie	500	1070	25.0
deluxe	1/4 pie	380	870	22.0
deluxe 'Pizza for One'	1 pie	580	1290	32.0
four cheese, original 'Pizza for One'	1 pie	540	1500	30.0
four cheese, zesty 'Pizza for One'	1 pie	550	1500	31.0
pepperoni	1/4 pie	370	940	21.0
pepperoni 'Pizza for One'	1 pie	545	1290	30.0
sausage	1/4 pie	375	900	22.0
sausage 'Pizza for One'	1 pie	570	1300	32.0
suprema	1/4 pie	380	970	24.0
suprema 'Pizza for One'	1 pie	680	1590	39.0
vegetable 'Pizza for One'	1 pie	490	1200	26.0

(Jeno's)

Food Name	Serv. Size	Total Cal.	Sod. MGS	Fat GMS
combination 'Crisp 'N Tasty'	1/2 pizza	280	680	15.0
pepperoni 'Crisp 'N Tasty'	1/2 pizza	280	710	15.0
pepperoni 'Pizza Pocket'	1 serving	370	790	20.0
sausage 'Crisp 'N Tasty'	1/2 pizza	280	640	15.0
sausage 'Pizza Pocket'	1 serving	360	660	19.0
sausage and pepperoni 'Pizza Pocket'	1 serving	360	710	20.0
supreme 'Pizza Pocket'	1 serving	370	720	19.0

(Oven Lovin')

Food Name	Serv. Size	Total Cal.	Sod. MGS	Fat GMS
cheese, microwave	1/2 pie	250	430	12.0
combination, microwave	1/2 pie	310	580	18.0
pepperoni, microwave	1/2 pie	300	620	17.0
sausage, microwave	1/2 pie	290	510	16.0
supreme, microwave	1/2 pie	310	570	18.0

Food Name	Serv. Size	Total Cal.	Sod. MGS	Fat GMS
(Pappalo's)				
pepperoni, 9 inch, traditional crust	1/2 pie	390	870	14.0
pepperoni, 12 inch, traditional crust	1/4 pie	350	700	11.0
pepperoni, pan pizza	1/6 pie	350	720	11.0
sausage, 9 inch, traditional crust	1/2 pie	380	680	13.0
sausage, 12 inch, traditional crust	1/4 pie	350	600	12.0
sausage, pan pizza	1/5 pie	350	530	11.0
sausage and pepperoni, 9 inch, traditional crust	1/2 pie	390	650	15.0
sausage and pepperoni, 12 inch, traditional crust	1/4 pie	360	730	12.0
sausage and pepperoni, pan pizza	1/5 pie	360	630	12.0
supreme, 9 inch, traditional crust	1/2 pie	400	700	16.0
supreme, 12 inch, traditional crust	1/4 pie	350	640	12.0
supreme, pan pizza	1/5 pie	340	610	12.0
three cheese, 9 inch, traditional crust	1/2 pie	350	640	11.0
three cheese, 12 inch, traditional crust	1/4 pie	310	440	7.0
three cheese, pan pizza	1/5 pie	310	490	8.0
(Pepperidge Farm)				
cheese, croissant pastry	1 pie	430	640	23.0
deluxe, croissant pastry	1 pie	440	790	23.0
pepperoni, croissant pastry	1 pie	420	690	22.0
(Tombstone)				
bacon, Canadian style, 'Original' 12 inch	3.6 oz	230	580	10.0
bacon cheeseburger, 'Special Order' 12 inch	4.7 oz	330	730	16.0
cheese, microwave, 7 inch	7.7 oz	500	940	24.0
cheese, 'Original' 9 inch	5.6 oz	380	730	17.0
cheese, 'Original' 12 inch	3.4 oz	230	460	10.0
cheese, w/hamburger, 'Original' 12 inch	3.7 oz	250	570	12.0
cheese, w/Italian sausage 'Italian Style Thincrust'	3.2 oz	220	490	13.0
cheese, w/pepperoni 'Italian Style Thincrust'	3 oz	230	540	14.0
cheese, w/pepperoni, 'Original' 12 inch	3.6 oz	260	620	14.0
cheese, w/sausage, mushrooms, 'Original' 12 inch	3.8 oz	240	570	11.0
cheese, w/sausage, 'Original' 12 inch	3.7 oz	240	590	11.0
cheese and hamburger, 'Original' 9 inch	6.3 oz	440	960	21.0
cheese and pepperoni, microwave, 7 inch	7.5 oz	550	1240	32.0
cheese and pepperoni, 'Original' 9 inch	6.3 oz	480	1100	26.0
cheese and sausage, 'Original' 9 inch	6.3 oz	420	1000	19.0
chicken, 'Light' 8 inch	4.5 oz	240	450	8.0
chicken deluxe 'Light' approx 1/2 pizza	3.7 oz	180	440	4.0
deluxe, 'Original' 9 inch	7.0 oz	440	1010	20.0
deluxe, 'Original' 12 inch	3.9 oz	240	570	11.0
four cheese 'Special Order'	4.3 oz	300	630	14.0

Food Name	Serv. Size	Total Cal.	Sod. MGS	Fat GMS
four meat 'Special Order'	4.6 oz	320	810	15.0
four meat, 'Special Order' 9 inch	3.9 oz	280	670	14.0
Italian sausage, microwave, 7 inch	8.0 oz	550	1210	32.0
Italian sausage 'Special Order'	4.5 oz	300	740	13.0
pepperoni, 'Double Top' w/double cheese, 12 inch	4.8 oz	360	920	20.0
pepperoni 'Light' 8 inch	4.0 oz	250	630	10.0
pepperoni 'Special Order'	4.4 oz	320	780	16.0
pepperoni 'Special Order' 9 inch	3.7 oz	280	650	14.0
pepperoni and sausage, 'Original' 9 inch	6.6 oz	490	1230	26.0
ranchero deluxe 'Mexican Style Thincrust'	3.4 oz	230	530	13.0
sausage, 'Double Top' w/double cheese, 12 inch	4.8 oz	330	860	16.0
sausage, w/pepperoni, 'Original' 12 inch	3.7 oz	260	640	13.0
sausage and pepperoni, 'Double Top' w/double cheese, 12 inch	4.8 oz	340	910	18.0
sausage and pepperoni, microwave, 7 inch	8 oz	570	1430	32.0
supreme 'Italian Style Thincrust'	3.38 oz	230	520	14.0
supreme, 'Light' 8 inch	4.6 oz	250	660	9.0
supreme, 'Light' 12 inch	4.5 oz	250	630	9.0
supreme, microwave, 7 inch	8.5 oz	550	1260	31.0
supreme, 'Original' 12 inch	3.8 oz	270	630	14.0
supreme 'Special Order'	4.4 oz	320	800	15.0
supreme, 'Special Order' 9 inch	4.0 oz	280	640	14.0
taco, microwave, 7 inch	8.4 oz	590	1460	34.0
three sausage, 'Special Order' 9 inch	3.8 oz	260	600	12.0
vegetable, 'Light' 8 inch	4.4 oz	240	500	8.0
vegetable, 'Light' 12 inch	4.3 oz	230	420	7.0
(Totino's)				
Canadian bacon 'Party Pizza'	1/2 pie	330	860	13.0
cheese 'Pan Pizza'	1/6 pie	290	440	10.0
cheese 'Party Pizza'	1/2 pie	290	530	10.0
cheese 'Party Pizza Family Size'	1/3 pie	320	580	11.0
combination 'Party Pizza'	1/2 pie	370	920	17.0
combination 'Party Pizza Family Size'	1/3 pie	400	990	18.0
hamburger 'Party Pizza'	1/2 pie	350	780	17.0
pepperoni 'Pan Pizza'	1/6 pie	330	620	15.0
pepperoni 'Party Pizza'	1/2 pie	380	980	19.0
pepperoni 'Party Pizza Family Size'	1/3 pie	410	1060	20.0
sausage 'Pan Pizza'	1/6 pie	320	500	13.0
sausage 'Party Pizza'	1/2 pie	370	800	17.0
sausage 'Party Pizza Family Size'	1/3 pie	410	870	18.0
sausage and pepperoni 'Pan Pizza'	1/6 pie	330	560	15.0

od Name	Serv. Size	Total Cal.	Sod. MGS	Fat GMS
ZZA CRUST, 'All Ready' (Pillsbury)	1/8 crust	90	170	1.0
ZZA CRUST MIX				
deep dish, prepared w/water, crust only (Martha White)	1 slice	110	110	<1.0
'Pouch Mix' (Gold Medal)	1/6 pkg	110	220	1.0
'Pouch Mix' (Robin Hood)	1/6 pkg	110	220	1.0
'Quick & Easy' (Chef Boyardee)	1/6 pkg	150	300	2.0
regular, prepared w/water, crust only (Martha White)	1 slice	100	125	2.0
ZZA DINNER, FROZEN				
cheese (Kid Cuisine)	6.85 oz	380	390	12.0
cheese 'Mega Meal' (Kid Cuisine)	9.7 oz	430	700	7.0
hamburger (Kid Cuisine)	6.85 oz	330	700	10.0
ZZA ENTRÉE, FROZEN				
cheese (Weight Watchers)	6.03 oz	300	310	7.0
deluxe combination 'Lowfat' (Weight Watchers)	7.32 oz	320	370	9.0
hamburger 'Looney Tunes Wile E. Coyote' (Tyson)	6 oz	310	630	11.0
pepperoni 'Looney Tunes Foghorn Leghorn' (Tyson)	6.35 oz	400	610	13.0
pepperoni 'Lowfat' (Weight Watchers)	6.08 oz	320	550	8.0
supreme, hand held 'Aussie Pie' (Mrs. Paterson's)	5.5 oz	470	880	27.0
ZZA MIX				
cheese 'Complete' (Chef Boyardee)	1/4 pkg	230	740	6.0
cheese, kit (Contadina)	4.94 oz	320	850	10.0
cheese '2 Complete' (Chef Boyardee)	1/8 pkg	210	650	5.0
pepperoni 'Complete' (Chef Boyardee)	1/4 pkg	250	870	9.0
pepperoni, kit (Contadina)	4.94 oz	370	980	16.0
pepperoni '2 Complete' (Chef Boyardee)	1/8 pkg	210	595	7.0
plain (Chef Boyardee)	1/4 pkg	180	640	3.0
sausage (Chef Boyardee)	1/4 pkg	270	930	10.0
ZZA ROLL, FROZEN				
cheese, approx 6 rolls (Jeno's)	3 oz	240	350	12.0
combination (Jeno's)	3 oz	220	230	9.0
hamburger, approx 6 rolls (Jeno's)	3 oz	240	280	13.0
pepperoni, approx 6 rolls (Jeno's)	3 oz	220	350	9.0
pepperoni and cheese, approx 6 rolls (Jeno's)	3 oz	230	390	13.0
pepperoni and cheese 'Microwave' 6 rolls (Jeno's)	3 oz	240	440	13.0
sausage (Jeno's)	3 oz	210	340	7.0
sausage and cheese 'Microwave' approx 6 rolls (Jeno's)	3 oz	250	440	13.0
sausage and pepperoni, approx 6 rolls (Jeno's)	3 oz	230	380	13.0
LANTAIN				
cooked	4 oz	132	6	0.2
cooked, sliced	1 cup	179	8	0.3
raw, approx 9.7 oz	1 med	218	7	0.7

Food Name	Serv. Size	Total Cal.	Sod. MGS	F G
raw, sliced	1 cup	181	6	0
raw, trimmed	1 oz	35	1	0
raw, trimmed, approx 9.7 oz	1 med	218	7	0
raw, untrimmed	1 lb	360	12	1
PLUM				
pitted	1 oz	16	tr	0
raw, sliced	1 cup	91	0	1
raw, 2 1/8-inch diam	1 med	36	0	0
untrimmed (Dole)	2 pieces	70	0	1
w/pits	1 lb	235	2	2
PLUM, JAPANESE				
peeled and seeded	1 oz	13	<1	0
raw, approx .6 oz	1 med	5	tr	<
untrimmed	1 lb	132	3	0
PLUM, PURPLE, CANNED				
halves or whole, unpeeled (S&W Nutradiet)	1/2 cup	52	0	0
in extra heavy syrup	1/2 cup	133	25	0.
in extra heavy syrup, pitted	4 oz	115	22	0
in extra heavy syrup, unpeeled, halves (S&W)	1/2 cup	135	25	0
in extra heavy syrup, unpeeled, whole (S&W)	1/2 cup	135	25	0
in extra heavy syrup, w/liquid	1 cup	264	50	0.
in extra heavy syrup, w/2.75 tbsp liquid	3 plums	134	25	0.
in heavy syrup	1/2 cup	115	25	0
in heavy syrup (Stokely)	1/2 cup	130	25	0
in heavy syrup, pitted	4 oz	101	22	0
in heavy syrup, w/liquid	1 cup	230	49	0.
in heavy syrup, w/2.75 tbsp liquid	3 plums	118	25	0
in juice	1/2 cup	73	2	<
in juice, pitted	4 oz	66	1	<.
in juice, whole (Featherweight)	1/2 cup	80	10	0
in light syrup	1/2 cup	79	25	0.
in light syrup (Stokely)	1/2 cup	100	20	0
in light syrup, pitted	4 oz	71	23	0.
in water	1/2 cup	51	1	<
in water, pitted	4 oz	46	1	<.
POI				
fresh	1/2 cup	134	14	0
fresh	1 oz	32	3	<.
POLENTA MIX, prepared (Fantastic Foods)	1/2 cup	106	246	2.
POLISH SAUSAGE				
	1 oz	92	248	8.

Food Name	Serv. Size	Total Cal.	Sod. MGS	Fat GMS
link, 10 inches long x 1 1/4 inch diam, 8 oz	1 large	739	1989	65.2
(Hillshire Farm) 'Links'	2 oz	190	520	17.0
(Hormel)	2 links	170	574	14.0
(OHSE)	1 oz	80	290	7.0
(OHSE) hot	1 oz	70	270	5.0
(Pilgrim's Pride)	3 oz	131	780	7.7
POLLACK, ALASKAN				
baked	4 oz	128	132	1.3
broiled	4 oz	128	132	1.3
microwaved	4 oz	128	132	1.3
raw	1 lb	365	449	3.6
raw	1 oz	23	28	0.2
POLLACK, ATLANTIC				
raw	1 lb	416	391	4.4
raw	3 oz	78	73	0.8
raw	1 oz	26	24	0.3
POLLACK, WALLEYE				
baked	4 oz	128	132	1.3
broiled	4 oz	128	132	1.3
dry-heat cooked	3 oz	96	99	1.0
microwaved	4 oz	128	132	1.3
raw	1 lb	365	449	3.6
raw	3 oz	69	84	0.7
raw	1 oz	23	28	0.2
POLLYFISH. See PARROTFISH.				
POMEGRANATE/Chinese apple				
raw, approx 3 3/8-inch diam	1 med	105	5	0.5
trimmed	1 oz	19	1	0.1
untrimmed	1 lb	172	8	0.8
POMEGRANATE JUICE (Knudsen & Sons)	8 oz	85	na	0.0
POMPANO, FLORIDA				
baked	4 oz	239	86	13.8
broiled	4 oz	239	86	13.8
dry-heat cooked	3 oz	179	65	10.3
microwaved	4 oz	239	86	13.8
raw	1 lb	745	294	42.9
raw	1 oz	46	18	2.7
POPCORN				
(NOTE: All popcorn is popped unless otherwise noted.)				
(Bachman)				
cheese flavor	.5 oz	90	165	6.0

Food Name	Serv. Size	Total Cal.	Sod. MGS	Fat GMS
'Lite'	.5 oz	50	35	1.0
regular	.5 oz	80	160	6.0
white cheddar cheese flavor	.5 oz	70	150	4.0
(Bearitos)				
cheese flavor 'Organic'	1 oz	137	122	8.0
'Organic 50% Less Oil'	.5 oz	70	70	3.0
'Organic Lite'	1 oz	132	39	6.9
'Organic No Salt'	1 oz	108	1	0.8
'Organic Traditional'	1 oz	140	85	9.2
(Bonnie Lee)				
w/oil and salt	1 oz	172	230	8.0
w/o oil and salt	1 oz	109	<1	1.0
(Cape Cod) white cheddar cheese flavor	.5 oz	80	150	5.0
(Clover Club) white cheddar cheese flavor	.5 oz	70	140	5.0
(Cracker Jack) caramel coated, w/peanuts	1 oz	120	85	3.0
(Estee) caramel coated	1 oz	140	55	3.0
(Frito Lay)				
cheese flavor	.5 oz	80	180	5.0
regular	.5 oz	70	200	3.0
(Jiffy Pop)				
butter flavor 'Pan Popcorn'	4 cups	130	270	6.0
'Pan Popcorn'	4 cups	130	270	6.0
(Jolly Time)				
white, air-popped	3 cups	60	2	<1.0
white, w/o salt	4 cups	75	2	1.0
yellow, air-popped	3 cups	60	2	<1.0
yellow, w/o salt	4 cups	75	2	1.0
(Keebler)				
honey caramel 'Pop Deluxe'	1 oz	120	180	3.0
white cheddar cheese flavor	1 oz	140	270	10.0
(Kettle Poppins)				
lightly salted	.5 oz	70	40	2.5
white cheddar	.5 oz	70	120	2.5
(Laura Scudder)				
'Tender Baby White Corn'	.5 oz	80	140	6.0
white cheddar cheese flavor	.5 oz	70	140	5.0
(Nature's Choice)				
caramel, original	1 oz	108	na	1.0
caramel, w/peanuts	1 oz	114	na	1.0
(Orville Redenbacher)				
caramel 'Ready-to-Eat'	1 oz	112	65	3.5

ood Name	Serv. Size	Total Cal.	Sod. MGS	Fat GMS
hot air 'Gourmet' prepared	3 cups	40	0	<1.0
original 'Gourmet' prepared	3 cups	80	0	4.0
white 'Gourmet'	3 cups	80	0	4.0
white cheddar cheese 'Ready-to-Eat'	1.058 oz	139	285	8.6
Pops-Rite)				
white, w/o salt, air popped	1 oz	100	na	2.0
white, w/o salt, oil popped	1 oz	220	na	15.0
yellow, w/o salt, air popped	1 oz	100	na	2.0
yellow, w/o salt, oil popped	1 oz	220	na	15.0
Smartfood) white cheddar cheese flavor	.5 oz	80	150	5.0
Ultra Slim Fast) butter flavor 'Lite 'N Tasty'	.5 oz	60	150	2.0
Vic's)				
caramel, lite 'Gourmet'	1/2 cup	60	50	2.0
white, lite 'Gourmet'	1 cup	35	15	2.0
white cheddar cheese, lite 'Gourmet'	2/3 cup	40	50	2.0
yellow cheddar cheese, lite 'Gourmet'	2/3 cup	40	60	2.0
Weight Watchers)				
butter	.66-oz pkg	90	100	3.0
caramel	.9-oz pkg	100	45	1.0
'Lightly Salted'	.66-oz pkg	80	65	4.0
white cheddar cheese flavor	.66-oz pkg	100	85	6.0
Wise)				
butter flavor, 1 cup	.5 oz	80	140	5.0
'Tender Baby White Corn'	.5 oz	80	140	6.0
'Tender Eating Baby Popcorn'	.5 oz	70	120	6.0
white cheddar cheese flavor	.5 oz	70	140	5.0

POPCORN, FROZEN

Orville Redenbacher)				
butter flavor 'Gourmet' microwave	3 cups	100	240	6.0
natural 'Gourmet' microwave	3 cups	100	200	6.0
Pillsbury)				
butter flavor	3 cups	210	480	13.0
'Original'	3 cups	210	420	13.0
'Salt-Free'	3 cups	170	na	7.0

POPCORN, MICROWAVE

(NOTE: All microwave popcorn is popped unless otherwise noted.)

Betty Crocker)				
butter flavor 'Pop•Secret'	1/4 bag	120	250	8.0
butter flavor 'Pop•Secret By Request'	1/3 bag	60	160	1.0
butter flavor 'Pop•Secret Light'	1/4 bag	90	160	4.0
butter flavor 'Pop•Secret Pop Qwiz'	1 bag	110	210	7.0

Food Name	Serv. Size	Total Cal.	Sod. MGS	Fa GM
butter flavor, salt-free 'Pop•Secret'	1/4 bag	120	5	7.
butter flavor, singles 'Pop•Secret'	1 bag	250	460	16.
butter flavor, singles 'Pop•Secret Light'	1 bag	180	310	8.
cheese flavor 'Pop•Secret'	1/3 bag	170	260	11.
natural 'Pop•Secret'	1/4 bag	120	250	8.
natural 'Pop•Secret By Request'	1/3 bag	60	170	1.
natural 'Pop•Secret Light'	1/4 bag	90	200	4.
natural 'Pop•Secret Pop Qwiz'	1 bag	110	220	7.
natural, singles 'Pop•Secret Light'	1 bag	170	440	7.
(Featherweight)				
butter flavor 'Low Salt'	3 cups	100	70	3.
'Natural Low Salt'	3 cups	80	0	1.
(Jiffy Pop)				
butter flavor	4 cups	140	270	7.
natural	4 cups	140	270	7.
(Jolly Time)				
butter flavor	3 cups	90	95	5.
butter flavor, light	3 cups	60	105	2.
cheddar flavor	3 cups	155	220	10.
natural	3 cups	120	125	7.
natural, light	3 cups	70	110	2.
(Orville Redenbacher)				
butter flavor 'Gourmet'	3 cups	100	240	6.
butter flavor, light 'Gourmet'	3 cups	70	110	3.
butter flavor, light, snack size	3 cups	70	90	3.
butter flavor, salt-free 'Gourmet'	3 cups	100	0	6.
butter flavor 'Smart•Pop'	3 cups	50	100	1.
butter flavor, snack size	3 cups	100	140	6.
butter toffee flavor 'Gourmet'	2 1/2 cups	210	85	12.
caramel flavor 'Gourmet'	2 1/2 cups	240	90	14.
cheddar cheese flavor 'Gourmet'	3 cups	130	280	8.
natural 'Gourmet'	3 cups	100	200	6.
natural, light 'Gourmet'	3 cups	70	115	3.
natural, salt-free 'Gourmet'	3 cups	100	0	6.
red herb and garlic flavor, 2 tbsp unpopped	1.27 oz	150	366	10.
sour cream 'n onion flavor 'Gourmet'	3 cups	160	270	12.
zesty butter flavor 'Reddenbutter' 2 tbsp unpopped	1.27 oz	148	259	10.
(Pillsbury)				
butter flavor	3 cups	210	410	13.
'Original'	3 cups	210	410	13.0

ood Name	Serv. Size	Total Cal.	Sod. MGS	Fat GMS
(Planters)				
butter flavor	3 cups	140	0	10.0
natural	3 cups	140	0	9.0
(Pop Weavers)				
butter flavor	4 cups	140	230	8.0
'Natural'	4 cups	140	230	8.0
(Pops-Rite)				
butter flavor	3 cups	90	140	5.0
'Natural'	3 cups	90	190	5.0
(Weight Watchers)	1-oz pkg	100	5	1.0
POPCORN OIL				
(Orville Redenbacher) popping	1 tbsp	120	0	14.0
(Planters)	1 tbsp	120	0	14.0
(Wesson) buttery flavor popping oil	1 tbsp	120	0	13.5
(Wesson) popping and topping oil 'Food Service'	1 tbsp	122	0	13.5
POPCORN SEASONING				
(McCormick/Schilling) 'Parsley Patch'	1 tsp	10	4	0.1
POPPY SEED				
whole	1 oz	151	6	12.6
whole	1 tbsp	47	2	3.9
whole	1 tsp	15	1	1.3
whole *(Durkee)*	1 tsp	15	0	<0.1
whole *(Laurel Leaf)*	1 tsp	15	0	<0.1
whole *(Spice Islands)*	1 tsp	13	<1	0.9
POPPY SEED OIL				
	1 cup	1927	0	218.0
	1 oz	251	0	28.4
	1 tbsp	120	0	13.6

PORK. See also HAM, CANNED; HAM, CURED; HAM, FRESH; HAM PATTY.

(NOTE: TRIMMED = Lean; separable fat removed. UNTRIMMED = Separable fat not removed.)

	Serv. Size	Total Cal.	Sod. MGS	Fat GMS
BACKFAT				
wholesale cuts, raw	1 lb	3683	50	402.3
wholesale cuts, raw	1 oz	230	3	25.1
BACKRIB				
Untrimmed				
raw	1 lb	1279	340	107.0
raw	1 oz	80	21	6.7
raw 'Gourmet' *(JM)*	5.5 oz	220	50	18.0
roasted	3 oz	315	86	25.1
BELLY				
wholesale cuts, raw	1 lb	2350	145	240.5

Food Name	Serv. Size	Total Cal.	Sod. MGS	Fat GMS
wholesale cuts, raw	1 oz	147	9	15.0
BOSTON BUTT				
Trimmed				
cured, medium fat, chopped, roasted	1 cup	340	1393	19.3
cured, medium fat, roasted	9.8 oz	678	2777	38.5
BRAINS				
braised	3 oz	117	77	8.1
in milk gravy (Armour)	2.75 oz	110	400	8.0
raw	1 oz	36	34	2.6
CENTER LOIN				
Trimmed				
braised	3 oz	172	53	7.1
broiled	3 oz	172	51	6.9
chopped, braised	1 cup	381	77	19.2
chopped, broiled	1 cup	323	109	14.7
chopped, roasted	1 cup	336	97	18.3
pan-fried	3 oz	197	73	8.9
pan-fried in vegetable oil	4 oz	302	96	14.0
raw	1 oz	45	19	2.0
roasted	3 oz	169	56	7.7
Untrimmed				
braised	3 oz	210	50	12.0
broiled	3 oz	204	49	11.1
chopped, braised	1 cup	496	71	35.5
chopped, broiled	1 cup	442	98	30.9
chopped, pan-fried in vegetable oil	1 cup	372	119	22.3
chopped, roasted	1 cup	427	90	30.5
pan-fried	3 oz	235	68	14.1
pan-fried in vegetable oil	4 oz	425	82	34.6
raw	1 oz	80	16	6.2
roasted	3 oz	199	54	11.4
CENTER RIB				
Trimmed				
braised	3 oz	175	35	8.0
broiled	3 oz	186	55	8.3
chopped, braised	1 cup	388	73	20.2
chopped, broiled	1 cup	361	94	20.9
chopped, pan-fried in vegetable oil	1 cup	360	70	21.4
chopped, roasted	1 cup	343	64	19.3
pan-fried	3 oz	185	44	9.2
pan-fried in vegetable oil	4 oz	291	57	17.4

od Name	Serv. Size	Total Cal.	Sod. MGS	Fat GMS
raw	1 lb	676	204	27.3
roasted	3 oz	190	40	9.5
Untrimmed				
braised	3 oz	213	34	12.8
broiled	3 oz	224	53	13.2
chopped, braised	1 cup	514	67	38.0
chopped, broiled	1 cup	480	85	36.9
chopped, pan-fried in vegetable oil	1 cup	546	63	46.2
chopped, roasted	1 cup	445	62	33.0
pan-fried	3 oz	225	43	14.4
pan-fried in vegetable oil	4 oz	442	51	37.4
raw	1 oz	82	11	6.6
roasted	3 oz	217	39	13.0
HITTERLINGS				
raw	1 oz	71	10	6.5
simmered	3 oz	258	33	24.4
HOP, BONELESS, 'America's Cut' *(JM)*	6 oz	330	90	20.0
OMPOSITE CUTS				
Trimmed				
loin and shoulder, cooked	3 oz	179	48	8.0
loin and shoulder, raw	1 lb	653	245	26.7
loin and shoulder, raw	1 oz	41	15	1.7
retail cuts, cooked	3 oz	232	53	14.6
retail cuts, raw	1 lb	980	249	67.8
retail cuts, raw	1 oz	61	16	4.2
roasted	3 oz	180	50	8.2
Untrimmed				
loin and shoulder, cooked	3 oz	214	48	12.6
loin and shoulder, raw	1 lb	907	231	58.5
loin and shoulder, raw	1 oz	57	14	3.7
raw	1 lb	1030	245	74.8
raw	1 oz	64	15	4.7
IDNEYS				
braised	1 cup	211	112	6.6
braised	3 oz	128	68	4.0
raw	1 oz	28	34	0.9
IVER				
braised	3 oz	140	42	3.7
fried	3 oz	205	94	9.8
raw	1 oz	38	25	1.0

Food Name	Serv. Size	Total Cal.	Sod. MGS	Fa GM
LOIN				
Trimmed				
blade, braised	3 oz	191	53	11.
blade, broiled	3 oz	199	68	11.
blade, chopped, braised	1 cup	438	113	28.
blade, chopped, broiled	1 cup	420	108	30.
blade, chopped, roasted	1 cup	391	95	27.
blade, pan-fried	3 oz	205	66	12.
blade, pan-fried in vegetable oil	4 oz	321	84	22.
blade, raw	1 lb	712	304	37.
blade, roasted	3 oz	210	25	12.
country-style ribs, braised	3 oz	199	54	11.
country-style ribs, raw	1 lb	712	304	37.
country-style ribs, raw	1 oz	45	19	2.
country-style ribs, roasted	3 oz	210	25	12.
whole, braised	3 oz	173	43	7.
whole, broiled	3 oz	178	54	8.
whole, chopped, braised	1 cup	382	105	20.
whole, chopped, broiled	1 cup	360	105	21.
whole, chopped, roasted	1 cup	336	97	19.
whole, raw	1 oz	44	18	2.
whole, roasted	3 oz	178	49	8.
whole or half, center cut, boneless (JM)	3 oz	190	50	13.
Untrimmed				
blade, braised	3 oz	275	47	21.
blade, broiled	3 oz	272	59	21.
blade, chopped, braised	1 cup	574	97	47.
blade, chopped, broiled	1 cup	550	94	47.
blade, chopped, roasted	1 cup	510	85	42.
blade, pan-fried	3 oz	291	57	23.
blade, pan-fried in vegetable oil	4 oz	469	69	41.
blade, raw	1 lb	1293	245	109.
blade, roasted	3 oz	275	25	20.
country-style ribs, braised	3 oz	252	50	18.
country-style ribs, raw	1 lb	1093	263	84.
country-style ribs, raw	1 oz	68	16	5.
country-style ribs, roasted	3 oz	279	44	21.
whole, braised	4 oz	417	74	31.
whole, broiled	3 oz	206	53	11.
whole, chopped, braised	1 cup	515	91	39.
whole, chopped, broiled	1 cup	484	92	38.

Food Name	Serv. Size	Total Cal.	Sod. MGS	Fat GMS
whole, chopped, roasted	1 cup	447	88	34.0
whole, raw	1 lb	898	227	57.1
whole, roasted	3 oz	211	50	12.4
LUNGS				
braised	3 oz	84	69	2.6
raw	1 oz	24	43	0.8
PANCREAS				
braised	3 oz	186	36	9.2
raw	1 oz	56	12	3.8
SHOULDER				
Trimmed				
arm picnic, braised	3 oz	211	87	10.4
arm picnic, chopped, braised	1 cup	347	143	17.1
arm picnic, chopped, roasted	1 cup	319	112	17.7
arm picnic, raw	1 lb	635	372	27.9
arm picnic, raw	1 oz	40	23	1.8
arm picnic, roasted	3 oz	194	68	10.7
Boston blade, braised	3 oz	232	64	13.2
Boston blade, broiled	3 oz	193	63	10.7
Boston blade, chopped, braised	1 cup	412	105	24.6
Boston blade, chopped, broiled	1 cup	384	118	25.8
Boston blade, chopped, roasted	1 cup	358	102	23.6
Boston blade, raw	1 oz	47	20	2.6
Boston blade, roasted	3 oz	197	75	12.2
whole, chopped, roasted	1 cup	341	107	21.0
whole, raw	1 lb	671	345	32.4
whole, raw	1 oz	42	22	2.0
whole, roasted	3 oz	195	64	11.5
whole, roasted, diced	1 cup	310	101	18.3
Untrimmed				
arm picnic, roasted	3 oz	269	59	20.4
Boston blade, braised	3 oz	271	59	18.5
Boston blade, broiled	3 oz	220	59	14.1
Boston blade, chopped, braised	1 cup	519	94	40.1
Boston blade, chopped, broiled	1 cup	490	105	39.8
Boston blade, raw	1 lb	989	286	71.8
Boston blade, roasted	3 oz	229	57	16.0
whole, chopped, roasted	1 cup	456	96	36.0
whole, diced, roasted	1 cup	394	92	28.9
whole, raw	1 lb	1070	295	81.6
whole, raw	1 oz	67	18	5.1

Food Name	Serv. Size	Total Cal.	Sod. MGS	Fat GMS
whole, roasted	3 oz	248	58	18.2
SIRLOIN				
Trimmed				
boneless, braised	3 ogz	149	39	5.6
boneless, broiled	3 oz	164	48	5.7
boneless, raw	1 lb	581	231	19.1
boneless, roasted	3 oz	168	48	7.0
braised	3 oz	167	45	7.7
broiled	3 oz	181	61	8.6
chopped, braised	1 cup	365	83	18.2
chopped, broiled	1 cup	340	84	19.0
chopped, roasted	1 cup	330	87	18.4
raw	1 oz	43	14	1.9
raw, approx 3.1 oz	1 chop	133	48	5.4
roasted	3 oz	184	54	8.8
Untrimmed				
boneless, braised	3 oz	161	39	7.1
boneless, broiled	3 oz	177	48	7.3
boneless, raw	1 lb	658	227	28.6
boneless, roasted	3 oz	176	48	8.0
braised	3 oz	208	43	12.8
broiled	3 oz	220	58	13.7
chopped, braised	1 cup	493	76	36.0
chopped, broiled	1 cup	463	77	35.4
chopped, roasted	1 cup	407	83	28.6
raw	1 oz	78	12	6.3
roasted	3 oz	222	51	13.6
SPARERIBS				
Untrimmed				
braised	3 oz	337	79	25.8
raw	1 lb	1297	345	107.0
raw	1 oz	81	22	6.7
raw 'Gourmet' *(JM)*	4.5 oz	250	70	22.0
TENDERLOIN				
Trimmed				
boneless *(JM)*	3 oz	120	40	5.0
broiled	3 oz	159	55	5.4
chopped or diced, roasted	1 cup	232	94	6.7
raw	1 lb	544	227	15.5
raw	1 oz	34	14	1.0
roasted	3 oz	139	48	4.1

Food Name	Serv. Size	Total Cal.	Sod. MGS	Fat GMS
Untrimmed				
broiled	3 oz	171	54	6.9
raw	1 lb	617	222	24.5
raw	1 oz	39	14	1.5
roasted	3 oz	147	47	5.1
TOP LOIN				
Trimmed				
braised	3 oz	172	36	7.3
broiled	3 oz	173	55	6.6
chopped, braised	1 cup	388	73	20.2
chopped, broiled	1 cup	361	94	20.9
chopped, pan-fried in vegetable oil	1 cup	360	70	21.4
chopped, roasted	1 cup	343	64	19.3
pan-fried	3 oz	191	48	8.9
pan-fried in vegetable oil	4 oz	291	57	17.4
raw	1 oz	46	13	2.1
roast, boneless, raw	1 lb	640	204	24.0
roast, boneless, raw	1 oz	40	13	1.5
roasted	3 oz	165	38	6.1
Untrimmed				
braised	3 oz	198	36	10.8
broiled	3 oz	195	54	9.6
chopped, braised	1 cup	533	66	40.8
chopped, broiled	1 cup	504	83	40.1
chopped, pan-fried in vegetable oil	1 cup	549	63	46.5
chopped, roasted	1 cup	462	62	35.2
pan-fried	3 oz	218	47	12.6
pan-fried in vegetable oil	3 oz	337	39	28.6
raw	1 oz	86	11	7.3
roast, boneless, raw	1 lb	866	195	52.7
roast, boneless, raw	1 oz	54	12	3.3
roasted	3 oz	192	37	9.7
PORK, CANNED				
	1 oz	95	365	8.6
approx .75 oz	1 slice	70	271	6.4
(Hormel)	3 oz	240	1056	21.0
(Hormel) chopped	3 oz	200	1073	16.0
PORK, CURED				
blade roll, untrimmed, diced, roasted	1 cup	402	1362	32.9
blade roll, untrimmed, diced, unheated	1 cup	377	1750	30.8
blade roll, untrimmed, roasted	4 oz	325	1103	26.6

Food Name	Serv. Size	Total Cal.	Sod. MGS	Fat GMS
blade roll, untrimmed, unheated	1 oz	76	354	6.2
boneless, blade roll, untrimmed, roasted	3 oz	244	827	20.0
boneless, blade roll, untrimmed, unheated	1 oz	76	354	6.2
PORK, GROUND				
cooked	3 oz	252	62	17.6
raw	1 oz	75	16	6.0
(JM)	3 oz	190	40	14.0
PORK, SALT, cured, raw	1 oz	212	404	22.8
PORK DINNER, FROZEN, chow mein 'Bi-Pack' (LaChoy)	8.642 oz	87	1218	3.2
PORK ENTRÉE				
Canned				
chow mein 'Bi-Pack' (LaChoy)	3/4 cup	80	970	3.0
sweet and sour (LaChoy)	3/4 cup	250	1540	4.0
Frozen				
barbecued back ribs 'Pork Classics' (John Morrell)	4.75 oz	240	480	17.0
barbecued chops, center cut 'Pork Classics' (John Morrell)	4.5 oz	230	410	9.0
barbecued loin, thin sliced 'Pork Classics' (John Morrell)	3 oz	150	440	6.0
barbecued spare ribs 'Pork Classics' (John Morrell)	4.5 oz	250	470	18.0
barbecued tenderloin 'Pork Classics' (John Morrell)	3 oz	130	220	5.0
breaded, steak (Hormel)	3 oz	220	(mq)	15.0
patty deluxe 'Looney Tunes Porky Pig' (Tyson)	6.5 oz	370	490	14.0
sweet and sour (Chun King)	13 oz	400	1460	5.0
PORK FAT				
separable fat from fully cooked ham, roasted	1 oz	167	177	17.5
separable fat from fully cooked ham, unheated	1 oz	164	143	17.4
separable fat from ham and arm picnic, roasted	3 oz	502	530	52.6
separable fat from ham and arm picnic, roasted	1 oz	168	177	17.5
separable fat from ham and arm picnic, unheated	1 oz	164	143	17.4
PORK RIND SNACK				
(Baken-ets)	1 oz	160	850	10.0
(Baken-ets) hot 'n spicy	1 oz	150	750	9.0
PORK SEASONING AND COATING MIX				
'Bag 'n Season' (Schilling)	1 pkg	103	3126	0.4
POT ROAST DINNER/ENTRÉE, FROZEN				
homestyle (Right Course)	9.25 oz	220	550	7.0
homestyle, w/browned potatoes (Stouffer's)	8 7/8 oz	280	690	11.0
Yankee (Budget Gourmet)	11 oz	380	690	21.0
Yankee (Healthy Choice)	11 oz	260	400	4.0
Yankee (Le Menu)	10 oz	330	700	13.0
Yankee 'Classics' (Armour)	10 oz	310	670	12.0

Food Name	Serv. Size	Total Cal.	Sod. MGS	Fat GMS
POT ROAST SEASONING MIX				
'Bag 'n Season' (Schilling)	1 pkg	55	3030	0.6
'Seasoning Blends' (Lawry's)	1 pkg	122	4008	0.7
POTATO				
Baked				
in skin	4 oz	124	9	0.1
in skin, pulp only	4 oz	105	6	0.1
in skin, skin only	2 oz	112	12	0.1
pulp	1/2 cup	57	3	0.1
Boiled				
in skin	2 oz	44	8	0.1
in skin, pulp only	4 oz	99	5	0.1
in skin, pulp only	1/2 cup	68	3	0.1
in skin, pulp only, approx 2.5 inch diam	1 potato	118	5	0.1
pulp only	4 oz	98	6	0.1
pulp only	1/2 cup	67	4	0.1
pulp only, approx 2.5 inch diam	1 potato	116	7	0.1
Hash brown, cooked in vegetable oil	4 oz	237	27	15.8
Microwaved				
in skin	4 oz	119	9	0.1
in skin, pulp only	4 oz	113	8	0.1
in skin, pulp only	1/2 cup	78	5	0.1
in skin, skin only	2 oz	75	9	0.1
Raw				
peeled	1 oz	22	2	<.1
pulp only, diced	1/2 cup	59	5	0.1
skin only	2 oz	33	6	0.1
unpeeled	1 lb	269	21	0.3
POTATO, CANNED				
(Stokely)	1/2 cup	50	360	0.0
(Veg•All)	1/2 cup	60	260	0.0
approx 1.2 oz	1 potato	21	(mq)	0.1
diced (Bush's Best)	1/2 cup	40	340	0.0
diced (Taylor's Brand)	1 cup	90	292	0.0
drained	4 oz	68	(mq)	0.2
drained	1/2 cup	54	234	0.2
drained, approx 1-inch diam	1 potato	21	91	0.1
new, extra small, whole (S&W)	1/2 cup	45	310	0.0
new, small, whole (IGA)	1/2 cup	45	300	0.0
new, whole, drained (Hunt's)	4 oz	70	230	<1.0
sliced (Bush's Best)	1/2 cup	40	340	0.0

Food Name	Serv. Size	Total Cal.	Sod. MGS	Fat GMS
sliced *(Taylor's Brand)*	1 cup	90	292	0.0
sliced, w/liquid *(Del Monte)*	1/2 cup	45	355	0.0
white, diced *(Allens)*	1/2 cup	45	360	<1.0
white, double diced *(Allens)*	1/2 cup	45	540	<1.0
white, sliced *(A&P)*	1/2 cup	45	320	<1.0
white, sliced *(Allens)*	1/2 cup	45	360	<1.0
white, sliced 'No Salt Added' *(Pathmark)*	1 cup	100	15	0.0
white, small, sliced *(Finast)*	1/2 cup	55	375	0.0
white, small, whole *(Finast)*	1/2 cup	55	375	0.0
white, whole *(A&P)*	1/2 cup	45	320	<1.0
white, whole 'No Salt Added' *(Pathmark)*	1 cup	100	15	0.0
whole *(Bush's Best)*	1/2 cup	40	340	0.0
whole, w/liquid	1 cup	120	903	0.5
whole, w/liquid	1/2 cup	60	452	0.2
whole, w/liquid *(Del Monte)*	1/2 cup	45	355	0.0
w/liquid	4 oz	45	341	0.2
POTATO, FINNISH YELLOW, raw *(Frieda's)*	3.5 oz	100	na	na
POTATO, FREEZE-DRIED				
hash brown, prepared *(Mountain House)*	1 cup	150	(mq)	0.0
POTATO, FROZEN				
fried	9 oz	419	58	16.5
fried, cottage cut, heated in oven	4 oz	247	51	9.3
fried, partially fried in oil, heated in oven	4 oz	252	35	9.9
fried, partially fried in oil, heated in oven	1.75 oz	111	15	4.4
hash brown, prepared in vegetable oil	4 oz	247	39	13.0
hash brown, w/butter sauce, prepared	4 oz	202	115	10.0
puffs, partially fried in oil, prepared	4 oz	252	846	12.2
whole, peeled	10 oz	221	71	0.5
whole, peeled, boiled, drained	4 oz	74	23	0.1
(A&P)				
fried, crinkle cut	3.5 oz	140	25	4.0
fried, regular	3.5 oz	140	25	4.0
fried, shoestring	3.5 oz	170	50	6.0
fried, steak fries	3.5 oz	140	30	4.0
hash brown	3.5 oz	80	20	0.0
morsels	3.5 oz	140	30	4.0
(Heinz)				
fried, crinkle cut 'Deep Fries'	3 oz	150	30	6.0
fried 'Deep Fries'	3 oz	160	20	6.0
fried, shoestring 'Deep Fries'	3 oz	200	20	10.0
hash brown, w/butter and onions 'Deep Fries'	3 oz	110	80	7.0

Food Name	Serv. Size	Total Cal.	Sod. MGS	Fat GMS
(MicroMagic)				
fried	3 oz	290	30	13.0
fried, skinny	3 oz	350	40	15.0
sticks 'Tater Sticks'	4 oz	390	620	22.0
(Ore-Ida)				
fried, cottage cut	3 oz	120	25	5.0
fried 'Country Style Dinner Fries'	3 oz	110	30	3.0
fried, crinkle cut 'Golden Crinkles'	3 oz	120	35	4.0
fried, crinkle cut 'Lites'	3 oz	90	35	2.0
fried, crinkle cut, microwave	3.5 oz	180	35	8.0
fried, crinkle cut 'Pixie Crinkles'	3 oz	140	40	6.0
fried 'Crisp Crowns'	3 oz	160	525	9.0
fried 'Crispers!'	3 oz	230	545	15.0
fried, French, extra crispy 'Nacho Crispers'	3 oz	180	280	10.0
fried, French 'Fast Fries'	3 oz	150	230	7.0
fried 'Golden Fries'	3 oz	120	35	4.0
fried 'Lites'	3 oz	90	30	2.0
fried, shoestring	3 oz	140	30	6.0
fried, shoestring 'Lites'	3 oz	90	25	4.0
fried, wedges 'Home Style Potato Wedges'	3 oz	100	45	3.0
fried, w/onions 'Crispy Crowns'	3 oz	170	570	9.0
hash brown 'Golden Patties'	2.5 oz	140	295	8.0
hash brown, microwave	2 oz	130	170	8.0
hash brown, shredded	3 oz	70	40	<1.0
hash brown 'Southern Style'	3 oz	70	35	<1.0
hash brown, w/cheddar 'Cheddar Browns'	3 oz	90	415	2.0
mashed, natural butter flavor, prepared w/2% milk	1/2 cup	170	230	5.0
mashed, natural butter flavor, unprepared	2.25 oz	100	140	3.0
puffs, bacon flavored 'Tater Tots'	3 oz	140	625	6.0
puffs 'Tater Tots'	3 oz	140	550	7.0
puffs 'Tater Tots' microwave	4 oz	200	670	9.0
puffs, w/onion 'Tater Tots'	3 oz	140	715	6.0
whole, small	3 oz	70	45	<1.0
(Quick 'n Crispy)				
fried, crinkle cut	4 oz	370	50	19.0
fried, shoestring	4 oz	390	50	20.0
fried, thin cuts	4 oz	370	50	19.0
wedges	4 oz	280	40	13.0
(Seabrook)				
diced and hash-shred	4 oz	80	41	0.0
fried	3 oz	120	25	4.0

Food Name	Serv. Size	Total Cal.	Sod. MGS	Fc GM
fried, cottage cut	2.8 oz	110	14	4.
fried, crinkle cut	3 oz	120	24	4.
fried, shoestring	3 oz	140	45	6.
white, whole, boiled	3.2 oz	60	5	0.
(Southern) white, whole	3.5 oz	69	20	0.

POTATO CHIPS AND SNACKS
(Allens)

barbecue flavor	1 oz	150	280	9.
hot flavor	1 oz	150	200	9.
potato sticks, shoestring, canned	1 oz	140	190	8.
potato sticks, shoestring, canned 'No Salt'	1 oz	140	10	8.
regular flavor	1 oz	160	270	10.

(Bachman)

'Kettle Cooked'	1 oz	140	115	8.
pasta snack chip 'Pastapazazz'	1 oz	150	340	9.
'Ridge'	1 oz	160	260	10.
'Ruffled'	1 oz	160	260	10.
Saratoga-style 'Kettle Cooked'	1 oz	140	115	8.
sour cream and onion flavor	1 oz	150	200	9.
'Unsalted'	1 oz	160	5	10.
vinegar flavor	1 oz	150	610	9.

(Barbara's Bakery)

herb and garlic flavor 'True Blues'	1 oz	140	120	9.
ripple	1 oz	150	250	10.
'True Blues'	1 oz	150	120	10.

(Barrel O'Fun)

	1 oz	150	160	10.0

(Cape Cod)

dill and sour cream flavor	1 oz	150	160	8.
dill and sour cream flavor 'No Salt'	1 oz	150	15	8.
'No Salt Added'	1 oz	150	0	8.0
regular flavor	1 oz	150	120	8.0
'Waves'	1 oz	150	120	8.

(Cottage Fries) 'No Salt Added'

	1 oz	160	5	11.

(Eagle)

barbecue flavor 'Extra Crunchy'	1 oz	150	220	8.0
barbecue flavor 'Extra Crunchy Louisiana'	1 oz	150	140	8.
barbecue flavor 'Thins'	1 oz	150	220	10.
'Eagle Thins'	1 oz	150	220	10.0
'Extra Crunchy'	1 oz	150	180	8.0
'Idaho Russet'	1 oz	150	180	8.
'Ridged Thins'	1 oz	150	220	10.

Food Name	Serv. Size	Total Cal.	Sod. MGS	Fat GMS
sour cream and onion flavor 'Ridged'	1 oz	150	280	10.0
(Eden Foods)				
brown rice chips	1 oz	130	197	5.0
sea vegetable chips	1 oz	130	200	5.0
wasabi snack chips	1 oz	130	200	4.0
(Featherweight) 'Low Salt'	1 oz	160	4	11.0
(Flavor Tree) sour cream and onion flavor potato sticks	1/4 cup	127	360	8.3
(Funyuns) rings, onion flavor, approx 11 rings	1 oz	140	275	6.0
(Great Snackers)				
barbecue flavor	1 serving	60	170	3.0
cheddar cheese flavor	1 serving	60	170	3.0
sour cream and onion flavor	.5 oz	70	140	3.0
toasted onion flavor	1 serving	60	120	3.0
(Hain)				
carrot chip	1 oz	150	160	9.0
carrot chip, barbecue	1 oz	140	160	8.0
carrot chip 'No Salt Added'	1 oz	150	30	7.0
(Health Valley)				
'Country'	1 oz	160	60	10.0
'Country Dip'	1 oz	160	60	10.0
'Country Dip No Salt Added'	1 oz	160	1	10.0
'Country Natural No Salt Added'	1 oz	160	1	10.0
'Country No Salt Added'	1 oz	160	1	10.0
'Country Ripple'	1 oz	160	60	10.0
'Country Ripple No Salt Added'	1 oz	160	1	10.0
'Natural'	1 oz	160	60	10.0
(Keebler)				
original flavor, lightly seasoned	1 oz	140	190	7.0
sour cream and onion flavor	1 oz	140	260	7.0
(Kettle Chips)				
jalapeño jack flavor	1 oz	150	110	9.0
lightly salted	1 oz	150	80	9.0
New York cheddar flavor	1 oz	150	100	9.0
no salt	1 oz	150	10	9.0
organically grown, w/sea salt	1 oz	150	80	9.0
salsa w/mesquite flavor	1 oz	150	120	9.0
sea salt and vinegar flavor	1 oz	150	120	9.0
yogurt and green onion flavor	1 oz	150	120	9.0
(King Kold)				
au gratin flavor	1 oz	150	220	8.0
barbecue flavor 'BBQ'	1 oz	140	360	8.0

Food Name	Serv. Size	Total Cal.	Sod. MGS	Fat GMS
dill flavor	1 oz	150	340	8.0
onion-garlic flavor	1 oz	150	420	9.0
regular flavor	1 oz	150	160	9.0
'Rip-L'	1 oz	150	150	9.0
sour cream and onion flavor	1 oz	150	220	10.0
(Lay's)				
barbecue flavor, approx 15-20 chips	1 oz	150	270	9.0
barbecue flavor 'Kansas City Style' approx 15-20 chips	1 oz	150	270	9.0
Cajun flavor 'Crunch Tators Amazin Cajun'	1 oz	150	150	8.0
cheddar cheese flavor, approx 15-20 chips	1 oz	150	1	10.0
'Flamin' Hot' approx 15-20 chips	1 oz	150	190	9.0
jalapeño flavor 'Crunch Tators Hoppin' Jalapeño'	1 oz	140	200	7.0
mesquite flavor 'Crunch Tators Mighty Mesquite'	1 oz	150	135	8.0
original flavor, approx 15-20 chips	1 oz	150	170	10.0
original flavor 'Crunch Tators' approx 16 chips	1 oz	150	120	8.0
salt and vinegar flavor, approx 15-20 chips	1 oz	150	390	10.0
sour cream and onion flavor, approx 15-20 chips	1 oz	160	220	10.0
tangy ranch flavor, approx 15-20 chips	1 oz	160	210	10.0
'Unsalted'	1 oz	150	10	10.0
(Louise's)				
mesquite barbecue flavor, fat-free	1 oz	100	200	<1.0
original flavor, fat-free	1 oz	100	200	<1.0
vinegar and salt flavor, fat-free	1 oz	100	200	<1.0
(Mr. Phipps)				
tater crisps, barbecue flavor	.5 oz	60	160	2.0
tater crisps, sour cream and onion flavor	.5 oz	60	150	2.0
(Munchos) plain, approx 16 chips	1 oz	160	230	10.0
(Nabisco)				
baked, cheddar cheese flavor, cracker chips 'Zings'	.5 oz	70	140	3.0
baked, ranch flavor, cracker chips 'Zings'	.5 oz	70	140	3.0
cracker chips, baked 'Zings'	.5 oz	70	115	3.0
(O'Boisies)				
regular flavor	1 oz	150	180	9.0
sour cream and onion flavor	1 oz	150	190	9.0
(Planters)				
potato sticks	1 oz	160	170	10.0
potato sticks, barbecue flavor	1 oz	160	220	10.0
(Poore Brothers)				
barbecue flavor	1 oz	150	60	10.0
Cajun flavor	1 oz	140	55	8.0
dill pickle flavor	1 oz	140	95	8.0

Food Name	Serv. Size	Total Cal.	Sod. MGS	Fat GMS
grilled steak and onion flavor	1 oz	140	110	8.0
jalapeño flavor	1 oz	140	100	9.0
Parmesan and garlic flavor	1 oz	140	80	9.0
regular flavor	1 oz	140	40	8.0
salt and vinegar flavor	1 oz	140	125	9.0
unsalted	1 oz	140	5	8.0
(Pringle's)				
barbecue flavor 'Light'	1 oz	150	125	8.0
cheese flavor 'Cheez-ums'	1 oz	170	200	13.0
French onion flavor 'Idaho Rippled'	1 oz	170	175	12.0
'Idaho Rippled'	1 oz	170	150	12.0
'Light'	1 oz	150	120	8.0
ranch flavor 'Light'	1 oz	150	135	8.0
'Regular'	1 oz	170	170	13.0
sour cream and onion flavor	1 oz	170	135	12.0
taco and cheddar flavor 'Idaho Rippled'	1 oz	170	160	12.0
(Ray's)				
taro chips, salted	1 oz	139	167	6.0
taro chips, unsalted	1 oz	139	15	6.0
(Ruffles)				
barbecue flavor	1 oz	150	320	9.0
Cajun flavor 'Cajun Spice'	1 oz	150	240	10.0
cheddar and sour cream flavor	1 oz	150	260	9.0
'Choice' 40% less fat, approx 16 chips	1 oz	130	130	6.0
'Light Choice' 1/3 less fat	1 oz	130	140	6.0
mesquite barbecue flavor 'Mesquite Grille'	1 oz	160	260	10.0
ranch flavor	1 oz	160	240	10.0
regular flavor	1 oz	150	190	10.0
sour cream and onion flavor	1 oz	150	240	9.0
(Schlotzsky's) barbecue, deli style	1 oz	150	115	6.0
(Snacktime)				
jalapeño flavor 'Krunchers!'	1 oz	150	270	9.0
'Krunchers!'	1 oz	150	170	9.0
mesquite barbecue flavor 'Krunchers!'	1 oz	150	200	9.0
(Spicer's)				
barbecue wheat flavor, for weight control	1 oz	100	75	5.0
natural flavor, for weight control	1 oz	100	65	4.0
sour cream and onion flavor, for weight control	1 oz	100	150	4.0
(Sun Chips)				
multi-grain snacks, French onion flavor	1 oz	140	120	7.0
multi-grain snacks, harvest cheddar flavor	1 oz	140	125	7.0

Food Name	Serv. Size	Total Cal.	Sod. MGS	Fat GMS
multi-grain snacks, original flavor	1 oz	150	100	8.0
(Tato Skins)				
potato skins, baked	1 oz	150	160	8.0
potato skins, cheese and bacon flavor	1 oz	150	180	8.0
potato skins, sour cream and chives flavor	1 oz	150	180	8.0
(Westbrae)				
no salt	1 oz	150	10	8.0
'Ripple'	1 oz	150	100	8.0
salted	1 oz	160	100	10.0
(Wise)				
barbecue flavor	1 oz	150	240	10.0
barbecue flavor 'Ridgies'	1 oz	150	240	10.0
hot flavor	1 oz	160	290	11.0
'New York Deli'	1 oz	160	120	11.0
onion-garlic flavor	1 oz	150	250	10.0
'Plain'	1 oz	150	190	10.0
'Ridgies'	1 oz	150	190	10.0
'Ridgies Super Crispy'	1 oz	150	220	10.0
rings, onion flavor	1 oz	130	360	5.0
'Rippled'	1 oz	150	190	10.0
sour cream and onion flavor 'Ridgies'	1 oz	160	240	11.0
(Zapp's)				
Cajun flavor 'Lite Kettle'	1 oz	150	94	8.0
Cajun flavor 'Original Kettle'	1 oz	150	94	8.0
jalapeño flavor 'Original Kettle'	1 oz	150	85	8.0
'Lite Kettle'	1 oz	150	45	8.0
'Lite Kettle No Salt Added'	1 oz	150	<1	8.0
mesquite barbecue flavor 'Lite Kettle'	1 oz	150	87	8.0
mesquite barbecue flavor 'Original Kettle'	1 oz	150	87	8.0
'Original Kettle'	1 oz	150	45	8.0
'Original Kettle No Salt Added'	1 oz	150	<1	8.0
sour cream and onion flavor 'Lite Kettle'	1 oz	150	79	8.0
POTATO DISH, CANNED, au gratin *(Pantry Express)*	1/2 cup	120	430	5.0
POTATO DISH, FROZEN				
au gratin 'Family Side Dish' *(Freezer Queen)*	4 oz	100	440	2.0
au gratin 'For One' *(Birds Eye)*	5.5 oz	240	590	13.0
au gratin 'One Serving' *(Green Giant)*	5.5 oz	200	560	10.0
au gratin, side dish *(Stouffer's)*	5.75 oz	170	670	9.0
baked, butter 'Twice Baked' *(Ore-Ida)*	5 oz	200	350	9.0
baked, cheddar cheese 'Twice Baked' *(Ore-Ida)*	5 oz	190	420	7.0
baked, ranch 'Twice Baked' *(Ore-Ida)*	5 oz	180	320	6.0

Food Name	Serv. Size	Total Cal.	Sod. MGS	Fat GMS
baked, sour cream and chives 'Twice Baked' (Ore-Ida)	5 oz	180	360	6.0
baked, stuffed w/cheddar cheese (Oh Boy!)	6 oz	142	612	4.0
baked, stuffed w/cheese flavored topping (Green Giant)	5 oz	200	520	6.0
baked, stuffed w/real bacon (Oh Boy!)	6 oz	116	641	3.0
baked, stuffed w/sour cream and chives (Green Giant)	5 oz	230	580	10.0
baked, stuffed w/sour cream and chives (Oh Boy!)	6 oz	129	418	5.0
baked, topped w/salsa and cheese (Ore-Ida)	5.6 oz	160	350	4.0
cheddared, 'Side Dish' (Budget Gourmet)	5.5 oz	230	450	13.0
cheddared, w/broccoli 'Side Dish' (Budget Gourmet)	5 oz	130	340	4.0
fried, 'Country Style Dinner Fries' (Ore-Ida)	3 oz	110	30	3.0
fried, w/onions 'Crispy Crowns' (Ore-Ida)	3 oz	170	570	9.0
garden casserole, low-fat, 'Quick Meals' (Healthy Choice)	9.25 oz	180	360	4.0
hash brown, w/butter and onions, 'Deep Fries' (Heinz)	3 oz	110	80	7.0
hash brown, w/cheddar, 'Cheddar Browns' (Ore-Ida)	3 oz	90	415	2.0
nacho, 'Side Dish' (Budget Gourmet)	5 oz	180	360	10.0
new, in sour cream sauce, 'Side Dish' (Budget Gourmet)	5 oz	120	300	6.0
'O'Brien' (Ore-Ida)	3 oz	60	25	<1.0
puffs, w/bacon-flavored vegetable protein, 'Tater Tots' (Ore-Ida)	3 oz	140	625	6.0
puffs, w/onion, 'Tater Tots' (Ore-Ida)	3 oz	140	715	6.0
scalloped, side dish (Stouffer's)	5.75 oz	130	610	6.0
shredded, w/cheese sauce and vegetables, 'Singles' (Stokely)	4.5 oz	130	480	6.0
sliced, w/cheddar cheese sauce and bacon, 'Singles' (Stokely)	4.5 oz	150	460	5.0
three cheese, 'Side Dish' (Budget Gourmet)	5.75 oz	230	410	11.0
wedges, hot and spicy, 'Texas Crispers' (Ore-Ida)	3 oz	180	250	10.0
w/broccoli and cheese flavor sauce, 'One Serving' (Green Giant)	5.5 oz	130	720	5.0
w/broccoli and cheese sauce, 'Family Side Dish' (Freezer Queen)	5.5 oz	140	79	3.0
POTATO DISH, MICROWAVE				
au gratin, 'Microwave Shelf Pack' (Green Giant)	1/2 cup	120	430	5.0
scalloped, microwave cup (Lunch Bucket)	7.5 oz	160	770	7.0
scalloped, w/ham, micro cup (Hormel)	7.5 oz	260	810	16.0
POTATO DISH MIX				
and cheese, au gratin 'Potatoes & Cheese' (Kraft) prepared	1/2 cup	130	570	5.0
and cheese, broccoli au gratin (Kraft) prepared	1/2 cup	150	530	5.0
broccoli au gratin 'Potato Medleys' (Betty Crocker) dry	1/5 pkg	110	550	1.0

Food Name	Serv. Size	Total Cal.	Sod. MGS	Fat GMS
broccoli au gratin 'Potato Medleys' *(Betty Crocker)* prepared w/margarine and 2% milk	1/2 cup	140	590	4.0
cheddar, w/mushrooms 'Potato Medleys' *(Betty Crocker)* dry	1/5 pkg	110	490	1.0
cheddar, w/mushrooms 'Potato Medleys' *(Betty Crocker)* prepared w/margarine and whole milk	1/2 cup	140	530	4.0
scalloped, w/broccoli 'Potato Medleys' *(Betty Crocker)* dry	1/5 pkg	100	460	2.0
scalloped, w/broccoli 'Potato Medleys' *(Betty Crocker)* prepared	1/2 cup	140	500	5.0
scalloped, w/green beans and mushrooms *(Betty Crocker)* dry	1/5 pkg	110	460	2.0
scalloped, w/green beans and mushrooms *(Betty Crocker)* prepared	1/2 cup	140	500	5.0
'SpudFlakes' *(Martha White)* prepared w/2% milk	1/3 cup	120	345	6.0
w/cheese, scalloped, and ham *(Kraft)* prepared	1/2 cup	150	510	5.0
w/cheese, scalloped 'Potatoes & Cheese' *(Kraft)* prepared	1/2 cup	140	500	5.0
w/cheese, sour cream and chive *(Kraft)* prepared	1/2 cup	150	610	5.0
w/two cheeses 'Potatoes & Cheese' *(Kraft)* prepared	1/2 cup	130	540	4.0
POTATO ENTRÉE, FROZEN				
baked, chicken divan *(Weight Watchers)*	11.25 oz	280	480	7.0
baked, homestyle turkey *(Weight Watchers)*	11.25 oz	230	510	7.0
baked, vegetable primavera *(Weight Watchers)*	11.15 oz	320	500	9.0
baked, w/broccoli and cheddar *(Lean Cuisine)*	10 3/8 oz	290	590	9.0
baked, w/broccoli and cheese *(Weight Watchers)*	10.5 oz	270	570	6.0
baked, w/broccoli and ham *(Weight Watchers)*	11.5 oz	240	520	5.0
baked, w/cheese sauce and broccoli 'Light & Healthy' *(Budget Gourmet)*	10.5 oz	300	740	10.0
baked, w/sour cream *(Lean Cuisine)*	10 3/8 oz	230	570	5.0
POTATO FLOUR				
	1/2 cup	316	31	0.7
	1 oz	100	10	0.2
POTATO MIX				
AU GRATIN				
(Betty Crocker) prepared w/margarine and skim milk	1/2 cup	150	600	5.0
(Fantastic Foods) prepared w/whole milk	1/2 cup	156	440	4.0
(Fantastic Foods) prepared w/whole milk and salted butter	1/2 cup	196	495	8.0
(French's) tangy, prepared	1/2 cup	130	480	5.0
(General Mills) dry	1/6 pkg	100	520	1.0
(General Mills) homestyle, w/broccoli, dry	1/6 pkg	90	490	1.0

Food Name	Serv. Size	Total Cal.	Sod. MGS	Fat GMS
(General Mills) homestyle, w/broccoli, prepared w/margarine and 2% milk	1/2 cup	140	550	6.0
(General Mills) prepared w/margarine and 2% milk	1/2 cup	150	580	6.0
(Idahoan) prepared	1/2 cup	130	475	5.0
(Pillsbury) 'Specialty' tangy, dry	1/6 pkg	90	470	1.0
(Pillsbury) tangy, prepared w/butter and whole milk	1/2 cup	140	520	6.0
CASSEROLE *(French's)* cheddar and bacon, prepared	1/2 cup	130	390	5.0
COUNTRY STYLE				
(Fantastic Foods) prepared	1/2 cup	85	316	0.3
(Fantastic Foods) prepared w/salted butter	1/2 cup	118	362	4.0
HASH BROWN				
(Betty Crocker) w/onions, prepared	1/6 pkg	110	40	1.0
(Betty Crocker) w/onions, prepared w/margarine	1/2 cup	160	100	6.0
(General Mills)	1/6 pkg	110	25	<1.0
(General Mills) prepared w/margarine	1/2 cup	160	100	6.0
(Idahoan) herb and butter, dry	1/6 pkg	90	425	2.0
(Idahoan) prepared w/unsalted butter	1/2 cup	140	50	7.0
(Idahoan) 'Quick One-Pan' prepared	1/2 cup	140	400	7.0
JULIENNE				
(General Mills) dry	1/6 pkg	90	520	1.0
(General Mills) prepared w/margarine and 2% milk	1/2 cup	130	580	5.0
MASHED				
(Betty Crocker) bacon and cheddar 'Twice Baked' dry	1/6 pkg	110	500	2.0
(Betty Crocker) bacon and cheddar 'Twice Baked' prepared	1/2 cup	210	600	11.0
(Betty Crocker) butter, herbed 'Twice Baked' dry	1/6 pkg	100	440	2.0
(Betty Crocker) butter, herbed 'Twice Baked' prepared	1/2 cup	220	540	13.0
(Betty Crocker) cheddar, mild, w/onion 'Twice Baked' dry	1/6 pkg	100	540	2.0
(Betty Crocker) cheddar, mild, w/onion 'Twice Baked' prepared	1/2 cup	190	640	11.0
(Betty Crocker) cheddar cheese 'Potato Buds' dry	1/12 pkg	110	440	2.0
(Betty Crocker) cheddar cheese 'Potato Buds' prepared	1/2 cup	180	510	9.0
(Betty Crocker) cheddar cheese 'Potato Buds' reduced fat recipe, dry	1/12 pkg	140	480	5.0
(Betty Crocker) 'Potato Buds' prepared	1/2 cup	130	360	6.0
(Betty Crocker) 'Potato Buds' prepared w/o added salt	1/2 cup	130	90	6.0
(Country Store) prepared	1/3 cup	70	10	0.0
(General Mills) American cheese, homestyle, dry	1/6 pkg	100	560	1.0
(General Mills) American cheese, homestyle, prepared w/margarine and 2% milk	1/2 cup	150	620	6.0
(General Mills) cheddar and bacon, dry	1/6 pkg	100	480	1.0

Food Name	Serv. Size	Total Cal.	Sod. MGS	Fat GMS
(General Mills) cheddar and bacon, prepared w/margarine and 2% milk	1/2 cup	150	540	6.0
(General Mills) cheddar cheese, homestyle, dry	1/6 pkg	90	470	1.0
(General Mills) cheddar cheese, homestyle, prepared w/margarine and 2% milk	1/2 cup	150	530	6.0
(Hungry Jack) 'Flakes' prepared	1/2 cup	140	380	7.0
(Idahoan) cheddar, spicy, dry	1/6 pkg	90	450	1.0
(Idahoan) cheddar, spicy, prepared	1/2 cup	140	500	5.0
(Pillsbury) cheddar and bacon 'Specialty' dry	1/6 pkg	90	430	1.0
(Pillsbury) cheddar and bacon 'Specialty' prepared w/butter and whole milk	1/2 cup	140	480	6.0
SCALLOPED				
(Betty Crocker) cheesy, dry	1/6 pkg	90	500	1.0
(Betty Crocker) cheesy, prepared	1/2 cup	140	560	5.0
(Betty Crocker) dry	1/6 pkg	90	520	1.0
(Betty Crocker) prepared	1/2 cup	140	580	5.0
(Betty Crocker) sour cream and chives, dry	1/6 pkg	100	460	2.0
(Betty Crocker) sour cream and chives, prepared	1/2 cup	140	520	5.0
(Betty Crocker) w/ham, dry	1/5 pkg	100	470	1.0
(Betty Crocker) w/ham, prepared	1/2 cup	160	540	6.0
(French's) creamy Italian, prepared	1/2 cup	120	430	3.0
(French's) crispy top, w/savory onion mix, prepared	1/2 cup	140	430	5.0
(French's) real cheese, prepared	1/2 cup	140	380	5.0
(French's) sour cream and chives, prepared	1/2 cup	150	550	7.0
(General Mills) dry	1/6 pkg	90	510	1.0
(General Mills) prepared w/margarine and 2% milk	1/2 cup	140	570	5.0
(General Mills) smoky cheddar, dry	1/6 pkg	100	520	1.0
(General Mills) smoky cheddar, prepared w/margarine and 2% milk	1/2 cup	140	580	5.0
(General Mills) sour cream and chive	1/6 pkg	100	460	2.0
(General Mills) sour cream and chive, prepared w/margarine and 2% milk	1/2 cup	150	520	6.0
(General Mills) w/ham, dry	1/5 pkg	100	550	1.0
(General Mills) w/ham, prepared w/margarine and 2% milk	1/2 cup	170	620	7.0
(Idahoan) prepared	1/2 cup	140	425	5.0
(Idahoan) prepared w/o added salt, w/unsalted butter	1/2 cup	140	55	7.0
(Idahoan) sour cream and chives, dry	1/6 pkg	90	340	2.0
(Idahoan) sour cream and chives, prepared	1/2 cup	130	400	5.0
(Pillsbury) sour cream and chives 'Specialty,' dry	1/6 pkg	100	450	2.0
(Pillsbury) sour cream and chives, 'Specialty,' prepared w/butter and whole milk	1/2 cup	150	500	6.0

Food Name	Serv. Size	Total Cal.	Sod. MGS	Fat GMS
STUFFED				
(Betty Crocker) sour cream and chives 'Twice Baked,' dry	1/6 pkg	90	480	2.0
(Betty Crocker) sour cream and chives 'Twice Baked' prepared	1/2 cup	200	570	11.0
WESTERN				
(Arrowhead Mills) flakes	2 oz	140	24	0.0
(Barbara's Bakery) dry	4 oz	389	63	1.0
(French's) creamy, prepared	1/2 cup	130	520	4.0
(General Mills) cheesy homestyle, dry	1/6 pkg	100	500	2.0
(General Mills) cheesy homestyle, prepared w/margarine and 2% milk	1/2 cup	150	560	6.0
(General Mills) potato buds, dry	1/8 pkg	70	20	0.0
(General Mills) potato buds, prepared	1/2 cup	130	360	6.0
(General Mills) potato buds, prepared w/o salt	1/2 cup	130	90	6.0
(Hungry Jack) flakes	13.3 oz	70	25	0.0
(Hungry Jack) flakes, prepared w/margarine, 2% milk, and water	1/2 cup	130	85	6.0
(Hungry Jack) flakes, prepared w/margarine, 2% milk, salt, and water	1/2 cup	130	260	6.0
(Idaho) granules	13.3 oz	60	30	0.0
(Idaho) granules, prepared	1/2 cup	130	320	6.0
(Idaho) granules, prepared w/margarine, 2% milk, and water	1/2 cup	120	85	5.0
(Idaho) granules, prepared w/margarine, 2% milk, salt, and water	1/2 cup	120	190	5.0
(Idaho Spuds) flakes	13.3 oz	70	40	0.0
(Idaho Spuds) flakes, prepared	1/2 cup	140	380	7.0
(Idaho Spuds) flakes, prepared w/margarine, 2% milk, and water	1/2 cup	130	105	6.0
(Idaho Spuds) flakes, prepared w/margarine, 2% milk, salt, and water	1/2 cup	130	370	6.0
(Idahoan) dry	1/3 cup	80	15	0.0
(Idahoan) 'Complete' dry	1/3 cup	100	310	2.0
(Pillsbury) cheesy 'Specialty' dry	1/6 pkg	100	490	2.0
(Pillsbury) cheesy 'Specialty,' prepared w/butter and whole milk	1/2 cup	150	540	6.0
(Pillsbury) creamy white sauce, 'Specialty,' dry	1/6 pkg	100	410	2.0
POTATO PANCAKE				
(Idaho) 3-inch diam each, prepared	3 cakes	90	420	2.0
(Kosher Empire) frozen, triangle, latkes w/onions	2 oz	77	108	2.4
(Pillsbury) 'Specialty'	1/8 pkg	70	400	0.0

Food Name	Serv. Size	Total Cal.	Sod. MGS	Fat GMS
(Pillsbury) 'Specialty' prepared w/water and egg, 3-inch diam each	3 cakes	90	420	2.0
POTATO SALAD, CANNED				
(Joan of Arc) German	1/2 cup	120	550	3.0
(Joan of Arc) homestyle	1/2 cup	340	1070	22.0
(Read) German	1/2 cup	120	550	3.0
(Read) homestyle	1/2 cup	340	1070	22.0
POTATO SALAD SEASONING *(Tone's)*	1 tsp	5	1498	0.2
POTATO STARCH *(Featherweight)*	1 cup	620	51	1.0
POTATO STICKS. See POTATO CHIPS AND SNACKS.				
POTTED MEAT SPREAD. See also LUNCHEON MEAT, CANNED; SANDWICH SPREAD.				
beef	1 cup	558	2925	43.2
chicken	1 cup	558	2925	43.2
turkey	1 cup	558	2925	43.2
(Hormel)	1 oz	53	280	4.0
(Hormel)	1 tbsp	30	145	2.0
(Libby's)	1.83 oz	110	320	9.0
POULTRY SEASONING				
dry	1 oz	87	8	2.1
dry	1 tbsp	11	1	0.3
dry	1 tsp	5	0	0.1
PRESERVES. See also FRUIT SPREAD; JAM; JELLY; MARMALADE.				
APPLE BUTTER				
(Bama)	2 tsp	25	5	0.0
(Knudsen & Sons) organic	2 tbsp	25	0	0.0
(Lucky Leaf)	4 oz	200	15	1.0
(Musselman's)	4 oz	200	15	1.0
(Smucker's) 'Autumn Harvest'	1 tsp	12	0	0.0
(Smucker's) cider	1 tsp	12	0	0.0
(Smucker's) natural	1 tsp	12	0	0.0
(Smucker's) 'Simply Fruit'	1 tsp	16	0	0.0
(Smucker's) spiced	1 tsp	12	0	0.0
(Tap'n Apple)	1 oz	45	<1	<.1
(White House)	1 oz	50	5	0.0
APRICOT				
(Knott's Berry Farm)	1 tsp	18	0	0.0
(Polaner)	2 tsp	35	5	0.0
APRICOT-PINEAPPLE				
(Knott's Berry Farm)	1 tsp	18	0	0.0
(Knudsen & Sons)	2 tsp	35	na	<1.0
BING CHERRY *(Knott's Berry Farm)*	1 tsp	18	0	0.0

Food Name	Serv. Size	Total Cal.	Sod. MGS	Fat GMS
BLACK CHERRY *(Knudsen & Sons)*	2 tsp	35	na	<1.0
BLACKBERRY				
(Knott's Berry Farm) seedless	1 tsp	18	0	0.0
(Knudsen & Sons)	2 tsp	35	na	<1.0
(Knudsen & Sons) organic	2 tsp	25	na	<1.0
(Polaner) seedless	2 tsp	35	5	0.0
BLUEBERRY				
(Knott's Berry Farm)	1 tsp	18	0	0.0
(Knudsen & Sons)	2 tsp	35	na	<1.0
(Knudsen & Sons) organic	2 tsp	25	na	<1.0
(Polaner)	2 tsp	35	5	0.0
BOYSENBERRY				
(Knott's Berry Farm)	1 tsp	18	0	0.0
(Knudsen & Sons)	2 tsp	35	na	<1.0
CONCORD GRAPE *(Knudsen & Sons)*	2 tsp	35	na	<1.0
KADOTA FIG *(Knott's Berry Farm)*	1 tsp	18	0	0.0
PEACH				
(Bama)	2 tsp	30	5	0.0
(Knudsen & Sons)	2 tsp	35	na	<1.0
(Polaner)	2 tsp	35	5	0.0
PINEAPPLE *(Polaner)*	2 tsp	35	5	0.0
RED CHERRY *(Knott's Berry Farm)*	1 tsp	18	0	0.0
RED RASPBERRY				
(Knott's Berry Farm) seedless	1 tsp	18	0	0.0
(Knudsen & Sons)	2 tsp	35	na	<1.0
(Knudsen & Sons) organic	2 tsp	25	na	<1.0
(Polaner)	2 tsp	35	5	0.0
(Polaner) seedless	2 tsp	35	5	0.0
(Smucker's) natural ingredients	1 tsp	18	0	0.0
STRAWBERRY				
(Bama)	2 tsp	30	5	0.0
(Knott's Berry Farm) pure, seedless	1 tsp	18	0	0.0
(Knudsen & Sons)	2 tsp	35	na	<1.0
(Knudsen & Sons) organic	2 tsp	25	na	<1.0
(Polaner)	2 tsp	35	5	0.0
(Smucker's) natural ingredients	1 tsp	18	0	0.0
PRETZELS				
(A & Eagle)	1 oz	110	570	2.0
(Bachman) 'Nutzels'	1 oz	110	470	2.0
(Bachman) 'Petite'	1 oz	110	410	2.0
(Bachman) 'Petite Sodium Free'	1 oz	110	2	2.0

Food Name	Serv. Size	Total Cal.	Sod. MGS	Fat GMS
(Estee) 'Unsalted'	5 pretzels	25	5	<1.0
(Featherweight) 'Low Salt'	20 pretzels	110	30	1.0
(Mister Salty) 'Juniors'	1 oz	110	500	2.0
(Pepperidge Farm) 'Goldfish'	1 oz	110	160	3.0
(Rokeach) 'Baldies Unsalted'	1 oz	110	30	0.0
(Rold Gold) 'Tiny Tim'	1 oz	110	610	1.0
BAVARIAN				
(Barbara's Bakery) 1 oz	2 pretzels	110	200	<1.0
(Barbara's Bakery) no salt added, 1 oz	2 pretzels	110	10	<1.0
(Rold Gold) 1 oz	3 pretzels	120	430	2.0
BEER (Quinlan)	1 oz	110	446	1.4
BRAIDS (Keebler) 'Butter Pretzels'	1 oz	110	620	1.0
CHEDDAR (Combos)	10 nuggets	143	335	5.8
CHIPS				
'Mr. Phipps' (Nabisco) lightly salted, .5 oz	8 chips	60	200	1.0
'Mr. Phipps' (Nabisco) original, .5 oz	8 chips	60	310	1.0
'Mr. Phipps' (Nabisco) sesame, .5 oz	8 chips	60	250	2.0
DUTCH STYLE				
	7.5-oz pkg	831	3578	9.6
	1 pretzel	62	269	0.7
(Estee) 'Unsalted'	2 pretzels	110	30	<1.0
(Mister Salty) 1 oz	2 pretzels	110	440	1.0
(Rokeach)	1 oz	110	na	0.0
(Rokeach) 'Unsalted'	1 oz	110	30	0.0
HARD				
(Bachman)	1 oz	110	290	<1.0
(Bachman) unsalted	1 oz	110	50	<1.0
plain, made w/unenriched flour, salted	10 twists	322	5	20.8
plain, made w/unenriched flour, unsalted	10 twists	229	1029	2.1
plain, salted	10 twists	229	1029	2.1
plain, unsalted	10 twists	229	173	2.1
whole wheat	2 oz	205	115	1.5
HONEYSWEET (Barbara's Bakery) 1 oz	2 pretzels	110	200	<1.0
KNOTS (Keebler) 'Butter Pretzels'	1 oz	110	530	1.0
LOGS				
(Bachman)	1 oz	110	470	2.0
(Quinlan)	1 oz	103	388	0.8
MINIS				
(Barbara's Bakery) 1 oz	17 pretzels	110	290	<1.0
(Barbara's Bakery) no salt added, 1 oz	17 pretzels	110	10	<1.0
(Mister Salty) 1 oz	22 pretzels	110	450	1.0

Food Name	Serv. Size	Total Cal.	Sod. MGS	Fat GMS
NINE-GRAIN *(Barbara's Bakery)* 1 oz	2 pretzels	110	200	<1.0
OAT BRAN *(Quinlan)*	1 oz	115	156	1.5
PARTY				
(Delicious)	1 oz	110	500	1.0
(Rokeach) 'Party Cannister'	1 oz	110	na	1.0
RICE BRAN, 'No-Salt' *(Quinlan)*	1 oz	101	52	2.3
RINGS				
(Bachman)	1 oz	110	410	2.0
(Mister Salty)	1 oz	110	510	2.0
(Mister Salty) butter flavor	1 oz	110	570	2.0
RODS				
(Bachman)	1 oz	110	240	2.0
(Rold Gold)	1 oz	110	550	2.0
(Seyfert's) butter flavor	1 oz	110	530	1.0
STICKS				
(Delicious)	1 oz	110	500	1.0
(Mister Salty)	1 oz	110	620	1.0
(Mister Salty) butter flavor	1 oz	110	620	1.0
(Mister Salty) fat-free	1 oz	110	380	<1.0
(Mister Salty) very thin, 1 oz	92 sticks	110	600	3.0
(Pepperidge Farm) 'Snack Sticks'	8 sticks	120	430	3.0
(Quinlan)	1 oz	105	538	0.6
(Rold Gold)	1 oz	110	760	1.0
THINS				
(Bachman)	1 oz	110	410	2.0
(Bachman) 'Thin'n Light'	1 oz	110	410	2.0
(Quinlan)	1 oz	104	765	0.6
(Quinlan) tiny	1 oz	109	601	1.5
(Quinlan) tiny 'No-Salt'	1 oz	115	10	1.6
(Quinlan) 'Ultra Thins'	1 oz	106	618	0.6
(Rold Gold) baked, 33% less sodium 'Fat Free'	1 oz	110	340	0.0
TREATS *(Bachman)*	1 oz	110	410	2.0
TWISTS				
(Bachman)	1 oz	110	410	2.0
(Delicious)	1 oz	110	500	1.0
(Mister Salty) .5 oz	5 twists	110	580	2.0
(Mister Salty) fat-free, 1 oz	9 twists	110	380	<1.0
(Rold Gold) thin, 1 oz	10 twists	110	470	1.0
(Rold Gold) tiny, 1 oz	15 twists	110	420	1.0
(Ultra Slim Fast)	1 oz	100	460	1.0

Food Name	Serv. Size	Total Cal.	Sod. MGS	Fat GMS
PRICKLY PEAR				
raw, trimmed	1 oz	12	1	0.1
raw, trimmed, approx 4.8 oz	1 fruit	42	5	0.5
raw, untrimmed	1 lb	140	18	1.7
PROSCIUTTO. See LUNCHEON MEAT, HAM.				
PRUNE				
dehydrated	4 oz	384	6	0.8
dehydrated, cooked	4 oz	128	2	0.3
Canned				
in heavy syrup, w/liquid	1 cup	246	7	0.5
in heavy syrup, w/liquid	1/2 cup	123	3	0.2
in heavy syrup, w/2 tbsp liquid	5 fruits	90	3	0.2
pitted, in heavy syrup, w/liquid	4 oz	119	3	0.2
PRUNE, DRIED				
pitted	1 cup	385	6	0.8
pitted	4 oz	271	5	0.6
pitted, approx 3 oz	10 fruits	201	3	0.4
pitted, cooked, stewed, sweetened	4 oz	141	2	0.2
pitted, cooked, stewed, unsweetened	4 oz	121	2	0.3
(Del Monte)	2 oz	120	10	0.0
(Del Monte) 'Moist Pak'	2 oz	120	10	0.0
(Del Monte) pitted	2 oz	140	10	0.0
(Dole)	2 oz	140	10	1.0
(Mariani) pitted, premium	1/4 cup	140	10	0.0
(SunSweet)	2 oz	120	10	0.0
(SunSweet) pitted	2 oz	140	10	0.0
PRUNE JUICE				
	6 oz	136	8	0.1
(Del Monte) 'Unsweetened'	6 oz	120	10	0.0
(J. Hungerford) 100% juice	9.03 oz	178	10	0.0
(Knudsen & Sons) organic	8 oz	170	na	0.0
(Lucky Leaf)	6 oz	150	0	0.0
(Mott's)	6 oz	130	8	0.0
(Mott's) country style	6 oz	130	7	0.0
(Pathmark) 'All Natural'	6 oz	120	10	0.0
(Pathmark) w/prune pulp 'Homestyle'	6 oz	130	10	0.0
(S&W) 'Unsweetened'	6 oz	120	20	0.0
(SunSweet)	6 oz	130	20	0.0
PRUNE WHIP				
cold	1 cup	203	213	0.3
hot	1 cup	140	148	0.2

ood Name	Serv. Size	Total Cal.	Sod. MGS	Fat GMS
PUDDING, FROZEN				
butterscotch *(Rich's)*	3 oz	130	130	6.0
chocolate *(Rich's)*	3 oz	140	135	7.0
vanilla *(Rich's)*	3 oz	130	160	6.0
PUDDING, READY-TO-SERVE				
ALMOND *(Rice Dream)* 'Dream Pudding,' non-dairy, low fat	4 oz	150	30	2.0
BANANA				
(Del Monte) 'Pudding Cup'	5 oz	180	285	5.0
(Lucky Leaf)	4 oz	150	110	5.0
(Musselman's)	4 oz	150	110	5.0
(Rice Dream) 'Dream Pudding,' non-dairy, fat-free	4 oz	120	5	0.0
(Snack Pack)	4.25 oz	145	180	6.0
(Snack Pack)	4 oz	158	163	5.7
BUTTERSCOTCH				
(Crowley)	4.5 oz	150	210	3.0
(Del Monte) 'Pudding Cup'	5 oz	180	285	5.0
(Featherweight)	1/2 cup	100	160	1.0
(Lucky Leaf)	4 oz	170	135	7.0
(Musselman's)	4 oz	170	135	7.0
(Rice Dream) 'Dream Pudding,' non-dairy, fat-free	4 oz	120	5	0.0
(Snack Pack)	4.25 oz	170	210	6.0
(Snack Pack)	4 oz	153	211	5.7
(Swiss Miss)	4 oz	156	182	5.6
(Ultra Slim Fast) 'Lite 'N Tasty'	4 oz	100	230	<1.0
(White House)	3.5 oz	113	195	3.0
BUTTERSCOTCH-CHOCOLATE-VANILLA SWIRL *(Jell-O)*	4 oz	180	140	5.0
CARAMELLO *(Hershey's)*	4 oz	180	170	6.0
CAROB *(Rice Dream)* 'Dream Pudding' non-dairy, fat-free	4 oz	130	30	0.0
CHOCOLATE				
(Crowley)	4.5 oz	190	100	3.0
(Del Monte) 'Pudding Cup'	5 oz	190	280	6.0
(Del Monte) 'Pudding Snack Light'	4.25 oz	100	85	1.0
(Estee)	1/2 cup	70	85	<1.0
(Featherweight)	1/2 cup	100	110	1.0
(Hershey's)	4 oz	180	260	5.0
(Jell-O) 'Free'	4 oz	100	200	0.0
(Jell-O) 'Light Pudding Snacks'	4 oz	100	125	2.0
(Jell-O) 'Pudding Snacks'	5.5 oz	230	170	8.0
(Jell-O) 'Pudding Snacks'	4 oz	170	130	6.0
(Lucky Leaf)	4 oz	180	100	7.0
(Musselman's)	4 oz	180	100	7.0

Food Name	Serv. Size	Total Cal.	Sod. MGS	Fat GMS
(Pathmark) 'No Frills'	5 oz	200	140	8.0
(Rice Dream) 'Dream Pudding,' non-dairy, fat-free	4 oz	170	30	0.0
(Snack Pack)	4.25 oz	160	125	5.0
(Snack Pack)	4 oz	161	178	5.9
(Snack Pack) fat-free	4 oz	96	212	0.4
(Snack Pack) 'Light'	4 oz	100	120	2.0
(Swiss Miss)	4 oz	166	177	5.7
(Swiss Miss) fat-free	4 oz	99	154	0.4
(Swiss Miss) 'Light'	4 oz	100	120	(mq)
(Swiss Miss) sundae	4 oz	220	140	7.0
(White House)	3.5 oz	120	130	4.0
CHOCOLATE FUDGE				
(Del Monte) 'Pudding Cup'	5 oz	190	260	6.0
(Jell-O) 'Light Pudding Snacks'	4 oz	100	125	1.0
(Jell-O) 'Pudding Snacks'	4 oz	170	130	6.0
(Lucky Leaf)	4 oz	180	105	8.0
(Musselman's)	4 oz	180	105	8.0
(Snack Pack)	4.25 oz	165	125	6.0
(Snack Pack)	4 oz	158	178	5.9
(Swiss Miss)	4 oz	175	207	5.6
(Swiss Miss) fat-free	4 oz	103	151	0.3
(Swiss Miss) 'Light'	4 oz	100	120	1.0
CHOCOLATE FUDGE-MILK CHOCOLATE SWIRL (Jell-O)	4 oz	170	135	6.0
CHOCOLATE-ALMOND (Hershey's)	4 oz	180	210	6.0
CHOCOLATE-CARAMEL SWIRL				
(Jell-O) 'Pudding Snacks'	4 oz	170	130	6.0
(Snack Pack)	4 oz	165	178	5.9
(Snack Pack) 4 pack	4 oz	170	180	6.0
(Swiss Miss)	4 oz	165	178	5.9
CHOCOLATE-MARSHMALLOW				
(Snack Pack)	4.25 oz	165	125	6.0
(Snack Pack)	4 oz	155	124	5.9
CHOCOLATE-MINT SWIRL (Jell-O) 'Free'	4 oz	100	220	0.0
CHOCOLATE-PEANUT BUTTER SWIRL				
(Snack Pack)	4 oz	169	173	6.3
(Snack Pack) 4 pack	4 oz	170	180	7.0
CHOCOLATE-VANILLA SWIRL				
(Hershey's) 'Kisses'	4 oz	180	210	6.0
(Hershey's) 'Kisses Free'	4 oz	100	180	0.0
(Jell-O) combo 'Light Pudding Snacks'	4 oz	100	125	2.0
(Jell-O) 'Free'	4 oz	100	220	0.0

Food Name	Serv. Size	Total Cal.	Sod. MGS	Fat GMS
(Jell-O) 'Pudding Snacks'	5.5 oz	240	180	8.0
(Jell-O) 'Pudding Snacks'	4 oz	170	135	6.0
CHOCOLATE-VANILLA-CHOCOLATE SWIRL *(Swiss Miss)*	4 oz	172	163	6.0
COCONUT				
(Rice Dream) 'Dream Pudding,' non-dairy, low fat	4 oz	150	10	2.0
LEMON				
(Rice Dream) 'Dream Pudding,' non-dairy, fat-free	4 oz	120	5	0.0
(Snack Pack)	4.25 oz	150	75	4.0
(Snack Pack)	4 oz	138	85	2.8
(White House)	3.5 oz	152	65	1.0
MILK CHOCOLATE				
(Jell-O) 'Pudding Snacks'	4 oz	170	135	6.0
(Snack Pack)	4 oz	166	166	5.9
(Snack Pack) 4 pack	4 oz	160	170	6.0
(Swiss Miss)	4 oz	166	166	2.9
MILK CHOCOLATE-CHOCOLATE FUDGE SWIRL *(Jell-O)*	4 oz	170	135	6.0
RICE				
(Crowley)	4.5 oz	125	80	2.0
(Lucky Leaf)	4 oz	120	95	3.0
(Musselman's)	4 oz	120	95	3.0
(White House)	3.5 oz	111	135	3.0
S'MORES SWIRL				
(Snack Pack)	4 oz	154	129	5.6
(Snack Pack) 4 pack	4 oz	150	125	6.0
TAPIOCA				
(Crowley)	4.5 oz	135	70	1.0
(Del Monte) 'Pudding Cup'	5 oz	180	250	4.0
(Jell-O) 'Pudding Snacks'	4 oz	170	140	4.0
(Lucky Leaf)	4 oz	140	95	6.0
(Musselman's)	4 oz	140	95	6.0
(Snack Pack)	4.25 oz	160	200	4.0
(Snack Pack)	4 oz	151	134	5.7
(Snack Pack) fat-free	4 oz	94	185	0.4
(Snack Pack) 'Light'	4 oz	100	105	2.0
(Swiss Miss)	4 oz	138	180	3.9
(Swiss Miss) fat-free	4 oz	99	151	0.3
(Swiss Miss) 'Light'	4 oz	100	105	2.0
(White House)	3.5 oz	131	105	6.0
VANILLA				
(Crowley)	4.5 oz	140	130	3.0
(Del Monte) 'Pudding Cup'	5 oz	180	285	5.0

Food Name	Serv. Size	Total Cal.	Sod. MGS	Fat GMS
(Del Monte) 'Pudding Snack Light'	4.25 oz	100	200	1.0
(Estee)	1/2 cup	70	65	<1.0
(Featherweight)	1/2 cup	100	150	2.0
(Jell-O) 'Free'	4 oz	100	250	0.0
(Jell-O) 'Light Pudding Snacks'	4 oz	100	130	2.0
(Jell-O) 'Pudding Snacks'	5.5 oz	250	190	9.0
(Jell-O) 'Pudding Snacks'	4 oz	180	140	7.0
(Lucky Leaf)	4 oz	170	135	7.0
(Musselman's)	4 oz	170	135	7.0
(Pathmark) 'No Frills'	5 oz	200	150	8.0
(Snack Pack)	4.25 oz	170	180	6.0
(Snack Pack)	4 oz	158	141	5.7
(Snack Pack) fat-free	4 oz	93	167	0.4
(Swiss Miss)	4 oz	156	181	5.6
(Swiss Miss) fat-free	4 oz	98	162	0.4
(Swiss Miss) 'Light'	4 oz	100	110	2.0
(Swiss Miss) sundae	4 oz	175	174	6.8
(Ultra Slim Fast) 'Lite 'N Tasty'	4 oz	100	230	<1.0
(White House)	3.5 oz	111	135	3.0
VANILLA-CHOCOLATE SWIRL (Jell-O) 'Pudding Snacks'	4 oz	180	140	6.0
PUDDING MIX. See also PUDDING/PIE FILLING MIX.				
BANANA				
(Jell-O) 'Instant' prepared	1/2 cup	160	410	4.0
(Jell-O) 'Instant Sugar-free' prepared w/2% milk	1/2 cup	80	390	2.0
BANANA CREAM				
(Jell-O) 'Microwave' prepared	1/2 cup	150	220	4.0
(Royal) 'Instant' prepared	1/2 cup	180	390	5.0
(Royal) prepared	1/2 cup	160	210	4.0
BUTTER ALMOND (Royal) toasted 'Instant' prepared	1/2 cup	170	350	4.0
BUTTER PECAN (Jell-O) 'Instant' prepared	1/2 cup	170	410	5.0
BUTTERSCOTCH				
(D-Zerta) low calorie, prepared w/skim milk	1/2 cup	70	65	0.0
(Featherweight) 'Instant' prepared	1/2 cup	100	190	0.0
(Featherweight) prepared	1/2 cup	12	6	0.0
(Jell-O) 'Instant' prepared	1/2 cup	160	450	4.0
(Jell-O) 'Instant Sugar-free' prepared w/2% milk	1/2 cup	90	390	2.0
(Jell-O) 'Microwave' prepared	1/2 cup	170	180	4.0
(Jell-O) prepared	1/2 cup	170	190	4.0
(Royal) 'Instant' prepared	1/2 cup	180	390	5.0
(Royal) 'Instant Sugar-free' prepared w/2% milk	1/2 cup	100	470	2.0
(Royal) prepared	1/2 cup	160	210	4.0

Food Name	Serv. Size	Total Cal.	Sod. MGS	Fat GMS
CHOCOLATE				
(D-Zerta) low calorie, prepared w/skim milk	1/2 cup	60	70	0.0
(Featherweight) 'Instant' prepared	1/2 cup	110	190	0.0
(Featherweight) prepared	1/2 cup	12	0	0.0
(Jell-O) 'Cook 'n Serve Sugar-free' prepared w/skim milk	1/2 cup	70	160	3.0
(Jell-O) 'Cook 'n Serve Sugar-free' prepared w/2% milk	1/2 cup	90	160	3.0
(Jell-O) 'Instant' prepared	1/2 cup	180	480	4.0
(Jell-O) 'Instant Sugar-free' prepared w/2% milk	1/2 cup	90	380	3.0
(Jell-O) 'Microwave' prepared	1/2 cup	170	190	5.0
(Jell-O) prepared	1/2 cup	160	170	4.0
(Royal) dark and sweet, prepared	1/2 cup	180	150	4.0
(Royal) 'Instant' prepared	1/2 cup	190	390	4.0
(Royal) 'Instant Sugar-free' prepared w/2% milk	1/2 cup	110	480	3.0
(Royal) prepared	1/2 cup	180	150	4.0
(Weight Watchers) 'Instant' prepared w/skim milk	1/2 cup	90	420	1.0
CHOCOLATE FUDGE				
(Jell-O) 'Instant' prepared	1/2 cup	180	440	5.0
(Jell-O) 'Instant Sugar-free' prepared w/2% milk	1/2 cup	100	330	3.0
(Jell-O) prepared	1/2 cup	160	170	4.0
CHOCOLATE-CHOCOLATE CHIP (Royal) prepared	1/2 cup	190	390	4.0
CHOCOLATE-MINT (Royal) 'Instant' prepared	1/2 cup	190	390	4.0
COCONUT, TOASTED (Royal) 'Instant' prepared	1/2 cup	170	350	4.0
COCONUT CREAM (Jell-O) 'Instant' prepared	1/2 cup	180	320	6.0
EGG				
(Jell-O) custard 'Americana' prepared	1/2 cup	160	200	5.0
(Royal) custard, prepared	1/2 cup	150	115	5.0
FLAN				
(Jell-O) prepared	1/2 cup	150	65	4.0
(Royal) w/caramel sauce, prepared	1/2 cup	150	115	5.0
FRENCH VANILLA				
(Jell-O) 'Instant' prepared	1/2 cup	160	400	4.0
(Jell-O) prepared	1/2 cup	170	190	4.0
KEY LIME (Royal) prepared	1/2 cup	160	120	3.0
LEMON				
(Featherweight) custard, prepared	1/2 cup	40	40	0.0
(French's) prepared	1/2 cup	110	110	1.0
(Jell-O) 'Instant' prepared	1/2 cup	170	360	4.0
(Royal) 'Instant' prepared	1/2 cup	180	350	5.0
(Royal) prepared	1/2 cup	160	120	3.0
MILK CHOCOLATE				
(Jell-O) 'Instant' prepared	1/2 cup	180	470	5.0

Food Name	Serv. Size	Total Cal.	Sod. MGS	Fat GMS
(Jell-O) 'Microwave' prepared	1/2 cup	160	190	5.0
(Jell-O) prepared	1/2 cup	160	170	4.0
PISTACHIO				
(Jell-O) 'Instant' prepared	1/2 cup	170	410	5.0
(Jell-O) 'Instant Sugar-free' prepared w/2% milk	1/2 cup	90	390	3.0
(Royal) nut 'Instant' prepared	1/2 cup	170	350	4.0
RASPBERRY *(Salada)* pudding and pie glaze, prepared	1/2 cup	130	5	0.0
RICE *(Jell-O)* 'Americana' prepared	1/2 cup	170	160	4.0
STRAWBERRY *(Salada)* pudding and pie glaze, prepared	1/2 cup	130	5	0.0
VANILLA				
(D-Zerta) low calorie, prepared w/skim milk	1/2 cup	70	65	0.0
(Featherweight) custard, prepared	1/2 cup	40	40	0.0
(Featherweight) 'Instant' prepared	1/2 cup	100	190	0.0
(Featherweight) prepared	1/2 cup	12	6	0.0
(Jell-O) 'Cook 'n Serve Sugar-free' prepared w/skim milk	1/2 cup	60	200	2.0
(Jell-O) 'Cook 'n Serve Sugar-free' prepared w/2% milk	1/2 cup	80	200	2.0
(Jell-O) 'Instant' prepared	1/2 cup	170	410	4.0
(Jell-O) 'Instant Sugar-free' prepared w/2% milk	1/2 cup	90	390	2.0
(Jell-O) 'Microwave' prepared	1/2 cup	160	180	4.0
(Jell-O) prepared	1/2 cup	160	200	4.0
(Jell-O) tapioca 'Americana' prepared	1/2 cup	160	170	4.0
(Royal) 'Instant' prepared	1/2 cup	180	390	5.0
(Royal) 'Instant Sugar-free' prepared w/2% milk	1/2 cup	100	470	2.0
(Royal) prepared	1/2 cup	160	210	4.0
(Royal) tapioca, prepared	1/2 cup	160	150	4.0
PUDDING/PIE FILLING MIX. See also PUDDING MIX.				
BANANA *(Jell-O)* instant, sugar-free, prepared w/2% milk	1/2 cup	80	390	2.0
BANANA CREAM				
(Jell-O) instant, prepared	1/2 cup	160	410	4.0
(Jell-O) microwave, prepared	1/2 cup	150	220	4.0
(Jell-O) prepared, w/o crust	1/6 pie	100	160	3.0
(Royal) dry	1 serving	80	110	0.0
(Royal) instant, dry	1 serving	90	390	0.0
BUTTER PECAN *(Jell-O)* instant, prepared	1/2 cup	170	410	5.0
BUTTERSCOTCH				
(D-Zerta) reduced calorie, prepared	1/2 cup	70	65	0.0
(Jell-O) instant, prepared	1/2 cup	160	450	4.0
(Jell-O) instant, sugar-free, prepared w/2% milk	1/2 cup	90	390	2.0
(Jell-O) microwave, prepared	1/2 cup	170	180	4.0
(Jell-O) prepared	1/2 cup	170	190	4.0
(Nabisco) 'My•T•Fine' prepared	1/2 cup	90	190	0.0

od Name	Serv. Size	Total Cal.	Sod. MGS	Fat GMS
(Royal) instant, dry	1 serving	90	400	0.0
(Royal) prepared	1/2 cup	90	180	0.0
HERRY-VANILLA *(Royal)* instant, dry	1 serving	90	300	0.0
HOCOLATE				
(D-Zerta) reduced calorie, prepared	1/2 cup	60	70	0.0
(Jell-O) instant, prepared	1/2 cup	180	480	4.0
(Jell-O) instant, sugar-free, prepared w/2% milk	1/2 cup	90	380	3.0
(Jell-O) microwave, prepared	1/2 cup	170	190	5.0
(Jell-O) prepared	1/2 cup	160	170	4.0
(Jell-O) sugar-free, prepared w/2% milk	1/2 cup	90	160	3.0
(Nabisco) 'My•T•Fine' prepared	1/2 cup	100	135	0.0
(Royal) dark and sweet, instant, dry	1 serving	110	460	0.0
(Royal) dark and sweet, prepared	1/2 cup	90	95	0.0
(Royal) instant, dry	1 serving	110	450	0.0
(Royal) instant, sugar-free, prepared	1/2 cup	50	420	0.0
(Royal) prepared	1/2 cup	90	90	0.0
HOCOLATE FUDGE				
(Jell-O) instant, prepared	1/2 cup	180	440	5.0
(Jell-O) instant, sugar-free, prepared w/2% milk	1/2 cup	100	330	3.0
(Jell-O) prepared	1/2 cup	160	170	4.0
(Nabisco) 'My•T•Fine' prepared	1/2 cup	100	140	0.0
HOCOLATE-ALMOND				
(Nabisco) 'My•T•Fine' prepared	1/2 cup	100	135	1.0
(Royal) instant, prepared	1/2 cup	120	440	1.0
HOCOLATE-CHOCOLATE CHIP *(Royal)* instant, dry	1 serving	110	390	1.0
HOCOLATE-PEANUT BUTTER CHIP *(Royal)* instant, dry	1 serving	110	480	1.0
OCONUT, TOASTED *(Royal)* instant, prepared	1/2 cup	100	450	2.0
OCONUT CREAM				
(Jell-O) instant, prepared	1/2 cup	180	320	6.0
(Jell-O) prepared, w/o crust	1/6 pie	110	140	4.0
GG *(Royal)* custard, prepared	1/2 cup	60	75	0.0
LAN				
(Jell-O) prepared	1/2 cup	150	65	4.0
(Royal) caramel custard, prepared	1/2 cup	60	55	0.0
RENCH VANILLA				
(Jell-O) instant, prepared	1/2 cup	160	400	4.0
(Jell-O) prepared	1/2 cup	170	190	4.0
EMON				
(Jell-O) instant, prepared	1/2 cup	170	360	4.0
(Nabisco) 'My•T•Fine' dry	1 serving	90	170	0.0
(Royal) instant, dry	1 serving	90	320	0.0

Food Name	Serv. Size	Total Cal.	Sod. MGS	F G
MILK CHOCOLATE				
(Jell-O) instant, prepared	1/2 cup	180	470	5
(Jell-O) microwave, prepared	1/2 cup	160	190	5
(Jell-O) prepared	1/2 cup	160	170	4
PISTACHIO				
(Jell-O) instant, prepared	1/2 cup	170	410	5
(Jell-O) instant, sugar-free, prepared w/2% milk	1/2 cup	90	390	3
(Royal) instant, dry	1 serving	90	360	1
STRAWBERRY (Royal) instant, dry	1 serving	100	330	0
TAPIOCA (Nabisco) 'My•T•Fine' dry	1 serving	80	160	0
VANILLA				
(D-Zerta) reduced calorie, w/aspartame, prepared	1/2 cup	70	65	0
(Jell-O) instant, prepared	1/2 cup	170	410	4
(Jell-O) instant, sugar-free, prepared w/2% milk	1/2 cup	90	390	2
(Jell-O) microwave, prepared	1/2 cup	160	180	4
(Jell-O) prepared	1/2 cup	160	200	4
(Jell-O) sugar-free, w/aspartame, prepared w/2% milk	1/2 cup	80	200	2
(Nabisco) 'My•T•Fine' prepared	1/2 cup	90	120	0
(Royal) instant, dry	1 serving	90	325	0
VANILLA-CHOCOLATE CHIP (Royal) instant, dry	1 serving	90	350	1
PUFF PASTRY, FROZEN				
sheet (Pepperidge Farm)	1/4 sheet	260	290	17
shell, mini (Pepperidge Farm)	1 shell	50	40	4
shell, patty (Pepperidge Farm)	1 shell	210	180	15
shell, ready to bake	1 shell	259	117	17
shell, ready to bake	1 oz	156	71	10
PUMPKIN				
boiled, drained	4 oz	23	1	0
boiled, drained, mashed	1/2 cup	24	1	0
raw, 1-inch cubes	1/2 cup	15	1	0
raw, trimmed	1 oz	7	<1	<
raw, untrimmed	1 lb	83	3	0
PUMPKIN, CANNED				
	1/2 cup	41	6	0
w/winter squash	4 oz	39	6	0
(Del Monte)	1/2 cup	35	10	0
(Libby's)	1/2 cup	42	6	0
(Libby's) solid pack	1/2 cup	42	6	0
(Stokely)	1/2 cup	40	15	0
PUMPKIN FLOWER				
boiled, drained	4 oz	17	7	0

od Name	Serv. Size	Total Cal.	Sod. MGS	Fat GMS
boiled, drained	1/2 cup	10	4	0.1
raw	1 cup	5	2	0.0
raw, trimmed	1 oz	4	1	<.1
raw, trimmed	1/2 cup	3	1	<.1
raw, untrimmed	1 lb	23	7	0.1
JMPKIN LEAF				
boiled, drained	4 oz	24	9	0.2
boiled, drained	1/2 cup	7	3	0.1
raw	1/2 cup	4	2	0.1
raw, trimmed	1 oz	5	3	0.1
raw, untrimmed	1 lb	36	20	0.7
JMPKIN PIE SPICE				
dried	1 tbsp	19	3	0.7
dried	1 tsp	6	1	0.2
JMPKIN SEED				
dried	1 lb	1817	59	153.9
roasted	1 lb	2021	82	88.0
roasted	1 cup	285	12	12.4
roasted, approx 85 seeds	1 oz	127	5	5.5
w/squash seeds, roasted	1 cup	285	12	12.4
w/squash seeds, roasted	1 oz	127	5	5.5
JMPKIN SEED, SHELLED				
dried	1 cup	747	24	63.3
dried, approx 142 kernels	1 oz	154	5	13.0
roasted	1 cup	1184	40	95.6
roasted	1 oz	148	5	12.0
w/squash seed kernels, dried	1 cup	747	25	63.3
w/squash seed kernels, dried, approx 142 kernels	1 oz	154	5	13.0
w/squash seed kernels, roasted	1 cup	1185	41	95.6
w/squash seed kernels, roasted	1 oz	149	6	12.0
JNCH. See also FRUIT PUNCH; and individual listings.				
(J. Hungerford)	9.03 oz	133	2	0.0
(Squeezit) 'Mean Green Puncher'	6.75 oz	100	5	0.0
(Squeezit) 'Rockin Red Puncher'	6.75 oz	110	5	0.0
JRPLESAURUS REX DRINK MIX				
(Kool-Aid) sugar-free, w/NutraSweet, prepared	8 oz	4	5	0.0
(Kool-Aid) sugar-sweetened, prepared	8 oz	80	5	0.0
(Kool-Aid) unsweetened, prepared w/sugar	8 oz	100	5	0.0
(Kool-Aid) unsweetened, prepared w/o sugar	8 oz	2	5	0.0
JRSLANE/pussley				
boiled, drained	4 oz	20	50	0.2

Food Name	Serv. Size	Total Cal.	Sod. MGS
boiled, drained	1/2 cup	10	26
raw	1 cup	7	19
raw, trimmed	1 oz	5	13
raw, trimmed	1/2 cup	4	10
raw, untrimmed	1 lb	56	156

Q

Food Name	Serv. Size	Total Cal.	Sod. MGS
QUAIL / bobwhite			
breast meat only, raw	1 oz	35	16
meat and skin, raw	1 oz	54	15
raw	1 oz	34	29
QUAIL GIBLETS, raw	3.5 oz	176	70
QUICHE			
(Nancy's) Classic French, Monterey jack and swiss, w/bacon	1 quiche	520	670	3?
(Nancy's) French baked, broccoli, cheddar	1 quiche	490	750	3?
QUINCE			
raw, trimmed	1 med	52	4
raw, trimmed	1 oz	16	1
raw, untrimmed	1 lb	158	11
QUINOA, WHOLE GRAIN			
dry	1/2 cup	318	18
dry	1 oz	106	na
dry (Ancient Harvest)	1/4 cup	159	8
dry (Eden Foods)	2 oz	200	30
dry (Quinoa)	1/4 cup	159	8
steam-rolled, flakes (Ancient Harvest)	1/3 cup	105	5
steam-rolled, flakes (Quinoa)	1/3 cup	105	5
QUINOA FLOUR, WHOLE GRAIN			
non-gluten (Ancient Harvest)	1/4 cup	132	10
non-gluten (Quinoa)	1/4 cup	132	10
QUINOA PASTA. See PASTA.			
QUINOA SEED (Arrowhead Mills)	2 oz	200	3

R

Food Name	Serv. Size	Total Cal.	Sod. MGS	Fat GMS
RABBIT				
Domesticated				
raw	1 lb	617	186	25.2
raw	1 oz	38	11	1.5
roasted	3 oz	167	40	6.8
roasted, diced	1 cup	216	52	8.8
stewed	3 oz	175	31	7.2
stewed, diced	1 cup	288	52	11.8
Wild				
raw	1 lb	517	227	10.5
raw	1 oz	32	14	0.7
stewed	3 oz	147	38	3.0
stewed, diced	1 cup	242	63	4.9
RADICCHIO				
raw	1 med	2	2	0.0
raw, shredded	1/2 cup	5	4	0.1
RADISH				
fresh *(Dole)*	7 med	20	35	0.0
raw, sliced	1/2 cup	10	14	0.3
raw, 1 inch long, 3/4 inch diam	10 radishes	8	11	0.2
raw, trimmed	1 oz	5	7	0.2
raw, untrimmed	1 lb	68	98	2.2
RADISH, BLACK/winter radish				
raw, trimmed	1 lb	77	82	0.5
raw, trimmed	1 oz	5	5	<.1
RADISH, ORIENTAL. See DAIKON.				
RADISH, WHITE ICICLE				
raw	1 med	2	3	0.0
raw, sliced	1/2 cup	7	8	0.1
raw, trimmed	1 oz	4	5	<.1
raw, untrimmed	1 lb	41	47	0.3
RAG GOURD. See GOURD, DISHCLOTH.				
RAINBOW PUNCH *(Kool-Aid)* 'Koolers'	8.45 oz	130	10	0.0
RAINBOW PUNCH MIX				
(Kool-Aid) sugar-sweetened	8 oz	80	20	0.0
(Kool-Aid) unsweetened, prepared w/sugar	8 oz	100	0	0.0
(Kool-Aid) unsweetened, prepared w/o sugar	8 oz	2	0	0.0
RAINBOW SMELT. See SMELT, RAINBOW.				

Food Name	Serv. Size	Total Cal.	Sod. MGS	Fat GMS
RAISIN				
Dark				
seedless	1 cup packed	495	20	0.8
seedless	1 cup	435	17	0.7
seedless	1 oz	85	3	0.1
seedless *(Cinderella)* Thompson	1/2 cup	250	15	0.0
seedless *(Dole)*	1/2 cup	260	25	0.0
seedless *(Finast)*	.5 oz	45	5	0.0
seedless *(Sun•Maid)*	1/2 cup	290	15	0.0
seedless *(Sun•Maid)* California sun-dried, 100% natural	1/2 cup	250	10	0.0
w/seeds	1 cup packed	488	46	0.9
w/seeds	1 cup	429	41	0.8
w/seeds	1 oz	84	8	0.2
w/seeds *(Sun•Maid)* Muscat	1/2 cup	270	25	1.0
Golden				
seedless	1 lb	1368	54	2.1
seedless	1 cup packed	498	20	0.8
seedless	1 cup	438	17	0.7
seedless	1 oz	86	3	0.1
seedless *(Del Monte)* natural	3 oz	250	15	0.0
seedless *(Dole)*	1/2 cup	260	25	0.0
w/seed *(Del Monte)*	3 oz	260	10	0.0
w/seed *(Dole)*	1/2 cup	250	25	0.0
w/seed *(Sun•Maid)* California	1/2 cup	250	10	0.0
RASPBERRY /bramble				
trimmed	1 pint	153	0	1.7
trimmed	1 cup	60	0	0.7
trimmed	1 oz	14	tr	0.2
untrimmed	1 lb	215	1	2.4
untrimmed	1 pint	154	tr	1.7
Canned				
red, in heavy syrup	4 oz	103	3	0.1
red, in heavy syrup, solid and liquid	1/2 cup	116	4	0.2
Frozen				
red, in light syrup *(Birds Eye)* 'Quick Thaw Pouch'	5 oz	100	0	1.0
red, sweetened, unthawed	10 oz	293	3	0.5
red, sweetened, unthawed	1 cup	258	3	0.4
sweetened	10 oz	291	1	0.5
sweetened	1/2 cup	128	1	0.2
sweetened	4 oz	117	1	0.2

Food Name	Serv. Size	Total Cal.	Sod. MGS	Fat GMS
RASPBERRY DRINK, W/CRANBERRY				
(A&P)	6 oz	110	0	<1.0
(Finast)	6 oz	110	10	0.0
(Pathmark)	6 oz	110	10	0.0
(Pathmark) 'Sodium Free'	6 oz	110	0	0.0
RASPBERRY JUICE				
(Apple & Eve) w/cranberry	6 oz	90	10	0.0
(Dole) blend 'Pure & Light Country Raspberry'	6 oz	87	15	0.2
(Santa Cruz Natural) red, organic	8 oz	120	na	<1.0
(Smucker's) red 'Naturally 100%'	8 oz	120	10	0.0
RASPBERRY JUICE COCKTAIL (Welch's) 'Orchard,' bottled	10 oz	160	10	0.0
RASPBERRY JUICE FLOAT (Knudsen & Sons)	8 oz	130	na	0.0
RASPBERRY LEMONADE				
(Knudsen & Sons)	8 oz	110	na	0.0
(Santa Cruz Natural) organic	8 oz	60	na	<1.0
(Santa Cruz Natural) 'Sparkling' organic	8 oz	85	na	<1.0
RASPBERRY NECTAR (Knudsen & Sons)	8 oz	120	na	0.0
RASPBERRY PUNCH MIX				
(Kool-Aid) sugar-sweetened, prepared	8 oz	80	25	0.0
(Kool-Aid) unsweetened, prepared w/sugar	8 oz	100	25	0.0
(Kool-Aid) unsweetened, prepared w/o sugar	8 oz	2	25	0.0
RASPBERRY SYRUP (Knudsen & Sons)	1 oz	75	na	<1.0
RASPBERRY TOPPING, fat-free (Smucker's) 'Light'	2 tbsp	55	0	0.0
RASPBERRY-PEACH JUICE (Knudsen & Sons)	8 oz	115	na	0.0
RAVIOLI ENTRÉE				
CANNED				
Beef				
(Chef Boyardee) 'Sir Chomps'	7.5 oz	170	690	3.0
(Chef Boyardee) w/meat sauce 'Smurfs'	7.5 oz	230	1160	5.0
(Estee)	7.5 oz	230	100	11.0
(Finast) w/sauce	7.5 oz	250	1165	10.0
(Franco-American) w/meat sauce 'RavioliO's'	7.5 oz	250	920	8.0
(Nalley's)	7.5 oz	180	1040	3.0
(Pathmark) bite size, w/tomato sauce 'No Frills'	7.5 oz	180	890	4.0
(Pathmark) w/tomato sauce 'No Frills'	7.5 oz	180	890	4.0
Cheese				
(Buitoni) w/sauce	7.5 oz	190	790	6.0
(Chef Boyardee) 'Sir Chomps'	7.5 oz	170	740	1.0
(Pathmark) w/tomato sauce 'No Frills'	7.5 oz	185	790	6.0
Chicken				
(Buitoni) meat, w/sauce	7.5 oz	180	890	4.0

Food Name	Serv. Size	Total Cal.	Sod. MGS	Fa GM
(Chef Boyardee)	7.5 oz	180	1100	4.
(Chef Boyardee) mini	7.5 oz	220	1090	8.
FROZEN				
(Celentano)	6.5 oz	380	510	11.
(Celentano) mini	4 oz	250	210	5.
Cheese				
(Amy's Kitchen) organic	1 cup	215	346	5.
(Buitoni)	4 oz	360	220	8.
(Healthy Choice) baked	9 oz	250	420	2.
(Kid Cuisine) mini	8.75 oz	250	730	2.
(Lean Cuisine) w/tomato sauce	8.5 oz	240	590	8.
(Smart Ones) Florentine	8.5 oz	130	540	1.
(Ultra Slim Fast)	12 oz	330	770	3.
(Weight Watchers) baked	9 oz	240	370	6.
MICROWAVE				
(Kid's Kitchen) mini microwave cup	7.5 oz	230	870	6.
Beef				
(Chef Boyardee)	7.5 oz	190	1160	4.
(Chef Boyardee) 'Main Meals' microwave cup	10.5 oz	290	na	4.
(Hormel) w/tomato sauce micro cup	7.5 oz	247	951	11.
(Libby's) w/sauce 'Diner' microwave cup	7.75 oz	240	890	5.
Cheese, w/meat sauce *(Chef Boyardee)*	7.5 oz	200	1010	3.
REFRIGERATED				
(Contadina) w/beef 'Fresh'	3 oz	270	250	11.
(Contadina) w/cheese 'Fresh'	3 oz	270	360	11.
(DiGiorno) w/Italian herb cheese, cooked	1 cup	280	490	10.
(DiGiorno) w/Italian sausage, cooked	1 cup	270	520	9.
RAZZLEBERRY JUICE *(Knudsen & Sons)*	8 oz	90	na	0.
RED BEAN, CANNED				
(A&P)	1/2 cup	120	400	<1.
(Allens)	1/2 cup	115	350	<1.
(Bush's Best)	1/2 cup	70	350	0.
(Green Giant)	1/2 cup	90	340	1.
(Joan of Arc)	1/2 cup	90	340	1.
(Van Camp's)	1 cup	194	928	0.
Small				
(B&M) baked style	8 oz	223	725	5.
(Hunt's)	4.48 oz	89	713	0.
RED CURRY BASE *(A Taste of Thai)*	1 tbsp	20	430	1.

RED PERCH. See OCEAN PERCH, ATLANTIC.
REDFISH. See OCEAN PERCH, ATLANTIC.

Food Name	Serv. Size	Total Cal.	Sod. MGS	Fat GMS
REFRIED BEANS, CANNED				
....	1/2 cup	135	534	1.4
....	4 oz	121	481	1.2
(Del Monte)	1/2 cup	130	530	2.0
(Gebhardt)	4 oz	130	490	2.0
(Little Pancho)	1/2 cup	80	330	0.0
(Old El Paso)	1/4 cup	55	200	<1.0
(Rosarita)	4.5 oz	109	497	2.8
NO-FAT (Rosarita)	4.5 oz	92	481	0.5
ORGANIC				
(Bearitos)	1 oz	30	61	0.5
(Bearitos) no salt	1 oz	29	2	0.5
(Bearitos) spicy	1 oz	31	56	0.6
SPICY				
(Del Monte)	1/2 cup	130	480	2.0
(Old El Paso)	1/4 cup	35	280	1.0
(Rosarita)	4.5 oz	109	530	2.6
VEGETARIAN				
(Old El Paso) spicy	1/4 cup	70	730	1.0
(Rosarita)	4.5 oz	118	550	2.3
(Rosarita) spicy	4 oz	120	470	2.0
(Rosarita) w/canola oil	4 oz	100	480	2.0
(Rosarita) w/soybean oil	4 oz	100	480	2.0
W/BACON (Rosarita)	4.5 oz	116	489	3.1
W/CHEESE (Old El Paso)	1/4 cup	36	280	1.0
W/GREEN CHILIES				
(Little Pancho)	1/2 cup	80	330	0.0
(Old El Paso)	1/4 cup	49	252	<1.0
(Rosarita)	4.5 oz	110	495	2.9
W/JALAPEÑO (Gebhardt)	4.5 oz	106	380	3.0
W/NACHO CHEESE (Rosarita)	4.5 oz	122	482	3.1
W/ONION (Rosarita)	4.5 oz	114	508	2.8
W/SAUSAGE (Old El Paso)	1/4 cup	180	300	8.0
REFRIED BEANS, DRIED (Rosarita)	1/3 cup	123	469	4.5
REFRIED BEANS ENTRÉE (Chi-Chi's)	7.5 oz	250	930	11.0
REFRIED BEANS MIX				
(Fantastic Foods) instant, prepared w/o added ingredients	1/2 cup	157	400	2.0
(Fantastic Foods) instant, prepared w/2 tbsp salted butter	1/2 cup	207	469	8.0
RELISH. See also specific listings.				
CHOWCHOW				
sour, w/cauliflower, onion, mustard	1 cup	70	3211	3.1

Food Name	Serv. Size	Total Cal.	Sod. MGS	Fat GMS
sweet, w/cauliflower, onion, mustard	1 cup	284	1291	2.2
CRANBERRY-ORANGE				
canned	1/2 cup	246	44	0.1
canned	4 oz	202	36	0.1
DILL *(Vlasic)*	1 oz	2	415	0.0
HAMBURGER				
pickle	1/2 cup	157	1337	0.7
pickle	1 tbsp	19	164	0.1
(Heinz)	1 oz	40	255	0.0
HOT DOG				
pickle	1/2 cup	111	1331	0.6
pickle	1 tbsp	14	164	0.1
(Heinz)	1 oz	35	200	0.0
(Vlasic)	1 oz	40	255	1.0
INDIA				
(Heinz)	1 oz	35	215	0.0
(Vlasic)	1 oz	30	205	0.0
JALAPEÑO *(Old El Paso)*	2 tbsp	16	100	0.0
PICCALILLI				
(Claussen)	1 oz	26	170	0.3
(Heinz)	1 oz	30	145	0.0
(Vlasic) hot	1 oz	35	165	0.0
PICKLE				
sweet	1/2 cup	159	989	0.6
sweet	1 tbsp	20	122	0.1
(Claussen)	1 tbsp	14	90	0.2
SWEET				
	1 tbsp	21	107	0.1
chopped	1 cup	338	1744	1.5
chopped	1 tbsp	21	107	0.1
finely cut	1 cup	338	1744	1.5
finely cut	1 tbsp	21	107	0.1
(Heinz)	1 oz	35	205	0.0
(Vlasic)	1 oz	30	220	0.0
RHUBARB				
frozen	1/2 cup	14	1	0.1
frozen	4 oz	24	2	0.1
frozen, sweetened, cooked	4 oz	132	1	0.1
frozen, sweetened, cooked	1/2 cup	139	1	0.1
raw, diced	1/2 cup	13	2	0.1
raw, trimmed	1 oz	6	1	0.1

Food Name	Serv. Size	Total Cal.	Sod. MGS	Fat GMS
raw, untrimmed	1 lb	71	14	0.7
RICE, ARBORIO, dry *(Colavita)*	1 oz	100	5	0.0
RICE, BASMATI				
BROWN				
(Arrowhead Mills) long grain, dry	2 oz	200	3	1.0
(Fantastic Foods) cooked	1/2 cup	102	3	0.5
(Fantastic Foods) cooked, prepared w/1 tbsp salted butter	1/2 cup	115	20	2.0
WHITE				
(Fantastic Foods) cooked	1/2 cup	103	1	0.0
(Fantastic Foods) cooked, prepared w/1 tbsp salted butter	1/2 cup	116	18	1.0
(Texmati) long grain, cooked	1/2 cup	82	0	0.0
RICE, BROWN				
(Lundberg Family) cooked	1 cup	232	0	1.2
(Minute) instant	1/2 cup	120	5	1.0
(Uncle Ben's) precooked, prepared	1/2 cup	90	11	1.0
LONG GRAIN				
cooked	1/2 cup	109	5	0.9
cooked	4 oz	126	6	1.0
cooked *(Carolina)*	1/2 cup	110	0	0.0
cooked *(Mahatma)*	1/2 cup	110	10	0.0
cooked *(River)*	1/2 cup	110	na	0.0
cooked *(S&W)*	3.5 oz	119	0	0.0
cooked *(Uncle Ben's)*	2/3 cup	130	0	1.0
dry	1 oz	105	2	0.8
dry	1/2 cup	340	6	2.7
dry *(Arrowhead Mills)*	2 oz	200	3	1.0
quick-cooked *(S&W)*	3.5 oz	110	0	0.0
MEDIUM GRAIN				
cooked	4 oz	127	1	0.9
cooked	1/2 cup	110	1	0.8
dry	1/2 cup	344	4	2.5
dry	1 oz	103	1	0.8
dry *(Arrowhead Mills)*	2 oz	200	3	1.0
SHORT GRAIN *(Arrowhead Mills)* dry	2 oz	200	3	1.0
RICE, GLUTINOUS				
cooked	1/2 cup	116	6	0.2
cooked	4 oz	110	6	0.2
dry	1/2 cup	120	0	0.2
dry	1 oz	105	2	0.2

Food Name	Serv. Size	Total Cal.	Sod. MGS	Fa GM
RICE, WHITE				
LONG GRAIN				
cooked	1/2 cup	194	3	5.8
cooked	4 oz	111	3	0.2
cooked *(Carolina)*	1/2 cup	100	10	0.0
cooked *(Finast)*	1/2 cup	115	0	0.0
cooked *(Mahatma)*	1/2 cup	110	na	0.0
cooked *(River)*	1/2 cup	100	10	0.0
cooked *(S&W)*	3.5 oz	106	0	0.0
cooked *(Uncle Ben's)*	2/3 cup	130	0	1.0
cooked *(Water Maid)*	1/2 cup	100	10	0.0
raw, enriched	1/2 cup	336	5	0.6
raw, unenriched	1 oz	103	1	0.2
In cooking bag				
(Minute)	1/2 cup	90	0	0.0
(Success) enriched, cooked	1/2 cup	100	0	0.0
(Uncle Ben's)	1/2 cup	90	10	<1.0
Parboiled				
cooked	1/2 cup	100	3	0.2
cooked	4 oz	129	3	3.1
enriched, cooked	1/2 cup	100	3	0.2
unenriched, dry	1/2 cup	341	5	0.5
(Uncle Ben's) 'Converted'	2/3 cup	120	0	<1.0
Precooked or instant				
cooked *(Carolina)* 'Instant'	1/2 cup	110	na	0.0
cooked *(Minute)* 'Original'	2/3 cup	120	5	0.0
cooked *(Minute)* 'Premium'	2/3 cup	120	0	0.0
cooked *(Uncle Ben's)*	2/3 cup	120	10	<1.0
dry	1/2 cup	182	3	0.1
dry	1 oz	107	2	0.1
enriched, cooked	1/2 cup	80	2	0.1
MEDIUM GRAIN				
cooked	1/2 cup	345	5	0.5
cooked	4 oz	147	tr	0.2
dry	1 oz	102	<1	0.2
enriched, dry	1/2 cup	353	1	0.6
unenriched, cooked	1/2 cup	133	0	0.2
unenriched, dry	1/2 cup	353	1	0.6
SHORT GRAIN				
cooked	1/2 cup	333	1	0.5
cooked	4 oz	147	tr	0.2

Food Name	Serv. Size	Total Cal.	Sod. MGS	Fat GMS
dry	1/2 cup	130	0	0.2
dry	1 oz	101	<1	0.1
unenriched, cooked	1/2 cup	133	0	0.2
unenriched, dry	1/2 cup	358	1	0.5
RICE, WILD				
cooked	4 oz	115	3	0.4
cooked	1/2 cup	83	2	0.3
cooked *(Fantastic Foods)*	1/2 cup	83	0	0.0
dry	1/2 cup	286	6	0.9
dry	1 oz	101	2	0.3
RICE BEVERAGE				
almond 'Amazake' *(Grainaissance)*	8 oz	198	20	4.0
apricot 'Amazake' *(Grainaissance)*	8 oz	158	20	0.0
carob 'Lite' *(Rice Dream)*	8 oz	150	80	3.0
chocolate flavored *(Rice Dream)*	8 oz	190	80	3.0
cocoa-almond 'Amazake' *(Grainaissance)*	8 oz	198	20	4.0
mocha java 'Amazake' *(Grainaissance)*	8 oz	178	20	2.0
original flavor 'Amazake' *(Grainaissance)*	8 oz	148	20	0.0
original flavor 'Horchata' *(Don José)*	8 oz	70	95	4.0
sesame 'Amazake' *(Grainaissance)*	8 oz	198	20	1.0
strawberry 'Horchata' *(Don José)*	8 oz	70	95	3.5
vanilla 'Lite' *(Rice Dream)*	8 oz	120	80	2.0
vanilla pecan 'Amazake' *(Grainaissance)*	8 oz	198	20	4.0
RICE BRAN				
crude	1 oz	90	1	5.9
crude	1/3 cup	88	1	5.8
RICE BRAN OIL				
	1 cup	1927	0	218.0
	1 oz	251	0	28.4
	1 tbsp	120	0	13.6
(Hain)	1 tbsp	120	0	14.0
RICE CAKE				
(Lundberg Family) sodium-free, all flavors	1 cake	60	3	0.5
(Lundberg Family) very low sodium, all flavors	1 cake	60	30	0.5
APPLE CINNAMON				
(Hain) mini	1/2 cup	60	10	<1.0
(Quaker)	1 cake	40	0	0.0
(Quaker) mini	5 cakes	50	0	0.0
BARBEQUE *(Hain)* mini	.5 oz	70	50	3.0
BROWN RICE				
buckwheat	1 cake	34	10	0.3

Food Name	Serv. Size	Total Cal.	Sod. MGS	Fat GMS
buckwheat, unsalted	1 cake	35	2	0.3
corn	1 cake	35	26	0.3
multi-grain	1 cake	35	23	0.3
multi-grain, unsalted	1 cake	34	0	0.3
plain	1 cake	35	29	0.3
rye	1 cake	35	10	0.3
sesame seed	1 cake	35	20	0.3
sesame seed, unsalted	1 cake	35	0	0.3
unsalted	1 cake	34	26	0.3
CARAMEL CORN *(Quaker)* mini	5 cakes	50	35	0.0
CAROB COATED				
(Carafection) 'Mint Rice Crisps'	1 oz	139	26	7.0
(Carafection) 'Rice Crisps'	1 oz	139	26	7.0
CHEESE *(Hain)* mini	5 cakes	60	80	2.0
CINNAMON				
(Chico-San) sugar, mini	5 cakes	50	0	0.0
(Quaker) crunch, fat-free	1 cake	50	25	0.0
CORN *(Quaker)*	1 cake	35	53	0.2
DILL *(Lundberg Family)* creamy, mini	5 cakes	60	57	<1.0
FIVE-GRAIN *(Hain)*	1 cake	40	10	<1.0
HONEY NUT				
(Chico-San) unglazed, mini	4 cakes	60	35	1.0
(Hain) mini	.5 oz	60	30	<1.0
MUGWORT *(Grainaissance)* bake & serve 'Mochi'	2 oz	140	2	1.3
MULTI-GRAIN				
(Chico-San) very low sodium	1 cake	35	30	0.0
(Pritikin) sodium-free	1 cake	35	0	0.0
(Pritikin) very low sodium	1 cake	35	30	0.0
(Quaker)	.32 oz	34	29	0.4
NACHO CHEESE				
(Hain) mini	.5 oz	70	90	2.0
(Lundberg Family) mini	5 cakes	57	116	<1.0
PLAIN				
(Chico-San) original	1 cake	35	30	0.0
(Grainaissance) organic bake & serve 'Mochi'	2 oz	140	2	1.3
(Hain)	1 cake	40	10	<1.0
(Hain) mini	.5 oz	60	20	<1.0
(Hain) mini, unsalted	.5 oz	60	5	<1.0
(Hain) unsalted	1 cake	40	5	<1.0
(Konriko) 'Original Unsalted'	1 cake	30	<1	0.0
(Pritikin) sodium-free	1 cake	35	0	0.0

Food Name	Serv. Size	Total Cal.	Sod. MGS	Fat GMS
(Pritikin) very low sodium	1 cake	35	35	0.0
(Quaker)	.32 oz	35	36	0.3
(Quaker) lightly salted	1 cake	35	35	0.0
(Quaker) unsalted	.32 oz	35	0	0.3
RAISIN-CINNAMON *(Grainaissance)* bake & serve 'Mochi'	2 oz	143	77	1.2
RANCH				
(Hain) mini	.5 oz	70	90	3.0
(Quaker)	1 cake	35	52	0.3
SESAME				
(Chico-San) original	1 cake	35	0	0.0
(Hain)	1 cake	40	10	<1.0
(Hain) unsalted	1 cake	40	5	<1.0
(Pritikin) sodium-free	1 cake	35	0	0.0
(Pritikin) very low sodium	1 cake	35	35	0.0
(Quaker)	.32 oz	35	36	0.3
(Westbrae) 'Double Sesame'	.28 oz	30	65	<1.0
SESAME-GARLIC				
(Grainaissance) bake & serve 'Mochi'	2 oz	143	25	1.9
(Westbrae)	.28 oz	30	55	<1.0
TERIYAKI				
(Hain) mini	.5 oz	50	75	<1.0
(Westbrae)	.28 oz	30	45	<1.0
WHEAT *(Quaker)*	1 cake	34	52	0.3
RICE DISH				
CANNED				
Fried *(LaChoy)*	4.903 oz	236	1024	1.1
Spanish				
(Featherweight)	7.5 oz	140	32	0.0
(Heinz)	7.25 oz	150	1045	5.0
(Old El Paso)	1/2 cup	70	400	1.0
(Van Camp's)	1 cup	160	1270	4.0
FREEZE-DRIED, w/chicken *(Mountain House)*	1 cup	400	241	13.0
FROZEN				
Country style *(Birds Eye)* 'International Rice Recipes'	3.3 oz	90	380	0.0
Florentine *(Green Giant)* 'Rice Originals'	1/2 cup	140	400	4.0
French style *(Birds Eye)* 'International Rice Recipes'	3.3 oz	110	610	0.0
Fried				
w/chicken *(Chun King)*	8 oz	260	1460	4.0
w/pork *(Chun King)*	8 oz	270	1210	6.0
Medley *(Green Giant)* 'Rice Originals'	1/2 cup	100	310	1.0
Mexican style, w/chicken *(Lean Cuisine)* 'Lunch Express'	9 1/8 oz	270	580	5.0

Food Name	Serv. Size	Total Cal.	Sod. MGS	Fat GMS
Oriental, w/vegetables *(Budget Gourmet)* 'Side Dish'	5.75 oz	210	310	10.0
Pilaf				
'Rice Originals' *(Green Giant)*	1/2 cup	110	530	1.0
w/green beans *(Budget Gourmet)* 'Side Dish'	5.5 oz	240	350	9.0
Spanish style *(Birds Eye)* 'International Rice Recipes'	3.3 oz	110	540	0.0
White and wild *(Green Giant)* 'Rice Originals'	1/2 cup	130	540	2.0
Wild, w/sherry *(Green Giant)* 'Microwave Garden Gourmet'	1 pkg	210	580	4.0
W/broccoli				
au gratin *(Birds Eye)* 'For One'	5.75 oz	180	430	6.0
in cheese flavored sauce *(Green Giant)*	1/2 cup	120	510	4.0
in cheese sauce *(Green Giant)* 'One Serving'	5.5 oz	180	550	6.0
'Rice Originals' *(Green Giant)*	1/2 cup	120	510	4.0
W/peas and mushrooms in sauce *(Green Giant)* 'One				
Serving'	5.5 oz	130	410	2.0
W/spinach in cheese sauce *(Green Giant)* 'Italian Blend'	1/2 cup	140	400	4.0
RICE DISH MIX				
(Arrowhead Mills)	2 oz	200	0	1.0
ALFREDO *(Country Inn)* prepared	1/2 cup	140	570	4.0
AMANDINE *(Hain)* '3-Grain Goodness' prepared	1/2 cup	130	260	5.0
BEEF BROCCOLI				
(Rice-A-Roni) 'Rice & Sauce'	1/4 pkg	120	530	0.0
(Rice-A-Roni) 'Rice & Sauce' prepared	1/2 cup	140	550	3.0
BEEF FLAVOR				
(Finast) dry mix	1.3 oz	130	780	1.0
(Lipton) 'Rice and Sauce' dry mix	1/2 cup	120	570	<1.0
(Lipton) 'Rice and Sauce' prepared w/1 tbsp butter	1/2 cup	150	600	3.0
(Mahatma) prepared	1/2 cup	100	340	1.0
(Minute) microwave, family size, dry mix	1 pkg	140	530	0.0
(Minute) microwave, family size, prepared w/salted butter	1/2 cup	160	560	3.0
(Minute) microwave, single size, dry mix	1 pkg	140	530	0.0
(Minute) microwave, single size, prepared w/salted butter	1/2 cup	150	550	2.0
(Rice-A-Roni) dry mix	1.13 oz	110	560	1.0
(Rice-A-Roni) prepared	1/2 cup	140	610	4.0
(Success) prepared	1/2 cup	100	370	0.0
W/mushrooms				
(Rice-A-Roni) dry mix	1.27 oz	120	710	<1.0
(Rice-A-Roni) prepared	1/2 cup	150	740	3.0
W/vermicelli *(Make-It-Easy)* dry mix	1.3 oz	130	(mq)	1.0
BROWN AND WILD				
(Success) prepared	1/2 cup	120	500	0.0
(Uncle Ben's) prepared	1/2 cup	130	500	1.0

Food Name	Serv. Size	Total Cal.	Sod. MGS	Fat GMS
Herb *(Arrowhead Mills)* 'Quick'	2 oz	140	128	1.0
Spanish style *(Arrowhead Mills)* 'Quick'	2 oz	150	145	1.0
Vegetable herb *(Arrowhead Mills)* 'Quick'	2 oz	150	85	1.0
W/mushrooms *(Uncle Ben's)* prepared	1/2 cup	130	500	1.0
CAJUN				
(Lipton) 'Rice and Sauce' dry mix	1/4 pkg	120	600	<1.0
(Lipton) 'Rice and Sauce' prepared w/1 tbsp butter	1/2 cup	150	630	3.0
CHICKEN FLAVOR				
(Finast) dry mix	1.6 oz	160	950	2.0
(Lipton) 'Rice and Sauce' dry mix	1/4 pkg	130	440	1.0
(Lipton) 'Rice and Sauce' prepared w/1 tbsp butter	1/2 cup	150	470	4.0
(Mahatma) prepared	1/2 cup	100	620	0.0
(Minute) microwave, family size, dry mix	1 pkg	130	640	1.0
(Minute) microwave, family size prepared w/salted butter	1/2 cup	160	670	4.0
(Minute) microwave, single size, dry mix	1 pkg	130	640	1.0
(Minute) microwave, single size, prepared w/salted butter	1/2 cup	150	660	3.0
(Rice-A-Roni) dry mix	1.13 oz	110	520	1.0
(Rice-A-Roni) prepared	1/2 cup	150	560	4.0
(Success) prepared	1/2 cup	110	420	2.0
Florentine				
(Rice-A-Roni) 'Savory Classics' dry mix	1.12 oz	108	874	0.8
(Rice-A-Roni) 'Savory Classics' prepared	1/2 cup	130	910	4.0
Honey-lemon, w/broccoli *(Suzi Wan)* prepared	7.5 oz	370	640	11.0
W/broccoli				
(Rice-A-Roni) dry mix	1.23 oz	120	670	1.0
(Rice-A-Roni) prepared	1/2 cup	150	710	3.0
(Suzi Wan) prepared	1/2 cup	120	500	1.0
W/creamy mushroom *(Country Inn)* prepared	1/2 cup	140	510	3.0
W/homestyle vegetables *(Country Inn)* prepared	1/2 cup	140	490	3.0
W/mushroom				
(Country Inn) 'Mushroom Royale' prepared	1/2 cup	120	560	1.0
(Rice-A-Roni) dry mix	1.17 oz	130	790	1.0
(Rice-A-Roni) prepared	1/2 cup	180	840	7.0
W/mushroom stock *(Country Inn)* prepared	1/2 cup	130	560	1.0
W/vegetables				
(Rice-A-Roni) dry mix	1.2 oz	120	760	<1.0
(Rice-A-Roni) prepared	1/2 cup	140	790	3.0
(Suzi Wan) prepared	1/2 cup	120	550	1.0
W/vegetables and vermicelli *(Make-It-Easy)* dry mix	1.3 oz	130	(mq)	1.0
DRUMSTICK				
(Minute) dry mix	1 pkg	120	650	0.0

Food Name	Serv. Size	Total Cal.	Sod. MGS	Fat GMS
(Minute) prepared w/salted butter	1/2 cup	150	690	4.0
FLORENTINE *(Country Inn)* prepared	1/2 cup	140	380	3.0
FRIED				
(Minute) dry mix	1 pkg	120	550	0.0
(Minute) prepared w/oil, w/o salt or butter	1/2 cup	160	550	5.0
(Rice-A-Roni) dry mix	1 oz	110	670	1.0
(Rice-A-Roni) prepared	1/2 cup	110	700	5.0
W/almonds				
(Rice-A-Roni) '1/2 less salt' dry mix	1/5 pkg	120	460	1.0
(Rice-A-Roni) '1/2 less salt' prepared	1/2 cup	130	470	2.0
JASMINE, soft *(A Taste of Thai)*	1/4 cup	160	0	0.0
HERB				
And butter				
(Lipton) 'Rice and Sauce' prepared w/1 tbsp butter	1/2 cup	150	470	5.0
(Rice-A-Roni) dry mix	1 oz	110	760	1.0
(Rice-A-Roni) prepared	1/2 cup	130	790	4.0
Au gratin				
(Country Inn) prepared	1/2 cup	140	450	3.0
(Success) prepared	1/2 cup	100	260	0.0
Wild rice and herbs *(Arrowhead Mills)*	1/4 pkg	140	220	1.0
LONG GRAIN AND WILD				
(Lipton) 'Rice and Sauce Original' dry mix	1/4 pkg	120	530	<1.0
(Lipton) 'Rice and Sauce Original' prepared w/1 tbsp butter	1/2 cup	150	560	3.0
(Mahatma) prepared	1/2 cup	100	480	0.0
(Minute) dry mix	1 pkg	120	530	0.0
(Minute) prepared w/salted butter	1/2 cup	150	570	4.0
(Minute) prepared w/o salt or butter	2/3 cup	120	0	0.0
(Near East) prepared	1/2 cup	130	430	4.0
(Rice-A-Roni) 'Original' dry mix	1.1 oz	110	620	0.0
(Rice-A-Roni) 'Original' prepared	1/2 cup	130	660	3.0
(Uncle Ben's) 'Fast Cooking' prepared	1/2 cup	100	410	<1.0
(Uncle Ben's) 'Fast Cooking' prepared w/salt and butter	1/2 cup	130	450	4.0
(Uncle Ben's) 'Original' prepared w/salt and butter	1/2 cup	120	520	2.0
(Uncle Ben's) 'Original' prepared w/o salt or butter	1/2 cup	100	500	<1.0
Mexican *(Old El Paso)* prepared	1/2 cup	140	370	2.0
Pilaf				
(Rice-A-Roni) dry mix	1 oz	100	510	0.0
(Rice-A-Roni) prepared	1/2 cup	130	550	3.0
W/chicken and almonds				
(Rice-A-Roni) dry mix	1.2 oz	120	660	1.0

Food Name	Serv. Size	Total Cal.	Sod. MGS	Fat GMS
(Rice-A-Roni) prepared	1/2 cup	140	690	4.0
W/chicken sauce				
(Uncle Ben's) prepared w/salt and butter	1/2 cup	160	680	5.0
(Uncle Ben's) prepared w/o salt or butter	1/2 cup	140	650	2.0
ORIENTAL				
(Hain) '3-Grain Goodness' prepared	1/2 cup	120	300	5.0
(Lipton) dry mix	1/4 pkg	120	330	<1.0
(Lipton) prepared w/1 tbsp butter	1/2 cup	150	360	3.0
PILAF				
(Casbah) dry mix	1 oz	90	(mq)	0.0
(Casbah) prepared	1/2 cup	90	(mq)	0.0
(Lipton) 'Rice and Sauce'	1/4 pkg	120	400	<1.0
(Lipton) 'Rice and Sauce' prepared w/1 tbsp margarine	1/2 cup	140	440	3.0
(Lipton) 'Rice and Sauce' prepared w/2 tbsp butter	1/2 cup	170	470	6.0
(Near East) prepared	1/2 cup	140	450	5.0
(Rice-A-Roni) dry mix	1.2 oz	120	570	0.0
(Rice-A-Roni) prepared	1/2 cup	150	550	4.0
(Success) prepared	1/2 cup	120	410	0.0
Beef flavored *(Near East)* prepared	1/2 cup	140	470	5.0
Brown rice				
(Quick Pilaf) Spanish, prepared w/o salt or butter	1/2 cup	98	314	0.7
(Quick Pilaf) Spanish, prepared w/2 tbsp salted butter	1/2 cup	136	369	5.0
(Quick Pilaf) w/miso, prepared w/o salt or butter	1/2 cup	105	240	1.0
(Quick Pilaf) w/miso, prepared w/2 tbsp salted butter	1/2 cup	145	295	5.5
Chicken flavored *(Near East)* prepared	1/2 cup	140	420	5.0
French				
(Minute) microwave, family size, dry mix	1 pkg	110	390	0.0
(Minute) microwave, family size, prepared w/salted butter	1/2 cup	130	420	3.0
(Minute) microwave, single size, dry mix	1 pkg	110	390	0.0
(Minute) microwave, single size, prepared w/salted butter	1/2 cup	120	410	2.0
Garden				
(Rice-A-Roni) 'Savory Classics' dry mix	1.12 oz	113	964	0.8
(Rice-A-Roni) 'Savory Classics' prepared	1/2 cup	140	1000	4.0
Lentil *(Near East)* prepared	1/2 cup	170	430	7.0
Nutted				
(Casbah) dry mix	1 oz	160	(mq)	2.0
(Casbah) prepared	1/2 cup	160	(mq)	2.0
Spanish				
(Casbah) dry mix	1 oz	90	(mq)	0.0
(Casbah) prepared	1/2 cup	90	(mq)	0.0
(Country Inn) w/vegetables, prepared	1/2 cup	120	280	1.0

Food Name	Serv. Size	Total Cal.	Sod. MGS	Fat GMS
Wheat *(Near East)* Spanish, prepared	1/2 cup	150	380	6.0
RIB ROAST				
(Minute) dry mix	1 pkg	120	680	0.0
(Minute) prepared w/salted butter	1/2 cup	150	720	4.0
RISOTTO				
(Rice-A-Roni) dry mix	1.5 oz	160	1070	1.0
(Rice-A-Roni) prepared	1/2 cup	200	1130	6.0
Chicken and cheese *(Country Inn)* prepared	1/2 cup	120	410	2.0
SPANISH STYLE				
(Arrowhead Mills) quick, dry mix	1/4 pkg	150	255	1.0
(Lipton) 'Rice and Sauce' dry mix	1/4 pkg	120	540	<1.0
(Lipton) 'Rice and Sauce' prepared w/1 tbsp butter	1/2 cup	140	570	3.0
(Mahatma) prepared	1/2 cup	100	190	0.0
(Near East) prepared	1/2 cup	170	540	7.0
(Rice-A-Roni) dry mix	.97 oz	110	950	1.0
(Rice-A-Roni) prepared	1/2 cup	150	1090	4.0
STROGANOFF				
(Rice-A-Roni) dry mix	1.35 oz	150	770	3.0
(Rice-A-Roni) prepared	1/2 cup	200	810	8.0
SWEET AND SOUR				
(Suzi Wan) 'Dinner Recipe' prepared	7.5 oz	220	240	1.0
(Suzi Wan) 'Dinner Recipe' prepared w/o butter	1/2 cup	130	460	1.0
(Suzi Wan) 'Dinner Recipe' prepared w/o butter or salt	7.5 oz	340	290	5.0
TERIYAKI				
(Suzi Wan) 'Dinner Recipe' prepared	7.5 oz	180	910	1.0
(Suzi Wan) 'Dinner Recipe' prepared w/o butter	1/2 cup	120	690	1.0
(Suzi Wan) 'Dinner Recipe' prepared w/o butter or salt	7.5 oz	360	970	12.0
THREE-FLAVOR *(Suzi Wan)* prepared	1/2 cup	120	570	1.0
W/ASPARAGUS				
Au gratin *(Country Inn)* prepared	1/2 cup	130	310	3.0
W/hollandaise sauce				
(Lipton) 'Rice & Sauce' dry mix	1/4 pkg	120	460	1.0
(Lipton) 'Rice and Sauce' prepared w/butter	1/2 cup	170	530	7.0
(Lipton) 'Rice and Sauce' prepared w/margarine	1/2 cup	150	500	4.0
W/BROCCOLI				
Amandine *(Country Inn)* prepared	1/2 cup	130	600	2.0
Au gratin				
(Country Inn) prepared	1/2 cup	130	300	3.0
(Rice-A-Roni) 'Savory Classics' dry mix	1.12 oz	129	372	3.4

Food Name	Serv. Size	Total Cal.	Sod. MGS	Fat GMS
(Rice-A-Roni) 'Savory Classics' prepared	1/2 cup	180	440	9.0
Stir-fry				
(Suzi Wan) prepared w/salt and butter	7.5 oz	370	800	15.0
(Suzi Wan) prepared w/o salt or butter	7.5 oz	200	750	3.0
W/cheddar cheese				
(Minute) microwave, dry mix	1 pkg	140	500	2.0
(Minute) microwave, prepared w/salted butter	1/2 cup	160	530	5.0
W/CAULIFLOWER, AU GRATIN				
(Country Inn) prepared	1/2 cup	130	570	3.0
(Rice-A-Roni) 'Savory Classics' dry mix	.5 oz	141	372	3.6
(Rice-A-Roni) 'Savory Classics' prepared	1/2 cup	170	410	7.0
W/CHEESE				
Cheddar				
(Rice-A-Roni) white, w/herbs, prepared	1 cup	130	940	5.0
(Rice-A-Roni) zesty 'Savory Classics' dry mix	1.3 oz	151	541	3.8
(Rice-A-Roni) zesty 'Savory Classics' prepared	1/2 cup	180	580	7.0
Parmesan				
(Rice-A-Roni) creamy, w/herbs 'Savory Classics' dry mix	1.22 oz	145	432	4.2
(Rice-A-Roni) creamy, w/herbs 'Savory Classics' prepared	1/2 cup	170	470	7.0
(Ultra Slim Fast) w/chicken flavored sauce, prepared	8 oz	240	1080	1.0
W/GREEN BEANS, AMANDINE				
(Country Inn) casserole, prepared	1/2 cup	120	370	2.0
(Rice-A-Roni) 'Savory Classics' dry mix	1.25 oz	152	416	4.8
(Rice-A-Roni) 'Savory Classics' prepared	1/2 cup	210	490	11.0
W/MUSHROOMS				
(Country Inn) creamy, w/wild rice, prepared	1/2 cup	140	310	3.0
(Lipton) 'Rice and Sauce' dry mix	1/4 pkg	120	550	<1.0
(Lipton) 'Rice and Sauce' prepared w/1 tbsp butter	1/2 cup	150	580	3.0
W/ORIENTAL STYLE SAUCE *(Ultra Slim Fast)* prepared	8 oz	240	900	1.0
W/VEGETABLES				
And cheddar				
(Lipton) dry mix	1/4 pkg	130	420	2.0
(Lipton) prepared w/1 tbsp margarine	1/2 cup	160	450	5.0
(Lipton) prepared w/2 tbsp butter	1/2 cup	180	490	7.0
Medley *(Country Inn)* prepared	1/2 cup	140	390	1.0
Spring vegetable and cheese				
(Arrowhead Mills) vegetable herb, dry mix	1/4 pkg	150	150	1.0
(Rice-A-Roni) 'Savory Classics' dry mix	1.22 oz	141	388	3.5
(Rice-A-Roni) 'Savory Classics' prepared	1/2 cup	170	420	7.0
YELLOW				
(Mahatma) prepared	1/2 cup	100	480	0.0

Food Name	Serv. Size	Total Cal.	Sod. MGS	Fat GMS
(Rice-A-Roni) dry mix	1.16 oz	110	730	0.0
(Rice-A-Roni) prepared	1/2 cup	140	780	4.0
(Success) prepared	1/2 cup	100	480	0.0
RICE FLOUR				
brown	1/2 cup	287	6	2.2
brown	1 oz	103	2	0.8
brown *(Arrowhead Mills)*	2 oz	200	3	1.0
brown *(Featherweight)*	1 cup	500	7	1.0
white	1/2 cup	289	0	1.1
white	1 oz	104	tr	0.4
RICE SEASONING *(Lawry's)* Mexican 'Seasoning Blends'	1 pkg	94	3246	2.0
RICE SYRUP *(Lundberg Family)* organic 'Sweet Dreams'	1 tbsp	42	2	<1.0
RIGATONI. See PASTA.				
RIGATONI ENTRÉE				
(Budget Gourmet) w/broccoli and chicken, in cream sauce, frozen	10.8 oz	290	710	7.0
(Chef Boyardee) microwave	7.5 oz	210	1080	6.0
(Chef Boyardee) 'Special Recipe' canned	7.5 oz	210	1040	6.0
(Healthy Choice) w/chicken 'Classics' frozen	12.5 oz	360	430	4.0
(Healthy Choice) w/meat sauce, frozen	9.5 oz	260	540	6.0
(Lean Cuisine) baked w/meat sauce and cheese, frozen	9.75 oz	250	430	8.0
(Stouffer's) w/meat sauce, homestyle, frozen	12 oz	400	860	13.0
ROAST BEEF ENTRÉE				
(Libby's) canned, w/gravy	6 oz	210	1030	8.0
(Top Shelf) frozen, tender	10 oz	240	880	6.0
ROAST BEEF HASH				
(Armour) canned	7.5 oz	350	1310	21.0
(Mary Kitchen) canned	7.5 oz	350	1142	22.0
(Stouffer's) frozen	10 oz	380	1340	22.0
ROAST BEEF LUNCHEON MEAT. See LUNCHEON MEAT.				
ROAST BEEF SPREAD, CANNED				
(Hormel)	.5 oz	31	(mq)	2.0
(Underwood)	2 1/8 oz	140	360	11.0
(Underwood) 'Light'	2 1/8 oz	90	210	6.0
(Underwood) mesquite-smoked	2 1/8 oz	126	300	11.0
ROCK-A-DILE RED DRINK				
(Kool-Aid) 'Kool Bursts'	6.75 oz	110	10	0.0
(Kool-Aid) 'Koolers'	8.45 oz	130	10	0.0
ROCK-A-DILE RED DRINK MIX				
(Kool-Aid) sugar-free w/NutraSweet, prepared	8 oz	4	0	0.0
(Kool-Aid) sugar-sweetened, prepared	8 oz	70	0	0.0

Food Name	Serv. Size	Total Cal.	Sod. MGS	Fat GMS
(Kool-Aid) unsweetened, prepared w/sugar	8 oz	100	0	0.0
(Kool-Aid) unsweetened, prepared w/o sugar	8 oz	2	0	0.0
ROCKFISH, PACIFIC, MIXED SPECIES				
baked, broiled, or microwaved	4 oz	137	87	2.3
baked, broiled, or microwaved	3 oz	103	65	1.7
raw	1 lb	427	272	7.1
raw	3 oz	80	51	1.3
raw	1 oz	27	17	0.4
ROE, MIXED SPECIES				
dry-heat cooked	3 oz	173	99	7.0
dry-heat cooked	1 oz	58	33	2.3
raw	1 lb	635	(mq)	29.1
raw	3 oz	119	77	5.5
raw	1 oz	39	25	1.8
raw	1 tbsp	22	(mq)	1.0
ROLL. See also BREAD; BUN; CROISSANT; ENGLISH MUFFIN.				
BUTTER *(Pillsbury)* 'Butterflake' refrigerated	1 roll	140	530	5.0
BUTTERMILK *(Wonder)* brown and serve	1 roll	80	140	2.0
CRESCENT				
(Pepperidge Farm) 'Deli Classic'	1 roll	110	150	6.0
(Pillsbury) refrigerated	1 roll	100	230	6.0
CLUB *(Pepperidge Farm)* 'Deli Classic' brown and serve	1 roll	100	190	1.0
DINNER				
egg	1-oz roll	87	155	1.8
oat bran	1-oz roll	67	117	1.3
rye	1-oz roll	81	253	1.0
wheat	1-oz roll	77	96	1.8
whole wheat	1-oz roll	75	136	1.3
(Arnold) 'Dinner Party' 24 per pkg	1 roll	51	81	1.2
(Awrey's)	1 roll	60	115	1.0
(Awrey's) 'Black Forest'	1 roll	50	110	1.0
(Awrey's) cracked wheat	1 roll	50	120	1.0
(Awrey's) crusty	1 roll	70	150	1.0
(Awrey's) poppy seed	1 roll	59	115	1.0
(Awrey's) sesame seed	1 roll	60	115	1.0
(Home Pride) wheat	1 roll	70	140	1.0
(Home Pride) white	1 roll	80	170	2.0
(Pepperidge Farm) country style 'Classic'	1 roll	50	90	1.0
(Pepperidge Farm) 'Old Fashioned'	1 roll	50	85	2.0
(Pepperidge Farm) 'Party'	1 roll	30	50	1.0
(Roman Meal)	1 roll	69	140	1.2

Food Name	Serv. Size	Total Cal.	Sod. MGS	Fat GMS
(Wonder)	1 roll	80	140	1.0
EGG *(Levy's)* 'Old Country Deli'	1-oz roll	146	431	2.8
FINGER *(Pepperidge Farm)* w/poppy seeds	1 roll	50	80	2.0
49ER				
(Colombo Brand) sour	1.2-oz roll	90	189	0.6
(Colombo Brand) sweet	1.2-oz roll	96	196	1.8
FRENCH STYLE				
	1 oz	79	173	1.2
(Du Jour) petite, brown and serve	1 roll	230	490	2.0
(Francisco) 'International'	1 roll	108	285	1.5
(Pepperidge Farm) 'Deli Classic' brown and serve, 3 per pkg	1/2 roll	120	250	1.0
(Pepperidge Farm) 'Deli Classic' 9 per pkg	1 roll	100	230	1.0
GEM STYLE *(Wonder)* brown and serve	1 roll	80	140	2.0
HARD	1 oz	83	154	1.2
HEARTH				
(Brownberry) 'Hearth' assorted	1 roll	124	247	2.3
(Pepperidge Farm) 'Hearth' brown and serve	1 roll	50	100	1.0
HOAGIE				
(Pepperidge Farm) soft 'Deli Classic'	1 roll	210	320	5.0
(Wonder)	1 roll	400	800	7.0
ITALIAN *(Du Jour)* crusty, brown and serve	1 roll	80	200	1.0
KAISER				
	1 oz	83	154	1.2
(Arnold) 'Francisco'	1 roll	184	338	2.9
(Brownberry) 'Hearth'	1 roll	152	318	2.8
LUIGI *(Colombo Brand)* 'Twin Pack'	2-oz roll	146	334	1.6
ONION *(Levy's)* 'Old Country Deli'	1-oz roll	153	380	1.9
PAN *(Wonder)*	1 roll	80	140	1.0
PARKER HOUSE				
(Bridgford)	1-oz roll	85	172	1.3
(Pepperidge Farm)	1 roll	60	80	1.0
POTATO *(Pepperidge Farm)* 'Hearty Classic'	1 roll	90	125	3.0
SANDWICH				
(Arnold) egg 'Dutch'	1 roll	123	203	3.3
(Awrey's) oat bran	1 roll	120	250	2.0
(Pepperidge Farm) onion, w/poppy seeds	1 roll	150	260	3.0
(Pepperidge Farm) potato	1 roll	160	260	4.0
(Pepperidge Farm) salad 'Deli Classic'	1 roll	110	150	4.0
(Pepperidge Farm) soft 'Family'	1 roll	100	190	2.0
(Pepperidge Farm) w/sesame seeds	1 roll	140	230	3.0

Food Name	Serv. Size	Total Cal.	Sod. MGS	Fat GMS
SOURDOUGH *(Pepperidge Farm)* French style	1 roll	100	240	1.0
STEAK				
(Colombo Brand) sour	2.6-oz roll	200	413	2.2
(Colombo Brand) sweet	2.6-oz roll	206	439	3.3
TWIST *(Pepperidge Farm)* golden 'Heat 'n Serve'	1 roll	110	150	5.0
ROLL, MIX				
(Dromedary) dry mix	1/8 pkg	209	363	2.0
(Dromedary) prepared	2 rolls	239	410	5.0
(Krusteaz) prepared	1 roll	150	190	3.0
(Pillsbury) prepared	2 rolls	270	420	17.0
(Pillsbury) 'Hot Roll Mix' dry mix	1/16 pkg	100	200	0.0
(Pillsbury) 'Hot Roll Mix' prepared	1 roll	120	210	2.0
ROLL, SWEET. See also BUN, SWEET; DANISH PASTRY.				
APPLE				
(Break Cake) 4.5 oz	2 rolls	380	460	5.0
(Break Cake) multi-pak, 1.4 oz	1 roll	120	150	2.0
APPLE CINNAMON, old fashioned *(Aunt Fanny's)* individual	2 oz	180	125	1.0
CARAMEL NUT *(Aunt Fanny's)* individual	2 oz	190	125	6.0
CHEESE	1 oz	102	101	5.2
CHERRY				
(Break Cake) 4.5 oz	2 rolls	400	390	3.0
(Break Cake) multi-pak, 1.4 oz	1 roll	130	125	2.0
CINNAMON				
(Aunt Fanny's) duos, individual	1.9 oz	180	150	5.0
(Aunt Fanny's) individual	2 oz	190	160	5.0
(Aunt Fanny's) rectangular 11-oz size	2 oz	181	64	4.0
(Awrey's) homestyle	1 roll	240	200	7.0
(Awrey's) swirl 'Grande'	1 roll	340	370	16.0
(Break Cake) 4.5 oz	2 rolls	420	430	10.0
(Break Cake) multi-pak, 1.3 oz	1 roll	120	125	3.0
(Hungry Jack) refrigerated dough w/icing, prepared	2 rolls	290	570	14.0
(Pillsbury) refrigerated dough w/icing, prepared	1 roll	110	260	5.0
CINNAMON NUT *(Break Cake)* 3 oz	2 rolls	330	220	11.0
CINNAMON RAISIN *(Aunt Fanny's)* rectangular 11-oz size	2 oz	181	83	3.0
DIXIE FRUIT ROLL *(Aunt Fanny's)* individual	2 oz	180	120	4.0
PECAN				
(Aunt Fanny's) rectangular 11-oz size	2 oz	184	79	4.0
(Break Cake) multi-pak, 1.3 oz	1 roll	120	120	3.0
RAISIN CINNAMON *(Break Cake)* multi-pak, 1.25 oz	1 roll	120	110	3.0
STRAWBERRY *(Aunt Fanny's)* rectangular 11-oz size	2 oz	190	140	4.0

Food Name	Serv. Size	Total Cal.	Sod. MGS	Fat GMS
ROLL, SWEET, FROZEN				
APPLE *(Weight Watchers)* sweet 'Microwave'	1/2 pkg	160	100	4.0
CHEESE *(Weight Watchers)* 'Microwave'	1/2 pkg	180	210	4.0
CINNAMON				
(Pepperidge Farm) 2 per pkg	1 roll	280	190	14.0
(Sara Lee) all butter	2-oz roll	230	220	11.0
(Sara Lee) all butter, w/icing packet	.5-oz pkt	50	0	0.0
(Weight Watchers) glazed	2.1 oz	180	170	5.0
STRAWBERRY *(Weight Watchers)* 'Microwave'	1/2 pkg	170	90	5.0
ROLL DOUGH, FROZEN				
unraised, enriched, 2 x 2 3/8 inches	1 roll	75	135	1.4
unraised, unenriched, 2 x 2 3/8 inches	1 roll	75	135	1.4
ROMAN BEAN. See CRANBERRY BEAN.				
ROOT BEER. See SOFT DRINKS AND MIXERS.				
ROOT BEER FLOAT *(Skipper's)*	1 serving	302	66	10.0
ROSEFISH. See OCEAN PERCH, ATLANTIC.				
ROSEMARY				
dried	1 oz	94	14	4.3
dried	1 tbsp	11	2	0.5
dried	1 tsp	4	1	0.2
dried *(Durkee)*	1 tsp	5	0	tr
dried *(Laurel Leaf)*	1 tsp	5	0	tr
dried *(Spice Islands)*	1 tsp	5	1	0.2
ROTINI. See PASTA.				
ROTINI ENTRÉE, FROZEN				
(Green Giant) cheddar 'Microwave Garden Gourmet'	1 pkg	230	570	10.0
(Mrs. Paul's) seafood 'Light'	9 oz	240	570	6.0
(Weight Watchers) three cheese, w/vegetables	9 oz	270	500	8.0
ROTINI ENTRÉE MIX				
(Velveeta) w/cheese and broccoli, dry mix	1/4 box	210	730	8.0
(Velveeta) w/cheese and broccoli, prepared	1/2 cup	210	730	8.0
RUCULO. See ARUGULA.				
RUGULA. See ARUGULA.				
RUM. See ALCOHOLIC BEVERAGES.				
RUTABAGA				
boiled, drained	4 oz	39	20	0.2
boiled, drained, cubed	1/2 cup	33	17	0.2
boiled, drained, mashed	1/2 cup	47	24	0.3
raw, cubed	1/2 cup	25	14	0.1
raw, trimmed	1 oz	10	6	0.1
raw, untrimmed	1 lb	140	77	0.8

Food Name	Serv. Size	Total Cal.	Sod. MGS	Fat GMS
RUTABAGA, CANNED (Allens) diced	1/2 cup	20	260	<1.0
RYE				
flakes	1/2 cup	281	5	2.1
flakes (Arrowhead Mills)	2 oz	190	1	1.0
whole grain	1 cup	567	10	4.2
whole grain	1 oz	95	2	0.7
whole grain (Arrowhead Mills)	2 oz	190	1	1.0
RYE CAKE (Quaker) 'Grain Cakes'	.32-oz piece	35	52	0.3
RYE FLOUR				
dark	1/2 cup	207	1	-1.7
dark	1 oz	92	<1	0.8
light	1/2 cup	187	1	0.7
light	1 oz	104	<1	0.4
medium	1/2 cup	181	2	0.9
medium	1 oz	100	1	0.5
(Arrowhead Mills) whole grain	2 oz	190	1	1.0
(Krusteaz)	1 cup	351	1	2.0
(Pillsbury) 'Bohemian Style' w/wheat flour	1 cup	400	0	1.0
(Pillsbury's Best)	1 cup	400	0	2.0
(Robin Hood) stone ground	1 cup	360	10	2.0
RYE WHISKEY. See ALCOHOLIC BEVERAGES.				

S

Food Name	Serv. Size	Total Cal.	Sod. MGS	Fat GMS
SABLEFISH / skil				
cooked	3 oz	213	61	16.7
raw	1 lb	886	254	69.4
raw	3 oz	166	48	13.0
raw	1 oz	55	16	4.3
raw, approx 6.8 oz	1/2 fillet	376	108	29.5
smoked	4 oz	291	836	22.8
smoked	3 oz	218	626	17.1
SACCHARIN. See SUGAR, ALTERNATIVE.				
SAFFLOWER OIL				
'Hi-Oleic' (Hain)	1 tbsp	120	0	14.0
high oleic (Spectrum Naturals)	1 tbsp	120	0	14.0
high oleic, unrefined (Spectrum Naturals)	1 tbsp	120	0	14.0
linoleic	1/2 cup	964	0	109.0
linoleic	1 tbsp	120	0	13.6

Food Name	Serv. Size	Total Cal.	Sod. MGS	Fat GMS
oleic	1/2 cup	964	0	109.0
oleic	1 tbsp	120	0	13.6
organic, unrefined *(Spectrum Naturals)*	1 tbsp	120	0	14.0
over 70% oleic	1 cup	1927	0	218.0
over 70% oleic	1 tbsp	124	0	14.0
SAFFLOWER SEED, dried, kernels	1 oz	147	1	10.9
SAFFLOWER SEED MEAL, partially defatted	1 oz	97	1	0.7
SAFFRON				
dried	1 oz	88	42	1.7
dried	1 tbsp	7	3	0.1
dried	1 tsp	2	1	0.0
SAGE				
ground	1 oz	89	3	3.6
ground	1 tbsp	6	0	0.3
ground	1 tsp	2	0	0.1
ground *(Durkee)*	1 tsp	3	0	tr
ground *(Laurel Leaf)*	1 tsp	3	0	tr
ground *(Spice Islands)*	1 tsp	4	<1	0.1
SALAD DRESSING				
BACON *(Kraft)* creamy 'Reduced Calorie'	1 tbsp	30	150	2.0
BACON AND TOMATO				
(Estee)	1 tbsp	8	35	<1.0
(Kraft)	1 tbsp	70	130	7.0
(Kraft) 'Reduced Calorie'	1 tbsp	30	150	2.0
BLUE CHEESE				
	1 cup	1235	2680	128.1
	1 tbsp	77	167	8.0
(Ayla's Organics) fat-free	2 tbsp	30	140	0.0
(Estee)	1 tbsp	8	50	<1.0
(Featherweight) 'Neu Bleu'	1 tbsp	4	110	0.0
(Hidden Valley Ranch) 'Lowfat'	1 tbsp	10	140	0.0
(Kraft) chunky	1 tbsp	60	230	6.0
(Kraft) chunky 'Reduced Calorie'	1 tbsp	30	240	2.0
(Kraft) 'Free'	1 tbsp	16	120	0.0
(Lawry's) 'Classic'	1 tbsp	186	385	2.0
(Litehouse) country, dressing and dip, refrigerated	1 tbsp	76	84	8.0
(Litehouse) 'Lite' dressing and dip, refrigerated	1 tbsp	33	86	3.0
(Litehouse) 'Original' dressing and dip, refrigerated	1 tbsp	77	82	8.0
(Roka)	1 tbsp	60	170	6.0
(Roka) 'Reduced Calorie'	1 tbsp	16	280	1.0
(S&W Nutradiet)	1 tbsp	25	200	2.0

Food Name	Serv. Size	Total Cal.	Sod. MGS	Fat GMS
(Skipper's) premium	1 pouch	222	240	23.0
(T. Marzetti)	1 tbsp	90	180	9.0
(T. Marzetti) chunky, refrigerated	1 tbsp	78	159	8.0
(T. Marzetti) 'Lite' refrigerated	1 tbsp	45	150	5.0
(Wish-Bone) chunky	1 tbsp	75	149	7.9
(Wish-Bone) chunky 'Lite'	1 tbsp	40	197	3.7
(Wish-Bone) chunky, lite 'Food Service'	.5 oz	40	200	4.0
(Wish-Bone) 'Healthy Sensation!'	.5 oz	20	140	na
BUTTERMILK				
(Hain) 'Old Fashioned'	1 tbsp	70	100	7.0
(Hollywood) 'Old Fashion'	1 tbsp	75	40	8.0
(Kraft) creamy	1 tbsp	80	120	8.0
(Kraft) creamy 'Reduced Calorie'	1 tbsp	30	125	3.0
(Seven Seas) 'Buttermilk Recipe'	1 tbsp	80	130	8.0
(T. Marzetti) and herbs	1 tbsp	95	150	10.0
(T. Marzetti) bacon, refrigerated	1 tbsp	93	127	10.0
(T. Marzetti) blue cheese, refrigerated	1 tbsp	90	161	10.0
CAESAR				
(Estee)	2 tbsp	8	130	<1.0
(Hain) creamy	1 tbsp	60	220	6.0
(Hain) creamy 'Low Salt'	1 tbsp	60	15	6.0
(Hollywood)	1 tbsp	70	65	7.0
(Kraft) golden	1 tbsp	70	180	7.0
(Lawry's) 'Classic'	1 tbsp	130	337	13.5
(Litehouse) dressing and dip, refrigerated	1 tbsp	57	84	6.0
(T. Marzetti)	1 tbsp	80	170	8.0
(T. Marzetti) house	1 tbsp	75	180	8.0
(T. Marzetti) refrigerated	1 tbsp	75	178	8.0
(Weight Watchers)	1 tbsp	4	200	0.0
(Wish-Bone)	1 tbsp	77	248	8.0
(Wish-Bone) w/olive oil 'Lite'	.5 oz	30	170	3.0
CALIFORNIA FRENCH				
(Catalina) nonfat 'Free'	1 tbsp	16	120	0.0
(T. Marzetti)	1 tbsp	90	100	6.0
(T. Marzetti) 'Fat-Free'	1 tbsp	16	140	0.0
(T. Marzetti) 'Light'	1 tbsp	40	180	3.0
CELERY SEED				
(T. Marzetti) and onion	1 tbsp	75	90	6.0
(T. Marzetti) refrigerated	1 tbsp	72	101	5.0
CHEESE				
(Featherweight)	1 tbsp	20	70	2.0

Food Name	Serv. Size	Total Cal.	Sod. MGS	Fat GMS
(Hain) vinaigrette	1 tbsp	55	130	6.0
(Hollywood)	1 tbsp	80	60	8.0
CHINESE VINEGAR *(Lawry's)* w/sesame and ginger 'Classic'	1 tbsp	145	325	15.0
CITRUS *(Hain)* tangy 'Canola'	1 tbsp	50	75	5.0
CREAMY				
(Estee)	1 tbsp	4	13	0.0
(Hain)	1 tbsp	80	100	8.0
(Hain) 'No Salt Added'	1 tbsp	80	25	8.0
(Hollywood)	1 tbsp	90	140	9.0
(Kraft) no oil 'Reduced Calorie'	1 tbsp	4	220	0.0
(Kraft) 'Reduced Calorie'	1 tbsp	25	120	2.0
(Kraft) w/real sour cream	1 tbsp	50	120	5.0
(Kraft) zesty	1 tbsp	50	260	5.0
(Kraft) zesty 'Reduced Calorie'	1 tbsp	20	230	2.0
(Lawry's) w/Parmesan cheese 'Classic'	1 oz	156	178	15.1
(Life) egg-free 'All Natural'	1 tbsp	39	4	4.0
(Pathmark)	1 tbsp	70	260	7.0
(Pathmark) zesty	1 tbsp	70	370	8.0
(Pathmark) zesty 'Reduced Calorie'	1 tbsp	6	190	0.0
(Rancher's Choice)	1 tbsp	90	140	10.0
(Rancher's Choice) 'Reduced Calorie'	1 tbsp	30	150	3.0
(S&W Nutradiet)	1 tbsp	10	180	1.0
(S&W Nutradiet) no oil	1 tbsp	2	290	0.0
(Seven Seas)	1 tbsp	70	240	7.0
(Wish-Bone)	1 tbsp	56	149	5.5
(Wish-Bone) 'Lite'	1 tbsp	26	148	2.0
(Weight Watchers) 'Single Serve' 1 packet	1 tbsp	9	430	0.0
CUCUMBER				
(Featherweight) creamy	1 tbsp	4	80	0.0
(Hain) dill, creamy	1 tbsp	80	210	8.0
(Kraft) creamy	1 tbsp	70	190	8.0
(Kraft) creamy 'Reduced Calorie'	1 tbsp	25	220	2.0
(Weight Watchers) creamy	1 tbsp	18	85	0.0
DIJON				
(Estee) creamy	1 tbsp	8	100	<1.0
(Featherweight) creamy	1 tbsp	20	80	2.0
(Great Impressions) mustard	1 tbsp	57	103	6.1
(Hain) vinaigrette	1 tbsp	50	180	5.0
(Hollywood) vinaigrette	1 tbsp	60	40	6.0
(Wish-Bone) vinaigrette 'Classic'	1 tbsp	60	171	6.1
(Wish-Bone) vinaigrette 'Lite Classic'	1 tbsp	30	176	2.8

Food Name	Serv. Size	Total Cal.	Sod. MGS	Fat GMS
DILL				
(Ayla's Organics) creamy, fat-free	2 tbsp	15	140	0.0
(Nasoya) creamy 'Vegi-Dressing'	1 tbsp	40	50	3.0
FRENCH				
(Ayla's Organics) fat-free	2 tbsp	10	150	0.0
(Catalina)	1 tbsp	60	180	5.0
(Catalina) 'Reduced Calorie'	1 tbsp	18	120	1.0
(Estee)	1 tbsp	4	10	0.0
(Estee) creamy	2 tbsp	10	130	0.0
(Featherweight)	1 tbsp	14	15	0.0
(Great Impressions) w/green pepper, low calorie	1 tbsp	64	188	5.2
(Hain) creamy	1 tbsp	60	80	6.0
(Hain) spicy mustard 'Canola'	1 tbsp	50	190	5.0
(Hollywood) creamy	1 tbsp	70	45	7.0
(Kraft)	1 tbsp	60	125	6.0
(Kraft) 'Miracle'	1 tbsp	70	240	6.0
(Kraft) nonfat 'Free'	1 tbsp	20	120	0.0
(Kraft) 'Reduced Calorie'	1 tbsp	20	120	1.0
(Litehouse) country herb, dressing and marinade, refrigerated	1 tbsp	54	196	5.0
(Pathmark) creamy	1 tbsp	60	90	5.0
(Pathmark) 'Reduced Calorie'	1 tbsp	20	160	1.0
(Pritikin) style, fat-free, sodium-free	1 tbsp	10	0	0.0
(S&W Nutradiet)	1 tbsp	18	120	0.0
(Seven Seas) creamy	1 tbsp	60	240	6.0
(Seven Seas) 'French! Light'	1 tbsp	35	210	3.0
(T. Marzetti) country	1 tbsp	72	110	6.0
(T. Marzetti) 'Frenchette'	1 tbsp	10	140	0.0
(T. Marzetti) honey, refrigerated	1 tbsp	74	115	6.0
(T. Marzetti) honey blue, refrigerated	1 tbsp	70	122	6.0
(T. Marzetti) honey 'Lite' refrigerated	1 tbsp	48	118	3.0
(T. Marzetti) 'Light'	1 tbsp	16	160	1.0
(Ultra Slim Fast) 'Cholesterol Free'	1 tbsp	20	105	<1.0
(Weight Watchers) low-calorie	1 tbsp	10	170	0.0
(Wish-Bone) creamy, garlic	1 tbsp	55	158	5.3
(Wish-Bone) 'Deluxe'	1 tbsp	60	83	5.4
(Wish-Bone) 'Deluxe Food Service'	1 tbsp	61	86	5.6
(Wish-Bone) garlic	1 tbsp	55	158	5.3
(Wish-Bone) 'Healthy Sensation!'	.5 oz	20	120	na
(Wish-Bone) 'Lite'	1 tbsp	31	70	2.5
(Wish-Bone) 'Lite Sweet 'n Spicy'	1 tbsp	18	110	0.5

Food Name	Serv. Size	Total Cal.	Sod. MGS	Fat GMS
(Wish-Bone) low-calorie 'Lite'	1 tbsp	30	67	2.5
(Wish-Bone) red, low-calorie 'Lite'	1 tbsp	17	155	0.4
(Wish-Bone) style 'Lite'	.5 oz	18	140	na
(Wish-Bone) style, lite 'Food Service'	.5 oz	30	75	3.0
(Wish-Bone) sweet 'n spicy	.5 oz	70	160	6.0
(Wish-Bone) sweet 'n spicy 'Lite'	.5 oz	18	130	na
FRUIT SALAD				
(Great Impressions) orange marmalade	1 tbsp	87	48	7.1
(Knott's Berry Farm)	1 tbsp	50	75	5.0
GARLIC				
(Ayla's Organics) and onion, fat-free	2 tbsp	10	140	0.0
(Ayla's Organics) creamy, fat-free	2 tbsp	30	140	0.0
(Estee) creamy	1 tbsp	2	10	0.0
(Hain) and sour cream	1 tbsp	70	100	7.0
(Kraft) creamy	1 tbsp	50	170	5.0
(Life) w/tofu 'All Natural' dressing and dip	1 tbsp	70	0	7.1
(Nasoya) herb 'Vegi-Dressing'	1 tbsp	40	50	3.0
(Pritikin) and herb, fat-free, sodium-free	1 tbsp	6	0	0.0
(T. Marzetti) Italian, refrigerated	1 tbsp	81	73	9.0
(Wish-Bone) creamy	1 tbsp	74	158	8.0
(Wish-Bone) Sierra	.5 oz	80	125	8.0
GINGER PLUM VINAIGRETTE *(Simply Delicious)*				
'Un-Dressing'	1 tbsp	36	199	4.0
HERB				
(Featherweight)	1 tbsp	6	5	0.0
(Featherweight) garden	1 tbsp	25	65	2.0
(Hain) savory 'No Salt Added'	1 tbsp	90	25	10.0
(Marie's) vinaigrette, fat-free 'Lite & Zesty'	1 tbsp	16	130	0.0
(Pritikin) vinaigrette, fat-free, sodium-free	1 tbsp	8	0	0.0
(Seven Seas) and spice 'Viva'	1 tbsp	60	170	6.0
(Seven Seas) and spice 'Viva Herbs & Spices! Light'	1 tbsp	30	200	3.0
(Simply Delicious) garlic vinaigrette 'Un-Dressing'	1 tbsp	43	132	4.0
(Wish-Bone) creamy 'Classics'	1 tbsp	70	228	7.3
HOMESTYLE				
(Dorothy Lynch)	1 tbsp	55	85	3.8
(Dorothy Lynch) 'Reduced Calorie'	1 tbsp	30	80	<1.0
HONEY AND SESAME *(Hain)*	1 tbsp	60	210	5.0
HONEY MUSTARD				
(Knott's Berry Farm) 'Peggy Jane's'	1 tbsp	60	40	6.0
(Litehouse) dressing and dip, refrigerated	1 tbsp	67	55	7.0
(Simply Delicious) vinaigrette 'Un-Dressing'	1 tbsp	41	122	4.0

Food Name	Serv. Size	Total Cal.	Sod. MGS	Fat GMS
(T. Marzetti) Dijon	1 tbsp	67	51	6.0
(T. Marzetti) Dijon, refrigerated	1 tbsp	68	103	6.0
(Wish-Bone) Dijon 'Healthy Sensation!'	1 tbsp	25	140	0.0
ITALIAN				
(Ayla's Organics) fat-free	2 tbsp	10	140	0.0
(Estee)	2 tbsp	4	130	0.0
(Featherweight)	1 tbsp	4	120	0.0
(Hain) 'Canola'	1 tbsp	50	150	5.0
(Hain) 'Traditional'	1 tbsp	80	330	8.0
(Hain) 'Traditional No Salt Added'	1 tbsp	60	20	6.0
(Hollywood)	1 tbsp	90	300	9.0
(Kraft) 'Deliciously Light'	1 tbsp	35	115	3.0
(Kraft) house	1 tbsp	60	115	6.0
(Kraft) house 'Reduced Calorie'	1 tbsp	30	115	2.0
(Kraft) nonfat 'Free'	1 tbsp	6	210	0.0
(Kraft) oil-free 'Reduced Calorie'	1 tbsp	4	220	0.0
(Kraft) 'Presto'	1 tbsp	70	150	7.0
(Kraft) zesty	1 tbsp	50	260	5.0
(Kraft) zesty 'Reduced Calorie'	1 tbsp	20	230	2.0
(Marie's) vinaigrette, fat-free 'Lite & Zesty'	1 tbsp	16	135	0.0
(Nasoya) 'Vegi-Dressing'	1 tbsp	40	50	3.0
(Ott's)	1 tbsp	80	87	9.1
(Pritikin) fat-free, sodium-free	1 tbsp	8	0	0.0
(Seven Seas) 'Free Viva'	1 tbsp	4	220	0.0
(Seven Seas) 'Viva'	1 tbsp	50	240	5.0
(Seven Seas) 'Viva Italian! Light'	1 tbsp	30	230	3.0
(Skipper's) gourmet	1 pouch	140	200	15.0
(Skipper's) lo-cal	1 pouch	17	680	1.0
(T. Marzetti) 'Fat-Free'	1 tbsp	5	270	0.0
(T. Marzetti) 'Frenchette'	1 tbsp	6	280	0.0
(T. Marzetti) gusto	1 tbsp	58	204	8.0
(T. Marzetti) 'Light'	1 tbsp	35	300	3.0
(T. Marzetti) w/olive oil	1 tbsp	60	220	7.0
(Ultra Slim Fast) 'Cholesterol Free'	1 tbsp	6	105	<1.0
(Wish-Bone)	1 tbsp	46	280	4.5
(Wish-Bone) blended	.5 oz	35	210	4.0
(Wish-Bone) 'Food Service'	.5 oz	45	290	5.0
(Wish-Bone) 'Healthy Sensation!'	1 tbsp	6	140	0.0
(Wish-Bone) 'Lite'	1 tbsp	7	212	0.3
(Wish-Bone) lite 'Food Service'	.5 oz	6	250	na
(Wish-Bone) 'Robusto'	1 tbsp	47	288	4.5

Food Name	Serv. Size	Total Cal.	Sod. MGS	Fa GM
(Weight Watchers) style	1 tbsp	6	200	0.
(Weight Watchers) style 'Single Serve' 1 packet	.75 oz	8	270	0.
ITALIAN, CREAMY				
(Estee)	2 tbsp	14	130	<1.0
(Kraft)	1 tbsp	60	115	6.
(Kraft) 'Deliciously Light'	1 tbsp	25	120	2.
(Kraft) 'Reduced Calorie'	1 tbsp	25	120	2.
(Kraft) w/real sour cream	1 tbsp	50	120	5.
(Litehouse) dressing and dip, refrigerated	1 tbsp	60	76	6.
(Seven Seas) 'Viva Creamy Italian! Light'	1 tbsp	45	230	4.
(T. Marzetti)	1 tbsp	80	100	8.
(Weight Watchers)	1 tbsp	12	85	0.
(Weight Watchers) whipped	1 tbsp	50	80	5.
(Wish-Bone)	.5 oz	60	150	6.
(Wish-Bone) 'Food Service'	.5 oz	25	140	na
(Wish-Bone) 'Lite'	.5 oz	25	140	na
LEMON TAHINI VINAIGRETTE *(Simply Delicious)*				
'Un-Dressing'	1 tbsp	43	170	4.
LIME CILANTRO VINAIGRETTE *(Simply Delicious)*				
'Un-Dressing'	1 tbsp	41	116	4.
MAYONNAISE TYPE. See also MAYONNAISE.				
(A&P)	1 tbsp	70	100	7.
(Bama)	1 tbsp	50	105	4.
(Finast)	1 tbsp	70	90	7.
(Kraft) 'Miracle Whip'	1 tbsp	70	85	7.
(Kraft) 'Miracle Whip Light'	1 tbsp	40	120	3.
(Kraft) nonfat 'Miracle Whip Free'	1 tbsp	15	105	0.
(P&Q)	1 tbsp	50	110	5.
(Pathmark) 'No Frills'	1 tbsp	50	120	5.
(Spin Blend)	1 tbsp	60	110	5.
(Spin Blend) cholesterol free	1 tbsp	40	110	4.
(Weight Watchers) whipped	1 tbsp	45	100	4.
(Weight Watchers) whipped, fat-free	1 tbsp	12	125	0.
(Weight Watchers) whipped, light	1 tbsp	50	100	5.
(Weight Watchers) whipped, low-sodium	1 tbsp	50	45	5.
OIL AND VINEGAR				
W/balsamic vinegar *(Great Impressions)*	1 tbsp	67	367	6.
W/olive oil				
(Kraft)	1 tbsp	70	210	8.
(Wish-Bone) Italian 'Classic'	1 tbsp	34	190	3.
(Wish-Bone) 'Lite Classic'	.5 oz	20	170	2.

Food Name	Serv. Size	Total Cal.	Sod. MGS	Fat GMS
(Wish-Bone) vinaigrette	1 tbsp	28	111	2.3
(Wish-Bone) vinaigrette 'Lite'	1 tbsp	16	111	0.9
W/red wine vinegar				
(Estee)	1 tbsp	2	10	0.0
(Featherweight)	1 tbsp	6	100	0.0
(Great Impressions)	1 tbsp	64	277	6.1
(Kraft)	1 tbsp	60	200	4.0
(Pathmark)	1 tbsp	70	235	7.0
(Seven Seas) 'Free'	1 tbsp	6	190	0.0
(Seven Seas) 'Viva'	1 tbsp	70	290	7.0
(Seven Seas) 'Viva Red Wine!'	1 tbsp	45	190	4.0
W/Cabernet *(Lawry's)* 'Classics'	1 tbsp	138	178	13.7
W/white wine vinegar *(Great Impressions)*	1 tbsp	63	242	6.6
ONION AND CHIVES				
(Kraft) creamy	1 tbsp	70	150	7.0
(Wish-Bone) 'Lite'	1 tbsp	37	164	3.3
ORIENTAL STYLE *(Featherweight)*	1 tbsp	20	75	2.0
PARMESAN *(Hidden Valley Ranch)* Italian 'Lowfat'	1 tbsp	16	140	1.0
PARMESAN PEPPERCORN				
(T. Marzetti)	1 tbsp	81	129	9.0
(T. Marzetti) refrigerated	1 tbsp	85	154	9.0
PEPPERCORN				
(Litehouse) dressing and dip, refrigerated	1 tbsp	67	66	7.0
(Simply Delicious) pink, vinaigrette 'Un-Dressing'	1 tbsp	40	148	4.0
(T. Marzetti) cracked, refrigerated	1 tbsp	62	135	7.0
(Weight Watchers) creamy	1 tbsp	8	85	0.0
POPPYSEED				
(Great Impressions)	1 tbsp	131	130	11.0
(Hain) 'Rancher's'	1 tbsp	60	105	7.0
(Knott's Berry Farm) 'Peggy Jane's'	1 tbsp	60	90	5.0
(Litehouse) dressing and dip, refrigerated	1 tbsp	65	83	6.0
(T. Marzetti)	1 tbsp	72	146	6.0
(T. Marzetti) refrigerated	1 tbsp	65	97	5.0
POTATO SALAD *(T. Marzetti)*	1 tbsp	80	170	7.0
RANCH				
(Hidden Valley Ranch) honey Dijon 'Lowfat'	1 tbsp	20	140	1.0
(Hidden Valley Ranch) original 'Light'	1 tbsp	40	140	4.0
(Kraft) nonfat 'Free'	1 tbsp	16	150	0.0
(Litehouse) country, dressing and dip, refrigerated	1 tbsp	61	75	7.0
(Litehouse) dressing and dip, refrigerated	1 tbsp	59	67	6.0
(Litehouse) jalapeño, dressing and dip, refrigerated	1 tbsp	60	80	6.0

Food Name	Serv. Size	Total Cal.	Sod. MGS	F... G...
(Litehouse) 'Lite' dressing and dip, refrigerated	1 tbsp	35	80	3
(Pritikin) fat-free, sodium-free	1 tbsp	16	0	0
(Seven Seas) 'Buttermilk Recipe Ranch! Light'	1 tbsp	50	135	5
(Seven Seas) 'Free'	1 tbsp	16	120	0
(Seven Seas) 'Viva'	1 tbsp	80	135	8
(Seven Seas) 'Viva Ranch! Light'	1 tbsp	50	125	5
(Skipper's) house	1 pouch	188	302	20
(T. Marzetti)	1 tbsp	90	92	2
(T. Marzetti) buttermilk, refrigerated	1 tbsp	93	127	10
(T. Marzetti) buttermilk 'Lite' refrigerated	1 tbsp	45	135	5
(T. Marzetti) Caesar	1 tbsp	95	150	10
(T. Marzetti) 'Fat-Free'	1 tbsp	12	220	0
(T. Marzetti) garden	1 tbsp	100	165	10
(T. Marzetti) honey Dijon	1 tbsp	89	100	9
(T. Marzetti) honey Dijon, refrigerated	1 tbsp	79	101	8
(T. Marzetti) 'Light'	1 tbsp	40	166	4
(T. Marzetti) Parmesan, refrigerated	1 tbsp	86	120	9
(T. Marzetti) peppercorn	1 tbsp	85	13	9
(T. Marzetti) peppercorn 'Fat-Free'	1 tbsp	14	173	0
(T. Marzetti) style	1 tbsp	90	100	6
(Weight Watchers) creamy	1 tbsp	25	100	0
(Weight Watchers) creamy 'Single Serve'	1 pkt	35	140	0
(Wish-Bone)	1 tbsp	78	156	8
(Wish-Bone) 'Food Service'	.5 oz	80	105	8
(Wish-Bone) 'Healthy Sensation!'	1 tbsp	16	140	0
(Wish-Bone) 'Lite'	1 tbsp	42	148	3
RED WINE VINAIGRETTE				
(Wish-Bone)	1 tbsp	51	216	3
(Wish-Bone) 'Lite'	.5 oz	20	140	2
ROMANO				
(T. Marzetti) cheese Italian	1 tbsp	80	135	8
(T. Marzetti) cheese Italian, refrigerated	1 tbsp	77	183	8
RUSSIAN				
(Ayla's Organics) fat-free	2 tbsp	10	140	0
(Featherweight)	1 tbsp	6	125	0
(Kraft)	1 tbsp	60	130	5
(Kraft) creamy	1 tbsp	60	150	5
(Kraft) 'Reduced Calorie'	1 tbsp	30	130	1
(Kraft) w/pure honey, low-calorie	1 tbsp	60	130	5
(S&W Nutradiet)	1 tbsp	25	120	1
(Weight Watchers) whipped	1 tbsp	50	80	5

Food Name	Serv. Size	Total Cal.	Sod. MGS	Fat GMS
(Wish-Bone)	1 tbsp	46	147	2.5
(Wish-Bone) 'Food Service'	1 tbsp	47	147	2.5
(Wish-Bone) 'Lite'	1 tbsp	22	126	0.6
SAN FRANCISCO *(Lawry's)* w/Romano cheese 'Classic'	1 oz	136	547	14.0
SANTA FE *(Wish-Bone)*	.5 oz	70	105	7.0
SESAME SEED				
(Ayla's Organics) toasted, fat-free	2 tbsp	20	190	0.0
(Nasoya) garlic 'Vegi-Dressing'	1 tbsp	40	50	3.0
(Wish-Bone) vinaigrette 'Food Service'	.5 oz	35	260	2.0
SOUR CREAM				
(Crowley) nondairy	1 oz	40	5	4.0
(Friendship) 'Sour Treat'	1 oz	36	15	3.0
SOUR CREAM AND CHIVES *(Litehouse)* vinaigrette, refrigerated	1 tbsp	63	72	7.0
SPINACH SALAD *(T. Marzetti)* refrigerated	1 tbsp	35	100	3.0
SWEET AND SAUCY *(T. Marzetti)*	1 tbsp	65	180	5.0
SWEET AND SOUR				
(T. Marzetti)	1 tbsp	72	100	6.0
(T. Marzetti) 'Fat-Free'	1 tbsp	20	130	0.0
(T. Marzetti) 'Light'	1 tbsp	45	105	3.0
(T. Marzetti) refrigerated	1 tbsp	72	99	6.0
SWISS CHEESE VINAIGRETTE *(Hain)*	1 tbsp	60	160	7.0
THOUSAND ISLAND				
(Estee)	1 tbsp	8	30	0.0
(Featherweight)	1 tbsp	18	70	0.0
(Hain)	1 tbsp	50	85	5.0
(Hollywood)	1 tbsp	60	15	6.0
(Kraft)	1 tbsp	60	150	5.0
(Kraft) and bacon	1 tbsp	60	100	6.0
(Kraft) nonfat 'Free'	1 tbsp	20	135	0.0
(Kraft) 'Reduced Calorie'	1 tbsp	20	135	1.0
(Litehouse) dressing and dip, refrigerated	1 tbsp	65	99	7.0
(S&W Nutradiet)	1 tbsp	25	105	2.0
(Seven Seas) creamy	1 tbsp	50	150	5.0
(Seven Seas) 'Thousand Island! Light'	1 tbsp	30	160	2.0
(Skipper's)	1 pouch	160	415	14.0
(T. Marzetti)	1 tbsp	74	120	7.0
(T. Marzetti) 'Fat-Free'	1 tbsp	17	172	0.0
(T. Marzetti) 'Frenchette'	1 tbsp	20	155	0.0
(T. Marzetti) 'Light'	1 tbsp	35	155	3.0
(T. Marzetti) refrigerated	1 tbsp	82	93	5.0

Food Name	Serv. Size	Total Cal.	Sod. MGS	Fat GMS
(Ultra Slim Fast) 'Cholesterol Free'	1 tbsp	18	95	<1.0
(Weight Watchers) whipped	1 tbsp	50	80	5.0
(Wish-Bone)	1 tbsp	63	158	5.6
(Wish-Bone) 'Food Service'	1 tbsp	40	107	3.2
(Wish-Bone) 'Healthy Sensation!'	.5 oz	20	135	na
(Wish-Bone) 'Lite'	1 tbsp	36	99	3.0
(Wish-Bone) lite 'Food Service'	.5 oz	20	140	na
TOMATO				
(Featherweight) zesty	1 tbsp	2	5	0.0
(Hain) vinaigrette, garden 'Canola'	1 tbsp	60	150	6.0
(Weight Watchers) vinaigrette	1 tbsp	8	150	0.0
VEGETABLE *(T. Marzetti)* dressing and dip, refrigerated	1 tbsp	88	120	10.0
VINTAGE *(Lawry's)* w/sherry wine 'Classic'	1 tbsp	110	415	10.5
WHITE WINE				
(Lawry's) w/Chardonnay 'Classic'	1 tbsp	153	178	15.7
(Marie's) fat-free 'Lite & Zesty'	1 tbsp	20	135	0.0
SALAD DRESSING MIX				
BACON *(Lawry's)* dry mix	1 pkg	65	1820	0.8
BLUE CHEESE				
(Hain) 'No Oil' prepared	1 tbsp	14	180	1.0
(Hidden Valley Ranch) dry mix	1 pkg	112	1931	2.0
(Weight Watchers) dry mix	1 tbsp	8	110	0.0
BLUE CHEESE AND HERBS *(Good Seasons)* dry mix	1 pkg	4	150	0.0
BUTTERMILK				
(Hain) 'No Oil' prepared	1 tbsp	11	150	<1.0
(Hidden Valley Ranch) original recipe, dry mix, .4 oz	1 pkg	25	2167	0.0
(Good Seasons) 'Farm Style' dry mix	1 pkg	4	95	0.0
CAESAR				
(Lawry's) dry mix	1 pkg	75	1962	3.1
(Hain) 'No Oil' prepared	1 tbsp	6	200	<1.0
CHEESE AND GARLIC				
(Good Seasons) dry mix	1 pkg	4	170	0.0
(Hain) 'No Oil' prepared	1 tbsp	6	180	<1.0
DILL *(Good Seasons)* 'Classic' dry mix	1 tbsp	2	150	0.0
FRENCH				
(Hain) 'No Oil' prepared	1 tbsp	12	340	0.0
(Weight Watchers) style, dry mix	1 tbsp	3	150	0.0
GARLIC AND HERBS *(Good Seasons)* dry mix	1 pkg	4	190	0.0
HERB				
(Good Seasons) 'Classic' dry mix	1 pkg	2	150	0.0
(Hain) 'No Oil' prepared	1 tbsp	2	140	0.0

Food Name	Serv. Size	Total Cal.	Sod. MGS	Fat GMS
(Hidden Valley Ranch) creamy, dry mix	1 pkg	76	1931	0.0
HONEY MUSTARD *(Good Seasons)* dry mix	1 tbsp	6	125	0.0
ITALIAN				
(Good Seasons) dry mix	1 pkg	2	170	0.0
(Good Seasons) 'Lite,' prepared	1 tbsp	25	180	3.0
(Good Seasons) mild, prepared	1 tbsp	70	190	8.0
(Good Seasons) 'No Oil,' prepared	1 tbsp	6	30	0.0
(Good Seasons) zesty, dry mix	1 pkg	2	120	0.0
(Good Seasons) zesty 'Lite,' prepared	1 tbsp	25	135	3.0
(Hain) 'No Oil,' prepared	1 tbsp	2	170	0.0
(Lawry's) dry mix	1 pkg	45	2255	0.2
(Lawry's) w/cheese, dry mix	1 pkg	74	1624	2.1
(Weight Watchers) dry mix	1 tbsp	2	140	0.0
ITALIAN, CREAMY *(Weight Watchers)* dry mix	1 tbsp	3	180	0.0
ITALIAN CHEESE				
(Good Seasons) dry mix	1 pkg	4	130	0.0
(Good Seasons) 'Lite' prepared	1 tbsp	25	135	3.0
LEMON AND HERBS *(Good Seasons)* dry mix	1 pkg	2	140	0.0
PEPPERCORN *(Hidden Valley Ranch)* original recipe, prepared	1 tbsp	58	110	3.0
RANCH				
(Good Seasons) dry mix	1 pkg	4	70	0.0
(Good Seasons) 'Lite' prepared	1 tbsp	30	115	2.0
(Hidden Valley Ranch) 'Original' dry mix	1 pkg	93	2211	1.0
(Hidden Valley Ranch) reduced calorie, dry mix	1 pkg	98	2301	2.0
(Hidden Valley Ranch) w/bacon, dry mix	1.2 oz	118	1953	2.0
RUSSIAN *(Weight Watchers)* dry mix	1 tbsp	4	120	0.0
SPICY PEANUT *(A Taste of Thai)* dry mix	1 tbsp	40	360	1.5
THOUSAND ISLAND				
(Hain) 'No Oil' prepared	1 tbsp	12	150	0.0
(Weight Watchers) dry mix	1 tbsp	4	140	0.0
SALAD MIX. See also PASTA DISH MIX; PASTA SALAD MIX.				
(Saco Foods) 'Easy Caesar' unprepared	.75 oz	98	246	7.0
SALAD SEASONING *(Schilling)* 'Salad Supreme'	1 tsp	11	2807	0.1
SALAD TOPPING				
(Salad Nibbler) crouton topping, buttermilk ranch	1 oz	128	241	5.0
(Salad Nibbler) crouton topping, seasoned cheddar	1 oz	129	224	6.0
(Special Edition) sesame salad nuggets	1 tbsp	35	115	2.5
(Special Edition) sesame salad nuggets, garlic and cheese	1 tbsp	40	130	2.5

SALAMI. See LUNCHEON MEAT.

SALISBURY STEAK DINNER. See BEEF DINNER, FROZEN.

SALISBURY STEAK ENTRÉE. See BEEF ENTRÉE, FROZEN; BEEF ENTRÉE, PACKAGED.

Food Name	Serv. Size	Total Cal.	Sod. MGS	Fat GMS
SALMON, ALTERNATIVE, smoked *(Mox Lox)*	1.5 oz	25	380	<1.0
SALMON, ATLANTIC				
Farmed				
dry-heat cooked	3 oz	175	52	10.5
raw	3 oz	156	50	9.2
Wild				
dry-heat cooked	3 oz	155	48	6.9
raw	3 oz	121	37	5.4
SALMON, CANNED				
CHUM				
(Bumble Bee)	1 cup	306	(mq)	11.4
(Bumble Bee) w/liquid	3.5 oz	160	490	8.0
COHO *(Deming's)* boiled	1/2 cup	140	450	5.0
MIXED *(Libby's)* skinless, boneless	3.25 oz	110	420	4.0
PINK				
Alaska, w/liquid *(Deming's)*	1/2 cup	140	450	6.0
chunk, skinless, boneless, in spring water				
(Chicken of the Sea)	2 oz	60	280	2.0
chunk, skinless, boneless, w/liquid *(Deming's)*	3.25 oz	120	420	5.0
skinless, boneless, w/liquid *(Bumble Bee)*	3.5 oz	120	420	5.0
solids, w/bone and liquid	3 oz	118	64	5.1
w/liquid	4 oz	158	628	6.9
w/liquid *(Bumble Bee)*	1 cup	310	851	13.0
w/liquid *(Bumble Bee)*	3.5 oz	160	490	8.0
w/liquid *(Del Monte)*	1/2 cup	160	660	7.0
w/liquid *(Featherweight)*	2 oz	70	45	3.0
w/liquid *(Libby's)*	7.75 oz	310	790	13.0
SOCKEYE				
(Bumble Bee)	1 cup	376	1148	20.5
(Libby's)	7.75 oz	380	760	21.0
Alaska *(Deming's)*	1/2 cup	170	450	9.0
Alaska, med *(Deming's)*	1/2 cup	150	450	7.0
blueback *(Rubinstein's)*	1/2 cup	170	450	9.0
blueback *(S&W Nutradiet)*	1/2 cup	188	45	11.0
blueback 'Fancy' *(S&W)*	1/2 cup	190	590	10.0
skinless, boneless, w/liquid *(Bumble Bee)*	3.5 oz	130	420	6.0
solids, w/bone, drained	3 oz	130	457	6.2
solids, w/bone, drained, w/o salt	3 oz	130	64	6.2
w/liquid *(Bumble Bee)*	3.5 oz	180	490	10.0
w/liquid *(Del Monte)*	1/2 cup	180	660	9.0

Food Name	Serv. Size	Total Cal.	Sod. MGS	Fat GMS
SALMON, CHINOOK/king/lox/smoked				
dry-heat cooked	3 oz	196	51	11.4
raw	1 lb	816	213	47.4
raw	3 oz	153	40	8.9
raw, approx 7 oz	1/2 fillet	356	93	20.7
smoked	3 oz	99	666	3.7
smoked, lox	4 oz	133	2268	4.9
smoked, lox	3 oz	99	1700	3.7
SALMON, CHUM/dog/keta				
dry-heat cooked	3 oz	131	54	4.1
raw	1 lb	544	449	17.1
raw	3 oz	102	43	3.2
raw	1 oz	34	14	1.1
raw, approx 7 oz	1/2 fillet	238	99	7.5
raw, fillet portions *(Peter Pan Seafoods)*	3.5 oz	120	50	3.8
raw, sides, w/pinbone *(Peter Pan Seafoods)*	3.5 oz	120	50	3.8
raw, solids, w/bone, drained, w/o salt	3 oz	120	64	4.7
raw, steaks *(Peter Pan Seafoods)*	3.5 oz	120	50	3.8
SALMON, COHO/silver				
Farmed				
dry-heat cooked	3 oz	151	44	7.0
raw	3 oz	136	40	6.5
Wild				
dry-heat cooked	3 oz	118	49	3.7
moist-heat cooked	3 oz	156	45	6.4
raw	1 lb	662	211	27.0
raw	3 oz	124	39	5.0
raw	1 oz	41	13	1.7
raw, approx 7 oz	1/2 fillet	289	91	11.7
SALMON, DOG. See SALMON, CHUM.				
SALMON, FROZEN, steak, w/o seasoning mix *(SeaPak)*	8-oz pkg	270	115	9.0
SALMON, HUMPBACK. See SALMON, PINK.				
SALMON, KETA. See SALMON, CHUM.				
SALMON, KING. See SALMON, CHINOOK.				
SALMON, PINK/humpback				
dry-heat cooked	3 oz	127	73	3.8
raw	1 lb	527	302	15.6
raw	3 oz	99	57	2.9
raw	1 oz	33	19	1.0
SALMON, RED. See SALMON, SOCKEYE.				
SALMON, REDEYE. See SALMON, SOCKEYE.				

Food Name	Serv. Size	Total Cal.	Sod. MGS	Fa GM
SALMON, SILVER. See SALMON, COHO.				
SALMON, SMOKED. See SALMON, CHINOOK.				
SALMON, SOCKEYE/ red/redeye				
dry-heat cooked	4 oz	245	75	12.
dry-heat cooked	3 oz	184	56	9.
raw	1 lb	763	211	38.
raw	3 oz	143	40	7.
raw	1 oz	48	13	2.
raw, approx 7 oz	1/2 fillet	333	93	17.
SALSA. See also SAUCE.				
(Hot Cha Cha) 'Texas'	1 oz	6	2	0.
(La Victoria) 'Brava'	1 tbsp	6	100	<1.
(La Victoria) 'Casera'	1 tbsp	4	80	<1.
(La Victoria) 'Supreme'	2 tbsp	10	220	0.
(La Victoria) 'Victoria'	1 tbsp	4	80	<1.
BURRITO (Del Monte)	1/4 cup	20	355	<1.
EXTRA CHUNKY (Rosarita) 'de Mexico Style'	2 tbsp	30	280	<1.
GREEN CHILI				
(Del Monte) mild	1/4 cup	20	590	0.
(Hain) hot	1/4 cup	22	480	0.
(La Victoria)	2 tbsp	10	150	0.
(Nabisco) hot	1 tbsp	6	190	0.
(Nabisco) medium 'Green Chile Salsa'	1 tbsp	6	190	0.
(Nabisco) mild 'Green Chile Salsa'	1 tbsp	8	190	0.
(Old El Paso) 'Thick 'n Chunky'	2 tbsp	3	270	0.
(Ortega) hot	1 oz	10	180	0.
(Ortega) medium	1 oz	8	180	0.
(Ortega) mild	1 oz	8	180	0.
(Rosarita) mild	1.093 oz	7	167	0.
(Territorial House)	.5 oz	4	80	<1.
HOT				
(Chi-Chi's)	1 oz	8	153	2.
(Enrico's) 'Chunky Style'	2 tbsp	8	34	0.
(Enrico's) 'Chunky Style No Salt Added'	2 tbsp	8	10	0.
(Old El Paso) 'Thick 'n Chunky'	2 tbsp	6	170	<1.
(Pablo's) 'Deli Style'	1 oz	10	250	0.
(Rosarita) chunky	3 tbsp	25	300	<1.
JALAPEÑO				
(La Victoria) green	1 tbsp	4	105	<1.
(La Victoria) red	1 tbsp	6	95	<1.

od Name	Serv. Size	Total Cal.	Sod. MGS	Fat GMS
EDIUM				
(Chi-Chi's)	1 oz	7	135	2.0
(Litehouse) 'Zesty'	1 tbsp	4	110	0.0
(Old El Paso) 'Thick 'n Chunky'	2 tbsp	6	170	<1.0
(Ortega) thick and chunky	1 tbsp	4	150	0.0
(Pace) 'Thick & Chunky'	2 tbsp	4	101	<1.0
(Rosarita) chunky	3 tbsp	25	350	<1.0
(Rosarita) 'Traditional'	1.093 oz	7	234	0.1
ILD				
(Chi-Chi's)	1 oz	7	116	2.0
(Enrico's) 'Chunky Style'	2 tbsp	8	34	0.0
(Enrico's) 'Chunky Style No Salt Added'	2 tbsp	8	10	0.0
(Hain)	1/2 cup	20	410	0.0
(Hunt's) 'Homestyle'	1.093 oz	27	236	0.2
(Old El Paso) 'Thick 'n Chunky'	2 tbsp	6	170	<1.0
(Pablo's) 'Deli Style'	1 oz	10	250	0.0
(Pace) and dip, mild 'Chunky'	2 tbsp	4	101	<1.0
(Pace) 'Thick & Chunky'	2 tbsp	4	101	<1.0
(Rosarita) 'Casa Mamita'	1.129 oz	7	170	0.1
(Rosarita) chunky	3 tbsp	25	340	<1.0
(Rosarita) roasted	1.093 oz	10	233	0.3
(Rosarita) 'Traditional'	1.093 oz	7	247	0.1
MELETTE (La Victoria)	1 tbsp	6	95	<1.0
ICANTE				
(Del Monte) hot	1/2 cup	20	385	0.0
(Del Monte) hot and chunky	1/4 cup	15	405	0.0
(La Victoria) medium	2 tbsp	5	180	0.0
(La Victoria) mild	2 tbsp	10	230	0.0
(LàCasita) mild, chunky	2 oz	16	226	0.0
(Old El Paso) hot	2 tbsp	10	160	<1.0
(Old El Paso) medium	2 tbsp	10	160	<1.0
(Old El Paso) mild	2 tbsp	10	160	<1.0
(Ortega)	1 oz	10	300	0.0
(Rosarita)	1.093 oz	7	247	0.1
ANCHERA				
(La Victoria)	1 tbsp	6	85	<1.0
(Ortega)	1 oz	12	250	0.0
OJA (Del Monte) mild	1/4 cup	20	510	0.0
ACO				
(Nabisco) 'Hot Thick and Smooth'	1 tbsp	8	105	0.0
(Nabisco) 'Medium Thick and Smooth'	1 tbsp	8	105	0.0

Food Name	Serv. Size	Total Cal.	Sod. MGS	Fc GM
(Nabisco) 'Mild Thick and Smooth'	1 tbsp	8	115	0.
(Ortega) hot	1 oz	10	300	0.
(Ortega) mild	1 oz	10	290	0.
(Rosarita) medium, chunky	3 tbsp	25	310	<1.
(Rosarita) mild	2 oz	27	304	0.
(Rosarita) mild, chunky	3 tbsp	25	300	<1.
TOMATILLO				
(Rosarita) green 'de Mexico Style'	2 tbsp	20	190	<1.
(Rosarita) medium	1.093 oz	8	188	0.
TRADITIONAL (Rosarita) 'de Mexico Style'	2 tbsp	12	350	0.
VERDE (Old El Paso) 'Thick 'n Chunky'	2 tbsp	10	135	<1.
VERY LOW SODIUM (Pritikin)	1/4 cup	25	15	0.
SALSIFY/oyster plant /vegetable oyster				
boiled, drained	4 oz	77	18	0.
boiled, drained, sliced	1/2 cup	46	11	0.
raw, sliced	1/2 cup	55	13	0.
raw, trimmed	1 oz	23	6	0.
raw, untrimmed	1 lb	325	79	0.
SALSIFY, BLACK/scorzonera				
raw	1 lb	372	91	0.
raw	1 oz	23	6	
SALT				
iodized (Morton)	1 tsp	0	2300	0.■
kosher (Morton)	1 tsp	0	1880	0.■
mixture 'Lite Salt' (Morton)	1 tsp	<1	1100	0.■
non-iodized (Morton)	1 tsp	0	2300	0.■
plain	1 cup	0	112398	0.■
plain	1 tbsp	0	6976	0.■
plain	1 tsp	0	2325	0.
sea (Hain)	1 tsp	0	2255	0.■
SALT, ALTERNATIVE				
Plain				
(Estee) 'Salt-It'	1/8 tsp	0	0	0.■
(Featherweight)	1/4 tsp	0	0	0.■
(Lawry's) 'Salt-Free'	1 tsp	10	2	0.
(Morton)	1 tsp	<1	<1	0.■
Seasoned				
(Estee) 'Seasoned Salt-It'	1/8 tsp	0	0	0.■
(Featherweight)	1/4 tsp	0	0	0.■
(Health Valley) all-purpose 'Instead of Salt'	1 tsp	11	3	0.
(Lawry's) 'Salt-Free'	1 tsp	3	7	<.

Food Name	Serv. Size	Total Cal.	Sod. MGS	Fat GMS
(Morton)	1 tsp	2	<1	<.1
SALT PORK, cured *(Hormel)*	2 oz	320	1800	33.0
SALT SEASONING				
(Lawry's)	1 tsp	4	1367	0.1
(Lawry's) 'Hot 'n Spicy'	1 tsp	3	79	0.1
(Lawry's) 'Lite'	1 tsp	8	357	<.1
(Morton)	1 tsp	4	1300	<.1
(Morton) 'Nature's Seasons'	1 tsp	3	1400	<.1
(Schilling)	1 tsp	4	980	na
(Schilling) 'Salt 'n Spice'	1 tsp	3	939	na
SANDWICH				
BEEF				
(Hot Pockets) frozen, pocket, and cheddar	5 oz	370	1390	17.0
(Lean Pockets) frozen, pocket, and broccoli	1 pkg	250	760	8.0
(Manwich) extra thick and chunky, prepared	1 sandwich	330	870	13.0
(Manwich) Mexican, prepared	1 sandwich	310	690	13.0
(Manwich) original, prepared	1 sandwich	320	590	13.0
(Manwich) 'Sloppy Joe' prepared	1 sandwich	310	620	13.0
(Tyson) frozen, barbecue, microwave	1 sandwich	200	600	2.7
CANADIAN BACON *(Quick Meal)* muffin, w/egg and cheese	4.5 oz	250	680	8.0
CHEESEBURGER				
(Kid Cuisine) frozen	6.25 oz	400	550	19.0
(Kid Cuisine) frozen, double 'Mega Meal'	9.1 oz	480	1040	20.0
(MicroMagic) frozen	4.75 oz	450	790	25.0
CHICKEN				
(Banquet) patties, breast meat 'Microwave'	4 oz	310	664	14.0
(BestFresh) breast, teriyaki, charbroiled	1 sandwich	490	1030	20.0
(BestFresh) w/cucumber yogurt dressing	1 sandwich	390	960	15.0
(Hot Pockets) frozen, pocket, and cheddar	5 oz	310	720	11.0
(Kid Cuisine)	8.2 oz	470	830	17.0
(Lean Pockets) frozen, pocket, Oriental	1 pkg	250	840	6.0
(Lean Pockets) frozen, pocket, Parmesan	1 pkg	270	750	6.0
(Lean Pockets) frozen, pocket, white meat only 'Fajita'	1 sandwich	250	810	6.0
(Lean Pockets) frozen, pocket, white meat only, glazed 'Supreme'	1 sandwich	240	630	7.0
(MicroMagic) frozen	4.5 oz	390	650	16.0
(Quick Meal)	4.3 oz	320	640	11.0
(Quick Meal) biscuit	4.2 oz	310	900	13.0
(Quick Meal) grilled	4.7 oz	300	620	9.0
(Tyson) boneless, grilled	3.5 oz	200	470	5.0
(Tyson) breast, boneless, grilled	3.5 oz	150	400	8.0

Food Name	Serv. Size	Total Cal.	Sod. MGS	Fat GMS
(Tyson) frozen, barbecue 'Microwave'	4 oz	230	510	6.0
(Tyson) frozen, breast 'Microwave'	3.5 oz	275	(mq)	12.0
(Tyson) frozen, mini 'Microwave'	3.5 oz	230	(mq)	5.0
(Ultimate 200) grilled	4 oz	200	420	5.0
EGG				
(Jimmy Dean) frozen, w/egg and cheese	1 biscuit	300	890	16.0
(Jimmy Dean) frozen, w/ham and cheese	1 biscuit	240	720	10.0
(Jimmy Dean) w/sausage and cheese	1 biscuit	390	1040	27.0
(Swanson) frozen, w/beefsteak and cheese 'Great Starts'	4.9 oz	360	730	20.0
(Swanson) frozen, w/Canadian bacon and cheese 'Great Starts'	5.2 oz	420	1845	22.0
(Swanson) frozen, w/Canadian bacon and cheese 'Great Starts'	4.1 oz	290	770	15.0
(Swanson) frozen, w/sausage and cheese 'Great Starts' ...	5.5 oz	460	1310	28.0
ENGLISH MUFFIN *(Weight Watchers)*	4 oz	240	540	8.0
FISH FILLET *(Quick Meal)*	5.2 oz	430	910	16.0
HAM AND CHEESE				
(Hot Pockets) frozen, pocket	5 oz	360	1320	16.0
(Owens) refrigerated 'Border Breakfasts'	2 oz	150	600	6.0
(Swanson) refrigerated, bagel 'Great Starts'	3 oz	240	600	8.0
(Ultimate 200) frozen, pocket	4 oz	200	490	6.0
(Weight Watchers) bagel	3 oz	210	460	6.0
HAMBURGER *(MicroMagic)* frozen	4 oz	350	500	18.0
HOT DOG				
(Kid Cuisine)	6.7 oz	450	880	19.0
(Kid Cuisine) 'Mega Meal'	8.25 oz	500	1260	25.0
OMELET				
(Weight Watchers) 'Classic'	3.84 oz	210	410	7.0
(Weight Watchers) 'Garden'	3.60 oz	210	480	6.0
PIZZA				
(Amy's Kitchen) frozen, pocket, cheese calzone, organic ..	4.5 oz	313	272	9.0
(Hot Pockets) frozen, pocket, pepperoni	5 oz	380	1240	17.0
(Hot Pockets) frozen, pocket, sausage	5 oz	360	590	16.0
(Lean Pockets) frozen, pocket 'Deluxe'	1 pkg	280	500	9.0
(Lean Pockets) frozen, pocket, sausage and pepperoni 'Deluxe'	1 sandwich	300	670	11.0
(Ultimate 200) pocket 'Deluxe'	4 oz	200	400	5.0
PORK *(Quick Meal)* barbecue	4.3 oz	350	550	14.0
RIB *(Swanson)* hot, smothered	10.25 oz	340	690	10.0

Food Name	Serv. Size	Total Cal.	Sod. MGS	Fat GMS
SAUSAGE				
(Jimmy Dean) refrigerated, microwave	1 sandwich	160	360	11.0
(Owens) refrigerated, biscuit 'Border Breakfasts'	2 oz	210	400	14.0
(Owens) refrigerated, biscuit, smoked 'Border Breakfasts'	2 oz	200	786	6.0
(Owens) refrigerated, biscuit, w/egg and cheese 'Border Breakfasts'	2.5 oz	250	500	15.0
(Quick Meal) biscuit	3.7 oz	350	870	22.0
(Quick Meal) biscuit, w/cheese	4.3 oz	420	1060	27.0
(Quick Meal) biscuit, w/egg	4.5 oz	350	780	21.0
(Quick Meal) muffin, w/egg and cheese	5.1 oz	76	143	4.0
(Swanson) frozen, biscuit, w/egg 'Great Starts'	4.7 oz	410	1180	22.0
(Weight Watchers) frozen, biscuit 'Microwave'	3 oz	220	560	11.0
SUBMARINE (BestFresh) 'Deluxe'	1 sandwich	790	2070	44.0
TURKEY				
(BestFresh) smoked	1 sandwich	580	1770	26.0
(Healthy Deli) w/corned beef 'Doubledecker'	1 oz	30	195	0.7
(Healthy Deli) w/ham 'Doubledecker'	1 oz	30	185	0.9
(Hot Pockets) pocket, frozen, w/ham and cheese	5 oz	320	780	11.0
(Lean Pockets) pocket, frozen, w/broccoli and cheese	1 sandwich	260	680	9.0
VEGETABLE				
(Ken & Robert's) pocket, barbecue style 'Truly Amazing'	5 oz	320	560	10.0
(Ken & Robert's) pocket, broccoli cheddar 'Truly Amazing'	5 oz	275	540	9.0
(Ken & Robert's) pocket, Greek style 'Truly Amazing'	5 oz	270	500	10.0
(Ken & Robert's) pocket, Indian style 'Truly Amazing'	5 oz	300	500	12.0
(Ken & Robert's) pocket, Oriental style 'Truly Amazing'	5 oz	295	572	12.0
(Ken & Robert's) pocket, pizza style 'Truly Amazing'	5 oz	315	620	12.0
(Ken & Robert's) pocket, Tex Mex style 'Truly Amazing'	5 oz	310	595	11.0
SANDWICH SEASONING MIX, dry (Manwich)	.25 oz	20	350	<1.0
SANDWICH SPREAD. See also LUNCHEON MEAT, CANNED; POTTED MEAT SPREAD.				
'Chub' (Oscar Mayer)	1 oz	67	273	4.7
pork and beef	1 oz	67	287	4.9
pork and beef	1 tbsp	35	152	2.6
SARDINE				
ATLANTIC				
in soybean oil, drained	3.75-oz can	191	465	10.5
in soybean oil, drained	2 oz	118	286	6.5
in soybean oil, drained, approx .8 oz	2 med	50	121	2.8
BRISLING, w/liquid (Underwood)	3.75-oz can	260	450	20.0
MAINE				
in mustard sauce, drained (Beach Cliff)	3 oz	227	350	18.0
in soybean oil, drained (Beach Cliff)	3 oz	240	20	20.0

Food Name	Serv. Size	Total Cal.	Sod. MGS	Fat GMS
in tomato sauce, drained (Beach Cliff)	3 oz	210	350	17.0
in water, drained (Beach Cliff)	3 oz	230	350	18.0
MIXED				
'Kippered Snacks' (Brunswick)	3.5 oz	185	610	14.0
in mustard sauce (Underwood)	3.75 oz	220	650	16.0
in oil (Featherweight)	1 7/8 oz	130	65	10.0
in soya oil, drained (Underwood)	3.75 oz	230	400	18.0
in Tabasco sauce, drained (Underwood)	3 oz	220	400	16.0
in tomato sauce (Del Monte)	1/2 cup	360	540	12.0
in tomato sauce (Underwood)	3.75 oz	220	500	16.0
in water (Featherweight)	1 7/8 oz	95	65	7.0
NORWAY				
in mild sardine oil, drained (Empress)	3.75-oz can	260	(mq)	20.0
in mild sardine oil, w/liquid (Empress)	3.75-oz can	460	(mq)	42.0
NORWEGIAN BRISLING (S&W)	1.5 oz	130	220	10.0
PACIFIC				
in tomato sauce, drained	13 oz	659	1532	44.3
in tomato sauce, drained	2 oz	101	235	6.8
in tomato sauce, drained, approx 1.3 oz	1 med	68	157	4.6
SAUCE. See also APPLESAUCE; BARBECUE SAUCE; CRANBERRY SAUCE; SALSA; TOMATO SAUCE.				
ALFREDO SAUCE				
(Betty Crocker) 'Recipe Sauces'	4 oz	190	650	17.0
(Contadina)	4 oz	350	500	34.0
(Contadina) 'Fresh' refrigerated	6 oz	540	620	53.0
(Contadina) 'Light' refrigerated	3.33 oz	150	460	10.0
(DiGiorno) reduced fat 'Lighter Varieties'	1/4 cup	180	580	11.0
(DiGiorno) refrigerated	2 oz	200	490	20.0
(Progresso) 'Authentic Pasta Sauces'	1/2 cup	340	1080	30.0
APPLE-APRICOT SAUCE (Lucky Leaf/Musselman's)				
'Fruit n' Sauce'	4 oz	90	20	0.0
APPLE-CHERRY SAUCE (Lucky Leaf/Musselman's)				
'Fruit n' Sauce'	4 oz	100	20	0.0
APPLE-CRANBERRY SAUCE (Lucky Leaf/Musselman's)				
'Fruit n' Sauce'	4 oz	80	15	0.0
APPLE-PEACH SAUCE (Lucky Leaf/Musselman's)				
'Fruit n' Sauce'	4 oz	90	20	0.0
APPLE-PINEAPPLE SAUCE (Lucky Leaf/Musselman's)				
'Fruit n' Sauce'	4 oz	110	20	0.0
APPLE-STRAWBERRY SAUCE (Lucky Leaf/Musselman's)				
'Fruit n' Sauce'	4 oz	100	20	0.0

Food Name	Serv. Size	Total Cal.	Sod. MGS	Fat GMS
BASIL-HERB SAUCE *(Golden Dipt)* 'Nature Bay'	2 grams	8	36	0.0
BEARNAISE SAUCE *(Great Impressions)*	2 tbsp	192	148	21.0
BEEF SAUCE				
(Ragu) barbecue 'Beef Tonight'	4 oz	70	580	<1.0
(Ragu) skillet lasagna 'Beef Tonight'	4 oz	60	630	1.0
(Ragu) Stroganoff 'Beef Tonight'	4 oz	130	770	12.0
BOLOGNESE SAUCE				
(Contadina)	5 oz	130	500	7.0
(Contadina) 'Fresh' refrigerated	7.5 oz	230	600	11.0
(Progresso) 'Authentic Pasta Sauces'	1/2 cup	150	520	8.0
BROWN GRAVY SAUCE *(LaChoy)*	3.139 oz	284	400	0.1
BROWNING SAUCE *(Gravymaster)*	1 tsp	12	<1	tr
CACCIATORE SAUCE *(Recipe Sauces)*	3.9 oz	40	570	<1.0
CARBONARA SAUCE *(DiGiorno)* refrigerated	2 oz	200	380	19.0
CHARDONNAY SAUCE *(Golden Dipt)* 'Nature Bay'	1 oz	60	160	6.0
CHEDDAR CHEESE SAUCE				
(J. Hungerford) 'Stadium'	2.011 oz	80	500	5.0
(Lucky Leaf/Musselman's)	4 oz	220	1000	18.0
(Lucky Leaf/Musselman's) aged	4 oz	240	920	20.0
(Lucky Leaf/Musselman's) aged, mild	4 oz	200	790	18.0
(Lucky Leaf/Musselman's) aged, sharp	4 oz	230	850	17.0
CHEESE SAUCE				
(Snow's) Welsh rarebit	1/2 cup	170	460	11.0
(White House) aged	3.5 oz	213	810	18.0
CHICKEN SAUCE				
(Ragu) cacciatore 'Chicken Tonight'	4 oz	70	490	2.0
(Ragu) country French 'Chicken Tonight'	4 oz	140	730	12.0
(Ragu) creamy, primavera 'Chicken Tonight'	4 oz	90	650	6.0
(Ragu) creamy, w/mushrooms 'Chicken Tonight'	4 oz	110	650	10.0
(Ragu) herbed, w/wine 'Chicken Tonight'	4 oz	100	610	4.0
(Ragu) honey mustard, light 'Chicken Tonight'	4 oz	50	420	<1.0
(Ragu) sweet and sour 'Chicken Tonight'	4 oz	80	280	0.0
(Ragu) sweet and spicy, light 'Chicken Tonight'	4 oz	50	390	<1.0
CHILI SAUCE				
(Chef Boyardee) hot dog, w/beef	1 oz	30	140	1.0
(Del Monte) tomato	1/4 cup	70	835	0.0
(El Molino) green, mild	2 tbsp	10	210	0.0
(Featherweight)	1 tbsp	8	10	0.0
(Gebhardt) hot dog	2 tbsp	20	150	1.0
(Heinz)	1 oz	30	430	0.0
(Hunt's)	1.199 oz	35	393	0.1

Food Name	Serv. Size	Total Cal.	Sod. MGS	Fat GMS
(Las Palmas) red	1/2 cup	25	670	1.0
(Manwich) 'Chili Fixin's'	5.3 oz	110	900	<1.0
(S&W) 'Chili Makin's'	1/2 cup	100	782	1.0
(Wolf Brand) hot dog	1.25 oz	44	199	2.3
CHOCOLATE SAUCE *(Chocolate Mountain)*	2 tbsp	120	80	4.0
CLAM SAUCE				
Red				
(Buitoni)	5 oz	190	560	6.0
(Contadina) 'Fresh' refrigerated	7.5 oz	120	800	4.0
(Ferrara)	4 oz	70	320	2.0
(Progresso)	1/2 cup	70	560	3.0
White				
(Contadina) 'Fresh' refrigerated	6 oz	290	800	23.0
(Ferrara)	4 oz	80	570	5.0
(Progresso)	1/2 cup	110	280	8.0
COCKTAIL SAUCE				
(Del Monte)	1/4 cup	70	765	0.0
(Estee)	1 tbsp	10	35	<1.0
(Golden Dipt) extra hot	1 tbsp	20	210	0.0
(Golden Dipt) regular	1 tbsp	20	210	0.0
(Great Impressions)	1 tbsp	21	182	0.1
(Great Impressions) 'Brandy Glow'	1 tbsp	68	106	6.7
(Great Impressions) 'Low Salt'	1 tbsp	21	6	0.1
(Sauceworks)	1 tbsp	14	170	0.0
(Skipper's)	1 tbsp	20	216	0.0
(Stokely)	1 tbsp	18	90	0.0
CRANBERRY-ORANGE SAUCE				
(Ocean Spray) crushed, for chicken 'Cran•Fruit'	2 oz	90	10	0.0
CRANBERRY-RASPBERRY SAUCE				
(Ocean Spray) crushed, for chicken 'Cran•Fruit'	2 oz	90	10	0.0
CREOLE SAUCE				
(Enrico's) Cajun 'Light'	4 oz	76	284	2.8
(Golden Dipt) cooking sauce	1 oz	20	190	1.0
DIABLO SAUCE *(Escoffier)*	1 tbsp	20	160	0.0
DIJONAISSE SAUCE *(Golden Dipt)* cooking sauce	1 oz	52	130	4.0
ENCHILADA SAUCE				
(Gebhardt)	3 tbsp	25	170	1.0
(La Victoria)	1 cup	80	1520	5.0
(Rosarita)	3 oz	20	430	0.0
Green *(Old El Paso)*	2 tbsp	11	200	0.0

Food Name	Serv. Size	Total Cal.	Sod. MGS	Fat GMS
Hot				
(Del Monte)	1/2 cup	45	1090	0.0
(El Molino)	2 tbsp	16	100	1.0
(Las Palmas)	1/2 cup	25	670	1.0
(Old El Paso)	1/4 cup	30	250	1.0
(Ortega)	1 oz	12	280	0.0
Mild				
(Del Monte)	1/2 cup	45	1150	0.0
(Old El Paso)	1/4 cup	25	250	1.0
(Ortega)	1 oz	12	280	0.0
(Rosarita)	2.5 oz	25	230	1.0
FAJITA SAUCE (Tio Sancho) 'Skillet Sauce'	1 oz	14	590	0.5
FORESTIERA SAUCE (Contadina) 'Fresh' refrigerated	7.5 oz	270	830	9.0
FOUR CHEESE SAUCE				
(Contadina)	4 oz	300	400	27.0
(Contadina) 'Fresh' refrigerated	6 oz	470	500	45.0
(DiGiorno) refrigerated	2 oz	170	340	16.0
FRENCH WHITE SAUCE (Golden Dipt) cooking sauce	1 oz	55	210	4.0
GARLIC-CHILI PEPPER SAUCE (A Taste of Thai)	1 tbsp	10	220	0.0
GARLIC-HERB SAUCE (Golden Dipt) 'Nature Bay'	2 grams	8	87	0.0
GUAVA SAUCE, cooked	1/2 cup	43	5	0.2
HERB AND GARLIC SAUCE (Lawry's) w/lemon juice	1/4 cup	36	3688	0.4
HOLLANDAISE SAUCE (Great Impressions)	2 tbsp	192	107	21.0
HONEY SOY SAUCE				
(Golden Dipt) cooking sauce	1 oz	90	250	8.0
(Golden Dipt) 'Nature Bay'	1 oz	90	250	8.0
HORSERADISH SAUCE				
(Great Impressions)	1 tbsp	74	199	7.6
(Heinz)	1 tbsp	74	113	7.4
(Life) strong 'All Natural'	1/2 tbsp	7	2	<1.0
(Sauceworks)	1 tbsp	50	105	5.0
HOT DOG SAUCE (Just Rite)	2 oz	60	220	3.0
HOT PEPPER SAUCE				
(Gebhardt) 'Louisiana Style'	1/2 tsp	0	45	0.0
(Tabasco)	1/4 tsp	<1	9	tr
HOT SAUCE (Gebhardt)	1/2 tsp	<1	55	<1.0
JALAPEÑO CHEESE SAUCE				
(Pablo's) 'Deli Style'	1 oz	59	470	4.0
(White House)	3.5 oz	193	890	16.0
LEMON BUTTER-DILL SAUCE (Golden Dipt) cooking sauce	1 oz	110	180	10.0
LEMON-DILL SAUCE (Golden Dipt) 'Nature Bay'	1 oz	110	150	11.0

Food Name	Serv. Size	Total Cal.	Sod. MGS	Fat GMS
LOBSTER SAUCE *(Progresso)* rock	1/2 cup	120	430	8.0
MARINARA SAUCE				
(Angela Mia)	4.409 oz	47	503	1.5
(Buitoni)	1/2 cup	70	570	3.0
(DiGiorno) refrigerated	5 oz	110	680	6.0
(Millina's Finest) organic, fat-free	4 oz	48	210	0.5
(Millina's Finest) Zinfandel, organic, fat-free	4 oz	44	215	0.5
(Pathmark) 'All Natural'	1/2 cup	80	710	2.0
(Pathmark) 'No Frills'	1/2 cup	80	620	3.0
(Prego)	4 oz	100	620	6.0
(Progresso)	1/2 cup	90	520	5.0
(Progresso) 'Authentic Pasta Sauces'	1/2 cup	110	250	6.0
(Rokeach)	3 oz	60	257	2.0
(Westbrae)	4 oz	40	370	<1.0
(Westbrae) w/mushrooms	4 oz	50	380	29.0
MESQUITE SAUCE *(Lawry's)* w/lime juice	1/4 cup	24	4142	0.4
MUSHROOM SAUCE *(Quincy's)*	3 oz	27	366	<1.0
NACHO CHEESE SAUCE				
(J. Hungerford)	2.011 oz	120	440	9.0
(J. Hungerford) 'Stadium'	2.011 oz	80	410	5.0
(Kaukauna)	1 oz	80	330	6.0
(Lucky Leaf)	4 oz	220	1010	18.0
(Musselman's)	4 oz	220	1010	18.0
(Pablo's) 'Deli Style'	1 oz	59	470	4.0
(White House)	3.5 oz	193	890	16.0
NEWBURG SAUCE *(Snow's)* w/sherry	1/3 cup	120	520	8.0
ORANGE SAUCE *(LaChoy)* Mandarin	1 tbsp	24	38	tr
ORANGE-DIJON SAUCE *(Golden Dipt)* 'Nature Bay'	1 oz	110	200	9.0
OREGANO-HERB SAUCE *(Golden Dipt)* 'Nature Bay'	2 grams	6	88	0.0
PARMIGIANA SAUCE *(Betty Crocker)* 'Recipe Sauces'	3.9 oz	50	430	1.0
PASTA SAUCE/spaghetti sauce				
(Angela Mia)	4.409 oz	49	607	0.5
(Campbell's) 'Homestyle'	4 oz	40	360	0.0
(Enrico's) 'All Natural'	4 oz	60	345	1.0
(Hunt's) 'Homestyle'	4 oz	60	530	2.0
(Hunt's) 'Olde Country'	4 oz	60	560	2.0
(Progresso)	1/2 cup	110	660	5.0
(Ragu) 'Old World Style'	4 oz	80	740	4.0
(Ragu) 'Slow Cooked Homestyle'	4 oz	110	510	5.0
(Ragu) 'Thick & Hearty'	4 oz	100	460	3.0

Food Name	Serv. Size	Total Cal.	Sod. MGS	Fat GMS
Garden				
(Prego) combination	4 oz	80	420	2.0
(Pritikin) chunky	1/2 cup	50	30	0.0
(Ragu) harvest 'Todays Recipe'	4 oz	50	370	1.0
Garlic and herb				
(Healthy Choice)	4 oz	40	350	<1.0
(Hunt's) 'Classic'	4.409 oz	58	598	2.1
(Hunt's) 'Light'	4.409 oz	39	379	0.8
(Hunt's) 'Olde Country'	4.409 oz	63	522	2.7
Garlic and onion				
(Campbell's) extra	4 oz	50	320	<1.0
(Del Monte)	1/2 cup	70	430	2.0
(Healthy Choice) chunky	4 oz	40	350	0.0
(Prego)	4 oz	110	510	4.0
Italian				
(Campbell's)	4 oz	50	360	0.0
(Healthy Choice) vegetable, chunky	4 oz	40	350	0.0
(Hunt's) vegetable 'Olde Country'	4.409 oz	64	616	2.6
(Pastorelli) 'Italian Chef'	4 oz	81	430	3.0
(Ragu) 'Fresh Italian'	4 oz	90	490	3.0
(Ragu) garden combination 'Chunky Gardenstyle'	4 oz	110	500	5.0
Meat				
(Chef Boyardee) w/ground beef 'Jars'	4 oz	90	605	3.0
(Hunt's)	4.444 oz	65	604	2.3
(Hunt's) 'Homestyle'	4.409 oz	56	596	2.6
(Hunt's) 'Light'	4.409 oz	45	437	1.2
(Hunt's) 'Olde Country'	4.409 oz	56	474	2.6
(Ragu) 'Homestyle'	4 oz	110	510	5.0
Meat flavor				
(Chef Boyardee)	3.75 oz	80	650	3.0
(Chef Boyardee) 'Original'	3.75 oz	120	650	6.0
(Contadina) 'Original Recipe'	1/2 cup	100	430	3.2
(Del Monte)	1/2 cup	70	440	2.0
(Hunt's)	4 oz	70	570	2.0
(P&Q)	1/2 cup	70	510	2.0
(Pathmark) 'All Natural'	1/2 cup	80	790	3.0
(Pathmark) 'No Frills'	1/2 cup	90	620	5.0
(Prego)	4 oz	140	660	6.0
(Progresso)	1/2 cup	110	660	5.0
(Weight Watchers)	1/3 cup	50	440	1.0

Food Name	Serv. Size	Total Cal.	Sod. MGS	Fat GMS
Meatless				
(Chef Boyardee) 'Jars'	4 oz	60	790	1.0
(P&Q)	1/2 cup	70	540	1.0
(Pathmark) 'All Natural'	1/2 cup	70	710	2.0
(Pathmark) 'No Frills'	1/2 cup	80	583	3.0
Mushroom				
(Campbell's)	4 oz	50	330	<1.0
(Campbell's) 'Healthy Request'	4 oz	50	330	<1.0
(Contadina) 'Original Recipe'	1/2 cup	90	430	2.3
(Del Monte)	1/2 cup	70	440	2.0
(Healthy Choice) chunky	4 oz	45	350	0.0
(Hunt's)	4.444 oz	65	604	2.3
(Hunt's) 'Homestyle'	4.409 oz	56	586	2.6
(Hunt's) 'Light'	4.409 oz	39	379	0.8
(Hunt's) 'Olde Country'	4.409 oz	53	542	2.7
(Prego) w/extra spice 'Extra Chunky'	4 oz	100	450	3.0
(Ragu) chunky 'Todays Recipe'	4 oz	50	370	1.0
(Ragu) 'Homestyle'	4 oz	110	530	2.0
(Ragu) super 'Chunky Gardenstyle'	4 oz	110	500	5.0
(Ragu) 'Thick & Hearty'	4 oz	100	460	3.0
Mushroom and green pepper				
(Enrico's) 'All Natural'	4 oz	60	345	1.0
(Enrico's) 'All Natural No Salt Added'	4 oz	60	30	1.0
(Prego) 'Extra Chunky'	4 oz	100	410	4.0
(Ragu) 'Chunky Gardenstyle'	4 oz	110	500	5.0
Mushroom and onion				
(Prego) 'Extra Chunky'	4 oz	100	490	4.0
(Ragu) 'Chunky Gardenstyle'	4 oz	110	560	5.0
Mushroom and tomato				
(DiGiorno) w/plum tomatoes, refrigerated	5 oz	100	240	1.0
(Millina's Finest) organic, fat-free	4 oz	45	198	0.5
(Prego) 'Extra Chunky'	4 oz	110	500	5.0
Mushroom flavor				
(Chef Boyardee)	3.75 oz	60	790	1.0
(Chef Boyardee) 'Jars'	4 oz	70	655	2.0
(Chef Boyardee) 'Original'	3.75 oz	80	680	3.0
(Enrico's)	4 oz	60	(mq)	1.0
(Enrico's) w/fresh mushrooms	4 oz	60	336	1.0
(Featherweight)	4 oz	60	310	1.0
(Hunt's)	4 oz	70	560	2.0
(P&Q)	1/2 cup	70	580	1.0

Food Name	Serv. Size	Total Cal.	Sod. MGS	Fat GMS
(Pathmark) 'All Natural'	1/2 cup	70	730	2.0
(Prego)	4 oz	130	630	5.0
(Progresso)	1/2 cup	110	630	5.0
(Weight Watchers)	1/3 cup	40	430	0.0
No salt added				
(Eden Foods) organic	4 oz	80	0	2.0
(Enrico's) 'All Natural No Salt Added'	4 oz	60	30	1.0
(Prego) 'No Salt Added'	4 oz	110	25	6.0
Original *(Pritikin)*	1/2 cup	60	35	1.0
Parmesan 'Classic' *(Hunt's)*	4.409 oz	50	634	2.1
Primavera				
(Progresso) creamy 'Authentic Pasta Sauces'	1/2 cup	190	410	17.0
(Westbrae)	4 oz	60	490	3.0
(Westbrae) no salt	4 oz	40	105	0.0
Sausage and green pepper *(Prego)* 'Extra Chunky'	4 oz	160	500	8.0
Sicilian *(Progresso)* 'Authentic Pasta Sauces'	1/2 cup	30	660	2.5
Sweet pepper and onion *(Millina's Finest)* organic, fat-free	4 oz	41	305	0.5
Three cheese *(Prego)*	4 oz	100	410	2.0
Tomato and basil				
(Hunt's) 'Classic'	4.409 oz	48	613	2.1
(Millina's Finest) organic, fat-free	4 oz	46	232	0.5
Tomato and herb				
(Ragu) 'Homestyle'	4 oz	110	510	5.0
(Ragu) 'Ragu Fine Italian'	4 oz	90	490	3.0
(Ragu) 'Today's Recipe'	4 oz	50	370	1.0
Tomato chunks *(Hunt's)* 'Chunky Style'	4 oz	50	470	<1.0
Tomato-based				
(Prego) and basil	4 oz	100	370	2.0
(Prego) and onion 'Extra Chunky'	4 oz	110	490	5.0
Tomatoes, garlic, and onion *(Ragu)* 'Chunky Gardenstyle'	4 oz	110	500	5.0
Traditional				
(Contadina) 'Original Recipe'	1/2 cup	90	440	2.3
(Del Monte)	1/2 cup	70	430	2.0
(Healthy Choice)	4 oz	40	380	<1.0
(Hunt's) 'Homestyle'	4.409 oz	56	596	2.6
(Hunt's) 'Light'	4.409 oz	39	421	0.8
(Hunt's) 'Olde Country'	4.409 oz	53	542	2.7
(Hunt's) 'Traditional'	4 oz	70	530	2.0
Zinfandel wine *(Sutter Home)*	1/2 cup	100	520	5.0
PEPPER STEAK SAUCE *(Betty Crocker)* 'Recipe Sauces'	3.8 oz	50	270	2.0
PEPPER-DILL SAUCE *(Golden Dipt)* 'Nature Bay'	2 grams	8	96	0.0

Food Name	Serv. Size	Total Cal.	Sod. MGS	Fat GMS
PESTO SAUCE				
(Contadina) refrigerated 'Fresh'	2.33 oz	350	420	34.0
(DiGiorno) refrigerated	2.3 oz	340	430	32.0
PICANTE SAUCE				
(Estee)	2 tbsp	8	60	0.0
(Gebhardt)	1 tbsp	4	120	0.0
(Wise)	2 tbsp	12	130	0.0
All varieties				
(Old El Paso)	2 tbsp	8	310	<1.0
(Old El Paso) 'Chunky'	2 tbsp	7	270	0.0
Extra mild *(Pace)* 'Thick & Chunky'	2 tsp	3	111	0.1
Hot				
(Chi-Chi's)	1 oz	10	268	2.0
(Guiltless Gourmet)	1 oz	8	133	0.0
(Pace) 'Thick & Chunky'	2 tsp	3	111	0.1
(Rosarita) chunky	3 tbsp	18	515	<1.0
(Rosarita) zesty jalapeño	1.093 oz	8	246	0.2
Medium				
(Chi-Chi's)	1 oz	8	192	2.0
(Guiltless Gourmet)	1 oz	8	133	0.0
(Pace) 'Thick & Chunky'	2 tsp	3	111	0.1
(Rosarita) chunky	3 tbsp	16	650	(mq)
(Rosarita) zesty jalapeño	1.093 oz	9	254	0.2
Mild				
(Azteca)	1 tbsp	4	85	0.0
(Chi-Chi's)	1 oz	9	198	2.0
(Guiltless Gourmet)	1 oz	8	133	0.0
(Hunt's) 'Homestyle'	1.093 oz	11	256	0.2
(Pace) 'Thick & Chunky'	2 tsp	3	111	0.1
(Rosarita)	3.5 oz	45	1015	<1.0
(Rosarita) chunky	3 tbsp	25	630	<1.0
(Rosarita) zesty jalapeño	1.093 oz	8	239	0.1
PIZZA SAUCE				
(Angela Mia)	2.222 oz	27	190	0.6
(Angela Mia) super heavy 'Premium Choice'	2.258 oz	28	36	0.5
(Chef Boyardee) w/cheese	2.63 oz	70	385	4.0
(Chef Boyardee) w/cheese 'Jars'	3.88 oz	90	565	6.0
(Contadina) original 'Quick & Easy'	1/4 cup	30	330	1.0
(Contadina) 'Pizza Squeeze'	1/4 cup	30	330	1.0
(Contadina) w/Italian cheese	1/4 cup	30	380	1.0
(Contadina) w/pepperoni	1/4 cup	40	360	2.0

Food Name	Serv. Size	Total Cal.	Sod. MGS	Fat GMS
(Eden Foods) and pasta sauce, organic	4 oz	80	320	3.0
(Enrico's) 'Homemade Style All Natural'	4 oz	60	(mq)	1.0
(Enrico's) 'Homemade Style All Natural No Salt'	4 oz	60	30	1.0
(Hunt's)	2.363 oz	32	416	1.1
(Hunt's)	2.222 oz	21	251	0.5
(Pastorelli) 'Italian Chef'	4 oz	90	430	3.0
(Pizza Quick)	3 tbsp	35	330	2.0
(Pizza Quick) traditional	1.7 oz	35	330	2.0
PLUM SAUCE *(LaChoy)* tangy	1 oz	45	17	0.1
RIB SAUCE *(Dip 'n Joy)* 'Saucy Rib'	1 oz	60	250	0.0
RIGOLLETO SAUCE *(DiGiorno)* refrigerated	5 oz	110	660	8.0
ROBERT SAUCE *(Escoffier)* 'Sauce Robert'	1 tbsp	20	70	0.0
SANDWICH SAUCE				
(Hormel) 'Not-so-Sloppy Sloppy Joe'	2.24 oz	70	730	1.0
(Libby's) 'Sloppy Joe'	2.5 oz	45	na	<1.0
(Manwich)	2.5 oz	40	390	0.0
(Manwich) bold	2.222 oz	62	802	1.1
(Manwich) extra thick and chunky	2.5 oz	60	640	<1.0
(Manwich) Mexican	2.258 oz	26	552	0.2
(Manwich) Mexican 'Sloppy Joe'	2.5 oz	35	460	<1.0
(Manwich) thick and chunky	2.293 oz	44	737	0.5
SEAFOOD COCKTAIL SAUCE *(Heinz)*	1/4 cup	60	680	0.0
SEAFOOD SAUCE				
(Great Impressions) Creole	1 tbsp	21	182	0.1
(Great Impressions) dipping	1 tbsp	17	129	0.7
(Great Impressions) dipping, Polynesian	1 tbsp	38	127	<1.0
SEASONING SAUCE *(A Taste of Thai)*	1 tbsp	15	1760	0.0
SHOYU. See SOY SAUCE.				
SHRIMP SAUCE *(Tone's)* 'Craboil'	1 tsp	10	1	0.6
SOY SAUCE				
shoyu	1 tbsp	9	3314	tr
shoyu, low-sodium	1 tbsp	9	600	tr
tamari	1 tbsp	11	1005	<.1
(Eden Foods) shoyu, organic	1/2 tsp	2	140	0.0
(Eden Foods) shoyu, organic, reduced sodium	1/2 tsp	2	80	0.0
(Kikkoman)	1 tbsp	10	892	tr
(Kikkoman) 'Lite'	1 tbsp	11	600	tr
(LaChoy)	1 tsp	<1	429	0.0
(LaChoy) 'Lite'	1 tsp	<1	220	0.0
(Westbrae) mild	1/2 tsp	2	85	0.0
(Westbrae) organic	1/2 tsp	2	105	0.0

Food Name	Serv. Size	Total Cal.	Sod. MGS	Fat GMS
(Westbrae) tamari	1/2 tsp	2	170	0.0
(Westbrae) wheat-free	1/2 tsp	3	140	0.0
SPAGHETTI SAUCE. See PASTA SAUCE.				
STEAK SAUCE				
(A.1.)	1 tbsp	18	160	0.0
(A.1.) bold	1 tbsp	18	160	0.0
(Heinz) '57'	1 tbsp	16	190	0.0
(Heinz) hickory smoke '57'	1 tbsp	16	180	0.0
(Heinz) traditional	1 tbsp	12	200	0.0
(Hunt's)	1 tbsp	10	256	0.1
(Lea & Perrins)	1 oz	40	220	<1.0
STIR-FRY SAUCE				
(Kikkoman)	1 tsp	6	120	tr
(LaChoy) Mandarin	4.48 oz	71	851	0.2
(LaChoy) sweet and sour	4.797 oz	146	821	0.1
(LaChoy) Szechwan	4.55 oz	73	612	0.2
(Lawry's)	1/4 cup	120	1128	3.8
STROGANOFF SAUCE (Betty Crocker) 'Recipe Sauces'	4 oz	60	540	4.0
SWEET AND SOUR SAUCE				
(A Taste of Thai) tangy, hot	2 tbsp	30	95	0.0
(Betty Crocker) 'Recipe Sauces'	4.1 oz	130	360	0.0
(Contadina)	1/2 cup	150	430	3.0
(Great Impressions) Hawaiian	2 tbsp	102	<1	0.0
(Great Impressions) hot	2 tbsp	102	<1	0.0
(Great Impressions) regular	2 tbsp	102	<1	0.0
(Hickory Farms) Hawaiian	2 tbsp	102	2	0.0
(Hickory Farms) regular	2 tbsp	102	<1	0.0
(Kikkoman)	1 tbsp	18	63	0.0
(LaChoy)	1 tbsp	30	320	na
(LaChoy) duck sauce	1 tbsp	26	59	tr
(Lawry's)	1/4 cup	549	4056	7.5
(Sauceworks)	1 tbsp	25	50	0.0
SZECHUAN SAUCE (LaChoy) hot and spicy	1 oz	48	141	0.2
TACO SAUCE				
(Estee)	2 tbsp	14	25	0.0
(Hain) and dip	4 tbsp	25	350	1.0
(Lawry's) 'Sauce'n Seasoner'	1/4 cup	40	636	0.6
(Old El Paso)	2 tbsp	15	300	0.0
(Rosarita)	.1764 oz	2	40	0.0
Chunky (Lawry's)	1/4 cup	22	549	0.4
Green (La Victoria)	1 tbsp	0	90	0.0

ood Name	Serv. Size	Total Cal.	Sod. MGS	Fat GMS
Hot				
(Chi-Chi's)	1 oz	18	254	2.0
(Del Monte)	1/4 cup	15	440	0.0
(Old El Paso)	2 tbsp	10	130	<1.0
(Ortega)	1 oz	12	210	0.0
Medium				
(Heinz)	1 tbsp	6	(mq)	0.0
(Old El Paso)	2 tbsp	10	130	<1.0
Mild				
(Del Monte)	1/2 cup	15	480	0.0
(Enrico's) 'No Salt Added'	2 tbsp	14	25	0.0
(Heinz)	1 tbsp	6	(mq)	0.0
(Old El Paso)	2 tbsp	10	130	<1.0
(Ortega)	1 oz	12	220	0.0
Red				
(El Molino) mild	2 tbsp	10	170	0.0
(La Victoria)	1 tbsp	5	80	0.0
Thick, chunky (Chi-Chi's)	1 oz	12	140	2.0
Western style (Ortega)	1 oz	8	180	0.0
TAMARI SAUCE. See SOY SAUCE.				
TARTAR SAUCE				
(Best Foods)	1 tbsp	70	220	8.0
(Best Foods) reduced fat	1 tbsp	30	210	2.0
(Golden Dipt)	1 tbsp	70	100	7.0
(Golden Dipt) 'Lite'	1 tbsp	50	40	4.0
(Great Impressions)	1 tbsp	86	76	9.0
(Heinz)	2 tbsp	140	240	14.0
(Hellmann's)	1 tbsp	70	220	8.0
(Kraft) nonfat 'Free'	1 tbsp	10	120	0.0
(Life) egg-free 'All Natural'	1 tbsp	38	2	4.0
(Sauceworks)	1 tbsp	50	85	5.0
(Sauceworks) natural lemon and herb flavor	1 tbsp	70	85	8.0
(Skipper's)	1 tbsp	65	102	7.0
(Weight Watchers)	1 tbsp	35	80	3.0
TERIYAKI SAUCE				
(Betty Crocker) 'Recipe Sauces'	3.9 oz	60	860	<1.0
(Golden Dipt) ginger marinade	1 oz	120	920	7.0
(Kikkoman)	1 tbsp	15	630	tr
(Kikkoman) 'Baste & Glaze'	1 tbsp	27	420	tr
(LaChoy)	1/2 tsp	5	290	<1.0
(LaChoy) basting sauce	1/2 tsp	2	110	<1.0

Food Name	Serv. Size	Total Cal.	Sod. MGS	Fat GMS
(LaChoy) 'Lite'	1/2 tsp	5	85	<1.0
(LaChoy) 'Sauce and Marinade'	1 oz	30	1640	0.0
(LaChoy) stir-fry sauce	4.621 oz	105	1152	0.1
(LaChoy) thick and rich	1 oz	41	509	0.1
(Lawry's) barbecue marinade	1/8 cup	82	6115	1.1
(Lawry's) w/pineapple juice	1/4 cup	72	7100	0.4
VEGETABLE SAUCE				
(Contadina) refrigerated, garden 'Light'	.5 oz	50	620	0.0
WORCESTERSHIRE SAUCE				
(French's) regular	1 tbsp	10	160	0.0
(French's) smoky	1 tbsp	10	160	0.0
(Heinz)	1 tsp	0	55	0.0
(Lea & Perrins)	1 tsp	5	55	<1.0
(Lea & Perrins) white wine	1 tsp	4	40	<1.0
(Life) 'All Natural'	1/2 tbsp	5	2	<1.0
SAUCE MIX				
ALFREDO SAUCE				
(French's) 'Pasta Toss' dry mix	2 tsp	25	310	2.0
(Lawry's) 'Pasta Alfredo' dry mix	1 pkg	226	3222	13.3
BEARNAISE SAUCE dry mix	.9-oz pkg	90	841	2.2
BEEF SAUTÉ SAUCE *(Lipton)* golden, dry mix	1/6 pkg	120	520	2.0
CHEESE SAUCE				
(French's) prepared	1/4 cup	80	430	4.0
(McCormick/Schilling) dry mix	1/4 pkg	35	477	1.5
(McCormick/Schilling) nacho, dry mix	1/4 pkg	42	409	1.5
CHICKEN SAUCE				
(Lawry's) southwest 'Seasoning Blends' dry mix	1 pkg	71	3947	0.3
(McCormick/Schilling) cacciatore 'Sauce Blends' dry mix	1 pkg	132	1092	4.8
(McCormick/Schilling) Creole 'Sauce Blends' dry mix	1 pkg	140	1084	4.8
(McCormick/Schilling) curry 'Sauce Blends' dry mix	1 pkg	152	1288	5.6
(McCormick/Schilling) Dijon 'Sauce Blends' dry mix	1 pkg	156	1414	6.8
(McCormick/Schilling) mesquite marinade 'Sauce Blends' dry mix	1 pkg	132	2068	3.0
(McCormick/Schilling) teriyaki 'Sauce Blends' dry mix	1 pkg	172	1380	3.6
CURRY SAUCE, prepared	1/2 cup	135	638	7.4
HOLLANDAISE SAUCE *(McCormick/Schilling)* dry mix	1/4 pkg	51	170	3.8
LEMON BUTTER SAUCE *(Weight Watchers)* dry mix	1 tbsp	6	90	0.0
MUSHROOM SAUCE dry mix	1-oz pkg	99	1766	2.7
PASTA SAUCE				
(Estee) prepared w/margarine and skim milk	4 oz	60	30	1.0
(Featherweight) prepared w/margarine and skim milk	4 oz	60	310	1.0

Food Name	Serv. Size	Total Cal.	Sod. MGS	Fat GMS
(French's) cheese and garlic 'Pasta Toss' dry mix	2 tsp	25	320	2.0
(French's) Italian 'Pasta Toss' dry mix	2 tsp	25	340	2.0
(French's) Italian style, prepared	5/8 cup	100	790	4.0
(French's) Romanoff 'Pasta Toss' dry mix	2 tsp	30	310	2.0
(French's) w/mushrooms, prepared	5/8 cup	100	1050	4.0
(Lawry's) 'Rich & Thick' dry mix	1 pkg	147	2172	2.2
(Lawry's) w/imported mushrooms, dry mix	1 pkg	143	2015	1.5
(McCormick/Schilling) dry mix	1/4 pkg	32	615	0.3
(Prego) prepared w/margarine and skim milk	4 oz	130	630	5.0
(Ragu) prepared w/margarine and skim milk	4 oz	80	740	4.0
PEANUT SAUCE (A Taste of Thai) dry mix	2 tbsp	25	115	0.5
PESTO SAUCE (French's) 'Pasta Toss' dry mix	2 tsp	20	280	1.0
SANDWICH SAUCE (Manwich) dry mix	.2469 oz	22	351	0.1
SEAFOOD SAUCE (Progresso) prepared	1/2 cup	110	445	6.0
SOUR CREAM SAUCE (McCormick/Schilling) dry mix	1/4 pkg	44	272	2.8
STROGANOFF SAUCE				
(Lawry's) dry mix	1 pkg	123	2814	0.3
(Natural Touch) prepared	4 oz	90	na	3.0
SWEET AND SOUR SAUCE	2-oz pkg	220	584	0.1
TACO SAUCE (Tio Sancho) 'Dinner Kit' dry mix	2-oz pkg	62	750	0.2
TERIYAKI SAUCE dry mix	1.6-oz pkg	130	4784	0.9
WHITE SAUCE prepared	1/2 cup	121	398	6.7
SAUERKRAUT, CANNED				
(A&P)	1/2 cup	20	800	<1.0
(Allens) w/liquid, shredded	1/2 cup	21	880	<1.0
(Bush's Best) 'Bavarian Kraut'	1/2 cup	60	400	0.0
(Bush's Best) 'Kraut' deli style	1/2 cup	20	680	0.0
(Bush's Best) 'Kraut' shredded	1/2 cup	20	680	0.0
(Claussen)	1/2 cup	17	517	0.2
(Del Monte)	1/2 cup	25	775	0.0
(Eden Foods) organic	1/2 cup	25	580	<1.0
(Finast)	1/2 cup	30	800	0.0
(Pathmark)	1/2 cup	20	880	0.0
(Snow Floss)	1/2 cup	28	780	0.0
(Stokely) 'Bavarian'	1/2 cup	30	780	0.0
(Stokely) w/liquid, shredded and chopped	1/2 cup	20	810	0.0
(Vlasic) 'Old Fashioned'	1 oz	4	280	0.0
SAUERKRAUT JUICE				
canned	1 cup	24	1905	0.0
canned or bottled (Biotta)	6 oz	21	1482	0.1
canned or bottled (S&W)	5 oz	14	1120	0.0

Food Name	Serv. Size	Total Cal.	Sod. MGS	Fat GMS
SAUSAGE. See also individual listings.				
(Hickory Farms) 'Safari'	1 oz	98	343	9.0
(Hillshire Farm) 'Country Recipe'	2 oz	180	490	16.0
(Hormel)	3 oz	290	(mq)	27.0
(JM) .5-oz patties, cooked	1 patty	70	170	6.0
(JM) raw	1 oz	130	180	14.0
(Jones Dairy Farm)	1 patty	155	281	14.4
(Jones Dairy Farm) 'Golden Brown'	1 patty	155	250	14.7
(Jones Dairy Farm) 'Golden Brown' mild	1 link	100	150	9.8
(Jones Dairy Farm) 'Golden Brown' spicy	1 link	100	159	9.5
Brown and serve				
(Eckrich) 'Lean Supreme Heat 'n Serve'	2 links	120	440	10.0
(Hormel)	2 links	140	430	13.0
(Hormel) uncooked	2 links	180	411	17.0
(Jones Dairy Farm) 'Light'	1 link	60	150	4.1
(Swift) 'Country Recipe'	1 link	130	240	12.0
(Swift) 'Country Recipe'	1 patty	130	240	12.0
(Swift) microwave	1 link	120	270	12.0
(Swift) 'Premium Original'	1 link	130	260	12.0
(Swift) 'Premium Original'	1 patty	120	270	12.0
(Swift) smoked flavor	1 link	120	280	11.0
Roll				
(Eckrich) minced	1-oz slice	80	300	7.0
(Jones Dairy Farm) 'Cello Roll'	1 slice	105	200	9.6
BEEF				
(Eckrich)	1 oz	100	270	9.0
(Eckrich) 'Lean Supreme'	1 oz	80	230	7.0
(Eckrich) 'Smok-Y-Links'	2 links	160	350	14.0
(Hillshire Farm) 'Bun Size'	2 oz	180	570	16.0
(Hillshire Farm) 'Flavorseal'	2 oz	180	490	16.0
(Jones Dairy Farm) 'Golden Brown'	1 link	75	159	6.1
(Oscar Mayer) 'Smokies' 1.5-oz links	1 link	124	429	11.0
(Swift) 'Premium Brown 'N Serve'	1 link	120	250	12.0
BEEF AND CHEDDAR (Hillshire Farms) 'Flavorseal'	2 oz	190	500	15.0
CHEESE				
(Hormel) 'Smokie Cheezers'	2 links	168	623	15.0
(Oscar Mayer) 'Smokies'	1.5 oz	126	452	11.2
Hot				
(Eckrich) 'Smok-Y-Links'	2 links	150	360	14.0
(Hillshire Farm) 'Flavorseal'	2 oz	180	510	16.0
Maple-flavored (Eckrich) 'Smok-Y-Links'	2 links	160	390	14.0

Food Name	Serv. Size	Total Cal.	Sod. MGS	Fat GMS
W/ham *(Eckrich)* 'Smok-Y-Links'	2 links	160	500	15.0
HOT				
(JM) .5-oz patties, cooked	1 patty	70	170	6.0
(JM) patties, raw	1 oz	130	180	14.0
(OHSE) 'Hot Links'	1 oz	80	310	3.0
ITALIAN STYLE				
cooked	3 oz	268	765	21.3
cooked	2.4 oz	216	618	17.2
pork, cooked	1 oz	92	261	7.3
pork, raw	1 oz	98	207	8.9
raw	4 oz	391	826	35.4
raw	3.2 oz	315	665	28.5
Hot *(Hillshire Farm)* 'Links'	2 oz	180	(mq)	17.0
Mild *(Hillshire Farm)* 'Links'	2 oz	190	(mq)	17.0
Smoked *(Hillshire Farm)* 'Flavorseal'	2 oz	200	500	18.0
MAPLE-FLAVORED *(Swift)* brown and serve	1 link	120	260	12.0
NEW ENGLAND STYLE				
(Eckrich)	1 oz	35	370	1.0
(Light & Lean)	2 slices	90	(mq)	6.0
(Oscar Mayer) .8-oz slices	1 slice	29	291	1.3
PICKLED				
(Penrose) beer, .5-oz links	1 link	40	220	3.0
(Penrose) firecracker, 1.5-oz links	1 link	120	620	10.0
(Penrose) firecracker, .5-oz links	1 link	40	220	3.0
(Penrose) firecracker, giant, 2.1-oz links	1 link	170	870	14.0
(Penrose) hot, .5-oz links	1 link	40	220	3.0
(Penrose) Polish, .5-oz links	1 link	40	220	3.0
(Penrose) red hot, .5-oz links	1 link	40	220	3.0
POLISH STYLE				
	1 oz	92	248	8.1
10-inch sausage	1 link	740	1989	65.2
PORK				
4-inch links, cooked	1 link	48	168	4.1
4-inch links, raw	1 link	117	187	11.3
fresh, cooked	1 oz	105	367	8.8
fresh, raw	2 oz	238	380	23.0
patties, 1/4 inch x 3 7/8 inch diam, cooked	1 patty	100	349	8.4
patties, 1/4 inch x 3 7/8 inch diam, raw	1 patty	238	380	23.0
(Hormel) 'Little Sizzlers'	2 links	103	172	9.0
(Hormel) 'Little Sizzlers'	1 oz	130	192	13.0
(Hormel) 'Midget Links'	2 links	143	327	13.0

Food Name	Serv. Size	Total Cal.	Sod. MGS	Fat GMS
(Jimmy Dean) cooked	1 oz	120	240	11.0
(Jimmy Dean) links	2 links	180	380	17.0
(Jimmy Dean) 'Light'	1.2 oz	80	230	7.0
(Jimmy Dean) patties	1 patty	140	300	13.0
(JM) 'Tasty Link' cooked	1.4 oz	190	290	18.0
(JM) 'Tasty Link' raw	1.8 oz	260	380	26.0
(Jones Dairy Farm)	1 link	140	176	13.7
(Jones Dairy Farm) 'Golden Brown Light'	1 link	55	132	4.2
(Jones Dairy Farm) 'Light'	1 link	70	232	5.0
(Oscar Mayer) 'Little Friers' cooked	8.9 oz	989	2641	90.3
(Oscar Mayer) 'Little Friers' cooked	1 link	82	219	7.5
(Tyson) country, whole hog	3.5 oz	320	905	29.0
PORK AND BACON *(JM)* 'Tasty Link' raw	1.8 oz	220	340	21.0
PORK AND BEEF				
fresh, cooked	1 oz	112	228	10.3
fresh, 1/4 inch x 3 7/8-inch diam patties, cooked	1 patty	107	217	9.8
fresh, 2 inch x 3/4-inch diam links, cooked	1 link	51	105	4.7
smoked, 4 inch x 1 1/8-inch diam links	1 link	228	643	20.6
smoked, 2 inch x 3/4-inch diam links	1 link	54	151	4.8
smoked, w/flour and nonfat dry milk added, 4 inch x 1 1/8-inch diam links	1 link	182	741	14.6
smoked, w/flour and nonfat dry milk added, 2 inch x 3/4-inch diam links	1 link	43	174	3.4
smoked, w/nonfat dry milk added, 4 inch x 1 1/8-inch diam links	1 link	213	798	18.8
smoked, w/nonfat dry milk added, 2 inch x 3/4-inch diam links	1 link	50	188	4.4
SAGE *(Jimmy Dean)* cooked	1 oz	120	240	11.0
SMOKED				
(Eckrich) 'Lean Supreme'	1 oz	70	230	6.0
(Eckrich) 'Skinless'	1 link	180	420	16.0
(Hillshire Farm) 'Bun Size'	2 oz	180	570	16.0
(Hillshire Farm) 'Flavorseal'	2 oz	190	500	17.0
(Hillshire Farm) 'Links'	2 oz	190	520	18.0
(Hillshire Farm) 'Lite'	2 oz	160	(mq)	13.0
(Hormel) 'Smokies'	2 links	160	597	14.0
(OHSE)	1 oz	80	320	7.0
(Oscar Mayer) 'Big & Juicy Smokie Links' 2.7-oz links	1 link	227	757	20.5
(Oscar Mayer) 'Little Smokies' .3-oz links	1 link	27	92	2.5
(Oscar Mayer) 'Smokie Links' 1.5-oz links	1 link	126	426	11.3
(Pilgrim's Pride)	3 oz	144	890	9.1

Food Name	Serv. Size	Total Cal.	Sod. MGS	Fat GMS
SWEDISH STYLE *(Hickory Farms)*	1 oz	100	380	9.0
TURKEY				
(Butterball)	1 oz	50	250	4.0
(Jimmy Dean) 'Light'	1.2 oz	80	230	7.0
(Louis Rich) cooked	1 link	46	234	2.7
(Louis Rich) 85% fat-free, cooked	24 gm	45	235	3.0
(Norbest) 'Tasti-Lean' chub or links	1 oz	53	179	2.8
Breakfast type				
(Hudson's) ground	1 oz	65	180	5.3
(Louis Rich) 85% fat-free	1 oz	55	230	3.0
(Louis Rich) ground, cooked	1 oz	56	215	3.5
(Mr. Turkey)	1 oz	58	181	4.3
Smoked				
(Louis Rich)	1 oz	43	249	2.4
(Louis Rich) 90% fat-free	1 oz	40	250	2.0
(Louis Rich) w/cheese	1 oz	47	269	2.8
(Louis Rich) w/cheddar, 90% fat-free	1 oz	45	270	3.0
(Mr. Turkey)	1 oz	47	230	3.4
TURKEY AND PORK *(Jimmy Dean)* 'Light'	1.2 oz	80	230	7.0
W/BACON *(Swift)* brown and serve	1 link	120	270	11.0
W/HAM *(Swift)* brown and serve	1 link	130	260	13.0
SAUSAGE, ALTERNATIVE				
(Heartline) 'Italian Sausage Style'	2 oz	176	680	7.0
(Heartline) 'Pepperoni Style' lite	.5 oz	22	135	0.0
Canned *(Worthington)* 'Saucettes'	2 links	140	350	9.0
Frozen				
(Morningstar Farms) links, 'Breakfast Links'	3 links	190	500	14.0
(Morningstar Farms) patties, 'Breakfast Patties'	2 patties	190	710	12.0
(Worthington) links, 'Prosage'	3 links	190	570	14.0
(Worthington) patties, 'Prosage'	2 patties	210	780	14.0
(Worthington) roll, 'Prosage' 3/8-inch slice	2 slices	180	570	12.0
SAUSAGE, CANNED				
(Hormel) hot	1 patty	150	549	13.0
(Hormel) mild	1 patty	150	541	13.0
SAUSAGE SEASONING, pork *(Tone's)*	1 tsp	12	1	0.3
SAUSAGE STICK				
(Hickory Farms) 'Sportsman Stick'	1 oz	138	1075	10.0
BEEF				
(Pemmican) Pepperoni	1.1 oz	170	500	14.0
(Pemmican) Tabasco	1.1 oz	120	410	10.0
(Pemmican) Teriyaki	1.1 oz	150	410	11.0

Food Name	Serv. Size	Total Cal.	Sod. MGS	F G
SMOKED				
(Slim Jim) 'Big Slim'	.52 oz	80	220	7
(Slim Jim) 'Giant Slim'	1.1 oz	180	470	16
(Slim Jim) 'Jumbo Jim'	1 oz	150	430	12
(Slim Jim) 'Super Slim'	.7 oz	110	300	10
Mild (Slim Jim) 'Handi-Paks'	.31 oz	50	130	4
Nacho (Slim Jim) 'Super Slim'	.31 oz	40	160	3
Pepperoni (Slim Jim) 'Handi-Paks'	.31 oz	50	130	4
Spicy				
(Slim Jim) 'Handi-Paks'	.31 oz	50	130	4
(Pemmican)	.8 oz	110	410	10
Tabasco (Slim Jim) 'Handi-Paks'	.31 oz	50	130	4
SUMMER SAUSAGE				
Beef (Hickory Farms)	1 oz	100	345	8
Smoked (Slim Jim)	.5 oz	80	200	7
Teriyaki (Pemmican)	.8 oz	110	410	10
SAUSAGE TACO				
refrigerated (Owens) 'Border Breakfasts'	2.17 oz	190	345	12
SAVORY				
ground	1 oz	77	7	1
ground	1 tbsp	12	1	0
ground	1 tsp	4	0	0
ground (Durkee)	1 tsp	5	0	
ground (Laurel Leaf)	1 tsp	5	0	
ground (Spice Islands)	1 tsp	5	<1	0
SCALLION. See ONION, GREEN.				
SCALLOP, ALTERNATIVE				
canned (Worthington) 'Vegetable Skallops'	1/2 cup	90	430	2
canned (Worthington) 'Vegetable Skallops' no salt	1/2 cup	80	80	1
mixed species, made from surimi	3 oz	84	676	0
SCALLOP, MIXED SPECIES				
breaded, fried	4 oz	244	526	12
fried, frozen (Mrs. Paul's)	3 oz	200	410	8
raw	1 lb	400	730	3
raw	3 oz	75	137	0
raw	1 oz	25	46	0
SCALLOP SQUASH. See SQUASH, SCALLOP.				
SCRAPPLE				
	1 oz	60	268	3
(Jones Dairy Farm)	1 slice	65	165	3
SCOTCH. See ALCOHOLIC BEVERAGES.				

od Name	Serv. Size	Total Cal.	Sod. MGS	Fat GMS
CHAV. See SOUP.				
CREWDRIVER. See ALCOHOLIC BEVERAGES.				
CROD ENTRÉE, FROZEN				
baked 'Microwave Entrees' (Gorton's)	1 pkg	320	420	18.0
CUP/sea bream				
dry-heat cooked	3 oz	115	46	3.0
raw	1 lb	477	191	12.4
raw	3 oz	89	36	2.3
raw	1 oz	30	12	0.8
EA BASS. See BASS, SEA, MIXED SPECIES.				
EA BREAM. See SCUP.				
EA DEVIL. See MONKFISH.				
EA PERCH. See OCEAN PERCH, ATLANTIC.				
EA TROUT. See TROUT, SEA, MIXED SPECIES.				
EAFOOD ENTRÉE, CANNED. See individual listings.				
EAFOOD ENTRÉE, FROZEN. See also individual listings.				
(Armour) w/natural herbs 'Classics Lite'	10 oz	190	1020	2.0
(Budget Gourmet) Newburg	10 oz	350	660	12.0
(Budget Gourmet) scallop and shrimp 'Mariner'	11.5 oz	320	690	9.0
(Cajun Cookin') gumbo	17 oz	330	1330	7.0
(Gorton's) clam 'Crunchy Clam Strips' microwave, 5.8-oz pkg	2.9 oz	270	350	17.0
(Pillsbury) casserole 'Microwave Classic'	1 pkg	420	950	24.0
(Swanson) Creole, w/rice 'Homestyle Recipe'	9 oz	240	810	6.0
EAFOOD FRYING MIX				
(Golden Dipt)	2/3 oz	60	600	0.0
(Golden Dipt) fish fry	2/3 oz	60	430	0.0
(Golden Dipt) fish fry, Cajun style	2/3 oz	60	470	0.0
EAFOOD SALAD. See also individual listings.				
(Longacre) w/crabmeat 'Saladfest'	1 oz	45	130	3.0
EAFOOD SEASONING MIX				
(Featherweight)	1/4 pkg	18	10	0.0
(Golden Dipt) all-purpose	1/4 tsp	2	85	0.0
(Golden Dipt) blackened redfish	1/4 tsp	2	140	0.0
(Golden Dipt) fish, broiled	1/4 tsp	2	125	0.0
(Golden Dipt) lemon pepper	1/4 tsp	8	115	0.0
(Golden Dipt) shrimp and crab, Cajun style	1/4 tsp	2	200	0.0
(Schilling) Chesapeake Bay	1/2 tsp	2	202	0.1
EASONING AND COATING MIX. See also individual listings.				
(Golden Dipt) breading	1 oz	90	630	0.0
(Shake 'N Bake) country mild recipe	1/4 pkt	80	500	4.0

Food Name	Serv. Size	Total Cal.	Sod. MGS
(Shake 'N Bake) Italian herb recipe	1/4 pkt	80	610
For chicken			
(Oven Fry) 'Extra Crispy'	1/4 pkt	120	840
(Oven Fry) 'Home Style Flour Recipe'	1/4 pkt	90	980
(Shake 'N Bake) hot and spicy	1/4 pkt	80	380
(Shake 'N Bake) 'Original Barbecue Recipe'	1/4 pkt	90	840
(Shake 'N Bake) 'Original Recipe'	1/4 pkt	80	450
For fish *(Shake 'N Bake)* 'Original Recipe'	1/4 pkt	70	410
For pork			
(Oven Fry) 'Extra Crispy'	1/8 pkt	60	350
(Shake 'N Bake) hot and spicy	1/8 pkt	45	220
(Shake 'N Bake) 'Original Barbecue Recipe'	1/8 pkt	35	260
(Shake 'N Bake) 'Original Recipe'	1/8 pkt	40	310
SEAWEED			
Dried			
agar	1 oz	87	29
nori	1 lb	158	217
nori	1 oz	10	14
spirulina	1 oz	82	297
Raw			
agar	1 lb	116	40
agar	1 oz	7	3
Irish moss	1 lb	222	303
Irish moss	1 oz	14	19
kelp	1 lb	195	1056
kelp	100 gm	43	233
kelp	1 oz	12	66
laver	1 lb	158	217
laver	100 gm	35	48
laver	1 oz	10	14
spirulina	1 lb	120	444
spirulina	1 oz	8	28
wakame	1 lb	206	3957
wakame	1 oz	13	247
SELTZER. See SOFT DRINKS AND MIXERS.			
SEMOLINA			
enriched	1/2 cup	311	6
unenriched	1/2 cup	109	1
whole grain	1 cup	602	2
whole grain	1 oz	102	<1

Food Name	Serv. Size	Total Cal.	Sod. MGS	Fat GMS
SESAME BUTTER. See also TAHINI MIX.				
gourmet *(Roaster Fresh)*	1 oz	168	3	15.0
made from raw and stone ground kernels	1 oz	162	21	13.6
made from raw and stone ground kernels	1 tbsp	86	11	7.2
made from roasted kernels	1 oz	169	33	15.3
made from roasted kernels	1 tbsp	89	17	8.1
made from unroasted kernels	1 oz	172	0	16.0
made from unroasted kernels	1 tbsp	85	0	7.9
organic *(Arrowhead Mills)*	1 oz	170	<1	17.0
organic, Mid-Eastern *(Westbrae)*	2 tbsp	220	na	20.0
organic 'Natural' *(Westbrae)*	2 tbsp	220	35	19.0
paste	1 oz	169	3	14.4
paste	1 tbsp	95	2	8.1
SESAME FLOUR				
high-fat	1 oz	149	12	10.5
low-fat	1 oz	95	11	0.5
partially defatted	1 oz	108	12	3.4
SESAME MEAL, partially defatted	1 oz	161	11	13.6
SESAME OIL				
	1/2 cup	964	0	109.0
	1 oz	251	0	28.4
	1 tbsp	120	0	13.6
(Eden Foods) hot pepper	1 tbsp	120	0	14.0
(Eden Foods) toasted	1 tbsp	120	0	14.0
(Eden Foods) unrefined	1 tbsp	120	0	14.0
(Hain)	1 tbsp	120	0	14.0
(Spectrum Naturals)	1 tbsp	120	0	14.0
(Spectrum Naturals) unrefined	1 tbsp	120	0	14.0
SESAME SEASONING				
(Schilling) all-purpose 'Parsley Patch'	1 tsp	15	2	1.0
SESAME SEED/sim sim				
Decorticated				
dried	1 tbsp	47	3	4.4
dried	1 tsp	16	1	1.5
Kernels				
dried	1 cup	882	59	82.2
dried	1 oz	167	11	15.5
dried	1 tbsp	47	3	4.4
dried	1 tsp	16	1	1.5
dried *(Arrowhead Mills)*	1 oz	160	3	14.0
dried, toasted	1 oz	161	11	13.6

Food Name	Serv. Size	Total Cal.	Sod. MGS	Fat GMS
Whole				
dried	1 lb	2598	51	225.3
dried	1 cup	825	16	71.5
dried	1 oz	162	3	14.1
dried	1 tbsp	52	1	4.5
dried *(Arrowhead Mills)*	1 oz	160	4	14.0
dried *(Durkee)*	1 tsp	13	0	<0.1
dried *(Laurel Leaf)*	1 tsp	13	0	<0.1
roasted	1 oz	160	3	13.6
SESAME STICKS				
(Barbara's Bakery)	1 oz	130	255	4.0
(Flavor Tree)	1/4 cup	133	358	9.1
(Flavor Tree) 'No Salt'	1/4 cup	131	7	8.1
SHAKE 'N BAKE. See SEASONING AND COATING MIX.				
SHALLOT				
freeze-dried	1 oz	99	17	0.1
freeze-dried	1/4 cup	13	2	0.0
freeze-dried	1 tbsp	3	1	0.0
raw	100 gm	72	12	0.1
raw	1 tbsp	7	1	0.0
raw, trimmed	1 oz	20	3	<.1
raw, untrimmed	1 lb	287	48	0.4
SHARK				
Mako, boneless steak, raw *(Peter Pan Seafoods)*	3.5 oz	87	79	1.2
Mixed species				
batter-dipped, fried	3 oz	194	104	11.7
raw	1 lb	591	360	20.5
raw	3 oz	110	67	3.8
raw	1 oz	37	22	1.3
SHEANUT OIL				
	1/2 cup	964	0	109.0
	1 oz	251	0	28.4
	1 tbsp	120	0	13.6
SHEEPSHEAD/California sheepshead/fathead/redhead				
baked	6.6-oz fillet	234	136	3.0
baked	4 oz	143	83	1.8
baked	3 oz	107	62	1.4
broiled	6.6-oz fillet	234	136	3.0
broiled	4 oz	143	83	1.8
microwaved	6.6-oz fillet	234	136	3.0
microwaved	4 oz	143	83	1.8

Food Name	Serv. Size	Total Cal.	Sod. MGS	Fat GMS
raw	1 lb	490	324	10.9
raw	3 oz	92	60	2.0
raw	1 oz	31	20	0.7
roasted	4 oz	143	83	1.8
SHERBET. See also FRUIT BAR, FROZEN; ICE BARS AND DESSERTS; SORBET.				
all flavors (Sealtest)	1/2 cup	130	30	1.0
orange	1/2 cup	132	44	1.9
orange	1 oz	40	13	0.6
orange (Borden)	1/2 cup	110	40	1.0
orange (Darigold)	1/2 cup	120	25	1.0
vanilla-orange 'Cubic Scoops' (Sealtest)	4 oz	130	40	4.0
vanilla-red raspberry 'Cubic Scoops' (Sealtest)	4 oz	130	40	4.0
SHERBET BAR				
all flavors 'Fat-Free' (Fudgsicle)	1 bar	70	45	0.0
all flavors 'Sugar-Free' (Fudgsicle)	1 bar	35	50	1.0
chocolate (Fudgsicle)	1 bar	70	70	1.0
chocolate, w/nuts 'Sugar-Free Fudge Nut Dip' (Fudgsicle)	1 bar	130	40	8.0
orange	2.75-oz bar	91	30	1.3
w/cream, all flavors 'Sugar-Free' (Creamsicle)	1 bar	25	20	1.0
SHORT RIBS ENTRÉE, FROZEN				
(Armour) boneless 'Classics'	9.75 oz	380	790	16.0
(Stouffer's) in gravy	9 oz	350	900	20.0
(Tyson) 'Gourmet Selection'	11 oz	470	950	24.0
SHORTENING				
COMMERCIAL				
hydrogenated soybean oil and cottonseed oil	1 cup	1812	0	205.0
hydrogenated soybean oil and cottonseed oil	1 tbsp	113	0	12.8
lard and vegetable oil	1 cup	1845	0	205.0
lard and vegetable oil	1 tbsp	115	0	12.8
(Wesson) 'Crystal'	1 tbsp	122	0	13.5
(Wesson) 'Lo-Melt'	1 tbsp	122	0	13.5
(Wesson) 'Super'	1 tbsp	122	0	13.5
(Wesson) 'Wesgold'	1 tbsp	122	0	13.5
(Wesson) 'Wespour'	1 tbsp	122	0	13.5
For baking				
hydrogenated soybean, palm, and cottonseed oils	1 cup	1812	0	205.0
hydrogenated soybean, palm, and cottonseed oils	1 tbsp	113	0	12.8
For bread				
hydrogenated soybean oil and cottonseed oil	1 cup	1812	0	205.0
hydrogenated soybean oil and cottonseed oil	1 tbsp	113	0	12.8

Food Name	Serv. Size	Total Cal.	Sod. MGS	Fat GMS
For cakes and frostings				
hydrogenated soybean and cottonseed oils	1 cup	1812	0	205.0
hydrogenated soybean and cottonseed oils	1 tbsp	113	0	12.8
hydrogenated soybean oil	1 cup	1812	0	205.0
hydrogenated soybean oil	1 tbsp	113	0	12.8
For confectionery				
fractionated palm oil	1 cup	1927	0	218.0
fractionated palm oil	1 tbsp	120	0	13.6
hydrogenated coconut and/or palm kernel oil	1 cup	1812	0	205.0
hydrogenated coconut and/or palm kernel oil	1 tbsp	113	0	12.8
Heavy duty, for frying				
beef tallow and cottonseed oil	1 cup	1845	0	205.0
beef tallow and cottonseed oil	1 tbsp	115	0	12.8
hydrogenated palm oil	1 cup	1812	0	205.0
hydrogenated palm oil	1 tbsp	113	0	12.8
hydrogenated soybean and cottonseed oils	1 cup	1812	0	205.0
hydrogenated soybean and cottonseed oils	1 tbsp	113	0	12.8
hydrogenated soybean oil, 30% linoleic	1 cup	1812	0	205.0
hydrogenated soybean oil, 30% linoleic	1 tbsp	113	0	12.8
hydrogenated soybean oil, under 1% linoleic	1 cup	1812	0	205.0
hydrogenated soybean oil, under 1% linoleic	1 tbsp	113	0	12.8
Multi-purpose				
hydrogenated soybean and palm oils	1 cup	1812	0	205.0
hydrogenated soybean and palm oils	1 tbsp	113	0	12.8
HOUSEHOLD				
hydrogenated soybean and cottonseed oils	1 cup	1812	0	205.0
hydrogenated soybean and cottonseed oils	1 tbsp	113	0	12.8
hydrogenated soybean oil and palm oil	1 cup	1812	0	205.0
hydrogenated soybean oil and palm oil	1 tbsp	113	0	12.8
lard and vegetable oil	1 cup	1845	0	205.0
lard and vegetable oil	1 tbsp	115	0	12.8
(Crisco) vegetable	1 tbsp	110	0	12.0
(Crisco) vegetable, butter flavor	1 tbsp	110	0	12.0
(Finast) vegetable	1 tbsp	110	0	13.0
(Finast) vegetable, butter flavor	1 tbsp	110	0	12.0
(Wesson)	1 tbsp	100	0	12.0
SHOYU. See SAUCE, SOY.				
SHRIMP, ALTERNATIVE				
made from surimi	1 lb	458	3198	6.7
made from surimi	1 oz	29	200	0.4
made from surimi	3 oz	86	599	1.3

Food Name	Serv. Size	Total Cal.	Sod. MGS	Fat GMS
SHRIMP, MIXED SPECIES				
boiled	4 oz	112	254	1.2
boiled, .8-oz size	4 shrimp	22	49	0.2
breaded, fried	3 oz	206	292	10.4
breaded, fried	1.1 oz	73	103	3.7
breaded, fried, .8-oz size	4 shrimp	73	103	3.7
fried	4 oz	274	390	13.9
moist-heat cooked	3 oz	84	190	0.9
moist-heat cooked, .8-oz size	4 shrimp	22	49	0.2
poached	4 oz	112	254	1.2
poached, .8-oz size	4 shrimp	22	49	0.2
raw	1 lb	481	673	7.8
raw	3 oz	90	126	1.5
raw, .8-oz size	4 shrimp	30	41	0.5
steamed	4 oz	112	254	1.2
steamed, .8-oz size	4 shrimp	22	49	0.2
Canned				
drained	1 cup	154	216	2.5
drained	3 oz	102	144	1.7
drained	4 oz	136	192	2.2
drained (Louisiana Brand)	2 oz	58	(mq)	1.0
large, drained (ShopRite)	2 oz	50	720	1.0
SHRIMP CHOW MEIN, canned				
(LaChoy)	3/4 cup	35	940	1.0
(LaChoy) 'Bi-Pack'	8.536 oz	60	935	1.0
(LaChoy) 'Bi-Pack'	3/4 cup	50	860	1.0
SHRIMP COCKTAIL				
(Booth) w/garlic butter sauce and vegetable rice	10 oz	400	750	25.0
(Budget Gourmet) w/fettuccine	9.5 oz	375	660	20.0
(LaChoy) w/lobster sauce 'Fresh & Lite'	10 oz	240	946	6.2
(Mrs. Paul's) w/clams and linguini 'Light'	10 oz	240	750	5.0
(Sau-Sea)	4 oz	113	1020	1.0
(SeaPak) 'Super Valu' heat and serve	4 oz	210	730	4.0
SHRIMP ENTRÉE, FROZEN				
BAY, BABY (Armour) 'Classics Lite'	9.75 oz	220	890	6.0
BATTERED				
(SeaPak) 'Shrimp 'n Batter'	4 oz	260	470	15.0
(SeaPak) w/crabmeat stuffing	4 oz	260	780	13.0
BREADED				
(Gorton's) original seasoning	2.7 oz	200	450	12.0
(Gorton's) popcorn style	2.7 oz	220	450	14.0

Food Name	Serv. Size	Total Cal.	Sod. MGS	Fat GMS
(Gorton's) scampi seasoning	2.7 oz	210	440	12.0
(Mrs. Paul's) fried	3 oz	200	430	11.0
BUTTERFLY				
(Gorton's) 'Specialty'	4 oz	160	540	<1.0
(SeaPak) breaded 'Mikado'	4 oz	160	170	1.0
BUTTERFLY/ROUND (SeaPak) breaded	4 oz	150	(mq)	1.0
CAJUN STYLE (Mrs. Paul's) 'Light'	9 oz	230	740	5.0
CREOLE				
(Armour) 'Classics Lite'	11.25 oz	260	900	2.0
(Cajun Cookin')	12 oz	390	1130	11.0
(Healthy Choice)	11.25 oz	230	430	2.0
CRISP (Gorton's) 'Specialty'	4 oz	280	740	15.0
CRUNCHY				
(Gorton's) 'Crunchy Shrimp' microwave	2 oz	160	380	9.0
(Gorton's) whole 'Microwave Specialty'	5 oz	380	870	20.0
ETOUFFEE (Cajun Cookin')	17 oz	360	1170	9.0
FETTUCCINE ALFREDO (Booth)	10 oz	260	620	8.0
JAMBALAYA (Cajun Cookin')	12 oz	450	800	20.0
MARINARA				
(Healthy Choice)	10.5 oz	260	320	1.0
(Smart Ones) w/linguini	8 oz	150	390	<1.0
NEW ORLEANS, w/wild rice (Booth)	10 oz	230	950	5.0
ORIENTAL, w/pineapple rice (Booth)	10 oz	190	950	3.0
PRIMAVERA				
(Booth) w/fettucini	10 oz	200	760	3.0
(Mrs. Paul's) 'Light'	9.5 oz	180	840.	3.0
(Right Course)	9 5/8 oz	240	590	7.0
SCAMPI (Gorton's) 'Microwave Entrées'	1 pkg	390	470	30.0
STIR-FRY (Shanghai)	10.3 oz	170	1200	2.0
SHRIMP ENTRÉE, PACKAGED				
(Ultra Slim Fast) creole	12 oz	240	730	4.0
(Ultra Slim Fast) marinara	12 oz	290	880	3.0
SHRIMP PASTE, canned	1 tsp	13	10	0.7
SHRIMP SALAD				
(Longacre) 'Saladfest'	1 oz	45	150	3.0
(Longacre) 'Saladfest' w/seafood	1 oz	42	160	3.0

SICAMA. See JICAMA.

SILVER HAKE. See WHITING, MIXED SPECIES.

SIM SIM. See SESAME SEED.

SKIL. See SABLEFISH.

SKUNK CABBAGE. See CABBAGE, SKUNK.

Food Name	Serv. Size	Total Cal.	Sod. MGS	Fat GMS
SLIMEHEAD. See ORANGE ROUGHY.				
SLOPPY JOE SEASONING MIX				
(French's)	1/8 pkg	16	390	0.0
(Lawry's) 'Seasoning Blends'	1 pkg	126	3442	0.4
(Schilling)	1/4 pkg	26	750	0.5
SMELT, RAINBOW				
broiled	4 oz	141	87	3.5
dry-heat cooked	4 oz	141	87	3.5
dry-heat cooked	3 oz	105	65	2.6
microwaved	4 oz	141	87	3.5
raw	1 lb	440	272	11.0
raw	3 oz	82	51	2.1
raw	1 oz	27	17	0.7
SNACK. See CORN CHIPS AND SNACKS; POTATO CHIPS AND SNACKS; SNACK BAR; SNACK MIX.				
SNACK BAR. See also DIET BAR.				
(Barbara's Bakery)				
apple, real fruit, .5 oz	1 bar	50	0	0.0
apricot, real fruit, .5 oz	1 bar	50	0	0.0
cherry, real fruit, .5 oz	1 bar	50	0	0.0
grape, real fruit, .5 oz	1 bar	50	0	0.0
raspberry, real fruit, .5 oz	1 bar	50	1	0.0
(Bear Valley)				
carob-cocoa, food bar 'Pemmican'	3.75 oz	440	80	12.0
coconut almond, food bar 'Meal Pack'	3.75 oz	400	80	12.0
fruit 'n nut, food bar 'Pemmican'	3.75 oz	420	90	13.0
sesame lemon, food bar 'Meal Pack'	3.75 oz	410	85	13.0
(Carnation)				
chocolate chip, breakfast bar	1 bar	200	180	11.0
chocolate crunch, breakfast bar	1 bar	190	150	10.0
peanut butter chocolate chip, breakfast bar	1 bar	200	170	11.0
peanut butter crunch, breakfast bar	1 bar	190	180	10.0
(Earth Grains)				
banana apple walnut 'Bagel Power Bar'	1 bar	270	280	6.0
citrus almond w/mixed fruit 'Bagel Power Bar'	1 bar	260	280	4.0
fruit and nut 'Bagel Power Bar'	1 bar	240	280	3.0
(Glenny's)				
apple-cinnamon	1.25 oz	120	15	<1.0
caramel	1.25 oz	120	65	<1.0
chocolate	1.25 oz	120	20	<1.0
raspberry	1.25 oz	120	15	<1.0

Food Name	Serv. Size	Total Cal.	Sod. MGS	Fat GMS
(Health Valley)				
apple, fat-free	1 bar	140	10	0.0
'Apple Bakes'	1 bar	100	27	3.0
apricot, fat-free	1 bar	140	10	0.0
date, fat-free	1 bar	140	10	0.0
'Date Bakes'	1 bar	100	25	3.0
'Fruit & Fitness'	1 bar	200	234	3.0
'Oat Bran, Fig & Nut Bakes'	1 bar	110	18	3.0
oat bran, raisin, and cinnamon	1 bar	140	12	2.0
'Oat Bran Apricot Bakes'	1 bar	100	18	2.0
'Oat Bran Jumbo Fruit and Nut Bars'	1 bar	150	11	4.0
'Oat Bran Jumbo Fruit Bars'	1 bar	170	9	5.0
raisin, fat-free	1 bar	140	10	0.0
'Raisin Bakes'	1 bar	100	19	3.0
rice bran, almond, and date	1 bar	190	6	6.0
(Kudos)				
peaches and cream 'Pan Squares'	1 square	150	105	6.0
peanut butter and chocolate chip 'Pan Squares'	1 square	170	105	9.0
strawberry and cream cheese 'Pan Squares'	1 square	150	105	6.0
(Tiger's Milk) peanut butter and honey, carob coated	1 bar	160	90	5.0
(Weider)				
'Sportsfood Enerquench Bar'	1 bar	200	80	1.0
'Sportsfood Protein Bar'	1 bar	160	140	4.0
SNACK BAR MIX, PREPARED				
(Betty Crocker)				
caramel oatmeal 'Supreme Dessert'	1 bar	110	65	5.0
chocolate and toffee 'Supreme Dessert'	1 bar	110	55	4.0
chocolate peanut butter 'Supreme Dessert'	1 bar	110	100	5.0
date 'Classic'	1 bar	60	35	2.0
lemon-Sunkist 'Supreme Dessert' prepared w/4 eggs	1 bar	110	65	4.0
M&M cookie bars 'Supreme Dessert'	1 bar	110	80	5.0
raspberry 'Supreme Dessert'	1 bar	100	95	4.0
SNACK MIX				
(Doo Dads) original recipe, 1 oz	1/2 cup	129	360	5.2
(Flavor Tree)				
'Party Mix'	1/4 cup	163	407	11.0
'Party Mix No Salt'	1 1/2 cup	163	8	10.8
(Pepperidge Farm)				
cheese, super cheddar 'Goldfish Party Mix'	1 oz	140	330	7.0
'Classic'	1 oz	140	360	8.0
lightly smoked	1 oz	150	350	9.0

Food Name	Serv. Size	Total Cal.	Sod. MGS	Fat GMS
nutty deluxe, cashews and almonds 'Goldfish'	1/2 cup	180	330	9.0
original, honey roasted peanuts 'Goldfish'	1/2 cup	170	360	8.0
spicy	1 oz	140	340	8.0
(Ralston)				
barbecue 'Chex' 2/3 cup	1 oz	130	380	5.0
'Chex Traditional' 2/3 cup	1 oz	120	288	4.9
cool sour cream and onion 'Chex' 2/3 cup	1 oz	130	300	5.0
golden cheddar 'Chex' 2/3 cup	1 oz	130	300	5.0
nacho cheese 'Chex' 2/3 cup	1 oz	130	430	5.0
(Ritz) traditional, baked	1 oz	130	310	6.0
SNAPPER, RED, MIXED SPECIES				
broiled	4 oz	145	65	2.0
dry-heat cooked	4 oz	145	65	2.0
dry-heat cooked	3 oz	109	48	1.5
microwaved	4 oz	145	65	2.0
raw	1 lb	452	291	6.1
raw	3 oz	85	54	1.1
raw	1 oz	28	18	0.4
SNOW PEAS. See PEAS, SNOW.				
SOBA NOODLE. See NOODLE, JAPANESE.				
SODA. See SOFT DRINKS AND MIXERS.				
SOFT DRINKS AND MIXERS. See also WATER, SPARKLING, FLAVORED.				
(A&W)				
cream soda	1 oz	14	2	tr
cream soda, 'Diet'	1 oz	<1	4	<.1
root beer	1 oz	15	5	<.1
root beer, 'Diet'	1 oz	<1	4	tr
(Canada Dry)				
collins mixer	8 oz	80	17	0.0
ginger ale	8 oz	90	7	0.0
ginger ale, 'Golden'	8 oz	100	24	0.0
grape, 'Concord'	8 oz	130	21	0.0
half and half	8 oz	110	17	0.0
tonic	8 oz	90	7	0.0
whiskey sour mixer	8 oz	90	17	0.0
(Coca Cola)				
cherry cola	6 oz	76	4	0.0
cherry cola, 'Diet'	6 oz	<1	4	0.0
cola, caffeine-free	6 oz	77	4	0.0
cola, 'Classic'	6 oz	72	7	0.0
cola, diet, caffeine-free	6 oz	<1	4	0.0

Food Name	Serv. Size	Total Cal.	Sod. MGS	Fat GMS
cola, diet, w/caffeine	6 oz	<1	4	0.0
cola, w/caffeine	6 oz	77	4	0.0
(Dr. Diablo) cola	12 oz	140	14	0.0
(Dr. Pepper)				
cola	12 oz	150	18	0.0
cola, caffeine-free	12 oz	150	18	0.0
diet	12 oz	3	18	0.0
diet, caffeine-free	12 oz	3	18	0.0
(Fanta)				
ginger ale	6 oz	63	14	0.0
grape	6 oz	86	7	0.0
orange	6 oz	88	7	0.0
root beer	6 oz	78	10	0.0
(Fresca) citrus	6 oz	2	tr	0.0
(Health Valley)				
ginger ale	12 oz	153	30	1.0
root beer, 'Old Fashioned'	12 oz	120	12	1.0
root beer, sarsaparilla	12 oz	153	27	1.0
wild berry	12 oz	142	27	1.0
(Hires)				
cream soda, caffeine-free	6 oz	90	40	<1.0
cream soda, 'Diet' caffeine-free	6 oz	2	45	<1.0
root beer, caffeine-free	6 oz	90	55	<1.0
root beer, 'Diet' caffeine-free, w/NutraSweet	6 oz	2	70	<1.0
(Jolt) cola	6 oz	85	10	0.0
(Mello Yello)				
citrus	6 oz	87	14	0.0
citrus, diet	6 oz	3	<1	0.0
(Mountain Dew)				
citrus	12 oz	179	31	0.0
citrus, diet	12 oz	4	<1	0.0
(Mr. Pibb) cola	6 oz	71	10	0.0
(Mug)				
root beer	12 oz	168	39	0.0
root beer, 'Diet'	12 oz	4	39	0.0
(Natural 90 Diet) all flavors	6 oz	2	10	0.0
(Pathmark) cola, 'No Frills Sugar-free'	8 oz	0	(mq)	0.0
(Pepsi)				
cherry cola, 'Diet Wild Cherry'	12 oz	1	2	0.0
cherry cola, 'Wild Cherry'	12 oz	163	2	0.0
cola, caffeine-free	12 oz	160	2	0.0

Food Name	Serv. Size	Total Cal.	Sod. MGS	Fat GMS
cola, clear 'Diet Crystal' w/NutraSweet	6 oz	0	35	0.0
cola, diet, caffeine-free	12 oz	<1	2	0.0
cola, diet, w/caffeine	12 oz	<1	2	0.0
cola, 'Light'	12 oz	<1	2	0.0
cola, w/caffeine	12 oz	160	2	0.0
(Santa Cruz Naturals) ginger ale, organic 'Sparkling'	8 oz	155	na	<1.0
(Schweppes)				
blackberry, 'Royal'	6 oz	35	5	0.0
citrus, tropical 'Royal'	6 oz	35	5	0.0
club soda	6 oz	0	25	0.0
collins mixer	6 oz	75	51	0.0
ginger ale	6 oz	65	10	0.0
ginger ale, raspberry	6 oz	65	10	0.0
ginger ale, raspberry 'Diet'	6 oz	2	55	0.0
ginger ale, 'Sugar-free'	6 oz	2	39	0.0
ginger beer	6 oz	70	30	0.0
grape	6 oz	95	15	0.0
grapefruit	6 oz	80	28	0.0
kiwi-passion fruit, 'Royal'	6 oz	35	5	0.0
lemon, bitter	6 oz	82	13	0.0
lemon, sour	6 oz	79	12	0.0
lemon-lime	6 oz	72	30	0.0
orange, sparkling	6 oz	88	17	0.0
peaches and cream, 'Royal'	6 oz	35	5	0.0
root beer	6 oz	76	17	0.0
seltzer, all flavors	6 oz	0	5	0.0
seltzer, 'Low Sodium'	6 oz	0	7	0.0
seltzer, 'Sodium-free'	6 oz	0	5	0.0
strawberry-banana, 'Royal'	6 oz	35	5	0.0
tonic	6 oz	64	8	0.0
tonic, 'Diet'	6 oz	2	45	0.0
vanilla bean, 'Royal'	6 oz	35	5	0.0
Vichy water	6 oz	0	76	0.0
wild cherry, 'Royal'	6 oz	35	5	0.0
wild raspberry, 'Royal'	6 oz	35	5	0.0
(7•Up)				
cherry citrus	12 oz	148	32	0.0
cherry citrus, diet	12 oz	4	32	0.0
lemon-lime	12 oz	144	32	0.0
lemon-lime, diet	12 oz	4	32	0.0

Food Name	Serv. Size	Total Cal.	Sod. MGS	Fat GMS
(Shasta)				
apple, 'Yoshi Apple'	8 oz	130	30	0.0
berry, 'Luigi Berry'	8 oz	130	30	0.0
black cherry	12 oz	162	29	0.0
cherry, 'Princess Toadstool Cherry'	8 oz	130	30	0.0
cherry cola	12 oz	140	22	0.0
citrus mist	12 oz	170	19	0.0
club soda	12 oz	0	46	0.0
cola	12 oz	147	3	0.0
cola, 'Free'	12 oz	151	2	0.0
collins mixer	12 oz	118	23	0.0
cream soda, 'Creme'	12 oz	154	23	0.0
ginger ale	12 oz	120	23	0.0
grape	12 oz	177	34	0.0
lemon-lime	12 oz	146	19	0.0
orange	12 oz	177	28	0.0
red berry	12 oz	158	20	0.0
root beer	12 oz	154	31	0.0
strawberry	12 oz	147	36	0.0
tonic	12 oz	121	17	0.0
(Slice)				
lemon-lime	12 oz	150	69	0.0
lemon-lime, 'Diet'	12 oz	16	69	0.0
orange, 'Diet'	12 oz	12	2	0.0
orange, Mandarin	12 oz	193	<1	0.0
(Snapple)				
'Amazin' Grape'	8 oz	120	5	0.0
'Cherry Lime Rickey'	8 oz	110	0	0.0
'Creme D'Vanilla'	8 oz	130	0	0.0
'French Cherry'	8 oz	120	0	0.0
'Kiwi Peach'	8 oz	120	0	0.0
'Kiwi Strawberry'	8 oz	130	5	0.0
'Mango Madness'	8 oz	130	5	0.0
'Passion Supreme'	8 oz	120	0	0.0
'Peach Melba'	8 oz	120	0	0.0
'Raspberry'	8 oz	120	0	0.0
'Tru Root Beer'	8 oz	110	0	0.0
(Spree)				
cherry-lime	12 oz	158	2	0.0
cola	12 oz	147	1	0.0
ginger ale	12 oz	120	1	0.0

Food Name	Serv. Size	Total Cal.	Sod. MGS	Fat GMS
grapefruit	12 oz	154	1	0.0
lemon-lime	12 oz	154	1	0.0
lemon-tangerine	12 oz	165	1	0.0
lime, Mandarin	12 oz	154	1	0.0
root beer	12 oz	154	2	0.0
tropical blend	12 oz	146	2	0.0
(Sprite)				
lemon-lime	6 oz	71	23	0.0
lemon-lime, diet	6 oz	2	tr	0.0
(Squirt)				
citrus	1 oz	13	2	tr
citrus, 'Diet'	1 oz	<1	1	tr
citrus berry, 'Ruby Red'	8 oz	120	25	0.0
(Tab)				
cola, caffeine-free	6 oz	<1	4	0.0
cola, w/caffeine	6 oz	<1	4	0.0
(Vernor's)				
ginger	3.5 oz	40	4	0.1
ginger, 'Diet'	3.5 oz	<1	7	0.1
(Wink) grapefruit	8 oz	120	19	0.0
(Yoo-Hoo) chocolate	9 oz	140	130	1.0
SOLE				
dry-heat cooked	3 oz	99	89	1.3
raw	3 oz	77	69	1.0
SOLE, FROZEN				
Dinner *(Healthy Choice)* au gratin	11 oz	270	470	5.0
Entrée				
(Gorton's) in lemon butter 'Microwave Entrees'	1 pkg	380	560	24.0
(Gorton's) seafood stuffed 'Select' approx 5 oz	1 fillet	160	730	3.0
(Healthy Choice) w/lemon butter sauce	8.25 oz	230	430	4.0
Fillet				
(Booth) Atlantic	4 oz	90	180	1.0
(Gorton's) 'Fishmarket Fresh'	5 oz	110	140	1.0
(Mrs. Paul's) breaded 'Light'	1 fillet	240	450	10.0
(SeaPak)	4 oz	90	135	1.0
(Van de Kamp's) breaded 'Light'	1 fillet	250	480	12.0
(Van de Kamp's) 'Natural'	4 oz	100	105	2.0

SOMEN NOODLE. See NOODLE, JAPANESE.

SORBET. See also FRUIT BARS, FROZEN; ICE BARS AND DESSERTS; SHERBET.

(Baskin-Robbins)				
fruit whip	1 scoop	80	20	0.0

Food Name	Serv. Size	Total Cal.	Sod. MGS	Fat GMS
red raspberry	1 scoop	140	25	0.0
(Cascadian Farms)				
blackberry	1 oz	25	na	0.1
raspberry	1 oz	28	na	0.2
strawberry	1 oz	26	na	0.1
(Dole)				
Mandarin orange	4 oz	110	9	0.1
peach	4 oz	120	11	0.6
pineapple	4 oz	120	11	0.1
raspberry	4 oz	110	12	<.1
strawberry	4 oz	110	1	0.1
(Frusen Glädjé) raspberry	1/2 cup	140	10	0.0
(Häagen Dazs)				
blueberry, and vanilla ice cream	1/2 cup	190	35	8.0
Key lime, and vanilla ice cream	1/2 cup	200	30	7.0
lemon 'Ice Cream Shop'	4 oz	140	5	0.0
orange, and vanilla ice cream	1/2 cup	190	35	8.0
orange 'Ice Cream Shop'	4 oz	113	7	0.0
raspberry, and vanilla ice cream	1/2 cup	180	35	8.0
raspberry 'Ice Cream Shop'	4 oz	93	7	0.0
SORGHUM				
broomcorn, whole grain	100 gm	327	1	2.9
whole grain	1 cup	650	na	6.3
whole grain	1 oz	96	na	0.9
SORGHUM SYRUP				
	1/2 cup	424	na	0.0
	1 tbsp	53	na	0.0
SORREL				
boiled, drained	4 oz	23	3	0.7
raw, trimmed	1 oz	6	1	0.2
raw, trimmed, chopped	1/2 cup	15	3	0.5
raw, untrimmed	1 lb	70	13	2.2
SOUP, CANNED, CONDENSED				
(NOTE: Unless otherwise specified, PREPARED = prepared as directed w/water.)				
ASPARAGUS, CREAM OF				
prepared	1 cup	87	2.3	.7
prepared w/whole milk	8 oz	161	1042	8.2
unprepared	10.75 oz	210	2385	9.9
(Campbell's) prepared	8 oz	80	820	4.0
BEAN				
(Campbell's) 'Homestyle' prepared	8 oz	130	700	1.0

Food Name	Serv. Size	Total Cal.	Sod. MGS	Fat GMS
W/bacon				
(Campbell's) 'Healthy Request'	4 oz	140	470	4.0
(Campbell's) 'Healthy Request' prepared	8 oz	140	470	4.0
(Campbell's) prepared	8 oz	140	840	4.0
W/frankfurters				
prepared	1 cup	188	1093	7.0
unprepared	11.25 oz	455	2653	16.9
W/pork				
prepared	1 cup	172	951	5.9
unprepared	11.5 oz	418	2309	14.4
BEEF				
(Campbell's) prepared	8 oz	80	830	2.0
W/bouillon (Campbell's) prepared	8 oz	16	820	0.0
W/broth (Campbell's) prepared	8 oz	16	820	0.0
W/vegetables (Campbell's) 'Healthy Request'	4 oz	70	490	2.0
BEEF MUSHROOM				
prepared	1 cup	73	942	3.0
unprepared	10.75 oz	186	2358	7.3
BEEF NOODLE				
prepared	1 cup	83	952	3.1
unprepared	10.75 oz	204	2315	7.5
(Campbell's) prepared	8 oz	70	830	3.0
(Campbell's) 'Homestyle' prepared	8 oz	80	810	4.0
W/ground beef (Campbell's) prepared	8 oz	90	820	4.0
BLACK BEAN				
prepared	1 cup	116	1198	1.5
unprepared	11 oz	282	2910	3.7
BROCCOLI, CREAM OF				
(Campbell's) prepared	8 oz	80	790	5.0
(Campbell's) prepared w/whole milk	8 oz	140	850	7.0
CELERY, CREAM OF				
prepared	1 cup	90	949	5.6
prepared w/whole milk	1 cup	164	1009	9.7
unprepared	10.75 oz	220	2309	13.6
(Campbell's) prepared	8 oz	100	820	7.0
CHEESE				
prepared	1 cup	156	958	10.5
prepared w/whole milk	1 cup	231	1019	14.6
unprepared	11 oz	378	2331	25.4
Cheddar (Campbell's) prepared	8 oz	110	810	6.0

Food Name	Serv. Size	Total Cal.	Sod. MGS	Fat GMS
Nacho				
(Campbell's) prepared	8 oz	110	740	8.0
(Campbell's) prepared w/whole milk	8 oz	180	800	12.0
CHICKEN				
W/barley (Campbell's) prepared	8 oz	70	850	2.0
W/dumplings				
prepared	1 cup	96	860	5.5
unprepared	10.5 oz	235	2095	13.4
(Campbell's) 'Chicken 'n Dumplings' prepared	8 oz	80	960	3.0
W/rice				
prepared	1 cup	60	815	1.9
unprepared	10.5 oz	146	1982	4.7
(Campbell's) prepared	8 oz	60	790	3.0
(Campbell's) 'Healthy Request'	4 oz	60	480	2.0
(Campbell's) 'Healthy Request' prepared	8 oz	60	480	3.0
CHICKEN, CREAM OF				
prepared	1 cup	117	986	7.4
unprepared	10.75 oz	284	2397	17.9
(Campbell's) prepared	8 oz	110	810	7.0
(Campbell's) 'Healthy Request'	4 oz	70	490	2.0
(Campbell's) 'Healthy Request' prepared	8 oz	70	490	2.0
W/broccoli				
(Campbell's)	4 oz	110	710	7.0
(Campbell's) prepared	8 oz	110	710	7.0
CHICKEN BROTH				
prepared	1 cup	39	776	1.4
unprepared	10.75 oz	95	1909	3.2
(Campbell's) prepared	8 oz	30	710	2.0
CHICKEN GUMBO				
prepared	1 cup	56	954	1.4
unprepared	10.75 oz	137	2321	3.5
CHICKEN MUSHROOM				
prepared	1 cup	132	942	9.1
unprepared	10.75 oz	332	2358	22.3
Creamy (Campbell's) prepared	8 oz	120	920	8.0
CHICKEN NOODLE				
prepared	1 cup	75	1106	2.5
unprepared	10.5 oz	182	2256	5.5
(Campbell's) prepared	8 oz	60	900	2.0
(Campbell's) 'Healthy Request'	4 oz	60	460	2.0
(Campbell's) 'Healthy Request' prepared	8 oz	60	440	2.0

Food Name	Serv. Size	Total Cal.	Sod. MGS	Fat GMS
(Campbell's) 'Homestyle' prepared	8 oz	70	880	3.0
Broth and noodles *(Campbell's)* prepared	8 oz	45	860	1.0
Creamy				
(Campbell's)	4 oz	120	800	7.0
(Campbell's) prepared	8 oz	120	800	7.0
(Campbell's) prepared w/2% milk	8 oz	180	850	9.0
Curly noodle *(Campbell's)* prepared	8 oz	80	800	3.0
Double noodle in broth				
(Campbell's)	4 oz	90	700	2.0
(Campbell's) prepared	8 oz	90	700	2.0
Ring noodle *(Campbell's)* 'Noodle-O's' prepared	8 oz	70	820	2.0
CHICKEN VEGETABLE				
prepared	1 cup	75	945	2.8
unprepared	10.5 oz	182	2298	6.9
(Campbell's) prepared	8 oz	70	850	3.0
CHILI BEEF				
prepared	1 cup	170	1035	6.6
unprepared	11.25 oz	412	2514	16.0
(Campbell's) prepared	8 oz	140	840	5.0
CLAM CHOWDER				
Manhattan style				
prepared	1 cup	78	578	2.2
unprepared	10.75 oz	186	1394	5.4
(Campbell's) prepared	8 oz	70	820	2.0
(Campbell's) 'Seashore Soups'	4 oz	70	820	2.0
(Doxsee) prepared	7.5 oz	70	780	2.0
(Snow's)	3.75 oz	70	630	2.0
(Snow's) prepared	7.5 oz	70	780	2.0
New England style				
prepared	8 oz	95	915	2.9
prepared w/whole milk	8 oz	164	992	6.6
(Campbell's) prepared	8 oz	80	870	3.0
(Campbell's) prepared w/whole milk	8 oz	150	930	7.0
(Campbell's) 'Seashore Soups'	4 oz	80	870	3.0
(Gorton's) prepared w/whole milk	1/4 can	140	740	5.0
(Snow's)	3.75 oz	70	620	2.0
(Snow's) prepared w/whole milk	7.5 oz	140	670	6.0
CONSOMMÉ				
Beef	10.5 oz	72	1550	0.0
Beef, w/gelatin				
prepared	1 cup	29	637	0.0

Food Name	Serv. Size	Total Cal.	Sod. MGS	Fat GMS
unprepared	10.5 oz	71	1550	0.0
(Campbell's) prepared	8 oz	25	750	0.0
CORN, CREAM OF, GOLDEN				
(Campbell's)	4 oz	110	700	3.0
(Campbell's) prepared	8 oz	110	700	3.0
(Campbell's) prepared w/2% milk	8 oz	160	760	5.0
CORN CHOWDER, NEW ENGLAND				
(Snow's)	3.75 oz	80	590	2.0
(Snow's) prepared w/whole milk	7.5 oz	150	640	6.0
FISH CHOWDER, NEW ENGLAND				
(Snow's)	3.75 oz	60	560	2.0
(Snow's) prepared w/whole milk	7.5 oz	130	620	6.0
GREEN PEA				
prepared	1 cup	165	988	2.9
prepared w/whole milk	1 cup	239	1046	7.0
unprepared	11.25 oz	399	2399	7.1
(Campbell's) prepared	8 oz	160	820	3.0
MINESTRONE				
prepared	1 cup	82	911	2.5
unprepared	10.5 oz	203	2217	6.1
(Campbell's) prepared	8 oz	80	900	2.0
MUSHROOM				
Beefy *(Campbell's)* prepared	8 oz	60	960	3.0
Golden *(Campbell's)* prepared	8 oz	70	870	3.0
W/beef stock				
prepared	1 cup	85	969	4.0
unprepared	10.75 oz	207	2358	9.8
MUSHROOM, CREAM OF				
prepared	1 cup	129	1032	9.0
prepared w/whole milk	1 cup	203	1076	13.6
unprepared	10.75 oz	314	2470	23.1
(Campbell's) prepared	8 oz	100	820	7.0
(Campbell's) 'Healthy Request'	4 oz	60	480	2.0
(Campbell's) 'Healthy Request' prepared	8 oz	60	480	2.0
MUSHROOM BARLEY				
prepared	1 cup	73	891	2.3
unprepared	10.75 oz	186	2227	5.5
(Rokeach) prepared	1 cup	85	904	0.2
ONION				
prepared	1 cup	58	1053	1.7
unprepared	10.5 oz	137	2563	4.2

Food Name	Serv. Size	Total Cal.	Sod. MGS	Fat GMS
unprepared	8 oz	113	2116	3.5
French *(Campbell's)* prepared	8 oz	60	900	2.0
ONION, CREAM OF				
prepared	1 cup	107	927	5.3
prepared w/whole milk	1 cup	186	1004	9.4
unprepared	10.75 oz	268	2318	12.8
(Campbell's) prepared	8 oz	100	830	5.0
(Campbell's) prepared w/half water, half milk	8 oz	140	860	7.0
OYSTER STEW				
prepared	1 cup	58	981	3.8
prepared w/whole milk	1 cup	135	1041	7.9
unprepared	10.5 oz	143	2384	9.3
(Campbell's) prepared	8 oz	70	840	5.0
(Campbell's) prepared w/whole milk	8 oz	140	890	9.0
PASTA				
Alphabet *(Campbell's)* prepared	8 oz	80	800	3.0
Chicken and stars *(Campbell's)* prepared	8 oz	60	870	2.0
Teddy bears in chicken broth				
(Campbell's)	4 oz	60	770	1.0
(Campbell's) prepared	8 oz	60	770	1.0
PEPPER POT				
prepared	1 cup	104	971	4.6
unprepared	10.5 oz	250	2360	11.3
(Campbell's) prepared	8 oz	90	970	4.0
POTATO, CREAM OF				
prepared	1 cup	73	1000	2.4
prepared w/whole milk	1 cup	149	1061	6.4
unprepared	10.75 oz	180	2431	5.7
(Campbell's) prepared	8 oz	80	870	3.0
(Campbell's) prepared w/tofu, 1 tbsp oil	8 oz	120	900	4.0
SCOTCH BROTH				
prepared	1 cup	80	1012	2.6
unprepared	10.5 oz	197	2461	6.4
(Campbell's) prepared	8 oz	80	870	3.0
SEAFOOD CHOWDER, NEW ENGLAND				
(Snow's)	3.75 oz	60	640	2.0
(Snow's) prepared w/whole milk	7.5 oz	140	670	6.0
SHRIMP, CREAM OF				
prepared	1 cup	90	976	5.2
prepared w/whole milk	1 cup	164	1037	9.3
unprepared	10.75 oz	220	2373	12.6

Food Name	Serv. Size	Total Cal.	Sod. MGS	Fat GMS
(Campbell's) prepared	8 oz	90	810	6.0
(Campbell's) prepared w/whole milk	8 oz	160	860	10.0
(Campbell's) 'Seashore Soups'	4 oz	90	810	6.0
(Campbell's) 'Seashore Soups' prepared w/2% milk	4 oz	140	810	10.0
SPLIT PEA				
W/egg barley *(Rokeach)* prepared	1 cup	132	757	0.5
W/ham				
prepared	1 cup	190	1007	4.4
unprepared	11.5 oz	460	2445	10.7
W/ham and bacon *(Campbell's)* prepared	8 oz	160	780	4.0
STOCKPOT				
prepared	1 cup	99	1047	3.9
unprepared	11 oz	243	2546	9.5
TOMATO				
prepared	1 cup	85	871	1.9
prepared w/whole milk	1 cup	161	932	6.0
unprepared	10.75 oz	207	2120	4.7
(Campbell's) prepared	8 oz	90	680	2.0
(Campbell's) prepared w/whole milk	8 oz	150	740	4.0
(Campbell's) 'Healthy Request'	4 oz	90	430	2.0
(Campbell's) 'Healthy Request' prepared	8 oz	90	430	2.0
(Campbell's) 'Healthy Request' prepared w/half 2% milk, half water	8 oz	140	490	3.0
(Campbell's) 'Healthy Request' prepared w/skim milk	4 oz	130	490	2.0
(Campbell's) 'Healthy Request' prepared w/whole milk	8 oz	150	490	4.0
Italian, w/basil and oregano				
(Campbell's)	4 oz	90	740	0.0
(Campbell's) prepared	8 oz	90	740	0.0
Zesty *(Campbell's)* prepared	8 oz	100	760	2.0
TOMATO, CREAM OF				
(Campbell's) 'Homestyle' prepared	8 oz	110	810	3.0
(Campbell's) 'Homestyle' prepared w/whole milk	8 oz	180	860	7.0
TOMATO BEEF W/NOODLES				
prepared	1 cup	139	917	4.3
unprepared	10.75 oz	342	2230	10.4
TOMATO BISQUE				
prepared w/milk	1 cup	198	1109	6.6
unprepared	11 oz	300	2546	6.1
(Campbell's) prepared	8 oz	120	820	3.0
TOMATO RICE				
prepared	1 cup	119	815	2.7

Food Name	Serv. Size	Total Cal.	Sod. MGS	Fat GMS
unprepared	11 oz	290	1981	6.6
(Campbell's) 'Old Fashioned' prepared	8 oz	110	730	2.0
TURKEY NOODLE				
prepared	1 cup	68	815	2.0
unprepared	10.75 oz	168	1983	4.8
(Campbell's) prepared	8 oz	70	880	2.0
TURKEY VEGETABLE				
prepared	1 cup	72	906	3.0
unprepared	10.5 oz	179	2202	7.4
(Campbell's) prepared	8 oz	70	710	3.0
VEGETABLE				
(Campbell's) prepared	8 oz	90	830	2.0
(Campbell's) 'Homestyle' prepared	8 oz	60	880	2.0
(Campbell's) 'Old Fashioned' prepared	8 oz	60	880	2.0
Hearty, w/pasta				
(Campbell's)	4 oz	70	800	<1.0
(Campbell's) prepared	8 oz	70	800	<1.0
Vegetarian				
prepared	1 cup	72	822	1.9
unprepared	10.5 oz	176	2003	4.7
(Campbell's) prepared	8 oz	80	790	2.0
W/beef broth				
prepared	1 cup	82	810	1.9
unprepared	10.5 oz	197	1970	4.7
W/beef stock				
(Campbell's) 'Healthy Request'	4 oz	90	500	2.0
(Campbell's) 'Healthy Request' prepared	8 oz	90	500	2.0
VEGETABLE BEEF				
prepared	1 cup	78	956	1.9
unprepared	10.75 oz	192	2327	4.6
(Campbell's) prepared	8 oz	70	780	2.0
(Campbell's) 'Healthy Request' prepared	8 oz	70	470	2.0
WON TON (Campbell's) prepared	8 oz	40	850	1.0
SOUP, CANNED, READY-TO-SERVE				
BEAN				
(Grandma Brown's)	1 cup	190	700	3.4
W/ham				
(Campbell's) 'Chunky Old Fashioned'	11 oz	290	1110	9.0
(Campbell's) 'Chunky Old Fashioned'	9 5/8 oz	250	960	8.0
(Campbell's) 'Home Cookin'	9.5 oz	180	890	4.0
(Campbell's) 'Home Cookin'	10.75 oz	210	1000	4.0

Food Name	Serv. Size	Total Cal.	Sod. MGS	Fat GMS
(Healthy Choice)	7.5 oz	220	480	4.0
(Hormel) 'Hearty Soup'	7.5 oz	190	640	4.0
BEEF				
(Progresso)	10.5 oz	180	840	6.0
(Progresso)	9.5 oz	160	760	5.0
Bouillon	8 oz	17	782	0.5
Broth (College Inn)	7 oz	16	960	0.0
Chunky				
(Campbell's) 'Chunky'	10.75 oz	200	1100	5.0
(Campbell's) 'Chunky'	9.5 oz	170	970	4.0
Fat-free (Health Valley)	6.9 oz	10	290	0.0
Fat-free, no salt added (Health Valley)	6.9 oz	10	5	0.0
Hearty				
(Healthy Choice) 'Hearty Beef'	7.5 oz	120	580	2.0
(Progresso)	9.5 oz	160	820	4.0
Stroganoff style (Campbell's) 'Chunky'	10.75 oz	320	1230	16.0
W/barley				
(Progresso)	10.5 oz	150	870	5.0
(Progresso)	9.5 oz	140	780	4.0
W/minestrone				
(Progresso)	10.5 oz	180	1000	6.0
(Progresso)	9.5 oz	170	910	5.0
W/noodles (Progresso)	9.5 oz	170	1030	4.0
W/tomato juice	1 oz	11	40	0.0
W/vegetables				
(Lipton) 'Hearty Ones'	11 oz	229	921	3.0
(Progresso)	10.5 oz	170	880	3.0
(Progresso)	9.5 oz	150	790	3.0
W/vegetables and pasta				
(Campbell's) 'Home Cookin'	10.75 oz	140	1060	2.0
(Campbell's) 'Home Cookin'	9.5 oz	120	940	2.0
BERRY				
Blueberry (Great Impressions)	6 oz	95	92	0.3
Three berry (Great Impressions)	6 oz	107	90	0.2
BLACK BEAN				
(Health Valley)	7.5 oz	160	285	3.0
(Health Valley) 'No Salt Added'	7.5 oz	160	20	3.0
(Health Valley) w/vegetables, fat-free	7.5 oz	70	290	0.0
BORSCHT				
(Gold's)	8 oz	100	1280	0.0
(Rokeach)	1 cup	96	985	0.3

Food Name	Serv. Size	Total Cal.	Sod. MGS	Fat GMS
(Rokeach) 'Unsalted'	1 cup	103	50	0.3
Low-calorie				
(Gold's)	8 oz	20	1160	<1.0
(Manischewitz)	1 cup	20	725	0.0
(Rokeach) 'Diet'	1 cup	29	897	0.2
W/beets (Manischewitz)	1 cup	80	660	0.0
BROCCOLI, CREAM OF (Andersen's)	7.5 oz	170	670	8.0
CHERRY (Great Impressions)	6 oz	123	88	0.2
CHICKEN				
(Progresso) 'Homestyle'	9.5 oz	110	740	3.0
Broth				
(Campbell's) 'Healthy Request'	8 oz	16	470	0.0
(Campbell's) 'Low Sodium'	10.5 oz	30	85	1.0
(College Inn)	1 cup	35	1320	3.0
(College Inn)	7 oz	35	990	3.0
(College Inn) lower salt	7 oz	20	550	2.0
(Hain)	8.75 oz	70	870	6.0
(Health Valley) fat-free	6.9 oz	20	290	0.0
(Hain) 'No Salt Added'	8.75 oz	60	75	5.0
(Health Valley)	7.5 oz	35	410	2.0
(Health Valley) 'No Salt Added'	7.5 oz	35	0	2.0
(Pritikin) defatted	1 cup	18	160	1.0
(Progresso)	4 oz	8	360	0.0
(Swanson)	7.25 oz	30	900	2.0
(Swanson) 'Natural Goodness'	7.25 oz	20	580	1.0
Chunky				
(Campbell's) 'Chunky Old Fashioned'	10.75 oz	180	1220	5.0
(Campbell's) 'Chunky Old Fashioned'	9.5 oz	150	1070	4.0
(Healthy Choice) 'Hearty Chicken'	7.5 oz	150	530	5.0
Hearty				
(Progresso)	10.5 oz	130	960	4.0
(Progresso)	9.5 oz	130	900	4.0
Nuggets, w/vegetables and noodles				
(Campbell's) 'Chunky'	10.75 oz	190	1060	6.0
(Campbell's) 'Chunky'	9.5 oz	170	940	6.0
W/meatballs (Progresso) 'Chickarina'	9.5 oz	130	820	5.0
W/noodles				
(Campbell's) 'Home Cookin'	10.75 oz	140	1150	4.0
(Campbell's) 'Home Cookin'	9.5 oz	110	1020	3.0
(Campbell's) 'Low Sodium'	10.75 oz	170	90	5.0
W/ribbon pasta (Pritikin)	1 cup	80	180	1.0

Food Name	Serv. Size	Total Cal.	Sod. MGS	Fat GMS
W/rice				
(Campbell's) 'Chunky'	9.5 oz	140	1060	4.0
(Healthy Choice)	7.5 oz	140	510	4.0
(Hormel) 'Hearty Soup'	7.5 oz	110	890	2.0
W/wild rice *(Progresso)*	9.5 oz	120	850	3.0
CHICKEN, CREAM OF *(Progresso)*	9.5 oz	190	970	11.0
CHICKEN BARLEY *(Progresso)*	9.25 oz	100	740	2.0
CHICKEN GUMBO, w/sausage				
(Campbell's) 'Home Cookin'	10.75 oz	140	1090	4.0
(Campbell's) 'Home Cookin'	9.5 oz	120	960	3.0
CHICKEN MINESTRONE				
(Campbell's) 'Home Cookin'	10.75 oz	180	950	6.0
(Campbell's) 'Home Cookin'	9.5 oz	160	840	5.0
(Progresso)	10.5 oz	140	1060	4.0
(Progresso)	9.5 oz	130	870	3.0
CHICKEN MUSHROOM, CREAMY				
(Campbell's) 'Chunky'	10.5 oz	270	1280	19.0
(Campbell's) 'Chunky'	9 3/8 oz	240	1140	17.0
CHICKEN NOODLE				
(Hain)	9.5 oz	120	980	4.0
(Hain) 'No Salt Added'	9.5 oz	120	90	4.0
(Healthy Choice) 'Old Fashioned Chicken Noodle'	7.5 oz	90	520	3.0
(Hormel) 'Hearty Soup'	7.5 oz	110	690	3.0
(Lipton) 'Hearty Ones Homestyle'	11 oz	227	989	4.0
(Progresso)	10.5 oz	120	970	4.0
(Progresso)	9.5 oz	120	920	4.0
(Progresso) 'Healthy Classics'	8 oz	80	460	2.0
(Weight Watchers)	10.5 oz	80	1230	2.0
Chunky				
(Campbell's) 'Chunky'	10.75 oz	200	1140	7.0
(Campbell's) 'Chunky'	9.5 oz	180	1000	7.0
Hearty *(Campbell's)* 'Healthy Request'	8 oz	80	470	2.0
CHICKEN RICE				
(Campbell's) 'Home Cookin'	10.75 oz	150	1090	6.0
(Campbell's) 'Home Cookin'	9.5 oz	130	960	5.0
(Progresso)	10.5 oz	120	990	4.0
(Progresso)	9.5 oz	130	750	3.0
Chunky	8 oz	127	888	3.2
Hearty *(Campbell's)* 'Healthy Request'	8 oz	110	480	3.0
W/vegetables *(Progresso)* 'Healthy Classics'	8 oz	80	440	2.0

Food Name	Serv. Size	Total Cal.	Sod. MGS	Fat GMS
CHICKEN VEGETABLE				
(Hain)	9.5 oz	120	930	4.0
(Hain) 'No Salt Added'	9.5 oz	130	100	4.0
(Campbell's) 'Chunky'	9.5 oz	170	1080	6.0
(Campbell's) 'Chunky Low Sodium'	10.75 oz	240	95	11.0
(Campbell's) 'Home Cookin'	10.75 oz	180	970	4.0
(Pritikin)	1 cup	70	150	1.0
(Progresso)	9.5 oz	140	800	4.0
Chunky				
(Health Valley)	7.5 oz	125	425	2.0
(Health Valley) 'No Salt Added'	7.5 oz	125	60	2.0
Hearty (Campbell's) 'Healthy Request'	8 oz	120	420	3.0
CHILI BEEF				
(Campbell's) 'Chunky'	11 oz	290	1120	7.0
(Campbell's) 'Chunky'	9.75 oz	260	990	6.0
(Healthy Choice) thick and hearty	7.5 oz	150	560	1.0
CLAM CHOWDER				
Manhattan style				
(Campbell's) 'Chunky'	10.75 oz	160	1110	4.0
(Campbell's) 'Chunky'	9.5 oz	150	980	4.0
(Health Valley)	7.5 oz	110	510	2.0
(Health Valley) 'No Salt Added'	7.5 oz	110	60	2.0
(Progresso)	9.5 oz	120	800	2.0
New England style				
(Campbell's) 'Chunky'	10.75 oz	290	1200	17.0
(Campbell's) 'Chunky'	9.5 oz	260	1060	15.0
(Campbell's) 'Healthy Request'	8 oz	100	490	3.0
(Campbell's) 'Home Cookin'	10.75 oz	260	1240	18.0
(Gorton's) 'New England Style'	7.5 oz	140	720	5.0
(Hain)	9.25 oz	180	780	4.0
(Hormel) 'Hearty Soup'	7.5 oz	130	790	5.0
(Progresso)	10.5 oz	220	1050	12.0
(Progresso)	9.25 oz	220	950	12.0
(Weight Watchers)	7.5 oz	90	450	0.0
CORN AND VEGETABLE, fat-free (Health Valley)	7.5 oz	70	290	0.0
CORN CHOWDER				
(Campbell's) 'Chunky'	10.75 oz	340	1200	21.0
(Campbell's) 'Chunky'	9.5 oz	300	1060	19.0
(Progresso)	9.25 oz	200	840	10.0
CRAB	8 oz	76	1235	1.5

Food Name	Serv. Size	Total Cal.	Sod. MGS	Fat GMS
CREOLE				
(Campbell's) 'Chunky'	10.75 oz	240	910	8.0
(Campbell's) 'Chunky'	9.5 oz	220	800	7.0
ESCAROLE, in chicken broth (Progresso)	9.25 oz	30	1100	1.0
GAZPACHO	8 oz	56	1183	2.2
HAM AND BEAN				
(Campbell's) w/butterbeans 'Chunky'	10.75 oz	280	1180	10.0
(Progresso)	9.5 oz	140	950	2.0
LEMON (Great Impressions)	6 oz	90	109	<1.0
LENTIL				
(Health Valley)	7.5 oz	170	435	2.0
(Health Valley) 'No Salt Added'	7.5 oz	170	25	2.0
(Progresso)	10.5 oz	140	1000	4.0
(Progresso)	9.5 oz	140	840	4.0
(Progresso) 'Healthy Classics'	8 oz	120	420	1.0
Hearty				
(Campbell's) 'Home Cookin'	10.75 oz	170	930	2.0
(Campbell's) 'Home Cookin'	9.5 oz	140	820	1.0
Vegetarian				
(Hain)	9.5 oz	160	690	3.0
(Hain) 'No Salt Added'	9.5 oz	160	65	3.0
W/carrots, fat-free (Health Valley)	7.5 oz	70	290	0.0
W/ham	8 oz	139	1319	2.8
W/sausage (Progresso)	9.5 oz	170	840	8.0
MACARONI AND BEAN				
(Progresso)	10.5 oz	150	1020	4.0
(Progresso)	9.5 oz	140	920	5.0
MENUDO (Old El Paso)	1/2 can	476	770	52.0
MINESTRONE				
(Campbell's) 'Chunky'	9.5 oz	160	870	4.0
(Campbell's) 'Healthy Request'	8 oz	90	420	2.0
(Campbell's) 'Home Cookin'	10.75 oz	140	1220	3.0
(Campbell's) 'Home Cookin'	9.5 oz	120	1080	3.0
(Hain)	9.5 oz	170	1060	2.0
(Hain) 'No Salt Added'	9.5 oz	160	35	4.0
(Health Valley)	7.5 oz	130	637	3.0
(Health Valley) 'No Salt Added'	7.5 oz	130	80	3.0
(Health Valley) 'Real Italian Fat-Free'	7.5 oz	80	290	0.0
(Healthy Choice)	7.5 oz	160	520	2.0
(Hormel) 'Hearty Soup'	7.5 oz	100	460	1.0
(Lipton) 'Hearty Ones'	11 oz	189	821	3.2

Food Name	Serv. Size	Total Cal.	Sod. MGS	Fat GMS
(Progresso)	10.5 oz	120	930	3.0
(Progresso)	9.5 oz	130	1010	4.0
(Progresso) chunky, hearty	9.25 oz	110	740	2.0
(Progresso) chunky, zesty	9.5 oz	150	1130	8.0
(Progresso) 'Healthy Classics'	8 oz	120	490	2.0
MUSHROOM, CREAM OF				
(Campbell's) 'Low Sodium'	10.5 oz	210	55	14.0
(Hain)	9.25 oz	110	740	4.0
(Progresso)	9.25 oz	160	1120	10.0
(Weight Watchers)	10.5 oz	90	1250	2.0
MUSHROOM BARLEY				
(Hain)	9.5 oz	100	600	2.0
(Health Valley)	7.5 oz	100	394	2.0
(Health Valley) 'No Salt Added'	7.5 oz	100	20	2.0
PEPPER STEAK				
(Campbell's) 'Chunky'	9.5 oz	160	920	3.0
(Campbell's) 'Chunky'	10.75 oz	180	1050	3.0
POTATO, CREAM OF (Andersen's)	7.5 oz	200	630	10.0
POTATO LEEK				
(Health Valley)	7.5 oz	130	360	2.0
(Health Valley) 'No Salt Added'	7.5 oz	130	20	2.0
SCHAV (Gold's)	8 oz	25	1380	0.0
SIRLOIN BURGER				
(Campbell's) 'Chunky'	10.75 oz	220	1240	9.0
(Campbell's) 'Chunky'	9.5 oz	200	1090	8.0
SPLIT PEA				
(Andersen's)	7.5 oz	130	770	0.0
(Campbell's) 'Low Sodium'	10.75 oz	230	30	4.0
(Grandma Brown's)	1 cup	208	522	4.1
(Hain)	9.5 oz	170	970	1.0
(Hain) 'No Salt Added'	9.5 oz	170	40	1.0
(Progresso)	9.5 oz	160	1050	3.0
Green				
(Health Valley)	7.5 oz	190	276	0.3
(Health Valley) 'No Salt Added'	7.5 oz	190	25	0.3
(Hain) vegetarian	9.5 oz	170	970	1.0
(Hain) vegetarian 'No Salt Added'	9.5 oz	170	70	1.0
(Progresso)	10.5 oz	201	920	3.0
W/ham				
(Campbell's) 'Chunky'	10.5 oz	230	1080	6.0
(Campbell's) 'Chunky'	9.5 oz	210	950	5.0

Food Name	Serv. Size	Total Cal.	Sod. MGS	Fat GMS
(Campbell's) 'Home Cookin'	10.75 oz	230	1310	1.0
(Campbell's) 'Home Cookin'	9.5 oz	200	1150	1.0
(Healthy Choice)	7.5 oz	170	460	3.0
(Progresso)	10.5 oz	160	980	5.0
(Progresso)	9.5 oz	150	880	5.0
STEAK AND POTATO				
(Campbell's) 'Chunky'	10.75 oz	200	1140	5.0
(Campbell's) 'Chunky'	9.5 oz	170	1000	4.0
TOMATO				
(Health Valley)	7.5 oz	100	450	3.0
(Health Valley) 'No Salt Added'	7.5 oz	100	40	3.0
(Healthy Choice) 'Tomato Garden'	7.5 oz	130	510	3.0
(Progresso)	9.5 oz	120	1100	3.0
Beef, w/rotini *(Progresso)*	9.5 oz	170	930	6.0
Garden				
(Campbell's) 'Home Cookin'	10.75 oz	150	930	3.0
(Campbell's) 'Home Cookin'	9.5 oz	130	820	2.0
W/tomato pieces *(Campbell's)* 'Low Sodium'	10.5 oz	190	45	6.0
W/tortellini *(Progresso)*	9.25 oz	130	1040	5.0
TOMATO VEGETABLE, fat-free *(Health Valley)*	7.5 oz	50	290	0.0
TORTELLINI				
(Progresso)	9.5 oz	90	930	3.0
(Progresso) Creamy	9.25 oz	240	910	16.0
TURKEY	8 oz	135	923	4.4
TURKEY RICE				
(Hain)	9.5 oz	100	970	3.0
(Hain) 'No Salt Added'	9.5 oz	120	85	4.0
TURKEY VEGETABLE				
(Campbell's) 'Chunky'	9 3/8 oz	150	1060	6.0
(Weight Watchers)	10.5 oz	70	1020	2.0
VEGETABLE				
(Campbell's) 'Chunky'	10.75 oz	160	1100	4.0
(Campbell's) 'Chunky'	9.5 oz	150	970	4.0
(Health Valley)	7.5 oz	110	296	1.0
(Health Valley) 'No Salt Added'	7.5 oz	110	40	1.0
(Healthy Choice) 'Country Vegetable'	7.5 oz	120	540	1.0
(Progresso)	9.5 oz	80	1190	2.0
(Progresso) 'Healthy Classics'	8 oz	80	450	1.0
Country				
(Campbell's) 'Home Cookin'	10.75 oz	120	1070	2.0
(Campbell's) 'Home Cookin'	9.5 oz	100	940	2.0

Food Name	Serv. Size	Total Cal.	Sod. MGS	Fat GMS
(Hormel) 'Hearty Soup'	7.5 oz	90	730	2.0
Five bean, chunky				
(Health Valley)	7.5 oz	110	448	2.0
(Health Valley) 'No Salt Added'	7.5 oz	110	56	2.0
Fourteen garden vegetables, fat-free (Health Valley)	7.5 oz	50	260	0.0
Hearty (Campbell's) 'Healthy Request'	8 oz	90	480	1.0
Italian, w/pasta				
(Hain)	9.5 oz	160	910	5.0
(Hain) 'Low Sodium'	9.5 oz	140	90	6.0
Mediterranean (Campbell's) 'Chunky'	9.5 oz	170	1010	6.0
Vegetarian				
chunky (Weight Watchers)	10.5 oz	100	1250	2.0
(Hain)	9.5 oz	140	920	4.0
(Hain) 'No Salt Added'	9.5 oz	150	45	5.0
W/barley, fat-free (Health Valley)	7.5 oz	60	270	0.0
W/beef stock (Weight Watchers)	10.5 oz	90	1370	2.0
VEGETABLE BEEF				
(Campbell's) 'Chunky Low Sodium'	10.75 oz	180	90	5.0
(Campbell's) 'Chunky Old Fashioned'	10.75 oz	190	1100	6.0
(Campbell's) 'Chunky Old Fashioned'	9.5 oz	160	970	5.0
(Campbell's) hearty	8 oz	120	460	2.0
(Campbell's) 'Home Cookin'	10.75 oz	140	1160	3.0
(Campbell's) 'Home Cookin'	9.5 oz	120	1020	2.0
(Hormel) 'Hearty Soup'	7.5 oz	90	730	1.0
(Healthy Choice) 'Vegetable Beef'	7.5 oz	130	530	1.0
VEGETABLE BROTH				
(Hain)	9.5 oz	45	1180	0.0
(Hain) 'Low Sodium'	9.5 oz	40	85	<1.0
SOUP, FROZEN				
ASPARAGUS, CREAM OF				
(Kettle Ready)	6 oz	62	406	4.3
(Myers)	9.75 oz	152	992	8.0
BARLEY BEAN (Tabatchnick)	7.5 oz	130	217	2.0
BEAN				
Northern bean (Tabatchnick)	7.5 oz	164	240	2.0
Savory, w/ham (Kettle Ready)	6 oz	113	459	3.6
W/beef and vegetables, hearty (Kettle Ready)	6 oz	85	448	3.0
BLACK BEAN, w/ham (Kettle Ready)	6 oz	154	613	6.2
BROCCOLI, CREAM OF				
(Kettle Ready)	6 oz	94	417	7.2
(Myers)	9.75 oz	174	905	11.0

Food Name	Serv. Size	Total Cal.	Sod. MGS	Fat GMS
(Tabatchnick)	7.5 oz	90	285	4.0
CABBAGE *(Tabatchnick)*	7.5 oz	110	185	2.0
CAULIFLOWER, CREAM OF *(Kettle Ready)*	6 oz	93	445	7.0
CHEDDAR CHEESE, CREAM OF				
(Kettle Ready)	6 oz	158	616	12.5
(Kettle Ready) w/broccoli	6 oz	137	533	11.3
CHEESE, w/broccoli *(Myers)*	9.75 oz	325	1257	23.0
CHICKEN *(Tabatchnick)*	7.5 oz	65	255	2.0
CHICKEN, CREAM OF *(Kettle Ready)*	6 oz	98	668	6.2
CHICKEN GUMBO *(Kettle Ready)*	6 oz	94	473	3.5
CHICKEN NOODLE				
(Kettle Ready)	6 oz	94	569	3.0
(Myers)	9.75 oz	87	1046	5.0
CHILI				
(Kettle Ready)	6 oz	161	454	6.5
(Kettle Ready) jalapeño	6 oz	173	531	8.0
CLAM CHOWDER				
Boston *(Kettle Ready)*	6 oz	131	417	7.3
Manhattan style *(Kettle Ready)*	6 oz	69	549	2.6
New England style				
(Kettle Ready)	6 oz	116	373	6.5
(Myers)	9.75 oz	152	910	5.0
(Stouffer's)	8 oz	180	790	9.0
(Tabatchnick)	7.5 oz	98	255	2.0
CORN CHOWDER w/broccoli *(Kettle Ready)*	6 oz	102	323	5.0
LENTIL *(Tabatchnick)*	7.5 oz	170	240	2.0
MINESTRONE				
(Kettle Ready) hearty	6 oz	104	577	4.4
(Tabatchnick)	7.5 oz	137	265	2.0
MUSHROOM, CREAM OF				
(Kettle Ready)	6 oz	85	371	6.4
(Tabatchnick)	6 oz	75	325	2.0
MUSHROOM BARLEY				
(Tabatchnick)	7.5 oz	92	234	2.0
(Tabatchnick) 'No Salt'	7.5 oz	97	77	1.0
ONION, French *(Kettle Ready)*	6 oz	42	562	2.2
PEA				
(Tabatchnick)	7.5 oz	175	290	1.0
(Tabatchnick) 'No Salt'	7.5 oz	175	79	1.0
SEAFOOD BISQUE *(Myers)*	9.75 oz	163	1393	8.0

Food Name	Serv. Size	Total Cal.	Sod. MGS	Fat GMS
SPINACH, CREAM OF				
(Myers)	9.75 oz	174	905	11.0
(Stouffer's)	8 oz	210	1020	15.0
(Tabatchnick)	7.5 oz	85	200	2.0
SPLIT PEA W/HAM (Kettle Ready)	6 oz	155	483	4.4
TOMATO RICE (Tabatchnick)	6 oz	73	300	1.0
TOMATO TORTELLINI (Kettle Ready)	6 oz	122	447	5.4
VEGETABLE				
(Kettle Ready) garden	6 oz	85	296	3.0
(Tabatchnick)	7.5 oz	97	190	1.0
(Tabatchnick) 'No Salt'	7.5 oz	92	77	2.0
VEGETABLE BEEF (Myers)	9.75 oz	120	1030	6.0
ZUCCHINI (Tabatchnick)	6 oz	80	285	2.0
SOUP, MICROWAVE				
BEAN				
W/bacon and ham (Campbell's)	7.5 oz	230	830	5.0
W/ham, chowder (Hormel) 'Micro-Cup Hearty Soups'	1 pkg	191	664	3.0
BEEF, w/vegetable (Hormel) 'Micro-Cup Hearty Soups'	1 pkg	71	811	1.0
CHICKEN				
W/rice (Campbell's) 'Microwave'	7.5 oz	100	820	4.0
W/vegetables and rice (Hormel) 'Micro-Cup Hearty Soups'	1 pkg	114	1025	3.0
CHICKEN NOODLE				
(Campbell's) 'Microwave'	7.5 oz	100	870	4.0
(Hormel) 'Micro-Cup Hearty Soups'	1 pkg	108	686	3.0
(Lunch Bucket) microwave cup	7.25 oz	90	810	2.0
(Weight Watchers) microwave cup	7.5 oz	90	450	1.0
CHILI BEEF (Campbell's) 'Microwave'	7.5 oz	190	870	4.0
CLAM CHOWDER				
New England (Hormel) 'Micro-Cup Hearty Soups'	1 pkg	118	882	5.0
MINESTRONE (Hormel) 'Micro-Cup Hearty Soups'	1 pkg	104	903	2.0
NOODLE				
Beef flavor (Campbell's) 'Cup Microwave'	1.35 oz	130	1270	2.0
Chicken flavor (Campbell's) 'Cup Microwave'	1.35 oz	140	1340	3.0
Pork flavor, w/vegetables (Campbell's) 'Hearty Microwave'	1.7 oz	180	1320	2.0
W/chicken broth (Campbell's) 'Cup Microwave'	1.35 oz	130	1360	2.0
VEGETABLE, country x				
(Hormel) 'Micro-Cup Hearty Soups'	1 pkg	89	865	2.0
(Lunch Bucket) microwave cup	7.25 oz	70	740	1.0
VEGETABLE BEEF				
(Campbell's) 'Microwave'	7.5 oz	100	830	2.0
(Weight Watchers) microwave cup	7.5 oz	90	450	1.0

Food Name	Serv. Size	Total Cal.	Sod. MGS	Fat GMS
SOUP MIX				
(NOTE: Unless otherwise specified, PREPARED = prepared as directed w/water.)				
ASPARAGUS, prepared	8 oz	52	707	1.5
ASPARAGUS, CREAM OF, prepared	8 oz	58	800	1.7
BEAN W/BACON, prepared	1 cup	106	927	2.2
BEEF				
Beef flavor, w/noodles				
(Campbell's) 'Ramen Noodle' prepared	6 oz	160	890	1.0
(Estee) prepared	6 oz	20	140	<1.0
(Lipton) 'Cup-A-Soup' prepared	6 oz	44	746	0.7
(Lipton) 'Hearty' prepared	6 oz	107	698	1.4
Beef flavor, w/noodles and vegetables				
(Campbell's) prepared	6 oz	220	1600	2.0
Broth				
cubed	1 cube	6	864	0.1
cubed, prepared	6 oz	5	869	0.1
powder, prepared	8 oz	20	1362	0.7
Hearty (Soup Starter) 'Homestyle'	.945 oz	90	740	<1.0
Vegetable (Soup Starter) 'Homestyle'	.91 oz	90	790	<1.0
W/noodles (Ultra Slim Fast) 1 envelope, prepared	6 oz	45	700	<1.0
BEEF NOODLE, prepared	8 oz	40	1042	0.8
BLACK BEAN				
(Fantastic Foods) 'Jumpin' black beans, prepared	10 oz	170	490	1.0
BROCCOLI				
Creamy				
(Lipton) 'Cup-A-Soup' prepared	6 oz	62	610	2.4
(Lipton) 'Cup-A-Soup Food Service' prepared	6 oz	62	658	2.3
(Ultra Slim Fast) 1 envelope, prepared	6 oz	75	800	<1.0
Golden (Lipton) 'Cup-A-Soup Lite' prepared	6 oz	42	427	1.2
W/cheese (Lipton) 'Cup-A-Soup' prepared	6 oz	70	595	3.4
BOUILLON				
Beef flavor				
cubed	1 cube	6	864	0.1
cubed (Steero)	1 cube	6	930	<1.0
cubed (Wyler's)	1 cube	6	930	<1.0
instant (Featherweight)	1 tsp	18	10	1.0
instant (Lite-Line) 'Low Sodium'	1 tsp	12	5	<1.0
instant (Steero)	1 tsp	6	930	<1.0
instant (Weight Watchers) 'Broth Mix'	1 pkt	8	930	0.0
instant (Wyler's)	1 tsp	6	930	<1.0
powder	1 pkt	14	1019	0.5

Food Name	Serv. Size	Total Cal.	Sod. MGS	Fat GMS
powder, prepared	8 oz	19	1359	0.7
Brown				
(G. Washington's) 'Seasoning & Broth'	.14 oz	6	1015	0.0
(G. Washington's) 'Seasoning & Broth' kosher	.14 oz	6	1110	0.0
Chicken flavor				
cubed	1 cube	9	1152	0.2
cubed (Steero)	1 cube	8	990	<1.0
cubed (Wyler's)	1 cube	8	900	<1.0
instant (Featherweight)	1 tsp	18	5	1.0
instant (Lite-Line) 'Low Sodium'	1 tsp	12	5	<1.0
instant (Steero)	1 tsp	8	990	<1.0
instant (Weight Watchers) 'Broth Mix'	1 pkt	°8	990	0.0
instant (Wyler's)	1 tsp	8	900	<1.0
Golden				
(G. Washington's') 'Seasoning & Broth'	.13 oz	6	935	0.0
(G. Washington's) 'Seasoning & Broth' kosher	.13 oz	6	1015	0.0
Onion flavor				
(G. Washington's) 'Seasoning and Broth'	.18 oz	12	695	0.0
(Wyler's) instant	1 tsp	10	670	<1.0
Vegetable flavor				
(G. Washington's) 'Seasoning & Broth'	.18 oz	12	715	0.0
(Wyler's) instant	1 tsp	6	910	<1.0
CAULIFLOWER, prepared	8 oz	69	843	1.7
CELERY, prepared	8 oz	63	838	1.6
CHEESE				
(Fantastic Noodles) creamy cheddar w/noodles, prepared	7 oz	178	578	8.0
(Hain) cheese and broccoli, prepared	6 oz	310	980	22.0
(Hain) 'Savory Soup & Sauce Mix' prepared	6 oz	250	890	16.0
CHICKEN				
prepared	8 oz	107	1185	5.3
(Soup Starter) 'Homestyle'	.735 oz	70	770	<1.0
Broth				
cubed	1 cube	10	1152	0.2
cubed, prepared	6 oz	9	593	0.2
(Lipton) 'Cup-A-Soup' prepared	6 oz	20	605	0.6
Creamy, w/vegetables (Lipton) prepared	6 oz	93	708	3.1
Creamy, w/white meat (Campbell's) prepared	6 oz	90	1020	4.0
Florentine (Lipton) 'Lite'	6 oz	42	481	0.5
Hearty				
(Lipton) 'Country Style'	6 oz	69	688	1.1
(Lipton) 'Supreme' prepared	6 oz	107	848	5.9

Food Name	Serv. Size	Total Cal.	Sod. MGS	Fat GMS
Lemon (Lipton) 'Cup-A-Soup Lite' prepared	6 oz	48	419	0.4
W/corn (Lipton) 'Country' prepared	6 oz	133	704	5.5
W/noodles (Ultra Slim Fast) 1 envelope, prepared	6 oz	45	970	<1.0
CHICKEN, CREAM OF				
(Lipton) 'Cup-A-Soup' prepared	6 oz	84	757	4.4
(Lipton) 'Food Service' prepared	6 oz	84	840	4.4
CHICKEN LEEK				
creamy (Ultra Slim Fast) 1 envelope, prepared	6 oz	50	1070	<1.0
CHICKEN NOODLE				
prepared	1 cup	53	1284	1.2
(Campbell's) 'Lowfat Block' prepared	1 cup	160	940	1.0
(Campbell's) 'Quality Recipe' prepared	1 cup	100	710	2.0
(Campbell's) 'Ramen Noodle' prepared	1 cup	190	970	8.0
(Estee) 'Instant' prepared	6 oz	25	135	<1.0
(Lipton) 'Cup-A-Soup' prepared	6 oz	48	635	1.1
(Lipton) 'Supreme' prepared	6 oz	107	757	5.9
(Mrs. Grass) 'Chickeny Rich'	1/4 pkg	70	900	2.0
Creamy, hearty (Lipton) prepared	7 oz	179	639	8.2
Hearty				
(Lipton) prepared	1 cup	83	753	1.3
(Lipton) prepared	7 oz	118	655	1.5
W/meat				
(Campbell's) white meat	6 oz	90	770	2.0
(Lipton) 'Cup' prepared	6 oz	46	660	1.0
(Lipton) 'Value Pack' prepared	6 oz	46	660	1.0
(Lipton) white meat, diced, prepared	1 cup	81	795	1.8
W/rice (Lipton) prepared	6 oz	47	667	0.8
W/vegetables				
(Campbell's) prepared	1 cup	270	1470	10.0
(Campbell's) lowfat, prepared	1 cup	220	1500	2.0
(Lipton) 'Cup' prepared	6 oz	47	566	0.6
(Lipton) hearty, prepared	1 cup	75	687	1.6
CHICKEN RICE, prepared	8 oz	61	981	1.4
CHICKEN VEGETABLE, prepared	8 oz	50	807	0.8
CHILI PEPPER (A Taste of Thai) hot and sour, prepared	1 cup	40	1330	2.0
CLAM CHOWDER				
Manhattan style (Golden Dipt)	1/4 pkg	80	700	2.0
New England style (Golden Dipt)	1/4 pkg	70	680	2.0
CONSOMMÉ, w/gelatin, prepared	1 cup	17	3299	0.0
GINGER (A Taste of Thai) tangy coconut, prepared	1 cup	250	1050	1.5

Food Name	Serv. Size	Total Cal.	Sod. MGS	Fat GMS
GREEN PEA				
(Lipton) 'Cup-A-Soup' prepared	6 oz	113	553	4.2
(Lipton) 'Cup-A-Soup Food Service' prepared	6 oz	115	635	4.5
HERB *(Lipton)* savory, w/garlic 'Recipe Secrets' prepared	8 oz	35	490	<1.0
LEEK				
Creamy *(Ultra Slim Fast)* 1 envelope prepared	6 oz	80	780	<1.0
LENTIL *(Hain)* 'Savory Soup Mix' prepared	6 oz	130	810	2.0
LOBSTER BISQUE *(Golden Dipt)* prepared	1/4 pkg	30	560	1.0
MINESTRONE				
(Hain) 'Savory Soup Mix' prepared	6 oz	110	870	1.0
(Manischewitz) prepared	6 oz	50	160	<1.0
MUSHROOM				
(Estee) 'Instant' prepared	6 oz	40	115	2.0
(Hain) 'Savory Soup & Recipe Mix' prepared	6 oz	210	710	15.0
(Hain) 'Savory Soup & Recipe Mix No Salt Added' prepared	6 oz	250	180	20.0
Beef flavor *(Lipton)* prepared	1 cup	38	763	0.5
MUSHROOM, CREAM OF *(Lipton)* 'Cup-A-Soup' prepared	6 oz	71	756	3.2
NOODLE				
(Campbell's) 'Quality Soup & Recipe' prepared	1 cup	110	700	2.0
(Lipton) 'Cup-A-Soup Ring Noodle' prepared	6 oz	47	650	0.7
(Lipton) 'Giggle Noodle' prepared	1 cup	77	784	2.1
(Lipton) 'Ring-O-Noodle' prepared	1 cup	71	784	2.0
Beef flavor				
(Cup O'Noodles) prepared	1 cup	290	1490	14.0
(Oodles of Noodles) prepared	1 cup	390	1810	18.0
(Top Ramen) prepared	1 cup	390	1810	18.0
Beefy, w/vegetables *(Lipton)* prepared	1 cup	85	810	0.9
Chicken flavor				
(Cup O'Noodles) prepared	1 cup	300	1790	16.0
(Cup O'Noodles) 'Hearty' prepared	1 cup	300	1210	14.0
(Oodles of Noodles) prepared	1 cup	400	1910	18.0
(Top Ramen) prepared	1 cup	400	1910	18.0
Hearty *(Campbell's)* 'Quality Soup & Recipe' prepared	1 cup	90	840	1.0
Hearty, w/vegetables *(Lipton)* prepared	1 cup	75	687	1.6
Oriental				
(Campbell's) 'Ramen Noodle' prepared	1 cup	190	930	8.0
(Campbell's) 'Ramen Noodle Lowfat Block' prepared	1 cup	150	940	1.0
(Oodles of Noodles) prepared	1 cup	390	1660	18.0
(Top Ramen) prepared	1 cup	390	1660	18.0

Food Name	Serv. Size	Total Cal.	Sod. MGS	Fat GMS
Oriental, w/vegetables				
(Campbell's) 'Cup-A-Ramen' prepared	1 cup	270	1210	10.0
(Campbell's) 'Cup-A-Ramen Lowfat' prepared	1 cup	220	1400	2.0
Pork flavor				
(Campbell's) 'Ramen Noodle' prepared	1 cup	200	860	8.0
(Campbell's) 'Ramen Noodle Lowfat Block' prepared	1 cup	150	1140	1.0
(Oodles of Noodles) prepared	1 cup	390	2060	20.0
(Top Ramen) prepared	1 cup	390	2060	20.0
Pork flavor, w/old-fashioned vegetables				
(Cup O'Noodles) 'Hearty' prepared	6 oz	290	1250	15.0
Pork flavor, w/seafood *(Cup O'Noodles)* 'Hearty' prepared	1 cup	300	1170	15.0
Pork flavor, w/shrimp *(Cup O'Noodles)* prepared	1 cup	300	1480	14.0
W/chicken broth				
(Campbell's) 'Cup 2 Minute Soup' prepared	6 oz	90	910	2.0
(Campbell's) 'Double Noodle'	1.78 oz	200	770	2.0
(Campbell's) 'Double Noodle' prepared	8 oz	200	770	2.0
ONION				
(Campbell's) 'Quality Soup & Recipe' prepared	1 cup	30	700	0.0
(Estee) prepared	6 oz	25	140	<1.0
(Hain) 'Savory Soup, Dip & Recipe Mix' prepared	6 oz	50	900	2.0
(Hain) 'Savory Soup, Dip & Recipe Mix' no salt, prepared	6 oz	50	470	1.0
(Lipton) prepared	1 cup	20	632	0.2
(Lipton) 'Cup-A-Soup' prepared	6 oz	27	665	0.5
(Mrs. Grass) 'Soup & Dip Mix' prepared	1/4 pkg	35	1070	<1.0
Beefy *(Lipton)* prepared	1 cup	29	803	1.0
Creamy				
(Lipton) 'Cup-A-Soup' prepared	6 oz	70	678	3.2
(Ultra Slim Fast) 1 envelope, prepared	6 oz	45	1180	<1.0
Golden, w/chicken broth *(Lipton)* prepared	1 cup	62	716	1.5
Mushroom *(Lipton)* prepared	1 cup	41	684	0.9
ORIENTAL *(Lipton)* 'Cup-A-Soup Lite' prepared	6 oz	45	457	1.7
POTATO LEEK *(Hain)* 'Savory Soup Mix' prepared	6 oz	260	690	18.0
SPLIT PEA				
Green				
(Hain) 'Savory Soup Mix' prepared	6 oz	310	940	10.0
(Manischewitz) prepared	6 oz	45	320	<1.0
Fat-free, thick and creamy *(Fantastic Foods)* 'Splittin Pea'	10 oz	145	490	1.0
W/carrots *(Health Valley)*	7.5 oz	80	290	0.0
SEAFOOD CHOWDER *(Golden Dipt)*	1/4 pkg	70	730	2.0
SHRIMP				
Bisque *(Golden Dipt)* dry mix	1/4 pkg	30	570	1.0

Food Name	Serv. Size	Total Cal.	Sod. MGS	Fat GMS
W/vegetables				
(Campbell's) 'Cup-A-Ramen' prepared	1 cup	280	1190	10.0
(Campbell's) 'Lowfat' prepared	1 cup	230	1290	2.0
TOMATO				
(Estee) 'Instant' prepared	6 oz	40	95	<1.0
(Hain) 'Savory Soup & Recipe Mix' prepared	6 oz	220	770	14.0
(Lipton) 'Cup-A-Soup' prepared	6 oz	103	524	0.9
(Lipton) 'Cup-A-Soup Food Service' prepared	6 oz	100	563	0.9
Creamy *(Ultra Slim Fast)* 1 envelope, prepared	6 oz	60	990	<1.0
Creamy, w/herb *(Lipton)* 'Cup-A-Soup Lite' prepared	6 oz	66	305	0.3
Minestrone *(Cous•cous)*	10 oz	200	590	0.0
TOMATO VEGETABLE				
prepared	8 oz	56	1146	0.9
W/noodles *(Fantastic Noodles)* prepared	7 oz	158	434	8.0
VEGETABLE				
(Campbell's) 'Quality Soup & Recipe' prepared	1 cup	40	710	0.0
(Hain) 'Savory Soup Mix' prepared	6 oz	80	730	1.0
(Hain) 'Savory Soup Mix No Salt Added' prepared	6 oz	80	330	1.0
(Lipton) prepared	1 cup	39	640	0.5
(Manischewitz) prepared	6 oz	50	65	<1.0
Country *(Lipton)* prepared	1 cup	80	803	0.7
Curry, w/noodles *(Fantastic Noodles)* prepared	7 oz	150	472	7.0
Garden *(Lipton)* 'Lots-A-Noodles Cup-A-Soup' prepared	7 oz	123	720	1.5
Harvest				
(Lipton) 'Country Style' prepared	6 oz	95	569	1.2
(Lipton) 'Cup-A-Soup Country Style' prepared	6 oz	91	459	1.2
Hearty *(Ultra Slim Fast)* 1 envelope, prepared	6 oz	45	850	<1.0
Miso, w/noodles *(Fantastic Noodles)* prepared	7 oz	152	434	7.0
Noodle, w/meatballs *(Lipton)* 'Country Style' prepared	6 oz	95	764	1.6
Parmesan *(Cous•cous)*	10 oz	200	550	3.0
Spring *(Lipton)* 'Cup-A-Soup' prepared	6 oz	33	746	0.8
VEGETABLE BEEF, prepared	8 oz	53	1002	1.1
VIRGINIA PEA				
(Lipton) prepared	6 oz	113	664	4.1
(Lipton) 'Country Style' prepared	6 oz	148	828	6.4
SOUR CREAM				
	1 cup	493	123	48.2
	1 oz	61	15	5.9
	1 tbsp	26	6	2.5
(Bison)	1 oz	50	15	5.0
(Breakstone's)	1 tbsp	30	5	3.0

Food Name	Serv. Size	Total Cal.	Sod. MGS	Fa GM
(Crowley)	1 oz	50	15	5.
(Darigold)	1 tbsp	23	5	2.
(Friendship)	2 tbsp	55	15	5.
(Knudsen) 'Hampshire'	1 oz	60	10	6.
(Sealtest)	1 tbsp	30	5	3.
French onion (Crowley)	1 oz	50	130	5.0
Pasteurized, 100% natural (Alta•Dena)	1 oz	60	15	6.
W/acidophilus, cultured (Alta•Dena) 'Kefir'	1 oz	70	40	6.
W/chives (Land O'Lakes) 'Light'	2 tbsp	40	150	2.
HALF AND HALF				
(Breakstone's) 'Light Choice'	1 tbsp	25	10	2.0
(Sealtest) 'Light'	1 tbsp	25	10	2.0
Cultured	1 tbsp	20	6	1.8
LIGHT/LOW-FAT				
(Crowley)	1 oz	30	25	2.0
(Friendship) 'Lite Delite'	2 tbsp	35	25	2.0
(Knudsen)	1 oz	40	20	3.0
(Land O'Lakes) 'Light'	2 tbsp	40	35	2.0
(Naturally Yours) 'Real•Dairy' no fat	2 tbsp	15	15	0.0
(Weight Watchers)	2 tbsp	35	40	2.0
SOUR CREAM, ALTERNATIVE/NONDAIRY				
	1 cup	479	235	44.9
	1 oz	59	29	5.8
(Crowley) dressing	1 oz	40	5	4.0
(Pet)	1 tbsp	25	25	2.0
Cultured				
	1 cup	479	235	44.9
	1 oz	58	29	5.8
(Light n' Lively) nonfat	1 tbsp	10	30	0.0
SOY BEVERAGE				
(Edensoy) 'Extra' original	8.45 oz	140	110	4.0
(Edensoy) original	8.45 oz	140	120	4.0
(Health Valley) fat-free 'Soy Moo'	1 cup	110	25	0.0
(Soyamel) powdered mix, prepared	8 oz	130	210	7.0
(WestSoy) 'Lite' plain	8 oz	100	100	2.0
(WestSoy) 'Natural' original	8 oz	150	115	5.0
(WestSoy) 'Natural' unsweetened	8 oz	100	40	5.0
(WestSoy) 'Plus' plain	8 oz	150	140	5.0
ALMOND FLAVOR				
(WestSoy) 'Lite'	6 oz	160	140	4.0
(WestSoy) 'Natural'	6 oz	250	140	11.0

Food Name	Serv. Size	Total Cal.	Sod. MGS	Fat GMS
BANANA FLAVOR *(WestSoy)* 'Lite' creamy banana	6 oz	160	140	3.0
CAROB FLAVOR				
(Ah Soy)	6 oz	160	120	3.0
(Edensoy)	8.45 oz	160	125	5.0
(WestSoy) 'Plus'	8 oz	160	80	5.0
Malted				
(WestSoy) 'Lite'	6 oz	160	140	3.0
(WestSoy) 'Natural'	6 oz	270	120	11.0
CHOCOLATE FLAVOR *(Ah Soy)*	6 oz	160	120	3.0
COCOA FLAVOR				
(WestSoy) 'Lite'	8 oz	140	95	2.0
(WestSoy) 'Lite' w/mint	6 oz	160	140	3.0
COFFEE FLAVOR *(WestSoy)* 'Natural' java malted	6 oz	270	140	11.0
VANILLA FLAVOR				
(Ah Soy)	6 oz	160	140	5.0
(Edensoy) 'Extra'	8.45 oz	150	95	3.0
(Edensoy) 'Natural Vanilla'	8.45 oz	150	140	3.0
(WestSoy) 'Lite'	8 oz	110	80	2.0
(WestSoy) 'Lite' vanilla royale	6 oz	160	140	3.0
(WestSoy) 'Plus'	8 oz	150	120	5.0
All natural *(WestSoy)*	8 oz	120	140	2.5
Malted *(WestSoy)* 'Natural'	6 oz	250	140	11.0
SOY FLOUR				
defatted	1 oz	93	6	0.3
defatted, stirred	1/2 cup	165	10	0.6
full-fat	1 oz	124	4	5.9
full-fat *(Arrowhead Mills)*	2 oz	250	1	11.0
full-fat, roasted	1 oz	125	3	6.2
full-fat, roasted, stirred	1/2 cup	185	5	9.2
full-fat, stirred	1/2 cup	183	5	8.7
low-fat	1 oz	92	5	1.9
low-fat, stirred	1/2 cup	143	8	3.0
SOY MEAL				
defatted, raw	1/2 cup	207	2	1.5
defatted, raw	1 oz	96	1	0.7
SOY MILK. See SOY BEVERAGE.				
SOY PROTEIN CONCENTRATE				
acid wash extracted	1 oz	93	252	0.1
acid/water wash extracted	1 oz	94	255	0.1
alcohol extracted	1 oz	93	1	0.1

Food Name	Serv. Size	Total Cal.	Sod. MGS	Fat GMS
SOY PROTEIN ISOLATE				
....	1 oz	95	281	1.0
potassium type	1 oz	91	14	0.2
w/potassium	1 oz	96	14	1.0
w/sodium	1 oz	96	281	1.0
SOYBEAN				
Dried				
boiled	4 oz	196	1	10.2
boiled	1/2 cup	149	1	7.7
dry-roasted	1/2 cup	387	2	18.6
dry-roasted	1 oz	128	1	6.1
raw	1/2 cup	387	2	18.5
raw	1 oz	118	1	5.7
raw (Arrowhead Mills)	2 oz	230	2	10.0
roasted	1/2 cup	405	140	21.8
roasted	1 oz	134	46	7.2
Green				
boiled, drained	4 oz	160	na	7.3
boiled, drained	1/2 cup	127	13	5.8
raw	1/2 cup	188	19	8.7
raw, in pods	1 lb	353	na	16.4
raw, shelled	1 oz	42	na	1.9
Kernels, roasted/toasted				
whole	1 cup	489	4	25.9
whole	1 oz	129	1	6.8
Mature				
boiled	1/2 cup	149	1	7.7
dry-roasted	1/2 cup	387	2	18.6
raw	1/2 cup	387	2	18.5
roasted	1/2 cup	405	140	21.8
Mature, sprouted				
boiled, drained	1 cup	48	5	1.8
raw	1 lb	580	62	30.4
raw	1/2 cup	43	5	2.3
steamed	1/2 cup	38	5	2.1
stir-fried	3.5 oz	125	14	7.1
SOYBEAN, FERMENTED. See also MISO.				
natto	1/2 cup	187	6	9.7
natto	1 oz	60	2	3.1
SOYBEAN FLAKES (Arrowhead Mills)	2 oz	250	2	11.0

Food Name	Serv. Size	Total Cal.	Sod. MGS	Fat GMS
SOYBEAN LECITHIN OIL				
....	1/2 cup	964	0	109.0
....	1 oz	251	0	28.4
....	1 tbsp	120	0	13.6
SOYBEAN OIL				
....	1 cup	1927	0	218.0
hydrogenated	1 cup	1927	0	218.0
hydrogenated	1 oz	251	0	28.4
hydrogenated	1 tbsp	120	0	13.6
(Hain)	1 tbsp	120	0	14.0
(IGA)	1 tbsp	120	0	14.0
SOYBEAN-COTTONSEED OIL				
hydrogenated	1/2 cup	964	0	109.0
hydrogenated	1 oz	251	0	28.4
hydrogenated	1 tbsp	120	0	13.6
SPAGHETTI. See PASTA.				
SPAGHETTI ENTRÉE, CANNED				
W/beef *(Chef Boyardee)* 'Beef-O-Getti'	7.5 oz	220	1240	9.0
W/beef, in tomato sauce *(Chef Boyardee)*	7.5 oz	240	1120	9.0
W/frankfurters *(Van Camp's)* 'Spaghettee Weenee'	1 cup	243	1128	7.4
W/frankfurters, in tomato sauce *(Franco-American)*				
'SpaghettiOs'	7.5 oz	220	1000	9.0
W/meatballs				
(Estee)	7.5 oz	240	130	14.0
(Featherweight)	7.5 oz	160	400	3.0
(Nalley's)	7.5 oz	190	950	4.0
W/meatballs, in sauce *(Buitoni)*	7.5 oz	190	940	8.0
W/meatballs, in tomato sauce				
(Chef Boyardee)	7.5 oz	230	970	9.0
(Franco-American)	7 3/8 oz	220	870	8.0
(Franco-American) 'SpaghettiOs'	7 3/8 oz	220	950	9.0
(Pathmark) 'No Frills'	7.5 oz	200	860	8.0
W/tomato and cheese sauce *(Franco-American)*				
'SpaghettiOs'	7.5 oz	170	860	2.0
W/tomato sauce, rings *(Finast)*	7.5 oz	150	480	1.0
SPAGHETTI ENTRÉE, FREEZE-DRIED				
(Mountain House) w/meat and sauce, prepared	1 cup	260	(mq)	5.0
SPAGHETTI ENTRÉE, FROZEN				
Parmesan, w/Italian-style green beans *(Stouffer's)*	10.25 oz	240	810	9.0
W/beef *(Dining Lite)*	9 oz	220	440	8.0
W/beef sauce and mushrooms *(Le Menu)* 'LightStyle'	9 oz	280	450	6.0

Food Name	Serv. Size	Total Cal.	Sod. MGS	Fat GMS
W/Italian-style meatballs *(Swanson)* 'Homestyle Recipe'	13 oz	490	940	18.0
W/meat sauce				
(Banquet) 'Casserole'	8 oz	270	1250	8.0
(Freezer Queen) 'Single Serve'	10 oz	350	610	12.0
(Kid Cuisine)	9.25 oz	310	690	12.0
(Lean Cuisine)	11.5 oz	290	500	6.0
(Stouffer's)	12 7/8 oz	320	560	12.0
(Weight Watchers)	10 oz	240	490	7.0
W/meatballs				
(Banquet)	10 oz	290	580	10.0
(Morton)	10 oz	200	1090	3.0
(Stouffer's) 19.5-oz pkg	1/2 pkg	290	790	9.0
(Stouffer's) 12 5/8-oz pkg	1 pkg	440	960	16.0
(Swanson)	12.5 oz	390	1100	17.0
W/meatballs and sauce *(Lean Cuisine)*	9.5 oz	290	550	7.0
SPAGHETTI ENTRÉE, MICROWAVE				
(Lunch Bucket) 'Spaghetti 'n Meatsauce' microwave cup ...	7.5 oz	240	870	5.0
Rings *(Kid's Kitchen)* microwave cup	7.5 oz	180	930	1.0
Rings and franks in tomato sauce *(Kid's Kitchen)*				
microwave cup	7.5 oz	290	960	12.0
W/meatballs				
(Chef Boyardee) 'Microwave'	7.5 oz	230	1060	10.0
(Hormel) micro cup	7.5 oz	210	930	7.0
(Kid's Kitchen) microwave cup	7.5 oz	220	880	8.0
W/meatballs, in sauce *(Libby's)* 'Diner'	7.75 oz	190	870	3.0
SPAGHETTI ENTRÉE, PACKAGED				
Spaghettini *(Top Shelf)*	1 serving	240	1020	5.0
W/beef and mushroom sauce *(Ultra Slim Fast)*	12 oz	370	990	10.0
W/meat sauce *(Top Shelf)*	10 oz	260	980	6.0
SPAGHETTI ENTRÉE MIX				
(Kraft) 'Mild American Dinner' prepared	1 cup	300	630	7.0
(Kraft) 'Tangy Italian Style Dinner' prepared	1 cup	310	670	8.0
Low-fat, w/whole wheat noodles *(Fantastic Foods)*				
'All-O-Round'	10 oz	211	275	2.0
W/condensed meat sauce *(Chef Boyardee)*				
'Dinner' prepared	3.25 oz	250	595	6.0
W/meat sauce				
(Chef Boyardee) 'Dinner' prepared	7.9 oz	240	1155	3.0
(Kraft) 'Dinner' prepared	1 cup	360	880	14.0
W/mushroom sauce *(Chef Boyardee)* 'Dinner' prepared	7.9 oz	210	1085	1.0
SPAGHETTI SEASONING *(Tone's)*	1 tsp	11	469	<.1

Food Name	Serv. Size	Total Cal.	Sod. MGS	Fat GMS
SPAGHETTI SQUASH. See SQUASH, SPAGHETTI.				
SPAM. See LUNCHEON MEAT, CANNED.				
SPARE RIB SEASONING MIX, 'Bag 'n Season' *(Schilling)*	1 pkg	185	3690	1.5
SPINACH				
boiled, drained	4 oz	26	79	0.3
boiled, drained	1/2 cup	21	63	0.2
raw	10-oz pkg	62	224	1.0
raw *(Dole)*	3 oz	9	107	0.3
raw, chopped	1/2 cup	6	22	0.1
raw, chopped	1 oz	6	22	0.1
raw, untrimmed	1 lb	73	257	1.1
SPINACH, CANNED				
drained solids	1/2 cup	25	29	0.5
drained solids, no salt added	4 oz	26	31	0.6
w/liquid	4 oz	22	362	0.4
w/liquid, low-sodium	4 oz	22	85	0.4
(Allens)	1/2 cup	28	35	<1.0
(Allens) chopped	1/2 cup	28	330	<1.0
(Allens) sliced	1/2 cup	28	330	<1.0
(Allens) whole	1/2 cup	28	330	<1.0
(Bush's Best) chopped	1/2 cup	25	330	0.0
(Del Monte) chopped, w/liquid	1/2 cup	25	355	0.0
(Del Monte) whole, w/liquid	1/2 cup	25	355	0.0
(Del Monte) whole, w/liquid, 'No Salt Added'	1/2 cup	25	35	0.0
(Featherweight)	1/2 cup	35	30	1.0
(Finast)	1/2 cup	25	360	0.0
(Finast) 'No Salt Added'	1/2 cup	25	110	0.0
(Freshlike) cut	1/2 cup	20	340	0.0
(Freshlike) cut, water-packed, w/o salt	1/2 cup	20	20	0.0
(Freshlike) cut, water packed, w/o sugar or salt	1/2 cup	20	20	0.0
(Pathmark) 'No Frills'	1 cup	45	700	1.0
(Pathmark) 'No Salt Added'	1/2 cup	30	35	1.0
(Pathmark) whole	1/2 cup	30	370	1.0
(S&W) 'Premium Northwest'	1/2 cup	25	395	0.0
(Stokely)	1/2 cup	30	420	0.0
(Veg•All) cut	1/2 cup	20	340	0.0
SPINACH, FROZEN				
Chopped				
boiled, drained	10-oz pkg	62	189	0.5
boiled, drained	1/2 cup	27	82	0.2
unprepared	10-oz pkg	68	210	0.9

Food Name	Serv. Size	Total Cal.	Sod. MGS	Fat GMS
unprepared	1 cup	37	115	0.5
(A&P)	3.3 oz	20	90	<1.0
(Birds Eye)	3.3 oz	20	90	0.0
(Finast)	3.3 oz	20	70	0.0
(Frosty Acres)	3.3 oz	20	70	0.0
(Seabrook)	3.3 oz	20	70	0.0
(Southern)	3.5 oz	25	100	0.3
Creamed				
(Birds Eye) 'Combination Vegetables'	3 oz	60	310	4.0
(Green Giant)	1/2 cup	70	480	3.0
(Stouffer's)	4.5 oz	170	380	14.0
Leaf				
boiled, drained	10-oz pkg	62	189	0.5
boiled, drained	4 oz	32	98	0.2
unprepared	10-oz pkg	68	210	0.9
unprepared	1 cup	37	-115	0.5
(A&P)	3.3 oz	25	100	<1.0
(Birds Eye) 'Portion Pack'	3.2 oz	20	70	0.0
(Birds Eye) whole leaf	3.3 oz	20	90	0.0
(Finast)	3.3 oz	20	75	0.0
(Freshlike) cut	3.3 oz	20	75	0.0
(Frosty Acres)	3.3 oz	20	75	0.0
(Green Giant) cut, in butter sauce	1/2 cup	40	380	2.0
(Green Giant) 'Harvest Fresh'	1/2 cup	25	170	0.0
(Green Giant) 'Plain Polybag'	1/2 cup	25	100	0.0
(Seabrook) cut	3.3 oz	20	77	0.0
(Southern) whole	3.5 oz	25	100	0.3
(Veg•All) cut	3.3 oz	20	75	0.0
SPINACH, NEW ZEALAND				
boiled, drained	4 oz	14	121	0.2
boiled, drained, chopped	1/2 cup	11	96	0.2
raw, chopped	1/2 cup	4	36	0.1
raw, untrimmed	1 lb	47	425	0.7
SPINACH ENTRÉE, FROZEN				
au gratin (Budget Gourmet)	6 oz	120	410	5.0
creamed (Stouffer's)	4.5 oz	190	400	16.0
soufflé (Stouffer's)	6 oz	220	820	15.0
SPINACH SALAD, 'Sassy Spinach Kit' (Saco)	1/2 cup	157	437	11.0
SPIRULINA				
dried	100 gm	290	1048	7.7
dried	1 oz	82	297	2.2

Food Name	Serv. Size	Total Cal.	Sod. MGS	Fat GMS
raw	100 gm	26	98	0.4
SPLIT PEAS				
boiled	4 oz	134	2	0.4
boiled *(A&P)*	1 cup	220	15	<1.0
boiled, mature seeds	1/2 cup	116	2	0.4
raw	1 oz	97	4	0.3
raw, green *(Arrowhead Mills)*	2 oz	200	14	1.0
raw, mature seeds	1/2 cup	334	15	1.1
SPONGE GOURD. See GOURD, DISHCLOTH.				
SPORTS DRINK				
CHOCOLATE				
(Weider) 'Dynamic Muscle Builder'	11 oz	220	260	<1.0
(Weider) 'Dynamic Weight Gainer'	11 oz	280	320	2.0
(Weider) high-energy 'Protein Blast'	11.5 oz	270	240	<1.0
(Weider) 'Sports Line Power Shake' Dutch chocolate	11 oz	220	150	<1.0
FRUIT PUNCH *(Pro-formance)*	8 oz	99	0	0.0
GRAPE				
(Opti-Carb 140)	16 oz	140	9	0.0
(Pro-formance)	8 oz	99	0	0.0
LEMON				
(Knudsen & Sons) 'Isotonic Sports Beverage'	8 oz	60	35	0.0
(Pro-formance)	8 oz	99	0	0.0
LEMONADE				
(Power Burst) advanced performance beverage	8 oz	50	25	0.0
LEMON-LIME *(Shasta)* caffeine-free, 'Body Works'	8 oz	60	95	0.0
ORANGE				
(All Sport) caffeine-free	8 oz	70	55	0.0
(Gatorade)	8 oz	50	110	0.0
(Opti-Carb 140)	16 oz	140	9	0.0
(PowerAde)	8 oz	70	70	0.0
(Pro-formance)	8 oz	99	0	0.0
(Shasta) caffeine-free, 'Body Works'	8 oz	60	95	0.0
(10-K)	8 oz	60	55	0.0
SPORTS DRINK MIX				
(Tiger's Milk)				
'Breakfast Booster' dry	2 level tbsp	70	20	<1.0
'Energy Booster' dry	3 heap tbsp	120	10	<1.0
'Protein Booster' Dutch chocolate, dry	3 heap tbsp	90	140	<1.0
'Protein Booster' vanilla-orange creme, dry	3 heap tbsp	90	140	<1.0
(Weider)				
'Big' chocolate malt, sugar-free, dry	4 scoops	320	370	2.0

Food Name	Serv. Size	Total Cal.	Sod. MGS	Fat GMS
'Carbo Energizer' orange, dry	4 scoops	230	40	0.0
'Crash Weight Gain No. 7' vanilla, dry	4 heap tbsp	300	84	3.0
'Dynamic Body Shaper' Dutch chocolate, dry	2 scoops	110	170	<1.0
'Dynamic Muscle Builder' dry	3 heap tbsp	100	116	0.0
'Dynamic Muscle Builder' natural chocolate, dry	2 scoops	120	170	1.0
'Dynamic Muscle Builder' natural vanilla, dry	2 scoops	120	180	<1.0
'Dynamic Weight Gainer' Dutch chocolate, dry	4 scoops	320	400	<1.0
'Dynamic Weight Gainer' peanut butter, dry	4 scoops	330	390	2.0
'90 Plus' vanilla, sugar-free, dry	2 scoops	100	150	0.0
'N2itro-Fire' protein blend, dry	2 tbsp	110	100	1.0
'Victory Explosive Workout' citrus, dry	4 tbsp	190	50	0.0
SPREAD, VEGETARIAN				
	1 cup	953	(mq)	83.2
	1 oz	110	(mq)	9.6
	1 tbsp	60	(mq)	5.2
(Best Foods)	1 tbsp	50	170	5.0
(Hellmann's)	1 tbsp	50	170	5.0
(Kraft)	1 tbsp	50	95	5.0
SPREADS. See CHEESE SPREAD; SPREAD, VEGETARIAN; and individual listings.				
SPRING ONION. See ONION, GREEN.				
SPRINKLES				
milk chocolate (Snack Pack)	3.88 oz	178	156	6.3
vanilla chocolate (Snack Pack)	3.88 oz	166	132	6.1
SQUASH SEED. See PUMPKIN SEED.				
SQUASH, ACORN/table queen squash				
boiled, mashed	1/2 cup	41	4	0.1
boiled, mashed	4 oz	39	3	0.1
raw (Frieda's)	1 lb	249	45	0.5
raw (Frieda's)	1 oz	16	3	<.1
raw, approx 4-inch diam	1 squash	172	13	0.4
raw, cubes	1/2 cup	28	3	0.1
raw, trimmed	1 oz	11	1	<.1
raw, untrimmed	1 lb	138	11	0.3
SQUASH, BANANA				
baked (Frieda's)	1 lb	286	45	1.8
baked (Frieda's)	1 oz	18	3	0.1
SQUASH, BUTTERNUT				
baked	4 oz	45	5	0.1
baked, cubes	1/2 cup	41	4	0.1
boiled, mashed	1/2 cup	47	2	0.1
raw, cubes	1/2 cup	32	3	0.1

Food Name	Serv. Size	Total Cal.	Sod. MGS	Fat GMS
raw, trimmed	1 oz	13	1	<.1
raw, untrimmed	1 lb	172	15	0.4
SQUASH, CROOKNECK				
boiled, drained	4 oz	23	1	0.4
boiled, drained, slices	1/2 cup	18	1	0.3
canned, drained, no salt added	4 oz	15	6	0.1
canned, yellow, cut (Allens)	1/2 cup	16	230	<1.0
frozen, boiled, drained	4 oz	28	7	0.2
frozen, cooked (Kohl's)	4 oz	45	0	<1.0
frozen, yellow (Seabrook)	3.3 oz	18	1	0.0
frozen, yellow (Southern)	3.5 oz	21	20	0.1
raw, ends trimmed	1 oz	5	1	0.1
raw, slices	1/2 cup	12	1	0.2
raw, untrimmed	1 lb	84	7	1.1
SQUASH, HUBBARD				
baked	4 oz	57	9	0.7
baked, cubes	1/2 cup	51	8	0.6
boiled, mashed	1/2 cup	35	6	0.4
boiled, mashed	4 oz	34	6	0.4
raw, cubes	1/2 cup	23	4	0.3
raw, trimmed	1 oz	11	2	0.1
raw, untrimmed	1 lb	116	20	1.5
SQUASH, MARROW/vegetable marrow squash				
raw, trimmed	1 oz	4	na	<.1
SQUASH, SCALLOP/cymling/pattypan squash				
boiled, drained	4 oz	18	1	0.2
boiled, drained, mashed	1/2 cup	19	1	0.2
boiled, drained, slices	1/2 cup	14	1	0.2
raw, slices	1/2 cup	12	1	0.1
raw, trimmed	1 oz	5	<1	0.1
raw, untrimmed	1 lb	81	5	0.9
SQUASH, SPAGHETTI				
baked or boiled, drained	4 oz	33	20	0.3
baked or boiled, drained	1/2 cup	23	14	0.2
raw, cubes	1/2 cup	16	9	0.3
raw, trimmed	1 oz	9	5	0.2
raw, untrimmed	1 lb	106	55	1.8
SQUASH, STRAIGHTNECK, raw, slices	1/2 cup	12	1	0.2
SQUASH, SUMMER, all varieties				
boiled, drained	4 oz	23	1	0.4
boiled, drained, slices	1/2 cup	18	1	0.3

Food Name	Serv. Size	Total Cal.	Sod. MGS-	Fat GMS
raw, slices	1/2 cup	13	1	0.1
raw, trimmed	1 oz	6	1	0.1
raw, untrimmed	1 lb	87	8	0.9
SQUASH, WINTER, all varieties				
baked	4 oz	44	1	0.7
baked, cubes	1/2 cup	40	1	0.6
frozen, cooked *(Birds Eye)*	4 oz	45	0	0.0
frozen, cooked *(Seabrook)*	4 oz	45	2	0.0
raw, cubes	1/2 cup	21	2	0.1
raw, trimmed	1 oz	11	1	0.1
raw, untrimmed	1 lb	119	12	0.7
SQUID, MIXED SPECIES/calamari				
fried	3 oz	149	260	6.4
raw	1 lb	416	199	6.3
raw	3 oz	78	37	1.2
raw	1 oz	26	12	0.4
STEAK SEASONING 'Spice Blends' *(Schilling)*	1/4 tsp	1	273	(tr)
STIR-FRY ENTRÉE KIT				
(Tyson)	9 oz	230	480	9.0
(Tyson) 'Yoshida Oriental Sauce'	1.6 oz	100	1260	1.0
STIR-FRY SEASONING *(Gilroy)*	1 tsp	6	5	0.0
STRAIGHTNECK SQUASH. See SQUASH, STRAIGHTNECK.				
STRAWBERRY				
trimmed	1 pint	96	3	1.2
trimmed	1 cup	45	1	0.6
trimmed	1 oz	9	<1	0.1
untrimmed	1 lb	130	5	1.6
Canned, in heavy syrup	4 oz	104	5	0.3
Freeze-dried *(Mountain House)* prepared	1/4 cup	45	<1	0.0
Frozen				
in light syrup, halves 'Quick Thaw Pouch' *(Birds Eye)*	5 oz	90	5	0.0
in light syrup, whole *(Birds Eye)*	4 oz	80	0	0.0
sweetened, sliced	10-oz pkg	273	9	0.4
sweetened, sliced	1 cup	245	8	0.3
sweetened, sliced	4 oz	109	3	0.1
sweetened, sliced *(Finast)*	3.3 oz	125	5	0.0
sweetened, whole	10-oz pkg	222	3	0.4
sweetened, whole	1 cup	199	3	0.4
sweetened, whole	4 oz	88	1	0.2
unsweetened	20-oz pkg	198	11	0.6
unsweetened	1 cup	52	3	0.2

Food Name	Serv. Size	Total Cal.	Sod. MGS	Fat GMS
unsweetened	4 oz	40	2	0.1
STRAWBERRY-BANANA NECTAR (Kern's)	6 oz	110	0	0.0
STRAWBERRY COLADA. See ALCOHOLIC BEVERAGES.				
STRAWBERRY DAIQUIRI. See ALCOHOLIC BEVERAGES.				
STRAWBERRY DRINK				
(Snapple) 'Strawberry Passion Awareness' real fruit	8 oz	120	25	0.0
STRAWBERRY FLAVOR DRINK				
(Ensure) liquid nutrition	8 oz	250	200	8.8
(Ensure) liquid nutrition 'Plus'	8 oz	355	250	12.6
(Frostee)	8 oz	180	150	7.0
(Sego) 'Lite'	10 oz	150	390	4.0
(Sego) 'Very Strawberry'	10 oz	225	360	5.0
(Squeezit) 'Silly Billy Strawberry'	6.75 oz	90	5	0.0
(Tang)	8.45 oz	120	10	0.0
(10-K)	8 oz	60	55	0.0
STRAWBERRY FLAVOR DRINK MIX, PREPARED				
(Kool-Aid) presweetened	8 oz	80	0	0.0
(Nestlé) 'Quik' 2 1/2 heap tsp w/whole milk	8 oz	220	120	8.0
(Nestlé) 'Quik' 2 1/2 heap tsp w/2% milk	8 oz	200	120	5.0
(Nestlé) 'Quik' 2 1/2 heap tsp w/skim milk	8 oz	160	125	0.0
(Turbo Nutrition) weight gain protein powder, 2 oz w/whole milk	8 oz	360	420	9.0
(Wylers) 'Crystals'	8 oz	85	43	0.3
STRAWBERRY GUAVA JUICE (Knudsen & Sons)	8 oz	105	na	0.0
STRAWBERRY GUAVA NECTAR				
(Santa Cruz Natural) organic	8 oz	90	na	<1.0
STRAWBERRY JUICE DRINK				
(Knudsen & Sons) float	8 oz	130	na	0.0
(Tang) 'Fruit Box'	8.45 oz	120	10	0.0
(Wyler's) 'Fruit Slush'	4 oz	157	10	0.0
STRAWBERRY LEMONADE				
(Kern's)	6 oz	110	0	0.0
(Knudsen & Sons)	8 oz	90	na	0.0
(Santa Cruz Natural) organic	8 oz	60	na	<1.0
(Snapple)	8 oz	110	5	0.0
STRAWBERRY NECTAR				
(Knudsen & Sons)	8 oz	105	na	0.0
(Libby's)	6 oz	110	0	0.0
STRAWBERRY PUNCH DRINK				
(Arizona) 'Cowboy Cocktail'	8 oz	120	20	0.0

Food Name	Serv. Size	Total Cal.	Sod. MGS	Fat GMS
STRAWBERRY PUNCH MIX				
(Kool-Aid) sugar-sweetened, prepared	8 oz	80	0	0.0
(Kool-Aid) unsweetened, prepared w/sugar	8 oz	100	25	0.0
(Kool-Aid) unsweetened, prepared w/o sugar	8 oz	2	25	0.0
STRAWBERRY SYRUP				
(Knott's Berry Farm)	1 oz	120	0	0.0
(Knudsen & Sons)	1 oz	75	na	<1.0
(S&W) w/saccharin	1 tsp	4	25	0.0
STRAWBERRY TOPPING				
(Kraft)	1 tbsp	50	5	0.0
(Smucker's)	2 tbsp	120	0	0.0
(Smucker's) fat-free 'Light'	2 tbsp	55	0	0.0
STRING BEAN. See GREEN BEAN.				
STROGANOFF DINNER. See BEEF ENTRÉE.				
STRUDEL. See individual listings.				
STUFFED PEPPER				
(Celentano) sweet red, frozen	13 oz	350	810	20.0
(Stouffer's) green, w/beef in tomato sauce, frozen	7.75 oz	200	650	8.0
(Stouffer's) single serving	10 oz	220	1010	8.0
STUFFING				
(Betty Crocker)				
chicken, dry	1/6 pkg	110	530	1.0
traditional herb, dry	1/6 pkg	110	550	1.0
traditional herb, prepared w/salted butter	1/2 cup	190	640	9.0
(Brownberry)				
corn, dry	1 oz	103	350	1.6
herb, dry	1 oz	100	297	1.3
(Croutettes) dry	.7 oz	70	260	0.0
(General Mills)				
chicken, dry	1/6 pkg	110	530	1.0
chicken, prepared w/margarine	1/2 cup	180	620	9.0
traditional herb, dry	1/6 pkg	110	550	<1.0
traditional herb, prepared w/margarine	1/2 cup	180	640	8.0
(Golden Dipt)				
Cajun style, dry	1/4 cup	40	590	0.0
cheddar and French, dry	1/2 cup	80	580	3.0
garden herb, dry	1/4 cup	40	330	0.0
(Golden Grain)				
chicken, dry	1 oz	106	637	1.2
cornbread, dry	1 oz	105	774	1.0
herb and butter, dry	1 oz	104	713	1.1

Food Name	Serv. Size	Total Cal.	Sod. MGS	Fat GMS
w/wild rice, dry	1 oz	108	611	1.1
(Pepperidge Farm)				
apple and raisin 'Distinctive Stuffing' dry	1 oz	110	410	1.0
classic chicken 'Distinctive Stuffing' dry	1 oz	110	410	1.0
cornbread, dry	1 oz	110	320	1.0
country style, dry	1 oz	100	400	1.0
cube, dry	1 oz	110	400	1.0
herb, country garden 'Distinctive Stuffing' dry	1 oz	120	300	4.0
herb, dry	1 oz	110	380	1.0
vegetable, harvest, w/almonds 'Distinctive' dry	1 oz	110	250	3.0
wild rice and mushroom 'Distinctive Stuffing' dry	1 oz	130	310	5.0
(Stove Top)				
Americana San Francisco, prepared w/salted butter	1/2 cup	170	650	9.0
beef, prepared w/salted butter	1/2 cup	180	590	9.0
chicken flavor, prepared w/salted butter	1/2 cup	180	570	9.0
cornbread 'Flexible Serving' prepared w/salted butter	1/2 cup	170	580	9.0
cornbread, prepared w/salted butter	1/2 cup	170	570	9.0
cornbread, prepared w/salted margarine	1/2 cup	180	590	9.0
homestyle herb 'Flexible Serving' prepared w/salted butter	1/2 cup	170	520	9.0
long grain and wild rice, prepared w/salted butter	1/2 cup	180	560	9.0
mushroom and onion, prepared w/salted butter	1/2 cup	180	490	9.0
pork 'Flexible Serving' prepared w/salted butter	1/2 cup	170	630	9.0
pork, prepared w/salted butter	1/2 cup	170	570	9.0
savory herbs, prepared w/salted butter	1/2 cup	170	590	9.0
turkey, prepared w/salted butter	1/2 cup	170	640	9.0
turkey, prepared w/salted margarine	1/2 cup	180	630	9.0
STUFFING, FROZEN				
chicken 'Stuffing Originals' *(Green Giant)*	1/2 cup	170	670	7.0
cornbread 'Stuffing Originals' *(Green Giant)*	1/2 cup	170	660	6.0
mushroom 'Stuffing Originals' *(Green Giant)*	1/2 cup	150	780	7.0
wild rice 'Stuffing Originals' *(Green Giant)*	1/2 cup	160	540	7.0
STUFFING MIX, MICROWAVE				
broccoli and cheese, prepared w/salted butter *(Stove Top)*	1/2 cup	170	580	8.0
cornbread, homestyle, prepared w/salted butter *(Stove Top)*	1/2 cup	160	450	7.0
mushroom and onion, prepared w/salted butter *(Stove Top)*	1/2 cup	170	510	7.0
STURGEON, MIXED SPECIES				
baked	4 oz	153	(mq)	5.9
broiled	4 oz	153	(mq)	5.9

Food Name	Serv. Size	Total Cal.	Sod. MGS	Fat GMS
dry-heat cooked	3 oz	115	59	4.4
microwaved	4 oz	153	(mq)	5.9
raw	1 lb	478	(mq)	18.3
raw	3 oz	89	46	3.4
raw	1 oz	30	(mq)	1.1
smoked	4 oz	196	(mq)	5.0
SUCCOTASH				
boiled, drained	4 oz	130	19	0.9
boiled, drained	1/2 cup	110	16	0.8
raw	1 lb	451	19	4.6
raw	1 oz	28	1	0.3
Canned				
(S&W) 'Country Style'	1/2 cup	80	250	1.0
(Stokely)	1/2 cup	90	300	0.0
Frozen				
boiled, drained	4 oz	105	51	1.0
boiled, drained	1/2 cup	79	38	0.8
unprepared	1/2 cup	73	35	0.7
(Frosty Acres)	3.3 oz	100	47	0.0
(Seabrook)	3.3 oz	100	47	0.0
SUGAR, ALTERNATIVE				
(Equal) aspartame	1 pkg	4	0	0.0
(Featherweight) saccharin	1 tablet	0	8	0.0
(Featherweight) saccharin, liquid	3 drops	0	0	0.0
(Nutra Taste) saccharin	1 pkt	4	0	0.0
(NutraSweet) aspartame 'Spoonful'	1 tsp	2	0	0.0
(S&W Nutradiet) saccharin, liquid	1/8 tsp	0	0	0.0
(Sprinkle Sweet)	1 tsp	2	19	0.0
(Sugar Twin) saccharin	1 pkt	4	0	0.0
(Sugar Twin) saccharin 'Plus'	1 pkt	3	0	0.0
(Sweet 'n Low)	1 pkt	4	0	0.0
(Sweet One)	1 pkt	4	0	0.0
(Sweet Plus)	1 pkt	4	0	0.0
(Sweet•10)	1/8 tsp	0	2	0.0
(Weight Watchers) 'Sweet'ner'	1 pkt	4	30	0.0
SUGAR, BEET OR CANE. See also SUGAR, ALTERNATIVE; SUGAR, DEXTROSE; SUGAR, MAPLE; SUGAR, TURBINADO; SUGAR CANE BATON.				
BROWN				
dark, 'Old Fashioned' (Domino)	1 tsp	16	0	0.0
golden, fresh from Hawaii (C&H)	1 tsp	16	0	0.0
light, 'Brownulated' (Domino)	1 tsp	12	0	0.0

Food Name	Serv. Size	Total Cal.	Sod. MGS	Fat GMS
light, golden, packed (Domino)	1 tsp	16	0	0.0
packed	1 cup	827	86	0.0
packed	1 oz	106	1	0.0
unpacked	1 cup	545	57	0.0
CONFECTIONER'S/powdered				
sifted	1 cup	385	1	0.0
sifted	1 oz	109	<1	0.0
sifted, 10-X (Domino)	1/2 cup	240	0	0.0
unsifted	1 cup	462	1	0.0
unsifted	1 tbsp	31	tr	0.0
GRANULATED				
	1 cup	774	2	0.0
	1 oz	109	<1	0.0
	1 tsp	15	0	0.0
cubes 'Dots' (Domino)	1 cube	8	0	0.0
cubes, 1/2 inch	2 cubes	19	tr	0.0
juice, organic (Sucanat)	1 tsp	12	0	0.0
lumps, 1 1/8 x 3/4 x 5/16 inches	1 lump	19	tr	0.0
packet, approx .2 oz	1 pkt	23	tr	0.0
'Packets' (Domino)	1 pkt	16	0	0.0
SUPERFINE, instant dissolving (Domino)	1 tsp	16	0	0.0
SUGAR, DEXTROSE				
anhydrous	100 gm	366	0	0.0
anhydrous	1 oz	104	tr	0.0
crystallized	100 gm	335	0	0.0
crystallized	1 oz	95	tr	0.0
SUGAR, MAPLE				
	100 gm	354	11	0.2
	1-oz piece	100	3	0.1
SUGAR, TURBINADO (Hain)	1 tbsp	50	0	0.0
SUGAR APPLE/sweetsop				
raw, approx 2 7/8-inch diam	1 med	146	14	0.5
raw, pulp	1 cup	235	23	0.7
trimmed	1/2 cup	118	12	0.4
trimmed	1 oz	27	3	0.1
untrimmed	1 lb	236	24	0.7
SUGAR CANE BATON (Frieda's)	1 oz	21	na	0.1
SUGAR CANE JUICE	1 oz	21	na	tr
SUMMER SAUSAGE				
(Eckrich)	1-oz slice	80	320	7.0
(Hillshire Farm)	2 oz	180	670	16.0

Food Name	Serv. Size	Total Cal.	Sod. MGS	Fat GMS
(Hormel) 'Perma-Fresh'	2 slices	140	706	11.0
(Hormel) 'Tangy Chub'	1 oz	90	317	7.0
(Hormel) 'Thuringer'	1 oz	90	332	9.0
BEEF				
(Hillshire Farm)	2 oz	190	(mq)	17.0
(Hormel) 'Beefy'	1 oz	100	313	9.0
(Lean & Lite)	1 oz	43	(mq)	2.3
(Light & Lean)	2 slices	100	(mq)	8.0
(OHSE)	1 oz	75	340	5.0
(Oscar Mayer)	.8-oz slice	69	331	6.1
TURKEY *(Louis Rich)*	1-oz slice	55	326	3.9
W/CHEESE *(Hillshire Farm)*	2 oz	200	(mq)	18.0
SUN-DRIED TOMATOES, in oil and herbs *(Bella Sun Luci)*	2/3 oz	60	20	3.0
SUNFISH/calico bass/crappie/pumpkinseed				
dry-heat cooked	3 oz	97	88	0.8
raw	1 lb	404	368	3.2
raw	3 oz	76	68	0.6
raw	1 oz	25	23	0.2
SUNFLOWER OIL				
hydrogenated	1/2 cup	964	0	109.0
hydrogenated	1 oz	251	0	28.4
linoleic	1/2 cup	964	0	109.0
linoleic	1 oz	251	0	28.4
(Hain)	1 tbsp	120	0	14.0
(IGA)	1 tbsp	120	0	14.0
(Kroger)	1 tbsp	122	0	13.6
(Pathmark)	1 tbsp	130	0	14.0
(Spectrum Naturals)	1 tbsp	120	0	14.0
(Wesson)	1 tbsp	122	0	13.6
SUNFLOWER SEED KERNELS				
Dried				
	1 cup	821	4	71.4
	1 oz	162	1	14.1
in shell	1 lb	1397	8	121.4
(Arrowhead Mills)	1 oz	160	3	13.0
(Frito-Lay's)	1 oz	160	265	14.0
Dry-roasted				
	1 cup	745	4	63.7
	1 oz	165	1	14.1
salted	1 cup	745	998	63.7
salted	1 oz	165	221	14.1

Food Name	Serv. Size	Total Cal.	Sod. MGS	Fat GMS
(Fisher)	1 oz	170	200	15.0
(Fisher) in shell	1 oz	170	110	15.0
(Fisher) in shell, salted	1 oz	170	110	14.0
(Flavor House)	1 oz	180	200	15.0
(Pathmark)	1 oz	180	150	14.0
(Planters)	1 oz	160	170	14.0
Oil-roasted				
	1 cup	830	4	77.6
	1 oz	175	1	16.3
salted	1 cup	830	814	77.6
salted	1 oz	175	171	16.3
(Fisher)	1 oz	170	170	16.0
(Planters)	1 oz	170	135	15.0
Toasted				
	1 cup	829	4	76.1
	1 oz	176	1	16.1
salted	1 cup	829	821	76.1
salted	1 oz	176	174	16.1
(Fisher)	1 oz	170	0	14.0
SUNFLOWER SEED FLOUR				
partially defatted	1 cup	261	2	1.3
partially defatted	1 oz	92	1	0.5
partially defatted	1 tbsp	16	0	0.1
SUNSHINE JUICE, organic (Santa Cruz Natural)	8 oz	100	na·	1.0
SURIMI				
	3 oz	84	122	0.8
leg style 'Classic Seablends' 10% crab				
(Peter Pan Seafoods)	3.5 oz	85	890	0.4
leg style 'Standard Seablends' (Peter Pan Seafoods)	3.5 oz	88	845	0.4
salad style 'Classic Seablends Combo' 10% crab				
(Peter Pan Seafoods)	3.5 oz	85	890	0.4
salad style 'Standard Seablends Combo'				
(Peter Pan Seafoods)	3.5 oz	88	845	0.4
SURINAM CHERRY. See PITANGA.				
SWAMP CABBAGE. See CABBAGE, SKUNK.				
SWEDISH MEATBALL DINNER/ENTRÉE				
frozen dinner, 'Classics' (Armour)	11.25 oz	330	1140	18.0
frozen entrée, w/parsley noodles, gravy				
'Lean Cuisine' (Stouffer's)	9.25 oz	420	740	21.0
frozen entrée, w/pasta, gravy 'Lean Cuisine' (Stouffer's)	9 1/8 oz	290	550	8.0

Food Name	Serv. Size	Total Cal.	Sod. MGS	Fat GMS
SWEDISH TURNIP				
boiled, drained	4 oz	39	20	0.2
boiled, drained, cubed	1/2 cup	29	15	0.2
boiled, drained, mashed	1/2 cup	41	22	0.2
raw, cubed	1/2 cup	25	14	0.1
raw, trimmed	1 oz	10	6	0.1
raw, untrimmed	1 lb	140	77	0.8
SWEET AND SOUR DINNER (LaChoy)	4.48 oz	89	838	0.2
SWEET POTATO. See also YAM.				
baked in skin, pulp only	4 oz	117	11	0.1
baked in skin, pulp only, 5 inches long, 2 inches diam	1 potato	118	12	0.1
baked in skin, pulp only, mashed	1/2 cup	103	10	0.1
boiled, w/o skin	4 oz	119	15	0.3
boiled, w/o skin, mashed	1/2 cup	172	21	0.5
dehydrated flakes, dry	1 cup	455	217	0.7
dehydrated flakes, prepared w/water	1 lb	431	204	0.5
dehydrated flakes, prepared w/water	1 cup	242	115	0.3
raw, cubes	1 cup	140	17	0.4
raw, 5 inches long, 2 inches diam	1 potato	136	17	0.4
raw, trimmed	1 oz	30	4	0.1
raw, untrimmed	1 lb	343	44	1.0
SWEET POTATO, CANNED				
Candied				
(Joan of Arc)	1/2 cup	240	15	0.0
(Princella)	1/2 cup	240	15	0.0
(Royal Prince)	1/2 cup	240	15	0.0
(S&W)	1/2 cup	180	355	0.0
In extra heavy syrup (S&W) 'Southern'	1/2 cup	139	27	1.0
In heavy syrup				
(Joan of Arc)	1/2 cup	130	35	0.0
(Princella)	1/2 cup	130	35	0.0
(Royal Prince)	1/2 cup	130	35	0.0
In light syrup				
(Finast)	1/2 cup	110	45	<1.0
(Joan of Arc)	1/2 cup	110	25	0.0
(Princella)	1/2 cup	110	25	0.0
(Royal Prince)	1/2 cup	110	25	0.0
In pineapple-orange sauce				
(Joan of Arc)	1/2 cup	210	35	0.0
(Princella)	1/2 cup	210	35	0.0
(Royal Prince)	1/2 cup	210	35	0.0

Food Name	Serv. Size	Total Cal.	Sod. MGS	Fat GMS
In syrup				
(Allens) cut	1/2 cup	90	20	<1.0
(Allens) whole	1/2 cup	90	40	<1.0
(Joan of Arc)	1/2 cup	90	45	0.0
(Kohl's) cut	1/2 cup	110	30	<1.0
(Pathmark) 'No Frills'	1/2 cup	105	33	0.0
(Pathmark) 'Southern'	1 cup	230	100	0.0
(Princella)	1/2 cup	90	45	0.0
(Royal Prince)	1/2 cup	90	45	0.0
(Taylor's Brand) whole and cut	1 cup	240	56	0.0
In water (Allens) cut	1/2 cup	70	20	<1.0
SWEET POTATO, FROZEN				
unprepared, cubes	1/2 cup	84	5	0.2
(Mrs. Paul's) candied	4 oz	170	40	0.0
(Mrs. Paul's) candied, w/apples 'Sweets 'n Apples'	4 oz	160	60	0.0
SWEET POTATO LEAF				
raw, approx 12 1/4 inches long	1 leaf	6	1	0.1
raw, chopped	1 cup	12	3	0.1
raw, trimmed	1 oz	10	3	0.1
raw, untrimmed	1 lb	149	38	1.3
steamed	4 oz	39	15	0.3
steamed	1/2 cup	11	4	0.1

SWEETBREAD. See BEEF, PANCREAS; BEEF, THYMUS; LAMB, PANCREAS; VEAL, PANCREAS; VEAL, THYMUS.

SWEETENERS. See SUGAR, ALTERNATIVE; SUGAR, BEET OR CANE; SUGAR, MAPLE; SUGAR, TURBINADO.

SWEETSOP. See SUGAR APPLE.

Food Name	Serv. Size	Total Cal.	Sod. MGS	Fat GMS
SWISS CHARD/chard				
boiled, drained	4 oz	23	203	0.1
boiled, drained, chopped	1/2 cup	18	158	0.1
raw, chopped	1/2 cup	3	38	0.0
raw, trimmed	1 oz	5	60	0.1
raw, untrimmed	1 lb	81	888	0.8
SWISS STEAK DINNER				
frozen (Budget Gourmet)	11.2 oz	450	1110	22.0
frozen (Swanson)	10 oz	350	700	11.0
SWISS STEAK SEASONING MIX				
'Bag 'n Season' (Schilling)	1 pkg	81	2651	0.4
SWORDFISH				
baked	4 oz	176	130	5.8
broiled	4 oz	176	130	5.8

Food Name	Serv. Size	Total Cal.	Sod. MGS	Fat GMS
dry-heat cooked	3 oz	132	98	4.4
frozen, steaks, w/o seasoning mix *(SeaPak)*	6-oz pkg	210	155	7.0
microwaved	4 oz	176	130	5.8
raw	1 lb	548	408	18.2
raw	3 oz	103	77	3.4
raw	1 oz	34	26	1.1
raw *(Peter Pan Seafoods)*	3.5 oz	118	102	4.0

T

Food Name	Serv. Size	Total Cal.	Sod. MGS	Fat GMS
TABBOULEH MIX				
(Casbah) dry	1 oz	126	(mq)	1.0
(Fantastic Foods) prepared w/oil and tomatoes	1/2 cup	161	250	10.0
(Fantastic Foods) prepared w/o oil	1/2 cup	85	265	0.5
(Near East) prepared	1/2 cup	170	290	9.0
TABLE QUEEN SQUASH. See SQUASH, ACORN.				
TACO DIP. See DIP, TACO.				
TACO KIT				
(Natural Touch) vegetarian	2 tbsp	90	(mq)	2.0
(Old El Paso) prepared	1 taco	67	423	3.0
(Tio Sancho) 'Dinner Kit' prepared	1 taco	64	1	3.1
TACO SEASONING MIX				
(Hain)	1/10 pkg	10	200	0.0
(Lawry's) 'Seasoning Blends'	1 pkg	118	1441	1.1
(Old El Paso)	1 pkg	100	3570	1.0
(Old El Paso)	1/12 pkg	8	298	<1.0
(Schilling)	1/4 pkg	31	675	0.5
(Tio Sancho)	1.51 oz	132	2623	1.7
(Tio Sancho) 'Dinner Kit' taco seasoning	1.25 oz	104	2500	1.4
TACO SHELL				
(Azteca) corn	1 shell	60	65	3.0
(Azteca) flour	1 shell	200	130	12.0
(Chi-Chi's)	1 shell	140	5	7.0
(Gebhardt)	1 shell	50	<1	2.0
(Lawry's)	1 shell	50	123	2.1
(Lawry's) 'Super'	1 shell	86	210	3.6
(Old El Paso)	1 shell	50	50	3.0
(Old El Paso) 'Mini'	3 shells	70	60	4.0
(Old El Paso) 'Super Size'	1 shell	100	95	6.0

Food Name	Serv. Size	Total Cal.	Sod. MGS	Fat GMS
(Ortega)	1 shell	50	5	2.0
(Rosarita)	1 shell	50	<1	2.0
(Tio Sancho)	1 shell	64	1	3.1
(Tio Sancho) 'Super'	1 shell	94	2	4.7
TAFFY. See CANDY.				
TAHINI MIX				
(Arrowhead Mills) organic	1 oz	170	<1	17.0
(Casbah) dry	1 oz	25	(mq)	5.0
(Erewhon) 'Sesame Tahini'	2 tbsp	200	65	18.0
(Maranatha Natural) 'Sesame Tahini'	2 tbsp	210	20	19.0
(Westbrae) raw, organic	2 tbsp	210	0	19.0
(Westbrae) toasted, organic	2 tbsp	220	0	19.0
TAMALE				
(Derby) beef	2 tamales	160	570	7.0
(Gebhardt)	2 tamales	290	730	22.0
(Gebhardt) jumbo	2 tamales	400	1025	30.0
Canned				
(Derby) beef	6.561 oz	253	1034	17.4
(Gebhardt)	5.75 oz	269	770	20.7
(Gebhardt) beef	4 oz	230	620	17.0
(Gebhardt) jumbo	6.949 oz	332	930	25.2
(Hormel)	7.5 oz	280	990	20.0
(Hormel) beef	2 tamales	140	550	10.0
(Hormel) hot 'n spicy	7.5 oz	280	990	20.0
(Libby's) beef, w/sauce	7.5 oz	408	1200	30.2
(Old El Paso)	2 tamales	190	380	12.0
(Van Camp's) w/sauce	1 cup	293	1132	16.2
(Wolf Brand)	7.75 oz	328	1181	24.5
Frozen				
(Amy's Kitchen) 'Mexican' organic	8 oz	170	190	3.0
(Hormel) beef	1 tamale	140	555	7.0
(Patio) dinner	13 oz	470	1850	21.0
TAMALITO (Dennison's) in chili gravy, canned	7.5 oz	310	1395	16.0
TAMARIND/Indian date				
pulp	1 cup	287	34	0.7
'Tamarindos' (Frieda's)	3.5 oz	239	51	0.6
trimmed	1 oz	68	8	0.2
untrimmed	1 lb	369	43	0.9
TANGELO JUICE, fresh	100 gm	41	1	0.1
TANGERINE				
peeled, seeded	1 oz	12	<1	0.1

Food Name	Serv. Size	Total Cal.	Sod. MGS	Fat GMS
sections, w/o membrane	1/2 cup	43	2	0.2
untrimmed	1 lb	144	4	0.6
TANGERINE, CANNED				
in heavy syrup (S&W)	1/2 cup	76	10	0.0
in juice	4 oz	42	6	<.1
in light syrup	4 oz	69	7	0.1
in light syrup (A&P)	1/2 cup	80	0	<1.0
in light syrup (Dole)	1/2 cup	76	0	0.1
in light syrup (Empress)	5.5 oz	100	10	0.1
in light syrup (Finast)	5.5 oz	100	na	0.0
'Natural Style' (S&W)	1/2 cup	60	10	0.0
sections, in water (Featherweight)	1/2 cup	35	10	0.0
unsweetened (S&W Nutradiet)	1/2 cup	28	10	0.0
TANGERINE JUICE				
canned, sweetened	1 cup	125	2	0.5
canned, sweetened	1 oz	16	0	0.1
chilled 'Pure & Light Mandarin Tangerine' (Dole)	6 oz	97	20	0.1
fresh	1 cup	106	2	0.5
fresh	1 oz	13	0	0.1
frozen concentrate, sweetened, diluted w/3 vol water	1 cup	111	2	0.3
frozen concentrate, sweetened, diluted w/3 vol water	1 oz	14	0	0.0
frozen concentrate, sweetened, undiluted	6 oz	345	6	0.8
frozen or chilled (Minute Maid)	6 oz	90	0	0.0
TANGERINE ORANGE DRINK				
'Thirst Quencher Light' (Gatorade)	8 oz	25	80	0.0
TAPIOCA, PEARL				
dry	1 cup	518	2	0.0
dry	1 oz	97	tr	tr
TARO				
cooked	4 oz	161	11	0.1
cooked, slices	1/2 cup	94	10	0.1
raw, slices	1/2 cup	56	6	0.1
raw, trimmed	1 oz	30	3	0.1
raw, untrimmed	1 lb	419	43	0.8
TARO, TAHITIAN				
cooked	4 oz	50	61	0.8
cooked, slices	1/2 cup	30	37	0.5
raw, slices	1/2 cup	25	31	0.6
raw, trimmed	1 lb	181	227	4.4
raw, trimmed	1 oz	11	14	0.3

ood Name	Serv. Size	Total Cal.	Sod. MGS	Fat GMS
TARO LEAF				
raw	1 cup	12	1	0.2
raw, 11 x 6 1/2 inches	1 leaf	4	0	0.1
raw, trimmed	1 oz	12	1	0.2
raw, untrimmed	1 lb	115	8	2.0
steamed	4 oz	27	2	0.5
steamed	1/2 cup	18	1	0.3
TARO SHOOTS				
cooked	4 oz	16	2	0.1
cooked, slices	1/2 cup	10	1	0.1
raw, 15 x 5 inches	1 shoot	9	1	0.1
raw, slices	1/2 cup	5	0	0.0
raw, trimmed	1 oz	3	<1	<.1
raw, untrimmed	1 lb	45	4	0.4
TARPON, ATLANTIC				
raw	1 lb	422	(mq)	1.8
raw	1 oz	26	(mq)	0.1
TARRAGON				
ground	1 oz	84	18	2.1
ground	1 tbsp	14	3	0.4
ground	1 tsp	5	1	0.1
ground *(Durkee)*	1 tsp	10	0	<0.1
ground *(Laurel Leaf)*	1 tsp	10	0	<0.1
ground *(Spice Islands)*	1 tsp	5	1	0.1
TEA				
Brewed				
prepared w/distilled water	6 oz	2	0	0.0
prepared w/tap water	6 oz	2	5	0.0
(Celestial Seasonings) caffeine-free	8 oz	4	5	tr
(Nestea)	6 oz	0	0	0.0
Instant				
decaffeinated *(Lipton)*	6 oz	0	0	0.0
lemon flavor *(Lipton)*	6 oz	3	1	0.0
regular *(Lipton)*	6 oz	0	0	0.0
TEA, FLAVORED				
(Bigelow)				
'Chinese Fortune'	5.25 oz	1	<1	tr
'Cinnamon Stick'	5.25 oz	1	<1	tr
'Constant Comment'	5.25 oz	1	<1	tr
'Darjeeling'	5.25 oz	1	<1	tr
'Earl Grey'	5.25 oz	1	1	tr

Food Name	Serv. Size	Total Cal.	Sod. MGS	Fa G
'English Teatime'	5.25 oz	1	tr	
'Lemon Lift'	5.25 oz	1	<1	
'Plantation Mint'	5.25 oz	1	1	
'Raspberry Royale'	5.25 oz	1	<1	
(Celestial Seasonings)				
'Amaretto Nights'	8 oz	3	1	
apple spice 'Fruit & Tea'	8 oz	3	1	
'Bavarian Chocolate Orange'	8 oz	7	5	
'Cinnamon Vienna'	8 oz	2	2	
'Classic English Breakfast'	8 oz	3	<1	
'Darjeeling Gardens'	8 oz	3	<1	
'Extraordinary Earl Grey'	8 oz	3	<1	
'Irish Cream Mist'	8 oz	3	1	
lemon 'Fruit & Tea'	8 oz	3	<1	
mint, Swiss	8 oz	3	<1	
'Morning Thunder'	8 oz	3	<1	
orange spice 'Fruit & Tea'	8 oz	3	<1	
raspberry 'Fruit & Tea'	8 oz	2	<1	
(Nestea)				
apple spice	16 oz	180	50	0.
apple spice	6 oz	66	18	0.
lemon, natural	16 oz	180	50	0.
lemon, natural	6 oz	66	18	0.
lemon, natural, diet	16 oz	180	50	0.
lemon, natural, diet	6 oz	66	18	0.
peach	16 oz	180	50	0.
peach	6 oz	66	18	0.
raspberry	16 oz	180	50	0.
raspberry	6 oz	66	18	0.
tropical	16 oz	180	50	0.
tropical	6 oz	66	18	0.
(Tetley)				
'Apple Freeze'	8 oz	79	<1	0.
'Classic'	8 oz	69	<1	0.
'Classic Lemon'	8 oz	108	<1	0.
'Diet Lemon Frost'	8 oz	10	<1	0.
'Diet Raspberry Blizzard'	8 oz	10	<1	0.
'Lemon Frost'	8 oz	89	<1	0.
'Orange Glazier'	8 oz	79	<1	0.
'Peach Chiller'	8 oz	79	<1	0.
'Raspberry Blizzard'	8 oz	95	<1	0.

Food Name	Serv. Size	Total Cal.	Sod. MGS	Fat GMS
(Wyler's) 'Fruit Tea Punch'	12 oz	118	1	0.0
TEA, HERBAL				
(Bigelow)				
almond orange	5 oz	<1	<1	tr
'Apple Orchard'	5.25 oz	5	1	tr
apple spice	5 oz	<1	1	tr
chamomile	5 oz	<1	2	tr
chamomile mint	5 oz	<1	1	tr
cinnamon orange	5 oz	<1	<1	tr
cranberry apple	5 oz	1	1	tr
'Fruit & Almond'	5.25 oz	1	<1	tr
grains, roasted, w/carob	5 oz	3	1	tr
hibiscus and rose hips	5 oz	1	1	tr
'I Love Lemon'	5.25 oz	1	<1	tr
'Lemon & C'	5 oz	<1	<1	tr
'Mint Blend'	5 oz	<1	3	tr
'Mint Medley'	5.25 oz	1	<1	tr
'Orange & C'	5 oz	<1	<1	tr
'Orange & Spice'	5.25 oz	1	1	tr
peppermint	5 oz	<1	2	<.1
red raspberry	5 oz	1	<1	tr
spearmint	5 oz	<1	1	tr
'Specially Strawberry'	5 oz	1	<1	tr
'Sweet Dreams'	5.25 oz	1	1	tr
'Take-A-Break'	5.25 oz	1	1	tr
(Celestial Seasonings)				
'Almond Sunset'	8 oz	3	2	tr
chamomile	8 oz	2	5	tr
'Cinnamon Apple Spice'	8 oz	3	1	tr
'Cinnamon Rose'	8 oz	2	1	tr
'Country Peach Spice'	8 oz	3	3	tr
'Cranberry Cove'	8 oz	3	1	tr
'Emperor's Choice'	8 oz	4	2	<.1
'Ginseng Plus'	8 oz	3	4	tr
'Grandma's Tummy Mint'	8 oz	2	7	tr
'Lemon Mist'	8 oz	2	3	tr
'Lemon Zinger'	8 oz	4	1	tr
'Mandarin Orange Spice'	8 oz	5	2	tr
'Mellow Mint'	8 oz	2	4	tr
'Mint Magic'	8 oz	1	3	tr
'Mo's 24'	8 oz	2	4	tr

Food Name	Serv. Size	Total Cal.	Sod. MGS	
'Orange Zinger'	8 oz	5	1	
peppermint	8 oz	2	8	
'Raspberry Patch'	8 oz	4	1	
'Red Zinger'	8 oz	4	2	
'Roastaroma'	8 oz	11	4	<
'Sleepytime'	8 oz	5	2	
spearmint	8 oz	5	6	<
'Strawberry Fields'	8 oz	4	1	
'Sunburst C'	8 oz	3	6	
'Wild Forest Blackberry'	8 oz	2	1	
(Lipton)				
'Almond Pleasure'	8 oz	4	0	0
chamomile	8 oz	4	0	0
cinnamon apple	8 oz	2	0	0
'Citrus Sunset'	8 oz	4	0	0
'Gentle/Tangy Orange'	8 oz	4	0	0
'Lemon Soother'	8 oz	4	0	0
'Toasty Spice'	8 oz	6	0	0
TEA, ICED				
BOTTLE, BOX, OR CAN				
(Arizona)				
'Diet'	8 oz	4	15	0
'Diet' with lemon	8 oz	4	15	0
raspberry flavor, sun-brewed style	8 oz	95	20	0
(Lipton) w/lemon, aseptic box	8.45 oz	96	20	0
(Nestea)				
	8 oz	90	35	0
diet	8 oz	4	35	0
(Shasta)	12 oz	124	28	0
(Snapple)				
cranberry	8 oz	110	10	0
'Diet'	8 oz	0	10	0
lemon	8 oz	110	10	0
mango	8 oz	110	5	0
mint	8 oz	120	10	0
old fashioned	8 oz	80	10	0
orange	8 oz	110	10	0
peach	8 oz	110	10	0
peach 'Diet'	8 oz	0	10	0
raspberry	8 oz	120	10	0
raspberry 'Diet'	8 oz	0	10	0

Food Name	Serv. Size	Total Cal.	Sod. MGS	Fat GMS
strawberry	8 oz	100	10	0.0
w/lemon, 'Diet'	8 oz	4	15	<1.0
(Tetley)				
brewed	8 oz	74	20	0.0
brewed, w/lemon	8 oz	74	20	0.0
sweetened	8 oz	74	20	0.0
(Veryfine)				
peach kiwi flavored, brewed, 'Chillers'	8 oz	80	5	0.0
w/lemon	8 oz	80	10	0.0
PREPARED FROM MIX				
(Crystal Light)				
w/NutraSweet	8 oz	4	0	0.0
w/Nutrasweet, decaffeinated	8 oz	4	0	0.0
(Lipton)				
lemon flavor	6 oz	55	1	0.0
lemon flavor, decaffeinated	6 oz	55	<1	0.0
lemon flavor, w/NutraSweet	8 oz	5	2	0.0
'Sugar-free'	8 oz	1	6	0.0
'Sugar-free' decaffeinated	8 oz	1	5	0.0
(Nestea)				
'Ice Teasers' all flavors	8 oz	6	0	0.0
lemon flavor	8 oz	6	0	0.0
lemon flavor, sugar-free	8 oz	4	0	0.0
lemon flavor, sugar-free, decaffeinated	2 tsp	6	0	0.0
'100%'	8 oz	2	0	0.0
'100%' decaffeinated	8 oz	0	0	0.0
sugar-free	8 oz	6	5	0.0
w/sugar and lemon	8 oz	70	0	0.0
(Pathmark)				
lemon flavor, low-calorie	8 oz	4	0	0.0
lemon flavor, low-calorie, decaffeinated	8 oz	4	0	0.0
lemon flavor, sugar-sweetened, decaffeinated	2 tbsp	80	0	0.0
TEA FLAVORED DRINK *(10-K)*	8 oz	60	55	0.0
TEASEED OIL				
	1 cup	1927	0	218.0
	1 oz	251	0	28.4
	1 tbsp	120	0	13.6
TEFF FLOUR, whole-grain *(Arrowhead Mills)*	2 oz	200	6	1.0
TEFF SEED *(Arrowhead Mills)*	1/2 cup	165	5	6.4
TEMPEH	1 oz	56	2	2.2
TENDERGREEN. See MUSTARD SPINACH.				

Food Name	Serv. Size	Total Cal.	Sod. MGS	Fat GMS
TEQUILA. See ALCOHOLIC BEVERAGES.				
TERIYAKI MARINADE				
(Lawry's)	2 tbsp	72	7100	0.4
(Lawry's) barbecue	1/4 cup	164	12330	2.3
TERRAPIN, diamondback, raw	100 gm	111	50	3.5
THURINGER CERVELAT				
(Hillshire Farm)	2 oz	180	650	15.0
(Hormel) 'Old Smokehouse'	1 oz	90	328	8.0
(Hormel) 'Old Smokehouse Chub'	1 oz	100	332	9.0
(Hormel) 'Old Smokehouse Sliced'	1 oz	100	321	9.0
(Hormel) 'Viking Club Cervelat'	1 oz	90	325	8.0
(JM) beef	1-oz slice	80	340	7.0
(JM) 'Cervelat'	1-oz slice	70	260	6.0
THYME				
ground	1 oz	78	16	2.1
ground	1 tbsp	12	2	0.3
ground	1 tsp	4	1	0.1
ground (Durkee)	1 tsp	5	0	tr
ground (Laurel Leaf)	1 tsp	5	0	tr
ground (Spice Islands)	1 tsp	5	1	0.1
TOASTED SESAME OIL. See SESAME OIL.				
TOASTER BISCUIT. See BISCUIT, TOASTER.				
TOASTER MUFFIN/PASTRY. See MUFFIN/PASTRY, TOASTER.				
TOFFEE. See CANDY.				
TOFU/soybean curd cake				
raw	1 oz	22	2	1.4
raw	1/2 cup	94	9	5.9
Flavored				
Chinese five-spice (Nasoya)	5 oz	150	15	8.0
French, country herb (Nasoya)	5 oz	150	15	8.0
pasteurized (Frieda's)	4.2 oz	86	8	(mq)
Freeze-dried/koyadofu	1 oz	136	2	8.6
Fried	1 oz	77	5	5.7
Grilled/yakidofu	1 oz	25	5	1.7
Okara	1 oz	22	3	0.5
Salted and fermented/fuyu	1 oz	33	814	2.3
Silken (Mori-Nu)	1/2 pkg	90	50	4.0
TOFU PATTY, FROZEN				
garden (Natural Touch)	2.5-oz patty	90	260	4.0
okara (Natural Touch)	2.25-oz patty	160	420	10.0

Food Name	Serv. Size	Total Cal.	Sod. MGS	Fat GMS
TOFU SPREAD				
green chili 'Tofu Topper' canned *(Natural Touch)*	2 tbsp	50	(mq)	4.0
herb and spice 'Tofu Topper' canned *(Natural Touch)*	2 tbsp	50	(mq)	4.0
Mexican 'Tofu Topper' canned *(Natural Touch)*	2 tbsp	60	(mq)	5.0
TOM COLLINS. See ALCOHOLIC BEVERAGES.				
TOMATILLO/ground husk tomato				
fresh *(Frieda's)*	3.5 oz	25	na	0.5
raw	1 med	11	0	0.4
raw, chopped	1/2 cup	21	1	0.7
TOMATO. See also TOMATO, SUN-DRIED.				
Green				
raw, 2 3/5-inch diam	1 tomato	30	16	0.3
trimmed	1 oz	7	4	0.1
untrimmed	1 lb	99	55	0.8
Red				
boiled	1/2 cup	32	13	0.5
boiled	4 oz	31	12	0.5
raw, chopped	1/2 cup	19	8	0.3
raw, 2 3/5-inch diam, 4.75 oz	1 tomato	26	11	0.4
raw, trimmed	1 oz	6	3	0.1
raw, untrimmed	1 lb	88	36	1.4
stewed	1 cup	80	460	2.7
stewed	4 oz	90	516	3.0
TOMATO, CANNED				
(A&P)				
sliced	1/2 cup	35	350	<1.0
whole	1/2 cup	25	220	<1.0
(Angela Mia)				
chopped, 'Premium Choice'	4 oz	24	254	0.4
crushed	4 oz	25	463	0.2
crushed, chunky	4 oz	26	378	0.3
crushed, 'Premium Choice'	2.222 oz	29	25	0.4
(Contadina)				
crushed, in purée	1/2 cup	30	350	<1.0
Italian style	1/2 cup	35	250	<1.0
Italian style, pear	1/2 cup	25	220	<1.0
'Recipe Ready'	1/2 cup	25	570	0.2
stewed	1/2 cup	35	350	<1.0
stewed, Mexican style	1/2 cup	35	230	0.3
whole, peeled	1/2 cup	25	260	<1.0
w/jalapeños	1/2 cup	35	250	<1.0

Food Name	Serv. Size	Total Cal.	Sod. MGS	Fat GMS
(Del Monte)				
stewed	1/2 cup	35	355	0.0
stewed, 'No Salt Added'	1/2 cup	35	45	0.0
wedges, w/liquid	1/2 cup	30	355	0.0
whole, peeled, w/liquid	1/2 cup	25	220	0.0
(Eden Foods) crushed, organic, no salt added	4 oz	35	0	0.0
(Featherweight)	1/2 cup	20	<1	0.0
(Finast)				
sliced	1/2 cup	35	355	0.0
whole, peeled	1/2 cup	25	195	0.0
(Hunt's)				
choice cut	4 oz	19	278	0.0
crushed	4 oz	31	317	0.4
crushed, 'Angela Mia'	4 oz	35	260	<1.0
crushed, Italian flavored	4 oz	40	460	<1.0
diced, in juice	4 oz	19	477	0.1
diced, in juice, 'No Salt Added'	4 oz	20	8	0.1
diced, in purée	4 oz	23	304	0.2
diced, w/green chilies	.3527 oz	2	33	0.1
pear shaped	4.868 oz	21	285	0.1
pear shaped	4.832 oz	21	373	0.1
pear shaped	4.656 oz	20	360	0.1
pear shaped, Italian flavored	4 oz	20	320	<1.0
peeled, choice cut	4 oz	20	460	<1.0
stewed	4 oz	33	357	0.1
stewed, 'Food Service'	4 oz	29	262	0.1
stewed, Italian flavored	4 oz	35	400	<1.0
stewed, 'No Salt Added'	1/2 cup	35	20	0.0
whole	4 oz	20	415	0.0
whole, Italian flavored	4 oz	25	420	<1.0
whole, 'No Salt Added'	4 oz	20	20	0.0
whole, peeled	5.608 oz	24	433	0.3
whole, peeled	5.22 oz	22	333	0.1
whole, peeled	5.009 oz	22	387	0.1
whole, peeled	4.832 oz	21	373	0.1
whole, peeled, 'No Salt Added'	4.832 oz	21	9	0.1
(Old El Paso) w/green chilies	1/4 cup	14	480	0.0
(Ortega) w/jalapeños	1 oz	8	120	0.0
(Pathmark)				
crushed	1/2 cup	40	210	0.0
crushed, 'No Frills'	1 cup	90	510	0.0

Food Name	Serv. Size	Total Cal.	Sod. MGS	Fat GMS
'No Frills'	1 cup	50	440	0.0
sliced	1/2 cup	35	360	0.0
whole, peeled, 'No Salt Added'	1/2 cup	25	20	0.0
whole, peeled, w/tomato juice	1/2 cup	25	220	0.0
(S&W)				
aspic, supreme	1/2 cup	60	860	0.0
cut, peeled, 'Ready-Cut'	1/2 cup	25	220	0.0
diced, in rich purée	1/2 cup	35	290	0.0
Italian, sliced	1/2 cup	35	355	0.0
Mexican style	1/2 cup	40	360	0.0
sliced	1/2 cup	35	355	0.0
stewed, '50% Salt Reduced'	1/2 cup	35	180	0.0
whole, peeled	1/2 cup	25	220	0.0
whole, peeled, Italian-style pear, w/basil	1/2 cup	25	200	0.0
(S&W Nutradiet) whole	1/2 cup	25	20	0.0
(Stokely)				
stewed	1/2 cup	35	220	0.0
whole	1/2 cup	25	190	0.0
TOMATO, PICKLED, kosher *(Claussen)*	1 oz	5	330	0.0
TOMATO-BEEF COCKTAIL *(Beefamato)*	6 oz	80	240	0.0
TOMATO-CHILE COCKTAIL *(Snap-E-Tom)*	6 oz	40	980	0.0
TOMATO-CLAM COCKTAIL *(Clamato)*	6 oz	96	815	0.0
TOMATO JUICE				
(A&P)	6 oz	30	550	0.0
(Biotta)	6 oz	28	277	0.1
(Campbell's)	6 oz	40	540	0.0
(Featherweight)	6 oz	35	10	0.0
(Hunt's)	9.03 oz	33	608	0.2
(Hunt's)	7.16 oz	28	513	0.2
(Hunt's)	6 oz	30	640	0.0
(Hunt's)	5.467 oz	22	399	0.1
(Hunt's) 'No Salt Added'	6 oz	45	30	0.0
(Knudsen & Sons) organic	8 oz	50	na	0.0
(Libby's)	6 oz	35	500	0.0
(Pathmark)	6 oz	30	510	0.0
(Pathmark) frozen, diluted	6 oz	35	450	0.0
(S&W) 'California'	6 oz	35	600	0.0
(S&W Nutradiet)	6 oz	35	20	0.0
(Stokely)	4 oz	20	330	0.0
(Welch's)	6 oz	35	550	0.0

Food Name	Serv. Size	Total Cal.	Sod. MGS	Fa GM
TOMATO PASTE				
(Contadina)	2 oz	50	40	<1.
(Contadina) Italian style	2 oz	65	520	1.
(Hunt's)	1.164 oz	24	81	0.
(Hunt's) 'Food Service'	1.164 oz	24	101	0.
(Hunt's) Italian style	1.164 oz	25	255	0.
(Hunt's) 'No Salt Added'	1.164 oz	24	11	0.
(Hunt's) w/garlic	2 oz	50	440	<1.0
(Hunt's) w/garlic	1.164 oz	26	247	0.
TOMATO POWDER				
ground	1 oz	86	38	0.
ground	100 gm	302	134	0.
TOMATO PURÉE				
(Angela Mia)	2.187 oz	16	21	0.
(Contadina)	1/2 cup	40	35	<1.0
(Contadina) w/crushed tomatoes	1/2 cup	30	350	<1.0
(Hunt's)	2.187 oz	23	98	0.
(Hunt's) 'Food Service'	2.222 oz	26	22	0.
TOMATO SAUCE				
CANNED				
(A&P)	1/2 cup	45	600	<1.0
(Contadina)	1/2 cup	30	580	<1.0
(Del Monte)	1 cup	70	1330	1.0
(Finast)	1/2 cup	45	650	0.0
(Health Valley)	1 cup	70	460	0.5
(Hunt's)	4 oz	30	730	0.0
(Hunt's)	2.187 oz	16	360	0.2
(Pathmark)	1/2 cup	40	620	0.0
(S&W)	1/2 cup	40	620	0.0
(Stokely)	1/2 cup	30	810	0.0
Casera (Hunt's)	2.187 oz	22	293	0.1
Chunky				
(Hunt's) chili	2.222 oz	21	320	0.4
(Hunt's) 'Food Service'	2.187 oz	15	360	0.2
(Hunt's) Italian	2.222 oz	29	293	1.1
(Hunt's) Mexican	2.222 oz	19	369	0.4
(Hunt's) tomato	2.187 oz	13	405	0.1
Garden vegetable (Contadina)	5 oz	80	580	3.0
Herb flavored (Hunt's)	4 oz	70	470	2.0
Hot, Maya (Hunt's)	1.058 oz	6	174	0.2

ood Name	Serv. Size	Total Cal.	Sod. MGS	Fat GMS
Italian style				
(Contadina)	1/2 cup	30	670	<1.0
(Contadina) sausage	5 oz	110	570	6.0
(Hunt's)	4 oz	60	520	2.0
(Hunt's)	2.222 oz	26	251	0.5
(Rokeach)	3 oz	60	243	2.0
Low sodium (Rokeach)	3 oz	50	124	2.0
Marinara				
(Buitoni)	1/2 cup	70	570	3.0
(Contadina)	4 oz	80	460	4.0
(Pathmark) 'No Frills'	1/2 cup	80	620	3.0
(Rokeach)	3 oz	60	257	2.0
'Meatloaf Fixin's' (Hunt's)	2 oz	20	580	<1.0
No salt added				
(Del Monte)	1 cup	70	50	1.0
(Finast)	8 oz	90	10	0.0
(Health Valley)	1 cup	70	43	0.5
(Hunt's)	4 oz	35	25	0.0
(Hunt's)	2.187 oz	16	11	0.2
(Pathmark)	1/2 cup	45	25	0.0
Pesto (Contadina)	2.33 oz	350	440	34.0
Plum (Contadina)	5 oz	80	420	4.0
'Special'				
(Hunt's)	4 oz	35	320	0.0
(Hunt's)	2.187 oz	21	144	0.6
'Thick and Zesty' (Contadina)	1/2 cup	40	650	<1.0
W/bits (Hunt's)	4 oz	30	620	<1.0
W/garlic				
(Hunt's)	4 oz	70	480	2.0
(Hunt's)	2.258 oz	29	269	1.0
W/green chilies (Old El Paso)	1/4 cup	14	480	<1.0
W/herbs (Hunt's)	2.187 oz	33	255	1.3
W/jalapeños (Old El Paso)	1/4 cup	11	150	1.0
W/mushrooms (Hunt's)	4 oz	25	710	<1.0
W/onions				
(Del Monte)	1 cup	100	1150	1.0
(Hunt's)	4 oz	40	650	<1.0
REFRIGERATED				
(Contadina) 'Light'	.5 oz	50	570	0.0
(Contadina) marinara 'Fresh'	7.5 oz	100	700	4.0
(Contadina) plum w/basil 'Fresh'	7.5 oz	100	700	4.0

Food Name	Serv. Size	Total Cal.	Sod. MGS	Fa GM
TOMATOES, SUN-DRIED. See SUN-DRIED TOMATOES.				
TOMATOSEED OIL				
....	1/2 cup	964	0	109.
....	1 oz	251	0	28.
....	1 tbsp	120	0	13.
TONIC. See SOFT DRINKS AND MIXERS.				
TORTELLINI PASTA, NONDAIRY				
regular *(Tofutti)* frozen	2 oz	210	158	4.
spinach *(Tofutti)* frozen	2 oz	210	158	4.
TORTELLINI PASTA, REFRIGERATED				
CHEESE *(DiGiorno)* approx 1 cup cooked	1/3 pkg	270	240	6.0
CHICKEN AND HERB *(DiGiorno)* approx 1 cup cooked	1/3 pkg	240	230	5.
EGG				
w/cheese, 'Fresh' *(Contadina)*	4.5 oz	380	570	6.0
w/cheese, 'Fresh' *(Contadina)*	3 oz	260	310	6.0
w/chicken and prosciutto, 'Fresh' *(Contadina)*	4.5 oz	370	560	7.0
w/meat, 'Fresh' *(Contadina)*	4.5 oz	380	580	6.0
MOZZARELLA GARLIC *(DiGiorno)* approx 1 cup cooked	1/3 pkg	260	270	8.0
SAUSAGE, Italian, 'Fresh' *(Contadina)*	3 oz	260	290	7.0
SPINACH				
w/cheese, 'Fresh' *(Contadina)*	4.5 oz	380	590	6.0
w/cheese, 'Fresh' *(Contadina)*	3 oz	260	360	6.0
w/chicken and prosciutto, 'Fresh' *(Contadina)*	4.5 oz	340	580	7.0
w/meat, 'Fresh' *(Contadina)*	4.5 oz	380	610	6.0
W/CHICKEN AND PROSCIUTTO *(Contadina)*	3 oz	250	370	6.0
W/MEAT				
(Contadina) 'Fresh'	3 oz	260	380	6.0
(DiGiorno) approx 1 cup cooked	1/3 pkg	280	360	9.0
TORTELLINI DISH/ENTRÉE, FROZEN				
(Birds Eye) in tomato sauce 'For One'	5.5 oz	210	500	5.0
(Budget Gourmet) 'Side Dish'	5.5 oz	180	400	9.0
(Green Giant) marinara 'One Serving'	5.5 oz	260	660	9.0
(Green Giant) Provençal 'Microwave Garden Gourmet'	1 pkg	260	840	6.0
(Le Menu) and meat sauce 'LightStyle'	8 oz	250	480	8.0
(Stouffer's) in Alfredo sauce	8 7/8 oz	580	830	37.0
(Stouffer's) w/tomato sauce	9.25 oz	360	720	15.0
(Top Shelf) in marinara sauce	10 oz	211	663	3.0
(Top Shelf) w/shrimp and seafood	10 oz	278	1341	8.0
(Weight Watchers)	9 oz	310	570	6.0
TORTILLA, CORN				
(Azteca)	1 tortilla	45	10	0.0

Food Name	Serv. Size	Total Cal.	Sod. MGS	Fat GMS
(Old El Paso)	1 tortilla	60	170	1.0
TORTILLA, FLOUR				
(Azteca) 9-inch diam	1 tortilla	130	180	3.0
(Azteca) 7-inch diam	1 tortilla	80	110	2.0
(Mission) 'Light'	1 tortilla	70	280	1.0
(Old El Paso)	1 tortilla	150	360	3.0
Burrito style				
(Garcia's)	1 tortilla	220	220	5.0
(Mission) 'Premium'	1 tortilla	230	395	6.0
(Tyson)	1 tortilla	173	40	4.0
(Tyson) large, heat-pressed	1 tortilla	182	90	4.0
(Tyson) small, hand-stretched	1 tortilla	106	50	2.0
Fajita style				
(Fry's) extra soft	1 tortilla	100	160	2.0
(Garcia's)	1 tortilla	100	220	2.5
(Tyson)	1 tortilla	84	20	2.0
Taco size				
(Mission) soft	1 tortilla	150	255	4.0
(Tyson) soft	1 tortilla	121	30	3.0
TORTILLA CHIPS. See also CORN CHIPS AND SNACKS.				
(Bachman)				
nacho	1 oz	140	210	6.0
'No Salt'	1 oz	140	0	6.0
(Barbara's Bakery)				
yellow corn, organic	1 oz	140	120	7.0
yellow corn, organic, no salt added	1 oz	140	15	7.0
(Bearitos)				
blue corn 'Organic'	1 oz	146	29	7.0
blue corn 'Organic No Salt'	1 oz	137	3	6.5
yellow corn 'Organic'	1 oz	143	58	6.4
yellow corn 'Organic No Salt'	1 oz	148	2	7.2
(Bravos)				
nacho cheese flavored, jalapeño	1 oz	150	170	7.0
nacho cheese flavored, round, crispy	1 oz	150	180	8.0
nacho cheese flavored, strips	1 oz	140	220	7.0
(Buenitos)				
'Tortilla Chips'	1 oz	150	80	8.0
'Tortilla Chips, No Salt Added'	1 oz	150	1	8.0
(Doritos)				
'Cool Ranch'	1 oz	140	170	7.0
'Cool Ranch Light'	1 oz	120	240	4.0

Food Name	Serv. Size	Total Cal.	Sod. MGS	Fat GMS
'Jumpin' Jack'	1 oz	140	220	7.0
nacho cheese	1 oz	140	240	7.0
nacho cheese 'Light'	1 oz	120	290	4.0
salsa and cheese 'Thins'	1 oz	150	180	8.0
'Salsa Rio'	1 oz	140	190	7.0
taco	1 oz	140	250	7.0
toasted corn	1 oz	140	80	7.0
white corn, lightly salted 'Thins'	1 oz	140	135	7.0
(Eagle) ranch	1 oz	140	190	8.0
(Featherweight)				
'Low Salt'	1 oz	150	10	8.0
nacho	1 oz	150	45	8.0
(Guiltless Gourmet)				
white corn, baked, salted	1 oz	110	160	1.5
yellow corn, baked, salted	1 oz	110	140	1.5
yellow corn, baked, unsalted	1 oz	110	25	1.5
(Hain)				
sesame	1 oz	140	190	7.0
sesame, cheese	1 oz	160	270	8.0
sesame, 'No Salt Added'	1 oz	140	0	7.0
taco	1 oz	160	320	11.0
(Keebler)				
cinnamon crispaña, flour 'Chacho's'	1 oz	140	70	7.0
original, restaurant style 'Chacho's'	1 oz	140	180	7.0
(Kettle Ties)				
blue corn, lightly salted	1 oz	140	80	6.0
blue corn, no salt	1 oz	140	2	6.0
yellow corn, lightly salted	1 oz	140	80	7.0
yellow corn, no salt	1 oz	140	3	7.0
(La Famous)				
'No Salt Added'	1 oz	140	5	7.0
plain	1 oz	140	180	7.0
(Laura Scudder's)				
lightly salted 'Restaurant Style'	1 oz	140	90	7.0
nacho, jalapeño 'Strips'	1 oz	150	170	7.0
nacho, 'Triangles'	1 oz	140	220	7.0
picante 'Restaurant Style Strips'	1 oz	150	190	7.0
(Old El Paso)				
crispy	1 oz	150	105	8.0
white, round 'NaChips' low sodium	1 oz	160	5	9.0

Food Name	Serv. Size	Total Cal.	Sod. MGS	Fat GMS
(Planters)				
nacho cheese	1 oz	150	160	8.0
traditional	1 oz	150	150	8.0
(Slimchips) fat-free	.4 oz	44	60	<.5
(Tio Sancho)				
'Microwave Snacks'	4 oz	567	590	26.1
nacho	.5 oz	70	282	5.7
(Tostitos)				
nacho, sharp	1 oz	150	200	8.0
white corn, baked 'Cool Ranch'	1 oz	130	170	3.0
white corn, baked, no salt	1 oz	110	0	1.0
white corn, baked 'Original'	1 oz	110	140	1.0
(Wise) nacho cheese flavored, crispy, round	1 oz	150	180	8.0
TOSTACO SHELL *(Old El Paso)*	1 shell	100	10	5.0
TOSTADA SHELL				
(Lawry's)	1 shell	73	147	3.5
(Old El Paso)	1 shell	55	65	3.0
(Ortega)	1 shell	50	5	2.0
(Pancho Villa)	1 shell	55	65	3.0
(Rosarita)	1 shell	60	<1	3.0
(Tio Sancho)	1 shell	67	1	3.2
TOWEL GOURD. See GOURD, DISHCLOTH.				
TRAIL MIX				
(Harmony) 'Delux Super'	1/4 cup	150	35	7.0
(Harmony) nut and berry mix	1/4 cup	160	0	8.0
TRITICALE				
whole grain	1/2 cup	323	5	2.0
whole grain	1 oz	95	1	0.6
TRITICALE FLOUR				
whole grain	1/2 cup	220	1	1.2
whole grain	1 oz	96	<1	0.5
TROPICAL CITRUS DRINK				
chilled *(Five Alive)*	6 oz	90	20	0.0
frozen, prepared *(Five Alive)*	6 oz	90	0	0.0
TROPICAL FRUIT DRINK				
bottled 'Thirst Quencher' *(Gatorade)*	8 oz	50	110	0.0
mix 'Thirst Quencher' prepared *(Gatorade)*	8 oz	60	110	0.0
TROPICAL FRUIT JUICE				
bottled *(Juicy Juice)*	6 oz	110	10	0.0
boxed *(Juicy Juice)*	8.45 oz	150	10	0.0
TROPICAL LIME COOLER *(Knudsen & Sons)*	8 oz	130	na	0.0

Food Name	Serv. Size	Total Cal.	Sod. MGS	Fat GMS
TROPICAL NECTAR, can or bottle *(Kern's)*	6 oz	110	5	0.0
TROPICAL ORANGE DRINK, 'Fruit Box' *(Tang)*	8.45 oz	150	10	0.0
TROPICAL PASSION JUICE *(Knudsen & Sons)*	8 oz	80	na	0.0
TROPICAL PUNCH				
Can, bottle, or box				
(Knudsen & Sons)	8 oz	105	na	0.0
(Kool-Aid) 'Koolers'	8.45 oz	130	10	0.0
(Minute Maid)	6 oz	90	20	0.0
(Santa Cruz Natural) organic	8 oz	110	na	<1.0
Mix				
(Kool-Aid) sugar-free, w/NutraSweet, prepared	8 oz	4	10	0.0
(Kool-Aid) sugar-sweetened, prepared	8 oz	80	0	0.0
(Kool-Aid) unsweetened, prepared w/sugar	8 oz	100	0	0.0
(Kool-Aid) unsweetened, prepared w/o sugar	8 oz	2	0	0.0
TROPICAL SALAD *(Sun Fresh)* chilled, packed in light syrup	3.5 oz	88	39	0.9
TROUT, MIXED SPECIES				
dry-heat cooked	3 oz	161	57	7.2
raw	1 lb	673	236	30.0
raw	3 oz	126	44	5.6
raw	1 oz	42	15	1.9
raw, approx 2.8 oz	1 fillet	117	41	5.2
TROUT, RAINBOW				
farmed, dry-heat cooked	3 oz	144	36	6.1
farmed, raw	3 oz	117	30	4.6
wild, dry-heat cooked	3 oz	127	48	4.9
wild, raw	3 oz	101	26	2.9
wild, raw, approx 2.8 oz	1 fillet	189	49	5.5
TROUT, SEA, MIXED SPECIES				
raw	1 lb	472	263	16.4
raw	3 oz	88	49	3.1
raw	1 oz	29	16	1.0
TUMERIC. See TURMERIC.				
TUNA, ALBACORE. See TUNA, CANNED; TUNA, FROZEN.				
TUNA, ALTERNATIVE, frozen 'Tuno' *(Worthington)*	2 oz	100	310	7.0
TUNA, BLUEFIN				
dry-heat cooked	4 oz	209	57	7.1
dry-heat cooked	3 oz	156	43	5.3
raw	1 lb	652	177	22.2
raw	3 oz	122	33	4.2
raw	1 oz	41	11	1.4

Food Name	Serv. Size	Total Cal.	Sod. MGS	Fat GMS
TUNA, CANNED				
LIGHT				
In canola oil, chunk *(Chicken of the Sea)*	2 oz	160	250	12.0
In oil				
drained	3 oz	168	301	7.0
drained, approx 6 oz	1 can	339	605	14.0
w/o salt, drained	3 oz	168	43	7.0
w/o salt, drained, approx 6 oz	1 can	339	86	14.0
In pure vegetable oil, chunk, w/liquid *(Chicken of the Sea)*	2 oz	160	250	12.0
In soybean oil				
chunk, drained	1 oz	56	100	2.3
chunk, drained *(A&P)*	2 oz	150	310	13.0
chunk, drained *(Bumble Bee)*	2 oz	110	310	12.0
chunk, drained *(Finast)*	2 oz	150	310	13.0
chunk, drained *(Star-Kist)*	2 oz	150	310	13.0
chunk 'Fancy' drained *(S&W)*	2 oz	140	450	10.0
solid, drained *(Progresso)*	1/3 cup	150	400	13.0
solid, drained *(Star-Kist)*	2 oz	150	310	13.0
w/o salt, drained	1 oz	56	14	2.3
In spring water, chunk, w/liquid *(Chicken of the Sea)*	2 oz	60	250	1.0
In water				
chunk, drained *(Bumble Bee)*	2 oz	50	310	1.0
chunk, drained *(Finast)*	2 oz	60	310	<1.0
chunk, drained *(Pathmark)*	2 oz	70	310	2.0
chunk, drained *(Star-Kist)*	2 oz	60	310	<1.0
chunk, diet, drained *(Star-Kist)*	2 oz	65	35	<1.0
chunk 'Fancy' drained *(S&W)*	2 oz	60	500	1.0
chunk 'No Salt Added' drained *(Weight Watchers)*	2 oz	60	210	<1.0
chunk '60% Less Salt' drained *(Star-Kist)*	2 oz	65	120	1.0
drained	3 oz	111	303	0.4
drained	1 oz	37	101	0.1
drained, approx 6.3 oz	1 can	216	587	0.8
drained *(A&P)*	2 oz	60	310	<1.0
drained *(Empress)*	2 oz	60	310	1.0
solid, drained *(Star-Kist)*	2 oz	60	310	<1.0
solid 'Prime Catch' drained *(Star-Kist)*	2 oz	60	310	<1.0
w/o salt, drained	3 oz	111	43	0.4
w/o salt, drained	1 oz	37	14	0.1
w/o salt, drained, approx 6.3 oz	1 can	216	83	0.8

Food Name	Serv. Size	Total Cal.	Sod. MGS	Fat GMS
WHITE				
In oil				
drained	3 oz	158	337	6.9
drained, approx 6.3 oz	1 can	331	705	14.4
w/o salt, drained	3 oz	158	43	6.9
w/o salt, drained, approx 6.3 oz	1 can	331	89	14.4
In soybean oil				
chunk, drained	1 oz	53	112	2.3
chunk, drained (A&P)	2 oz	150	310	10.0
chunk, drained (Bumble Bee)	2 oz	110	310	12.0
chunk, drained (Star-Kist)	2 oz	140	310	10.0
solid, albacore, drained (Bumble Bee)	2 oz	100	310	8.0
solid, albacore, drained (Finast)	2 oz	145	320	10.0
solid, albacore, drained (S&W)	2 oz	160	450	12.0
solid, albacore, drained (Star-Kist)	2 oz	140	310	10.0
w/o salt, drained	1 oz	53	14	2.3
In spring water, solid, fancy albacore (Chicken of the Sea)	2 oz	60	250	1.0
In water				
chunk, diet, drained (Star-Kist)	2 oz	70	30	1.0
chunk, drained (A&P)	2 oz	100	310	5.0
chunk, drained (Bumble Bee)	2 oz	60	310	2.0
chunk '60% Less Salt' drained (Star-Kist)	2 oz	70	120	<1.0
drained	3 oz	116	333	2.1
drained, approx 6.1 oz	1 can	234	674	4.2
solid, albacore, drained (A&P)	2 oz	70	310	<1.0
solid, albacore, drained (Bumble Bee)	2 oz	60	310	2.0
solid, albacore, drained (Finast)	2 oz	70	310	1.0
solid, albacore, drained (Pathmark)	2 oz	70	310	2.0
solid, albacore, drained (Star-Kist)	2 oz	70	310	1.0
solid, albacore, drained (Weight Watchers)	2 oz	70	210	1.0
w/o salt, drained	3 oz	116	43	2.1
w/o salt, drained	1 oz	39	14	0.7
w/o salt, drained, approx 6.1 oz	1 can	234	86	4.2
TUNA, FROZEN				
(Peter Pan Seafoods) albacore, white, steaks, skinless, boneless, raw	3.5 oz	102	51	4.9
(Peter Pan Seafoods) yellowfin, steaks, skinless, boneless, raw	3.5 oz	131	61	4.1
(SeaPak) steak, w/o seasoning mix	6-oz pkg	180	65	2.0
TUNA, SKIPJACK/aku/arctic bonito/katsuo/oceanic bonito. See also BONITO.				
dry-heat cooked	3 oz	112	40	1.1

Food Name	Serv. Size	Total Cal.	Sod. MGS	Fat GMS
raw	1 lb	468	167	4.6
raw	3 oz	88	31	0.9
raw	1 oz	29	10	0.3
raw, approx 7 oz	1/2 fillet	204	73	2.0
TUNA, YELLOWFIN/ahi				
dry-heat cooked	3 oz	118	40	1.0
raw	1 lb	492	168	4.3
raw	3 oz	92	31	0.8
raw	1 oz	31	10	0.3
TUNA ENTRÉE, FROZEN				
noodle casserole *(Stouffer's)*	10 oz	280	1090	15.0
noodle casserole *(Weight Watchers)*	9 oz	230	550	7.0
pie *(Banquet)*	7 oz	540	810	33.0
TUNA ENTRÉE, MIX				
au gratin, dry mix *(Tuna Helper)*	1/5 pkg	180	800	5.0
buttery rice, dry mix *(Tuna Helper)*	1/5 pkg	160	830	2.0
cheesy noodle, dry mix *(Tuna Helper)*	1/5 pkg	160	810	4.0
creamy broccoli, dry mix *(Tuna Helper)*	1/5 pkg	200	800	4.0
fettuccine Alfredo, dry mix *(Tuna Helper)*	1/5 pkg	160	760	3.0
mushroom, creamy, dry mix *(Tuna Helper)*	1/5 pkg	140	580	1.0
noodle, creamy, dry mix *(Tuna Helper)*	1/5 pkg	210	790	8.0
pot pie, dry mix *(Tuna Helper)*	1/6 pkg	290	730	17.0
salad, dry mix *(Tuna Helper)*	1/5 pkg	140	580	1.0
tetrazzini, dry mix *(Tuna Helper)*	1/5 pkg	160	620	3.0
TUNA LUNCH KIT				
'Charlie's Lunch Kit' w/1 mayo packet *(Star-Kist)*	4.6 oz	290	780	15.0
'Charlie's Lunch Kit' w/2 mayo packets *(Star-Kist)*	5 oz	370	845	15.0
TUNA MIX				
classic Italian 'Tuna Mix-ins' dry mix *(Bumble Bee)*	1 oz	25	5	0.0
garden and herb 'Tuna Mix-ins' dry mix *(Bumble Bee)*	1 oz	25	5	0.0
lemon herb 'Tuna Mix-ins' dry mix *(Bumble Bee)*	1 oz	25	5	0.0
zesty tomato 'Tuna Mix-ins' dry mix *(Bumble Bee)*	1 oz	25	5	0.0
TUNA SALAD				
(Longacre)	1 oz	58	130	4.0
(Longacre) 'Saladfest'	1 oz	52	180	4.0
TUNA SALAD SPREAD *(Libby's)* 'Spreadables'	1.9 oz	80	220	5.0
TURBOT, DOMESTIC				
raw	1 lb	845	363	62.8
raw	1 oz	53	23	3.9
raw, approx 7.2 oz	1/2 fillet	380	163	28.2

Food Name	Serv. Size	Total Cal.	Sod. MGS	Fat GMS
TURBOT, EUROPEAN				
dry-heat cooked	3 oz	104	163	3.2
raw	1 lb	432	678	13.4
raw	3 oz	81	127	2.5
raw	1 oz	27	43	0.8
raw, approx 7.2 oz	1/2 fillet	194	306	6.0
TURKEY, ALL CLASSES				
BACK MEAT W/SKIN				
raw	1 lb	896	304	59.2
raw	1 oz	56	19	3.7
roasted	4 oz	276	83	16.3
BREAST MEAT W/SKIN				
raw	1 lb	720	272	32.0
raw	1 oz	45	17	2.0
roasted	4 oz	214	71	8.4
DARK MEAT ONLY				
raw	1 lb	560	352	19.2
raw	1 oz	35	22	1.2
roasted	1 cup	262	111	10.1
roasted	4 oz	212	90	8.2
DARK MEAT W/SKIN				
raw	1 lb	720	320	40.0
raw	1 oz	45	20	2.5
roasted	4 oz	251	86	13.1
LEG MEAT W/SKIN				
raw	1 lb	656	336	30.4
raw	1 oz	41	21	1.9
roasted	4 oz	236	87	11.1
LIGHT MEAT ONLY				
raw	1 lb	528	288	6.4
raw	1 oz	33	18	0.4
roasted	4 oz	178	73	3.7
roasted, diced	1 cup	220	90	4.5
LIGHT MEAT W/SKIN				
raw	1 lb	72.0	272	33.6
raw	1 oz	45	17	2.1
roasted	4 oz	223	71	9.4
NECK MEAT ONLY				
raw	1 lb	608	416	24.0
raw	1 oz	38	26	1.5
simmered	4 oz	204	64	8.2

Food Name	Serv. Size	Total Cal.	Sod. MGS	Fat GMS
SKIN ONLY				
raw	1 lb	1760	160	168.0
raw	1 oz	110	10	10.5
roasted	1 oz	125	15	11.2
WING MEAT W/SKIN				
raw	1 lb	896	256	56.0
raw	1 oz	56	16	3.5
roasted	4 oz	260	69	14.1
TURKEY, ALTERNATIVE				
(Worthington) roll, smoked, frozen	4 slices	180	820	12.0
(Worthington) sliced, smoked, frozen	4 slices	180	820	12.0
(Worthington) 'Turkee Slices' canned	2 slices	130	430	9.0
(Worthington) '209' canned, drained	2 slices	120	(mq)	8.0
TURKEY, BONELESS. See also LUNCHEON MEAT.				
BREAST				
(Butterball) 'Slice 'n Serve'	1 oz	35	230	1.0
(Longacre) 'Gourmet'	1 oz	35	300	1.0
(Longacre) 'Gourmet Low Salt'	1 oz	30	150	<1.0
(Longacre) 'Premium'	1 oz	30	250	1.0
(Longacre) 'Salt Watchers'	1 oz	32	10	<1.0
(Mr. Turkey)	1 oz	31	233	0.7
Barbecue seasoned (Butterball) Slice 'n Serve	1 oz	40	210	2.0
Browned				
(Longacre) glazed 'Gourmet'	1 oz	35	240	1.0
(Longacre) glazed 'Premium'	1 oz	30	300	1.0
(Longacre) roasted 'Gourmet'	1 oz	35	260	1.0
(Longacre) roasted 'Premium'	1 oz	30	300	1.0
Golden				
(Boar's Head)	1 oz	35	200	1.0
(Boar's Head) skinless	1 oz	30	(mq)	<1.0
Hickory smoked (Butterball) 'Slice 'n Serve'	1 oz	35	250	1.0
Honey roasted (Louis Rich)	1 oz	32	315	0.8
Lean, lite				
(Longacre) 'Deli'	1 oz	35	160	1.0
(Longacre) skinless 'Deli'	1 oz	35	160	<1.0
(Longacre) smoked 'Deli'	1 oz	35	160	1.0
Skinless				
(Longacre) 'Catering'	1 oz	35	280	<1.0
(Longacre) 'Gourmet'	1 oz	30	260	<1.0
(Longacre) 'Premium'	1 oz	30	250	<1.0
(Norbest) 'Blue Label'	1 oz	26	252	0.4

Food Name	Serv. Size	Total Cal.	Sod. MGS	Fat GMS
(Norbest) 'Norfresh'	1 oz	27	269	0.3
(Norbest) 'Norfresh Blue Label'	1 oz	24	253	0.3
(Norbest) 'Norfresh Yellow Label'	1 oz	24	284	0.5
(Norbest) 'Orange Label'	1 oz	26	239	0.2
(Norbest) salt-free 'Blue Label'	1 oz	33	13	0.3
(Norbest) 'Tan Label'	1 oz	24	354	0.5
(Norbest) 'Yellow Label'	1 oz	26	272	0.5
Smoked				
(Healthy Deli) 'Gourmet'	1 oz	31	170	0.5
(Hormel) 'Perma-Fresh'	2 slices	60	540	2.0
(Longacre)	1 oz	35	240	1.0
(Norbest) 'Gold Label'	1 oz	29	270	<.6
(OHSE)	1 oz	30	340	1.0
W/skin				
(Norbest) 'Blue Label'	1 oz	28	239	0.7
(Norbest) 'Norfresh Orange Label'	1 oz	26	256	0.3
(Norbest) 'Norfresh Yellow Label'	1 oz	25	244	0.5
(Norbest) 'Orange Label'	1 oz	28	232	0.3
(Norbest) prebrowned 'Orange Label'	1 oz	29	259	0.8
(Norbest) salt-free 'Blue Label'	1 oz	35	13	0.5
(Norbest) smoked 'Orange Label'	1 oz	30	284	0.5
(Norbest) 'Yellow Label'	1 oz	26	271	0.4
BREAST AND LIGHT MEAT				
(Longacre) browned and roasted	1 oz	40	240	2.0
(Longacre) 'Deli Chef'	1 oz	35	240	1.0
(Longacre) skinless 'Deli Chef'	1 oz	40	240	2.0
BREAST AND THIGH *(Norbest)* 'Blue Label'	1 oz	31	238	0.9
DARK MEAT *(Norbest)* ham flavor, hickory smoked	1 oz	39	335	2.2
OVEN COOKED *(OHSE)*	1 oz	30	190	1.0
ROLL				
(Norbest) white meat 'Orange Label'	1 oz	29	299	0.9
(Norbest) white and dark meat 'Orange Label'	1 oz	36	314	2.0
SMOKED *(Louis Rich)*	1 oz	32	284	1.0
W/PORK *(Healthy Favorites)* 'Breakfast Strips'	11 grams	18	145	1.0
TURKEY, CANNED				
(Hormel) chunk	6.75 oz	230	1278	10.0
(Hormel) chunk	2.5 oz	80	420	3.0
(Swanson) white	2.5 oz	80	260	1.0
(Tyson) 'Wholesale Club Item'	3.5 oz	120	360	3.0

Food Name	Serv. Size	Total Cal.	Sod. MGS	Fat GMS
TURKEY, FROZEN/REFRIGERATED				
BREAST				
Cooked				
(Land O'Lakes)	3 oz	100	55	1.0
(Longacre) 'Cook-N-Bag'	1 oz	38	85	<1.0
(Louis Rich)	1 oz	47	21	1.5
(Louis Rich) barbecue	1 oz	33	315	1.0
(Louis Rich) hen, w/o wings	1 oz	50	19	2.0
(Louis Rich) hickory smoked	1 oz	33	346	1.0
(Louis Rich) honey roasted	1 oz	33	318	0.8
(Louis Rich) oven roasted	1 oz	31	296	0.9
(Louis Rich) roast	1 oz	42	20	0.8
(Louis Rich) slices	1 oz	39	24	0.5
(Louis Rich) smoked	1 oz	33	268	1.0
(Louis Rich) steaks	1 oz	39	24	0.5
(Louis Rich) tenderloins	1 oz	39	24	0.5
(Mr. Turkey) barbecue, quarter 'Chub'	1 oz	34	251	1.0
(Mr. Turkey) oven roasted, quarter 'Chub'	1 oz	34	266	1.0
(Mr. Turkey) smoked, quarter 'Chub'	1 oz	35	263	1.0
(Tyson) skinless, boneless 'Wholesale Club Item'	3.5 oz	160	65	3.0
w/skin, roasted, broth pre-basted	4 oz	143	450	3.9
Raw				
(Longacre) 'Cook-N-Bag'	1 oz	27	120	<1.0
(Longacre) 'Ready-to-Cook'	1 oz	39	150	<1.0
(Norbest) steaks, cubed	4 oz	135	81	2.0
(Norbest) strips and tips 'Tasti-Lean'	4 oz	135	81	2.0
(Norbest) tenderloin 'Tasti-Lean Tenders'	4 oz	135	81	2.0
(Norbest) w/gravy	4 oz	115	492	2.4
CUTLET (Norbest) raw 'Tasti-Lean'	4 oz	135	81	2.0
DARK MEAT (Butterball) w/o skin, roasted, approx 3.5 oz	2 slices	195	90	10.0
DRUMSTICK				
(Land O'Lakes)	3 oz	120	85	5.0
(Louis Rich) cooked	1 oz	56	22	2.6
(Louis Rich) cooked 'Fresh Turkey Cuts'	1 oz	55	25	3.0
HINDQUARTER ROAST (Land O'Lakes)	3 oz	140	80	8.0
LIGHT AND DARK MEAT				
roasted, then seasoned	4 oz	176	771	6.6
seasoned raw, then roasted	1 lb	544	3075	10.0
seasoned raw, then roasted	1 oz	34	192	0.6
(Butterball) w/skin, roasted, approx 3.5 oz	2 slices	195	115	10.0
LIGHT MEAT (Butterball) w/o skin, roasted, approx 3.5 oz	2 slices	160	130	4.0

Food Name	Serv. Size	Total Cal.	Sod. MGS	Fat GMS
THIGH				
w/skin, roasted, pre-basted w/broth	4 oz	178	496	9.7
(Land O'Lakes)	3 oz	150	75	10.0
(Louis Rich) cooked	1 oz	64	20	3.7
(Louis Rich) cooked 'Fresh Turkey Cuts'	1 oz	65	20	4.0
WHOLE				
(Louis Rich) w/o giblets, cooked	1 oz	52	23	2.3
(Louis Rich) w/o giblets, cooked 'Fresh Whole Turkey'	1 oz	50	25	2.0
(Norbest) boneless, cooked	1 oz	42	105	1.5
(Norbest) boneless, smoked, cooked	1 oz	42	218	1.6
WING				
(Land O'Lakes)	3 oz	120	65	5.0
(Louis Rich) cooked	1 oz	54	20	2.7
(Louis Rich) cooked 'Drumettes'	1 oz	51	20	2.2
(Louis Rich) cooked 'Fresh Turkey Cuts'	1 oz	55	20	3.0
(Louis Rich) drumettes, cooked 'Fresh Turkey Cuts'	1 oz	50	20	2.0
(Louis Rich) portions, cooked	1 oz	54	17	2.9
(Louis Rich) portions, cooked 'Fresh Turkey Cuts'	1 oz	55	20	3.0
W/GRAVY (Norbest) raw	4 oz	115	600	2.7
YOUNG				
(Land O'Lakes)	3 oz	130	55	7.0
(Land O'Lakes) butter-basted	3 oz	140	135	8.0
(Land O'Lakes) self-basting, w/broth	3 oz	120	145	5.0
TURKEY, FRYER-ROASTER				
BACK MEAT ONLY				
raw	1 lb	544	288	16.0
raw	1 oz	34	18	1.0
roasted	4 oz	193	83	6.4
BACK MEAT W/SKIN				
raw	1 lb	688	272	336.0
raw	1 oz	43	17	2.1
roasted	4 oz	231	79	11.6
BREAST, MEAT ONLY				
raw	1 lb	496	224	3.2
raw	1 oz	31	14	0.2
roasted	4 oz	153	59	0.8
BREAST MEAT W/SKIN				
raw	1 lb	560	224	12.8
raw	1 oz	35	14	0.8
roasted	4 oz	174	60	3.6

Food Name	Serv. Size	Total Cal.	Sod. MGS	Fat GMS
DARK MEAT ONLY				
raw	1 lb	496	320	12.8
raw	1 oz	31	20	0.8
roasted	4 oz	184	90	4.9
roasted, diced	1 cup	227	111	6.0
DARK MEAT W/SKIN				
raw	1 lb	592	304	22.4
raw	1 oz	37	19	1.4
roasted	4 oz	206	86	8.0
LEG MEAT ONLY				
raw	1 lb	496	320	11.2
raw	1 oz	31	20	0.7
roasted	4 oz	180	92	4.3
LEG MEAT W/SKIN				
raw	1 lb	528	320	16.0
raw	1 oz	33	20	1.0
roasted	4 oz	193	91	6.1
LIGHT MEAT ONLY				
raw	1 lb	496	240	1.6
raw	1 oz	31	15	0.1
roasted	4 oz	159	64	1.3
roasted, diced	1 cup	196	78	1.6
LIGHT MEAT W/SKIN				
raw	1 lb	608	224	17.6
raw	1 oz	38	14	1.1
roasted	4 oz	186	65	5.2
SKIN ONLY				
raw	1 lb	1280	160	107.2
raw	1 oz	80	10	6.7
WING MEAT ONLY				
raw	1 lb	480	288	4.8
raw	1 oz	30	18	0.3
roasted	4 oz	185	88	3.9
WING MEAT W/SKIN				
raw	1 lb	720	256	35.2
raw	1 oz	45	16	2.2
roasted	4 oz	235	83	11.2
TURKEY, GROUND				
Cooked				
	4 oz	260	94	15.6
approx 2.9 oz	1 patty	193	88	10.8

Food Name	Serv. Size	Total Cal.	Sod. MGS	Fat GMS
yield from 1 lb raw	11.6 oz	754	273	45.5
(Hudson's)	1 oz	55	35	3.7
(Longacre)	1 oz	60	20	4.0
(Louis Rich) 85% fat-free	1 oz	60	30	3.0
(Louis Rich) 90% fat-free	1 oz	50	30	3.0
(Louis Rich) 90% fat-free, natural flavorings	1 oz	50	35	2.0
(Mr. Turkey)	1 oz	54	27	4.0
Raw				
	1 lb	676	426	37.5
	1 oz	40	27	2.1
(Norbest)	1 oz	45	34	2.6
(Louis Rich) w/natural flavoring	1 oz	50	33	2.2
TURKEY, YOUNG HEN				
BACK MEAT W/SKIN				
raw	1 lb	992	272	72.0
raw	1 oz	62	17	4.5
roasted	4 oz	288	78	17.7
BREAST MEAT W/SKIN				
raw	1 lb	752	256	38.4
raw	1 oz	47	16	2.4
roasted	4 oz	220	66	8.9
DARK MEAT ONLY				
raw	1 lb	592	336	22.4
raw	1 oz	37	21	1.4
roasted	4 oz	218	85	8.8
roasted, diced	1 cup	269	105	10.9
DARK MEAT W/SKIN				
raw	1 lb	784	304	46.4
raw	1 oz	49	19	2.9
roasted	4 oz	263	82	14.5
LEG MEAT W/SKIN				
raw	1 lb	688	320	33.6
raw	1 oz	43	20	2.1
roasted	4 oz	242	83	11.9
LIGHT MEAT ONLY				
raw	1 lb	528	272	8.0
raw	1 oz	33	17	0.5
roasted	4 oz	183	68	4.2
roasted, diced	1 cup	225	84	5.2
LIGHT MEAT W/SKIN				
raw	1 lb	752	256	36.8

Food Name	Serv. Size	Total Cal.	Sod. MGS	Fat GMS
raw	1 oz	47	16	2.3
roasted	4 oz	235	66	10.7
SKIN ONLY				
roasted	1 oz	137	12	12.6
WING MEAT W/SKIN				
raw	1 lb	960	224	62.4
raw	1 oz	60	14	3.9
roasted	4 oz	270	64	15.3
TURKEY, YOUNG TOM				
BACK MEAT W/SKIN				
raw	1 lb	81.6	320	51.2
raw	1 oz	51	20	3.2
roasted	4 oz	270	87	15.5
BREAST MEAT W/SKIN				
raw	1 lb	688	288	28.8
raw	1 oz	43	18	1.8
roasted	4 oz	214	76	8.4
DARK MEAT ONLY				
raw	1 lb	560	368	19.2
raw	1 oz	35	23	1.2
roasted	4 oz	210	93	7.9
roasted, diced	1 cup	259	115	9.8
DARK MEAT W/SKIN				
raw	1 lb	688	336	35.2
raw	1 oz	43	21	2.2
roasted	4 oz	245	91	12.3
LEG MEAT W/SKIN				
raw	1 lb	640	352	28.8
raw	1 oz	40	22	1.8
roasted	4 oz	234	91	10.9
LIGHT MEAT ONLY				
raw	1 lb	512	304	6.4
raw	1 oz	32	19	0.4
roasted	4 oz	175	77	3.3
roasted, diced	1 cup	216	95	4.1
LIGHT MEAT W/SKIN				
raw	1 lb	704	288	32.0
raw	1 oz	44	18	2.0
roasted	4 oz	217	76	8.7
SKIN ONLY				
raw	1 lb	1664	176	157.0

Food Name	Serv. Size	Total Cal.	Sod. MGS	Fat GMS
raw	1 oz	104	11	9.8
roasted	1 oz	120	17	10.6
WING MEAT W/SKIN				
raw	1 lb	848	272	51.2
raw	1 oz	53	17	3.2
roasted	4 oz	251	75	13.0
TURKEY BREAST				
BARBECUED *(Louis Rich)* skinless	1 oz	30	280	<1.0
HONEY ROASTED				
(Louis Rich) 95% fat-free	1-oz slice	35	315	1.0
(Louis Rich) skinless	1 oz	30	295	<1.0
OVEN ROASTED				
(Louis Rich) 'Carving Board'	22 grams	21	272	0.3
(Louis Rich) 'Fresh Turkey Cuts'	1 oz	45	20	2.0
(Louis Rich) 96% fat-free 'Deli-Thin'	1 slice	10	130	<1.0
(Louis Rich) 97% fat-free	1-oz slice	30	315	<1.0
(Louis Rich) 97% fat-free 'Deli-Thin'	1 slice	10	125	<1.0
(Louis Rich) roast 'Fresh Turkey Cuts'	1 oz	40	20	<1.0
(Louis Rich) skinless	1 oz	25	275	<1.0
(Louis Rich) slices 'Fresh Turkey Cuts'	1 oz	40	25	<1.0
(Louis Rich) steaks 'Fresh Turkey Cuts'	1 oz	40	25	<1.0
(Louis Rich) tenderloins 'Fresh Turkey Cuts'	1 oz	40	25	<1.0
SMOKED				
(Louis Rich) 'Carving Board'	10 grams	9	124	0.1
(Louis Rich) 96% fat-free	1 oz	35	270	1.0
(Louis Rich) 97% fat-free 'Deli-Thin'	1 slice	10	110	<1.0
(Louis Rich) 98% fat-free	1-oz slice	20	210	<1.0
(Louis Rich) skinless	1 oz	30	330	<1.0
TURKEY DINNER, FROZEN				
(Banquet)	10.5 oz	390	1110	20.0
(Banquet) 'Extra Helping'	19 oz	750	1980	42.0
(Morton)	10 oz	230	1300	6.0
(Swanson)	11.5 oz	350	1090	11.0
(Swanson) 'Hungry Man'	17 oz	550	1810	18.0
BREAST				
(Budget Gourmet) Dijon	11.2 oz	340	860	12.0
(Budget Gourmet) sliced	11.1 oz	290	1200	9.0
(Healthy Choice) medallions, w/vegetables 'Classics'	12.5 oz	350	480	6.0
(Le Menu) sliced, w/mushroom gravy	10.5 oz	300	1020	7.0
(Swanson) w/pasta	11.25 oz	310	670	9.0
DIVAN *(Le Menu)* 'LightStyle'	10 oz	260	420	7.0

Food Name	Serv. Size	Total Cal.	Sod. MGS	Fat GMS
SLICED				
(Freezer Queen)	10 oz	280	1210	8.0
(Le Menu) 'LightStyle'	10 oz	210	540	5.0
TETRAZZINI (Healthy Choice)	12.6 oz	340	490	6.0
W/DRESSING AND GRAVY				
(Armour) 'Classics'	11.5 oz	320	1280	12.0
(Banquet) w/dressing and gravy 'Healthy Balance'	11.25 oz	270	750	5.0
TURKEY ENTRÉE				
(Dinty Moore) w/dressing and gravy 'American Classics'	10 oz	290	910	5.0
(Hormel) and vegetables 'Health Selections' microwave cup	7.25 oz	220	420	2.0
(Libby's) w/dressing and gravy 'Diner' microwave cup	7 oz	170	830	7.0
(Mountain House) tetrazzini, freeze-dried, prepared	1 cup	200	(mq)	8.0
(Turkey by George) hickory barbecue	5 oz	190	840	5.0
(Turkey by George) Italian Parmesan	5 oz	170	860	5.0
(Turkey by George) lemon pepper	5 oz	160	830	4.0
(Turkey by George) mustard tarragon	5 oz	180	830	6.0
(Ultra Slim Fast) glazed, w/dressing	10.5 oz	340	570	5.0
(Ultra Slim Fast) medallions, in herb sauce	12 oz	280	950	6.0
TURKEY ENTRÉE, FROZEN				
À LA KING (Budget Gourmet) w/rice	10 oz	390	740	18.0
BREAST				
(Healthy Choice) sliced, w/dressing and gravy 'Classics'	10 oz	270	530	4.0
(Lean Cuisine) sliced, w/dressing	7 7/8 oz	200	590	5.0
(Lean Cuisine) sliced, w/mushroom sauce and rice	8 oz	230	540	7.0
(Stouffer's) roast, w/stuffing and gravy	7 7/8 oz	270	920	9.0
(Tyson) 'Gourmet Selections'	11.5 oz	380	1350	11.0
(Weight Watchers) stuffed	8.5 oz	270	520	8.0
CASSEROLE (Pillsbury) 'Microwave Classic'	1 pkg	430	880	25.0
CROQUETTES (Freezer Queen) breaded, w/gravy	7 oz	250	940	13.0
DIJON (Lean Cuisine)	9.5 oz	210	590	6.0
GLAZED (Le Menu) 'LightStyle'	8.25 oz	260	720	6.0
HOMESTYLE (Lean Cuisine) w/vegetables and pasta	9 3/8 oz	230	550	5.0
MEDALLIONS (Smart Ones) roasted, w/mushroom sauce	8.5 oz	200	440	1.0
PIE				
(Banquet)	7 oz	510	860	31.0
(Banquet) 'Supreme Microwave'	7 oz	430	740	27.0
(Mrs. Paterson's) w/broccoli 'Aussie Pie'	5.5 oz	460	790	26.0
(Stouffer's)	10 oz	410	750	24.0
(Swanson) 'Hungry Man'	16 oz	650	1470	36.0
(Swanson) 'Pot Pie'	7 oz	380	720	21.0

Food Name	Serv. Size	Total Cal.	Sod. MGS	Fat GMS
(Tyson)	9 oz	370	981	18.0
ROASTED *(Healthy Choice)* and mushrooms in gravy	8.5 oz	200	380	3.0
SLICED				
(Banquet) w/gravy 'Cookin' Bags'	5 oz	100	(mq)	6.0
(Banquet) w/gravy 'Family Entrees'	8 oz	150	(mq)	8.0
(Freezer Queen) w/dressing and gravy 'Single Serve'	9 oz	230	1130	5.0
(Freezer Queen) w/gravy 'Cook-In-Pouch'	5 oz	70	880	2.0
(Freezer Queen) w/gravy 'Family Suppers'	7 oz	110	1160	5.0
(Right Course) in mild curry sauce, w/rice pilaf	8.75 oz	320	570	8.0
TETRAZZINI *(Stouffer's)*	10 oz	400	960	23.0
W/DRESSING				
(Freezer Queen) w/dressing and gravy 'Deluxe Family'	7 oz	160	1130	5.0
(Tyson) 'Looney Tunes Elmer Fudd'	6.55 oz	260	510	7.0
W/DRESSING AND POTATOES				
(Swanson) 'Homestyle Recipe'	9 oz	290	1010	11.0
W/GRAVY *(Tyson)* 'Gourmet Selections'	9.5 oz	320	900	12.0
W/VEGETABLES *(Healthy Choice)* low fat 'Homestyle'	9.5 oz	230	470	3.0
WHITE MEAT *(Le Menu)* w/stuffing and gravy	8 oz	200	610	5.0
TURKEY FAT				
	1 cup	1846	0	204.6
	1 oz	255	0	28.3
	1 tbsp	115	0	12.8
TURKEY GIBLETS				
raw	1 oz	37	25	1.2
raw: 1 gizzard, 1 heart, and 1 liver, approx 8.6 oz	1 pkt	315	212	10.2
simmered	4 oz	189	67	5.8
simmered, chopped, or diced	1 cup	243	85	7.4
simmered, w/giblet fat	1 cup	242	86	7.4
TURKEY GIZZARD				
raw	1 oz	33	23	1.0
raw, approx 4 oz	1 gizzard	132	90	4.2
simmered	1 cup	236	78	5.6
simmered	4 oz	185	61	4.4
TURKEY HAM SALAD				
(Longacre)	1 oz	53	190	4.0
(Longacre) 'Saladfest'	1 oz	58	270	4.0
TURKEY LIVER				
raw	1 oz	39	27	1.1
raw, approx 3.6 oz	1 liver	140	98	4.1
simmered	1 cup	237	90	8.3
simmered	4 oz	192	73	6.7

Food Name	Serv. Size	Total Cal.	Sod. MGS	Fat GMS
TURKEY NUGGET *(Louis Rich)* 80% fat-free, breaded, cooked	3/4 oz	60	155	4.0
TURKEY SALAD				
(Longacre)	1 oz	70	200	5.0
(Longacre) 'Saladfest'	1 oz	68	180	5.0
TURKEY SEASONING MIX *(Schilling)* roast 'Bag'n Season'	1 pkg	146	1935	5.0
TURKEY SPREAD				
(Libby's) 'Spreadables'	1.9 oz	100	260	6.0
(Underwood) chunky 'Light'	2 1/8 oz	75	330	2.0
TURKEY STICK				
(Louis Rich) cooked, breaded, 80% fat-free	.95 oz	80	195	5.0
(Louis Rich) cooked, prepared	1 oz	81	197	5.0
(The Turkey Store) breast meat, cheese 'Gobble Stix'	1 stick	30	na	0.8
(The Turkey Store) breast meat, smoked 'Gobble Stix'	1 stick	25	na	0.2
TURMERIC				
ground	1 oz	100	11	2.8
ground	1 tbsp	24	3	0.7
ground	1 tsp	8	1	0.2
ground *(Durkee)*	1 tsp	9	0	tr
ground *(Laurel Leaf)*	1 tsp	9	0	tr
ground *(Spice Islands)*	1 tsp	7	<1	0.2
TURNIP				
boiled, drained	4 oz	20	57	0.1
boiled, drained, cubed	1/2 cup	14	39	0.1
boiled, drained, mashed	1/2 cup	21	58	0.1
raw, cubed	1/2 cup	18	44	0.1
raw, trimmed	1 oz	8	19	<.1
raw, untrimmed	1 lb	100	248	0.4
Canned				
(Allens) diced	1/2 cup	16	25	<1.0
(Stokely)	1/2 cup	20	350	0.0
Frozen				
boiled, drained	4 oz	26	41	0.3
mashed	3 1/3 oz	15	23	0.2
(Southern) diced	3.5 oz	17	50	0.2
TURNIP GREENS				
boiled, drained	4 oz	23	33	0.3
boiled, drained, chopped	1/2 cup	14	21	0.2
raw, chopped	1/2 cup	8	11	0.1
raw, untrimmed	1 lb	85	126	1.0

Food Name	Serv. Size	Total Cal.	Sod. MGS	Fat GMS
TURNIP GREENS, CANNED				
Chopped				
(Allens)	1/2 cup	21	15	<1.0
(Bush's Best)	1/2 cup	20	310	0.0
W/diced turnips				
(Allens) chopped	1/2 cup	19	15	<1.0
(Bush's Best)	1/2 cup	25	370	0.0
(Stokely)	1/2 cup	20	340	0.0
W/liquid	1/2 cup	16	324	0.4
TURNIP GREENS, FROZEN				
boiled, drained	10 oz	66	33	0.9
boiled, drained	4 oz	34	17	0.5
boiled, drained	1/2 cup	25	12	0.3
chopped	10 oz	62	34	0.9
chopped	1/2 cup	18	10	0.3
chopped (Frosty Acres)	3.3 oz	20	10	0.0
chopped (Seabrook)	3.3 oz	20	11	0.0
chopped (Southern)	3.5 oz	25	70	0.3
w/turnips	10 oz	60	51	0.5
w/turnips (Seabrook)	3.3 oz	20	na	0.0
w/turnips, boiled, drained	4 oz	19	17	0.2
TURNIP-ROOTED PARSLEY. See PARSLEY ROOT.				
TURNOVER. See also PASTRY.				
apple, frozen (Pepperidge Farm)	1 turnover	300	210	17.0
apple, refrigerated (Pillsbury)	1 turnover	170	320	8.0
blueberry, frozen (Pepperidge Farm)	1 turnover	310	230	19.0
cherry, frozen (Pepperidge Farm)	1 turnover	310	280	19.0
cherry, refrigerated (Pillsbury)	1 turnover	170	320	8.0
peach, frozen (Pepperidge Farm)	1 turnover	310	260	18.0
raspberry, frozen (Pepperidge Farm)	1 turnover	310	260	17.0
TUSK. See CUSK.				

U

Food Name	Serv. Size	Total Cal.	Sod. MGS	Fat GMS

UDON NOODLE. See NOODLE, JAPANESE.
ULTRA SLIM FAST. See DIET DRINK.
UMEBOSHI PLUM. See PLUM, JAPANESE.

V

Food Name	Serv. Size	Total Cal.	Sod. MGS	Fat GMS
VANILLA BAKING CHIPS (Hershey's)	1/4 cup	240	65	14.0
VANILLA EXTRACT, pure (Virginia Dare)	1 tsp	10	0	0.0
VANILLA FLAVOR DRINK, CANNED				
(Ensure) liquid nutrition	8 oz	250	200	8.8
(Ensure) liquid nutrition 'Plus'	8 oz	355	250	12.6
(Ensure) liquid nutrition, w/fiber	8 oz	260	200	8.8
(Sego) 'Lite'	10 oz	150	390	4.0
(Sego) 'Lite French Vanilla'	10 oz	150	390	4.0
(Sego) 'Very Vanilla'	10 oz	225	360	5.0
(Sustacal) liquid food, nutritionally complete	8 oz	240	220	5.5
VEAL				
(NOTE: TRIMMED = Lean; separable fat removed. UNTRIMMED = Separable fat not removed.)				
BRAINS				
braised	3 oz	116	133	8.2
pan-fried	3 oz	181	150	14.2
raw	1 oz	33	36	2.3
GROUND				
broiled	1 cup	200	96	8.8
broiled	3 oz	146	71	6.4
raw	1 cup	325	185	15.3
raw	1 oz	40	23	1.9
HEART				
braised	3 oz	158	49	5.7
raw	1 oz	31	22	1.1
simmered	4 oz	368	116	13.4
KIDNEYS				
braised	3 oz	139	94	4.8
raw	1 oz	28	50	0.9
LEG				
Trimmed				
braised	3 oz	173	57	4.3
pan-fried	3 oz	156	65	3.9
raw	1 oz	30	18	0.5
roasted	3 oz	127	58	2.9
Untrimmed				
braised	3 oz	179	57	5.4
pan-fried	3 oz	179	65	7.1
raw	1 oz	33	18	0.9

Food Name	Serv. Size	Total Cal.	Sod. MGS	Fat GMS
roasted	3 oz	136	58	4.0
LEG AND SHOULDER				
raw, trimmed	1 oz	31	23	0.7
trimmed, braised	3 oz	160	79	3.7
LIVER				
braised	3 oz	140	45	5.9
pan-fried	3 oz	208	112	9.7
raw	4 oz	152	70	5.0
raw	1 oz	38	17	1.2
LOIN				
Trimmed				
braised	3 oz	192	71	7.8
raw	1 oz	32	25	0.9
roasted	3 oz	149	82	5.9
stewed	4 oz	256	95	10.4
Untrimmed				
braised	3 oz	241	68	14.6
raw	1 oz	46	24	2.6
roasted	3 oz	184	79	10.5
stewed	4 oz	322	91	19.5
LUNGS				
braised	3 oz	88	48	2.2
raw	1 oz	25	30	0.6
PANCREAS				
braised	3 oz	218	58	12.4
raw	1 oz	51	19	3.7
RIB				
Trimmed				
braised	3 oz	185	84	6.6
raw	1 lb	544	431	17.6
raw	1 oz	34	27	1.1
roasted	3 oz	150	82	6.3
stewed	4 oz	247	112	8.9
Untrimmed				
braised	3 oz	213	81	10.6
raw	1 lb	735	404	40.9
raw	1 oz	45	25	2.5
roasted	3 oz	194	78	11.9
stewed	4 oz	285	108	14.2

Food Name	Serv. Size	Total Cal.	Sod. MGS	Fat GMS
SHOULDER, ARM				
Trimmed				
braised	3 oz	171	77	4.5
braised, approx 5.6 oz	1 steak	321	143	8.5
raw	1 oz	29	24	0.6
roasted	3 oz	139	77	4.9
roasted, approx 9.6 oz	1 steak	447	248	15.8
Untrimmed				
braised	3 oz	201	74	8.7
braised, approx 6.1 oz	1 steak	409	151	17.7
raw	1 oz	37	23	1.5
roasted	3 oz	156	77	7.0
SHOULDER, BLADE				
Trimmed				
braised	3 oz	168	86	5.5
diced, braised	1 cup	277	141	9.1
diced, roasted	1 cup	239	143	9.6
diced, stewed	1 cup	277	141	9.1
raw	1 lb	513	440	14.8
raw	1 oz	32	27	0.9
roasted	3 oz	145	87	5.8
stewed	4 oz	224	115	7.3
Untrimmed				
braised	3 oz	191	83	8.6
diced, braised	1 cup	315	137	14.1
diced, roasted	1 cup	260	140	12.1
diced, stewed	1 cup	315	137	14.1
raw	1 lb	585	431	23.6
raw	1 oz	36	27	1.5
roasted	3 oz	158	85	7.4
stewed	4 oz	255	111	11.4
SHOULDER, WHOLE				
Trimmed				
braised	3 oz	169	82	5.2
diced, braised	1 cup	279	136	8.5
diced, roasted	1 cup	238	136	9.3
diced, stewed	1 cup	279	136	8.5
raw	1 lb	508	417	13.6
raw	1 oz	31	26	0.8
roasted	3 oz	144	82	5.6
stewed	4 oz	226	110	6.9

Food Name	Serv. Size	Total Cal.	Sod. MGS	Fa GM
Untrimmed				
braised	3 oz	194	81	8.
diced, braised	1 cup	319	133	14.
diced, roasted	1 cup	258	134	11.
diced, stewed	1 cup	319	133	14.
raw	1 lb	590	413	24.
raw	1 oz	36	25	1.
roasted	3 oz	156	82	7.
stewed	4 oz	259	108	11.
SIRLOIN				
Trimmed				
braised	3 oz	173	69	5.
diced, braised	1 cup	286	113	9.
diced, roasted	1 cup	235	119	8.
diced, stewed	1 cup	286	113	9.
raw	1 lb	499	363	11
raw	1 oz	31	22	0.
roasted	3 oz	143	72	5.
stewed	4 oz	231	92	7.
Untrimmed				
braised	3 oz	214	67	11.
diced, braised	1 cup	353	111	18.
diced, roasted	1 cup	283	116	14.
diced, stewed	1 cup	353	111	18.
raw	1 lb	689	345	35.
raw	1 oz	43	21	2.
roasted	3 oz	172	71	8.
stewed	4 oz	286	90	14.
THYMUS				
braised	3 oz	148	56	3.
raw	1 oz	28	23	0.
TONGUE				
braised	3 oz	172	54	8.
raw	1 oz	37	23	1.
TOP ROUND				
Trimmed				
braised	4 oz	230	76	5.
diced, braised	1 cup	284	94	7.
diced, roasted	1 cup	210	95	4.
diced, stewed	1 cup	284	94	7.
pan-fried in vegetable oil	4 oz	208	87	5.

Food Name	Serv. Size	Total Cal.	Sod. MGS	Fat GMS
roasted	4 oz	170	77	3.8
stewed	4 oz	230	76	5.8
Untrimmed				
diced, roasted	1 cup	224	95	6.5
diced, stewed	1 cup	295	94	8.9
pan-fried in vegetable oil	4 oz	239	86	9.5
roasted	4 oz	181	77	5.3
stewed	4 oz	239	76	7.2
VEAL ENTRÉE, FROZEN				
MARSALA *(Le Menu)* 'LightStyle'	10 oz	230	700	3.0
PARMIGIANA				
(Armour) 'Classics'	11.25 oz	400	1320	22.0
(Le Menu)	11.5 oz	390	840	17.0
(Morton)	10 oz	260	1510	8.0
(Swanson)	12.25 oz	430	1010	20.0
(Swanson) 'Homestyle Recipe'	10 oz	330	960	13.0
(Swanson) 'Hungry Man'	18.25 oz	590	1840	26.0
(Ultimate 200)	8.2 oz	150	550	4.0
Breaded				
(Banquet) 'Cookin' Bags'	4 oz	230	(mq)	11.0
(Banquet) 'Family Entrées'	8 oz	370	(mq)	18.0
(Freezer Queen)	5 oz	220	560	12.0
(Freezer Queen) 'Cook-In-Pouch'	5 oz	220	560	12.0
(Freezer Queen) 'Deluxe Family Suppers'	7 oz	300	820	15.0
Platter *(Freezer Queen)*	10 oz	400	870	20.0
W/pasta Alfredo *(Stouffer's)* homestyle	9.25 oz	350	1060	15.0
STEAK				
(Hormel)	4 oz	130	(mq)	4.0
(Hormel) breaded	4 oz	240	(mq)	13.0
VEGETABLE. See individual listings.				
VEGETABLE DISH, CANNED. See also individual listings.				
Corn, beans, and carrots, w/pasta, in tomato sauce				
(Green Giant)	1/2 cup	80	330	2.0
Green beans, potatoes, and mushrooms, in sauce				
(Green Giant)	1/2 cup	50	430	2.0
Snap beans, potatoes, and mushrooms, in sauce				
(Green Giant)	1/2 cup	50	430	2.0
String beans, potatoes, and mushrooms, in sauce				
(Green Giant)	1/2 cup	50	430	2.0

Food Name	Serv. Size	Total Cal.	Sod. MGS	Fat GMS
VEGETABLE DISH, FROZEN. See also individual listings.				
Broccoli, cauliflower, carrots				
(Birds Eye) 'Butter Sauce'	3.3 oz	45	290	2.0
(Birds Eye) 'Cheese Sauce'	4.5 oz	110	410	5.0
(Birds Eye) 'Farm Fresh'	4 oz	35	40	0.0
(Green Giant) 'Butter Sauce'	1/2 cup	30	240	1.0
(Green Giant) in cheese sauce	1/2 cup	60	490	2.0
(Green Giant) 'One Serving'	1 pkg	30	40	0.0
(Stokely) 'Singles' w/baby carrots	3 oz	25	25	1.0
(Stokely) w/baby carrots, in cheese sauce	4 oz	70	180	3.0
Broccoli, cauliflower, peppers, w/red peppers 'Farm Fresh'				
(Birds Eye)	4 oz	30	25	0.0
Broccoli, corn, peppers, w/red peppers 'Farm Fresh'				
(Birds Eye)	4 oz	60	15	1.0
Broccoli, green beans, onions, peppers, w/pearl onions				
and red peppers (Birds Eye)	4 oz	35	15	0.0
Broccoli, peppers, bamboo shoots, mushrooms, w/red				
peppers (Birds Eye)	4 oz	30	20	0.0
Broccoli and carrots, w/rotini, in cheese sauce				
(Green Giant)	1 pkg	100	440	2.0
Brussels sprouts, cauliflower, carrots (Birds Eye)	4 oz	40	30	0.0
Cauliflower, broccoli, carrots, in cheese sauce				
(Freezer Queen)	5 oz	60	360	1.0
Cauliflower, carrots, snow peas, w/baby carrots and snow				
pea pods (Birds Eye)	4 oz	40	35	0.0
Cauliflower, zucchini, carrots, peppers, w/red peppers				
(Birds Eye)	4 oz	30	25	0.0
Peas, carrots, water chestnuts, w/sugar snap peas and				
baby carrots (Birds Eye)	3.2 oz	50	20	0.0
Zucchini, carrots, onions, mushrooms, w/pearl onions				
(Birds Eye)	4 oz	30	15	0.0
VEGETABLE ENTRÉE				
Chinese style, w/chicken, frozen (Budget Gourmet)	10 oz	280	590	7.0
Country style, w/beef tips (Ultra Slim Fast)	12 oz	230	960	5.0
Italian style, w/chicken, frozen (Budget Gourmet)	10.25 oz	310	690	8.0
Pot pie, frozen				
(Amy's Kitchen) organic	8 oz	347	260	16.0
(Morton) w/beef	7 oz	430	740	31.0
(Morton) w/chicken	7 oz	420	740	28.0
(Morton) w/turkey	7 oz	420	740	28.0
Stir-fry, frozen (Shanghai)	5.1 oz	75	510	1.0

Food Name	Serv. Size	Total Cal.	Sod. MGS	Fat GMS
VEGETABLE FLAKES *(French's)* dehydrated	1 tbsp	12	20	0.0
VEGETABLE JUICE				
cocktail, canned	6 oz	35	664	0.2
cocktail, canned	1/2 cup	23	442	0.1
(Biotta) 'Breuss Juice'	6 oz	67	147	0.1
(Biotta) 'Cocktail'	6 oz	50	497	0.1
(Knudsen & Sons) 'Very Veggie'	8 oz	40	na	0.0
(Knudsen & Sons) 'Very Veggie' low sodium	8 oz	40	32	0.0
(Knudsen & Sons) 'Very Veggie' organic	8 oz	40	na	0.0
(Knudsen & Sons) 'Very Veggie' spicy	8 oz	40	560	0.0
(Smucker's) hearty	8 oz	58	714	<.1
(Smucker's) hot and spicy	8 oz	58	650	<.1
(V•8)	6 oz	35	560	0.0
(V•8) 'Light'n Tangy'	6 oz	40	240	0.0
(V•8) 'No Salt Added'	6 oz	35	45	0.0
(V•8) 'Picante' mild	6 oz	35	520	0.0
(V•8) spicy hot	6 oz	35	650	0.0
(Veryfine) '100%'	6 oz	32	600	0.0
VEGETABLE MARROW SQUASH. See SQUASH, MARROW.				
VEGETABLE OIL. See also individual listings.				
(Crisco)	1 tbsp	120	0	14.0
(Finast)	1 tbsp	120	0	14.0
(Hain) 'All Blend'	1 tbsp	120	0	14.0
(Hain) w/garlic 'Garlic & Oil'	1 tbsp	120	0	14.0
(Kroger)	1 tbsp	122	0	13.6
(Pathmark)	1 tbsp	120	0	14.0
(Pathmark) 'No Frills'	1 tbsp	130	0	14.0
(Puritan)	1 tbsp	120	0	14.0
(Wesson)	1 tbsp	120	0	14.0
VEGETABLE OIL SPRAY. See COOKING SPRAY.				
VEGETABLE OIL SPREAD. See MARGARINE SPREAD.				
VEGETABLE OYSTER. See SALSIFY.				
VEGETABLE SPONGE. See GOURD, DISHCLOTH.				
VEGETABLE STICKS, breaded, frozen *(Farm Rich)*	4 oz	240	980	10.0
VEGETABLES, MIXED, CANNED				
drained	4 oz	53	169	0.3
drained	1/2 cup	39	122	0.2
w/liquid	4 oz	41	254	0.3
w/liquid	1/2 cup	40	355	0.0
(A&P) 'Eastern'	1/2 cup	45	330	<1.0
(A&P) 'No Salt Added'	1/2 cup	40	20	<1.0

Food Name	Serv. Size	Total Cal.	Sod. MGS	Fat GMS
(A&P) 'Western'	1/2 cup	40	380	<1.0
(Bush's Best) 'Mixed Greens'	1/2 cup	20	300	0.0
(Featherweight)	1/2 cup	40	25	0.0
(Finast)	1/2 cup	40	390	0.0
(Finast) 'No Salt Added'	1/2 cup	40	25	0.0
(Freshlike) water packed, w/o salt	1/2 cup	35	25	0.0
(Freshlike) water packed, w/o sugar or salt	1/2 cup	35	25	0.0
(Green Giant) 'Garden Medley'	1/2 cup	35	350	0.0
(Green Giant) 'Pantry Express'	1/2 cup	35	300	<1.0
(LaChoy) 'Chinese'	1/2 cup	12	30	0.1
(LaChoy) 'Chop Suey'	1/2 cup	9	330	0.1
(LaChoy) 'Fancy Mix'	1/2 cup	12	30	<1.0
(P&Q) 'Chunky Eastern'	1/2 cup	40	330	<1.0
(P&Q) 'Chunky Western'	1/2 cup	40	380	<1.0
(Pathmark)	1/2 cup	35	320	0.0
(Pathmark) 'No Salt Added'	1/2 cup	35	25	0.0
(S&W) 'Old Fashioned Harvest'	1/2 cup	35	380	0.0
(Stokely)	1/2 cup	40	300	0.0
(Stokely) 'No Salt or Sugar Added'	1/2 cup	40	25	0.0
(Veg•All) 'Homestyle Large Cut'	1/2 cup	35	380	0.0
(Veg•All) 'Lite'	1/2 cup	35	25	0.0
(Veg•All) 'Original'	1/2 cup	35	320	0.0
VEGETABLES, MIXED, FROZEN				
boiled, drained	10-oz pkg	162	96	0.4
boiled, drained	4 oz	67	40	0.2
boiled, drained	1/2 cup	54	32	0.1
(A&P)	3.3 oz	65	55	<1.0
(Birds Eye)	3.3 oz	60	40	0.0
(Birds Eye) 'Portion Pack'	3 oz	50	35	0.0
(Freshlike)	3.3 oz	70	45	0.0
(Frosty Acres)	3.3 oz	65	50	0.0
(Green Giant)	1/2 cup	40	40	0.0
(Green Giant) 'Harvest Fresh'	1/2 cup	40	125	0.0
(Green Giant) 'Plain Polybag'	1/2 cup	40	40	0.0
(Health Valley)	1/2 cup	68	39	0.0
(Seabrook)	3.3 oz	65	50	0.0
(Southern)	3.5 oz	69	60	0.0
(Stokely) 'Singles'	3 oz	60	40	1.0
(Veg•All)	3.3 oz	70	45	0.0
CALIFORNIA STYLE				
(A&P) 'California Blend'	3.3 oz	25	25	<1.0

Food Name	Serv. Size	Total Cal.	Sod. MGS	Fat GMS
(Freshlike) 'California Blend'	3.3 oz	30	20	0.0
(Green Giant) 'American Mixtures'	1/2 cup	25	40	0.0
(Veg•All) 'California Blend'	3.3 oz	30	20	0.0
CHINESE STYLE				
(Birds Eye) chow mein, w/Oriental sauce 'Custom Cuisine'	4.6 oz	80	570	2.0
(Birds Eye) chow mein, w/seasoned sauce	3.3 oz	90	370	4.0
(Birds Eye) 'Stir-Fry'	3.3 oz	35	540	0.0
CHUCKWAGON STYLE				
(Freshlike) 'Chuckwagon Blend'	3.3 oz	70	5	1.0
(Veg•All) 'Chuckwagon Blend'	3.3 oz	70	5	1.0
COUNTRY STYLE				
(Birds Eye) 'International Rice Recipes'	3.3 oz	90	380	0.0
(Freshlike) 'Country Blend'	3.3 oz	50	15	0.0
(Green Giant) 'American Mixtures Heartland'	1/2 cup	25	35	0.0
(Veg•All) 'Country Blend'	3.3 oz	50	15	0.0
DUTCH STYLE *(Frosty Acres)*	3.2 oz	30	30	0.0
FOR BEEF				
(Birds Eye) Oriental style, w/sauce	4.6 oz	90	350	4.0
(Birds Eye) w/cream mushroom 'Custom Cuisine'	4.6 oz	60	450	2.0
FOR CHICKEN				
(Birds Eye) w/tomato basil sauce	4.6 oz	110	360	3.0
(Birds Eye) w/wild rice, in white wine sauce	4.6 oz	100	510	2.0
FOR CHICKEN OR FISH *(Birds Eye)* w/Dijon mustard sauce	4.6 oz	70	310	3.0
FOR CHICKEN OR SHRIMP *(Birds Eye)* w/delicate herb sauce	4.6 oz	90	460	5.0
FOR SOUP				
(Freshlike)	3.3 oz	50	40	0.0
(Veg•All)	3.3 oz	50	40	0.0
FOR STEW				
(A&P)	4 oz	60	30	<1.0
(Freshlike) 5-ways	3.3 oz	50	40	0.0
(Freshlike) 4-ways	3.3 oz	50	40	0.0
(Frosty Acres)	3 oz	42	21	0.0
(Kohl's)	3.3 oz	50	30	<1.0
(Ore-Ida)	3 oz	60	40	<1.0
(Veg•All) 5-ways	3.3 oz	50	40	0.0
(Veg•All) 4-ways	3.3 oz	50	40	0.0
FRENCH STYLE *(Birds Eye)* 'International Recipes'	3.3 oz	110	610	0.0
IN BUTTER SAUCE				
(Finast)	3.3 oz	70	340	4.0
(Green Giant)	1/2 cup	60	300	2.0

Food Name	Serv. Size	Total Cal.	Sod. MGS	Fat GMS
ITALIAN STYLE				
(A&P) blend	3.3 oz	40	35	<1.0
(Birds Eye) 'International Recipes'	3.3 oz	100	490	5.0
(Freshlike) 'Italian Blend'	3.3 oz	30	20	0.0
(Freshlike) 'Italian Blend' food service	3.3 oz	25	20	0.0
(Veg•All) 'Italian Blend'	3.3 oz	30	20	0.0
(Veg•All) 'Italian Blend' food service	3.3 oz	25	20	0.0
JAPANESE STYLE				
(Birds Eye) 'International Recipes'	3.3 oz	90	420	5.0
(Birds Eye) 'Stir-Fry'	3.3 oz	30	510	0.0
LE SUEUR STYLE (Green Giant) 'Valley Combinations'	1/2 cup	70	400	2.0
MANHATTAN STYLE (Green Giant) 'American Mixtures'	1/2 cup	25	15	0.0
MIDWEST STYLE				
(Freshlike) 'Midwestern Blend'	3.3 oz	40	30	0.0
(Veg•All) 'Midwestern Blend'	3.3 oz	40	30	0.0
NEW ENGLAND STYLE				
(Birds Eye) 'International Recipes'	3.3 oz	130	430	7.0
(Green Giant) 'American Mixtures'	1/2 cup	70	75	1.0
ORIENTAL STYLE				
(A&P) blend	3.3 oz	25	15	<1.0
(Birds Eye) 'International Recipes'	3.3 oz	70	300	4.0
(Freshlike) 'Oriental Blend'	3.3 oz	25	10	0.0
(Frosty Acres)	3.2 oz	25	15	0.0
(Veg•All) 'Oriental Blend'	3.3 oz	25	10	0.0
SAN FRANCISCO STYLE				
(Birds Eye) 'International Recipes'	3.3 oz	100	400	5.0
(Green Giant) 'American Mixtures'	1/2 cup	25	35	0.0
SANTA FE STYLE (Green Giant) 'American Mixtures'	1/2 cup	70	0	1.0
SCANDINAVIAN STYLE				
(Freshlike) 'Scandinavian Blend'	3.3 oz	45	30	0.0
(Veg•All) 'Scandinavian Blend'	3.3 oz	45	30	0.0
SEATTLE STYLE (Green Giant) 'American Mixtures'	1/2 cup	25	35	0.0
SPANISH STYLE (Birds Eye) 'International Recipes'	3.3 oz	110	540	0.0
WESTERN STYLE (Green Giant) 'American Mixtures'	1/2 cup	60	25	2.0
WINTER VEGETABLES				
(A&P) blend	3.3 oz	24	190	<1.0
(Freshlike) 'Winter Blend'	3.3 oz	25	25	0.0
(Veg•All) 'Winter Blend'	3.3 oz	25	25	0.0
W/PASTA				
(Birds Eye) cheese tortellini, in tomato sauce 'For One'	5.5 oz	210	500	5.0
(Birds Eye) in Stroganoff sauce 'Custom Cuisine'	4.6 oz	120	700	5.0

Food Name	Serv. Size	Total Cal.	Sod. MGS	Fat GMS
(Birds Eye) in white cheese sauce 'Custom Cuisine'	4.6 oz	150	440	6.0
(Birds Eye) primavera style, w/seasoned sauce	3.3 oz	120	340	5.0
(Stokely) rotini, in cheddar cheese sauce 'Singles'	4 oz	100	380	3.0
(Stokely) shells, in Italian style sauce 'Singles'	4 oz	170	270	15.0
W/TERIYAKI SAUCE *(Stokely)* 'Singles'	4 oz	100	580	0.0
W/WHITE AND WILD RICE, pilaf *(Stokely)* 'Singles'	4 oz	80	290	0.0
VEGETABLES, MIXED, MICROWAVE				
(Green Giant) 'Microwave Shelf-Pack'	1/2 cup	35	300	<1.0
(Pantry Express) 'Microwave Shelf-Pack'	1/2 cup	35	300	<1.0
VEGETARIAN ENTRÉE. See also individual listings.				
(Amy's Kitchen) Salisbury steak, organic, frozen				
'Country Dinner' 11 oz 482		12.0	4.0	na
(Ken & Robert's) patty, frozen 'Truly Amazing'	2.5-oz patty	110	390	2.0
(LaChoy) chow mein, w/o meat, canned	3/4 cup	35	820	0.4
(Natural Touch) patty, frozen 'Dinner Entree'	3 oz	230	300	14.0
(Tofutti) tortellini, meatless, frozen	2 oz	220	110	2.0
(Worthington) roast, frozen 'Dinner Roast'	2 oz	120	440	8.0
VEGETARIAN ENTRÉE MIX. See also individual listings.				
(Tofu Classics) stroganoff, creamy, prepared w/tofu	1/2 cup	94	264	3.0
(Tofu Classics) stroganoff, creamy, prepared w/tofu and				
salted butter	1/2 cup	127	310	7.0

VEGETARIAN FOODS. See BACON, ALTERNATIVE; BEEF, ALTERNATIVE; BEEF JERKY, ALTERNATIVE; BURGER, VEGETARIAN; BURGER MIX, VEGETARIAN; CHICKEN, ALTERNATIVE; CRAB, ALTERNATIVE; FISH FILLET, ALTERNATIVE; HAM, ALTERNATIVE; LUNCHEON MEAT, ALTERNATIVE; MEAT, ALTERNATIVE; MEAT LOAF MIX, ALTERNATIVE; SAUSAGE, ALTERNATIVE; SCALLOP, ALTERNATIVE; SPREAD, VEGETARIAN; TUNA, ALTERNATIVE; TURKEY, ALTERNATIVE; VEGETARIAN ENTRÉE; and individual listings.

VIENNA SAUSAGE, CANNED				
beef and pork	1 oz	79	270	7.1
2 inches long, 7/8 inch diam	1 sausage	45	152	4.0
(Armour) chicken, in beef stock 'Premium' lite	2 oz	150	400	13.0
(Armour) hot and spicy	2.5 oz	190	860	17.0
(Armour) in barbecue sauce	2.5 oz	190	760	17.0
(Armour) in beef stock	2 oz	180	530	17.0
(Armour) in beef stock, lite	2 oz	150	400	13.0
(Armour) smoked	2 oz	180	530	17.0
(Hormel)	1 oz	69	225	7.0
(Hormel) chicken	1 oz	56	220	5.0
(Hormel) w/o broth	4 links	200	479	18.0
(Libby's) chicken, in beef broth	2 oz	130	560	10.0
(Libby's) in barbecue sauce	2.5 oz	180	420	15.0

Food Name	Serv. Size	Total Cal.	Sod. MGS	Fa GM
(Libby's) in beef broth	2 oz	160	330	15.0
VINE SPINACH/basella				
raw	1 lb	86	(mq)	1.4
raw	3.5 oz	19	24	0.3
VINEGAR				
APPLE CIDER				
	1 cup	34	2	0.0
	1 tbsp	2	0	0.0
(Great Impressions)	1 tbsp	7	<1	0.0
(Hain)	1 tbsp	2	1	0.0
(Heinz)	.51 oz	2	1	0.0
(Heinz) gourmet 'Decanter'	.51 oz	4	0	0.0
(Indian Summer)	1 cup	40	5	<1.0
(Lucky Leaf)	1 oz	4	0	0.0
(Musselman's)	1 oz	4	0	0.0
(Spectrum Naturals) filtered	1 tbsp	7	55	0.0
(Spectrum Naturals) unfiltered	1 tbsp	7	55	0.0
(White House)	1 oz	4	5	0.0
BROWN RICE				
(Spectrum Naturals) organic	1 tbsp	0	0	0.0
(Spectrum Naturals) organic, seasoned	1 tbsp	10	240	0.0
WHITE				
	1 cup	29	2	0.0
	1 tbsp	2	0	0.0
(Heinz)	1 tbsp	2	1	0.0
(Indian Summer)	1 cup	30	5	<1.0
(Lucky Leaf)	1 oz	4	0	0.0
(Musselman's)	1 oz	4	0	0.0
(Spectrum Naturals) organic	1 tbsp	0	0	0.0
WINE				
(Great Impressions) basil	1 tbsp	7	<1	0.0
(Great Impressions) paprika, hot	1 tbsp	6	<1	0.0
(Great Impressions) raspberry	1 tbsp	7	<1	0.0
(Heinz) gourmet 'Decanter'	.51 oz	4	0	0.0
(Heinz) tarragon, gourmet 'Decanter'	.51 oz	2	0	0.0
(Lucky Leaf) red	1 oz	0	0	0.0
(Musselman's) red	1 oz	0	0	0.0
(Regina) all varieties	1 oz	4	0	0.0
(Spectrum Naturals) garlic, organic	1 tbsp	0	0	0.0
(Spectrum Naturals) Italian herb, organic	1 tbsp	0	0	0.0
(Spectrum Naturals) raspberry, organic	1 tbsp	10	0	0.0

Food Name	Serv. Size	Total Cal.	Sod. MGS	Fat GMS
(Spectrum Naturals) red, organic	1 tbsp	0	0	0.0
(Spectrum Naturals) white, organic	1 tbsp	0	0	0.0
VITA JUICE (Knudsen & Sons)	8 oz	90	na	0.0

VODKA. See ALCOHOLIC BEVERAGES.

W

Food Name	Serv. Size	Total Cal.	Sod. MGS	Fat GMS
WAFFLE, FROZEN				
(Aunt Jemima) 'Original' 2.5 oz	1 waffle	173	591	5.6
(Downyflake)	2 waffles	120	420	3.0
(Downyflake) 'Crisp & Healthy'	1 waffle	80	180	1.0
(Downyflake) 'Hot-N-Buttery'	2 waffles	180	620	6.0
(Downyflake) 'Jumbo'	2 waffles	170	570	4.0
(Eggo) 'Homestyle'	1 waffle	120	250	5.0
(Eggo) 'Nutri-Grain'	1 waffle	130	250	5.0
(Roman Meal)	2 waffles	280	680	14.0
APPLE (Eggo) 'Fruit Top'	3.1 oz	190	250	6.0
APPLE CINNAMON				
(Aunt Jemima) 2.5 oz	1 waffle	176	616	5.6
(Downyflake) 'Crisp & Healthy'	1 waffle	80	180	1.0
(Eggo)	1 waffle	130	250	5.0
(Van's)	1 waffle	75	68	2.0
BLUEBERRY				
(Aunt Jemima) 2.5 oz	1 waffle	175	684	5.2
(Downyflake)	2 waffles	180	570	4.0
(Eggo)	1 waffle	130	250	5.0
(Eggo) 'Fruit Top'	3.1 oz	190	250	6.0
(Krusteaz) 1.2 oz	1 waffle	110	210	3.0
BUTTERMILK				
(Aunt Jemima) 2.5 oz	1 waffle	179	615	5.8
(Downyflake)	2 waffles	190	750	5.0
(Downyflake) 'Jumbo'	2 waffles	170	630	4.0
(Eggo)	1 waffle	120	250	5.0
(Krusteaz) 1.2 oz	1 waffle	100	190	2.0
GOLDEN (Krusteaz) 1.2 oz	1 waffle	100	190	2.0
HONEY ALMOND (Van's)	1 waffle	75	68	2.0
MULTIGRAIN				
(Downyflake)	2 waffles	250	500	4.0
(Van's)	1 waffle	75	68	2.0

Food Name	Serv. Size	Total Cal.	Sod. MGS	Fat GMS
OAT BRAN				
(Aunt Jemima)	2.5 oz	154	676	2.8
(Downyflake)	2 waffles	260	650	13.0
(Eggo) 'Common Sense'	1 waffle	110	220	4.0
(Eggo) w/fruit and nut 'Common Sense'	1 waffle	120	220	5.0
(Van's) 'Belgian'	1 waffle	89	124	2.0
ORIGINAL *(Van's)* 'Belgian'	1 waffle	86	54	2.0
PEACH *(Eggo)* 'Fruit Top'	3.1 oz	190	240	6.0
RAISIN BRAN *(Eggo)* 'Nutri-Grain'	1 waffle	130	250	5.0
RICE BRAN *(Downyflake)*	2 waffles	210	230	11.0
SEVEN GRAIN *(Van's)* 'Belgian'	1 waffle	88	81	2.0
STRAWBERRY				
(Eggo)	1 waffle	130	250	5.0
(Eggo) 'Fruit Top'	1 waffle	190	230	6.0
WHOLE-GRAIN WHEAT *(Aunt Jemima)*	1 waffle	154	676	2.8
WAFFLE BREAKFAST, FROZEN				
(Swanson) Belgian, w/sausage 'Great Starts'	2.85 oz	280	420	19.0
(Swanson) Belgian, w/strawberries and sausage	3.5 oz	210	240	8.0
(Swanson) w/bacon 'Great Starts'	2.2 oz	230	710	14.0
WAFFLE MIX. See PANCAKE/WAFFLE MIX.				
WAKAME. See SEAWEED.				
WALNUT, BLACK				
Dried				
	1 oz	172	0	16.1
chopped	1 cup	759	1	70.7
finely ground	1 cup	486	1	45.3
in shell	1 lb	661	2	61.6
Raw *(Planters)*	1 oz	180	0	17.0
Shelled *(Fisher)*	1 oz	170	0	16.0
WALNUT, ENGLISH				
Dried				
	1 lb	1310	21	126.3
halves	1 cup	642	10	61.9
halves, approx 14	1 oz	182	3	17.6
in shell	1 lb	1310	21	126.3
pieces or chips	1 cup	770	12	74.2
(Diamond)	1 oz	192	na	19.0
(Fisher) chopped	1 oz	180	0	18.0
(Fisher) ground	1 oz	180	0	18.0
(Planters) halves	1 oz	190	0	20.0
(Planters) pieces	1 oz	190	0	20.0

Food Name	Serv. Size	Total Cal.	Sod. MGS	Fat GMS
(Planters) whole	1 oz	190	0	20.0
Raw *(Fisher)*	1 oz	180	0	18.0
WALNUT, PERSIAN				
Dried, in shell	1 lb	1310	21	126.3
Dried, shelled				
halves	1 cup	642	10	61.9
halves, approx 14	1 oz	182	3	17.6
pieces or chips	1 cup	770	12	74.2
(Diamond)	1 oz	192	na	19.0
(Planters) halves	1 oz	190	0	20.0
(Planters) pieces	1 oz	190	0	20.0
(Planters) whole	1 oz	190	0	20.0
WALNUT OIL				
	1 cup	1927	0	218.0
	1 tbsp	120	0	13.6
(Hain)	1 tbsp	120	0	14.0
(Spectrum Naturals)	1 tbsp	120	0	14.0
WASABI	1/4 oz	24	2	<.1
WATER, BOTTLED				
(Perrier)	1 cup	0	2	0.0
(Perrier)	6.5-oz bottle	0	2	0.0
(Poland Spring)	1 cup	0	2	0.0
distilled *(Arrowhead)*	1 liter	0	0	0.0
drinking *(Arrowhead)*	1 liter	0	16	0.0
fluoridated *(Arrowhead)*	1 liter	0	16	0.0
mineral *(Perrier)*	1 liter	0	19	0.0
sparkling, natural, unflavored *(Clearly Canadian)*	6 oz	0	3	0.0
spring *(Arrowhead)*	1 liter	0	9	0.0
spring, Arizona Tule *(Arrowhead)*	1 liter	0	7	0.0
Vichy *(Schweppes)*	6 oz	0	76	0.0
WATER, SPARKLING, FLAVORED. See also SOFT DRINKS AND MIXERS.				
BLACK CHERRY				
'Refresher' *(Quest)*	10 oz	2	40	0.0
'Refresher' *(Quest)*	8 oz	2	35	0.0
BLACKBERRY, 'Mountain Blackberry' *(Clearly Canadian)*	6 oz	70	10	0.0
CHERRY, 'Wild Cherry' *(Clearly Canadian)*	6 oz	70	10	0.0
CHERRY-BLACKBERRY, w/juice *(Cascadia)*	6 oz	2	0	0.0
CRANBERRY, 'Coastal Cranberry' *(Clearly Canadian)*	6 oz	70	10	0.0
GRAPEFRUIT, w/juice *(Cascadia)*	6 oz	2	0	0.0
GUAVA-BERRY, w/juice *(Cascadia)*	6 oz	2	0	0.0
LEMONAID, w/juice *(Cascadia)*	6 oz	2	0	0.0

Food Name	Serv. Size	Total Cal.	Sod. MGS	Fat GMS
LEMON-LIME *(H2OH!)*	6 oz	0	0	0.0
LOGANBERRY, 'Western Loganberry' *(Clearly Canadian)*	6 oz	70	10	0.0
NATURAL BERRY *(H2OH!)*	6 oz	0	0	0.0
PEACH, 'Orchard Peach' *(Clearly Canadian)*	6 oz	70	10	0.0
PEACH-CITRUS				
'Refresher' *(Quest)*	10 oz	2	40	0.0
'Refresher' *(Quest)*	8 oz	2	35	0.0
RASPBERRY				
'Country Raspberry' *(Clearly Canadian)*	6 oz	70	10	0.0
'Refresher' *(Quest)*	10 oz	2	40	0.0
'Refresher' *(Quest)*	8 oz	2	35	0.0
RED RASPBERRY				
'Refresher' *(Quest)*	10 oz	2	40	0.0
'Refresher' *(Quest)*	8 oz	2	35	0.0
STRAWBERRY-KIWI				
'Refresher' *(Quest)*	10 oz	2	40	0.0
'Refresher' *(Quest)*	8 oz	2	35	0.0
TANGERINE-LIME				
'Refresher' *(Quest)*	10 oz	2	40	0.0
'Refresher' *(Quest)*	8 oz	2	35	0.0
WATER CHESTNUT, CHINESE/matai				
approx 1.7 oz	4 fruits	38	5	0.0
slices	1/2 cup	66	9	0.1
trimmed	1 oz	30	4	<.1
untrimmed	1 lb	369	50	0.4
Canned				
sliced, w/liquid	1/2 cup	35	6	0.0
w/liquid	4 oz	57	9	0.1
w/liquid	4 fruits	14	2	0.0
(LaChoy)	1.28 oz	18	3	<.1
(LaChoy) chopped	.6349 oz	9	2	0.1
(LaChoy) sliced	1/4 cup	18	3	<1.0
(LaChoy) sliced	.776 oz	11	3	0.1
(LaChoy) whole	4 fruits	14	2	<1.0
(LaChoy) whole	.6702 oz	10	2	0.1
WATERCRESS				
chopped	1/2 cup	2	7	0.0
fresh	1 sprig	0	1	0.0
trimmed	1 oz	3	12	<.1
untrimmed	1 lb	46	170	0.4

Food Name	Serv. Size	Total Cal.	Sod. MGS	Fat GMS
WATERMELON				
diced	1 cup	51	3	0.7
diced	1/2 cup	25	2	0.3
sliced, 1/16 of 10-inch-diam fruit	1 slice	154	10	2.1
trimmed	1 oz	9	1	0.1
untrimmed	1 lb	74	5	1.0
WATERMELON SEED, DRIED				
in hard coat	1 lb	935	166	79.5
kernels	1 cup	602	107	51.2
kernels	1 oz	158	28	13.4
WAX BEAN, CANNED				
(Allens)	1/2 cup	15	260	<1.0
(Del Monte) golden, cut	1/2 cup	20	355	0.0
(Del Monte) golden, French style	1/2 cup	20	355	0.0
(Stokely)	1/2 cup	20	360	0.0
(Stokely) 'No Salt or Sugar'	1/2 cup	20	5	0.0
WAX BEAN, FROZEN				
(Frosty Acres)	3 oz	25	1	0.0
(Seabrook) cut	3 oz	25	1	0.0
WAX GOURD. See GOURD, WAX.				
WELSH ONION. See ONION, WELSH.				
WELSH RAREBIT				
(Snow's) canned	1/2 cup	170	460	11.0
(Stouffer's) frozen	5 oz	270	460	20.0
WESTERN DINNER, FROZEN				
(Banquet)	11 oz	630	720	41.0
(Morton)	10 oz	290	1450	14.0
(Swanson)	11.5 oz	430	1060	19.0
WHALE, raw	100 gm	156	78	7.5
WHEAT, SPROUTED				
	1/3 cup	71	6	0.5
	1 oz	56	5	0.4
WHEAT, WHOLE GRAIN				
DURUM				
	1 cup	650	3	4.7
	1/2 cup	325	2	2.4
	1 oz	96	<1	0.7
HARD RED				
spring	1 cup	631	4	3.7
spring	1/2 cup	316	2	1.8
spring	1 oz	93	<1	0.5

Food Name	Serv. Size	Total Cal.	Sod. MGS	Fat GMS
spring or winter *(Arrowhead Mills)*	2 oz	190	1	1.0
winter	1 cup	628	4	3.0
winter	1/2 cup	314	2	1.5
winter	1 oz	93	<1	0.4
HARD WHITE				
	1 cup	656	na	3.3
	1/2 cup	328	2	1.6
	1 oz	97	na	0.5
SOFT RED				
for pastry *(Arrowhead Mills)*	2 oz	190	1	1.0
winter	1 cup	556	4	2.6
winter	1/2 cup	278	2	1.3
winter	1 oz	94	<1	0.4
SOFT WHITE				
	1 cup	571	na	3.3
	1/2 cup	286	2	1.7
	1 oz	96	na	0.6
WHEAT BRAN				
crude	1/2 cup	65	1	1.3
crude	1 oz	61	<1	1.2
crude	2 tbsp	15	0	0.3
crude *(Arrowhead Mills)*	2 oz	50	3	2.0
toasted *(Kretschmer)*	1 oz	57	2	2.3
unprocessed *(Quaker)*	2 tbsp	8	0	0.2
WHEAT CAKE				
(Quaker) 'Grain Cakes'	1 cake	34	52	0.3
(Quaker) lightly salted	1 cake	35	50	0.0
WHEAT FLAKES *(Arrowhead Mills)*	2 oz	210	1	1.0
WHEAT FLOUR				
RYE				
(Pillsbury's Best) medium-colored	1 cup	400	0	2.0
(Pillsbury's Best) w/wheat 'Bohemian Style'	1 cup	400	0	1.0
WHITE				
(Drifted Snow)	1 cup	400	0	1.0
(Softasilk)	1/4 cup	100	0	0.0
(Wondra)	1 cup	400	0	1.0
All-purpose				
enriched	1/2 cup	226	1	0.6
enriched	1 oz	103	<1	0.3
enriched, calcium-fortified	1/2 cup	226	1	0.6
(Ballard)	1 cup	400	0	1.0

Food Name	Serv. Size	Total Cal.	Sod. MGS	Fat GMS
(Ceresota)	4 oz	390	0	1.0
(Gold Medal)	1 cup	400	0	1.0
(Heckers)	4 oz	390	0	1.0
(Pillsbury's Best)	1 cup	400	0	1.0
(Red Band)	1 cup	390	0	1.0
(Robin Hood)	1 cup	400	0	1.0
(White Deer)	1 cup	400	0	1.0
All-purpose, unbleached				
enriched	1/2 cup	226	1	0.6
(Arrowhead Mills)	2 oz	200	1	1.0
(Gold Medal)	1 cup	400	0	1.0
(Pillsbury's Best)	1 cup	400	0	1.0
(Robin Hood)	1 cup	400	0	1.0
Bread				
enriched	1/2 cup	249	1	1.1
enriched	1 oz	102	<1	0.5
(Gold Medal) 'Better for Bread'	1 cup	400	0	1.0
(Pillsbury's Best)	1 cup	400	0	2.0
Cake				
enriched	1/2 cup	195	1	0.5
enriched	1 oz	103	<1	0.2
Self-rising				
enriched	1/2 cup	219	787	0.6
enriched	1 oz	100	360	0.3
(Aunt Jemima) enriched	1 oz	109	368	0.3
(Ballard)	1 cup	380	1290	1.0
(Gold Medal)	1 cup	380	1520	1.0
(Pillsbury's Best)	1 cup	380	1290	1.0
(Pillsbury's Best) unbleached	1 cup	380	1290	1.0
(Red Band)	1 cup	380	1520	1.0
(Robin Hood)	1 cup	380	1520	1.0
Shake and blend *(Pillsbury's Best)*	2 tbsp	50	0	0.0
Tortilla mix				
enriched	1/3 cup	150	250	3.9
enriched	1 oz	115	192	3.0
WHOLE GRAIN				
	1/2 cup	203	3	1.1
	1 oz	96	1	0.5
(Arrowhead Mills) pastry	2 oz	180	1	1.0
(Arrowhead Mills) stone ground	2 oz	200	1	1.0
(Ceresota)	4 oz	400	0	2.0

Food Name	Serv. Size	Total Cal.	Sod. MGS	Fat GMS
(Gold Medal)	1 cup	350	0	2.0
(Gold Medal) blend	1 cup	380	0	2.0
(Heckers)	4 oz	400	0	2.0
(Krusteaz)	1 cup	450	5	2.0
(Pillsbury's Best)	1 cup	400	10	2.0
WHEAT GERM				
crude	1/4 cup	104	3	2.8
crude	1 oz	102	3	2.8
toasted	1 cup	431	4	12.1
toasted	1 oz	108	1	3.0
(Arrowhead Mills) raw	2 oz	210	1	6.0
(Kretschmer)	1 oz	103	2	3.4
(Kretschmer) honey crunch	1 oz	105	2	2.8
WHEAT GERM OIL				
	1 cup	1927	0	218.0
	1 tbsp	120	0	13.6
(Spectrum Naturals) unrefined	1 tbsp	120	0	14.0
WHEAT GLUTEN *(Arrowhead Mills)* 'Vita 1' toasted	1 oz	100	1	1.0
WHEAT NUTS				
macadamia flavor, w/o salt	1 oz	176	13	16.0
other flavors, w/o salt	1 oz	184	26	17.7
unflavored, w/salt added	1 oz	177	143	16.4
WHEAT PILAF MIX, dry mix *(Casbah)*	1 oz	100	(mq)	0.0
WHELK				
moist-heat cooked	3 oz	234	350	0.7
raw	1 lb	623	934	1.8
raw	3 oz	116	175	0.3
raw	1 oz	39	54	0.1
WHEY				
Acid				
dry	1 cup	193	552	0.3
dry	1 oz	96	274	0.2
dry	1 tbsp	10	28	0.0
fluid	1 quart	235	473	0.9
fluid	1 cup	59	118	0.2
fluid	1 oz	7	14	<.1
Sweet				
dry	1 cup	512	1565	1.5
dry	1 oz	100	306	0.3
dry	1 tbsp	26	81	0.1
fluid	1 quart	263	526	3.5

Food Name	Serv. Size	Total Cal.	Sod. MGS	Fat GMS
fluid	1 cup	66	132	0.9
fluid	1 oz	8	15	0.1

WHIPPED TOPPING. See CREAM TOPPING.

WHISKEY. See ALCOHOLIC BEVERAGES.

WHITE BEAN

boiled	4 oz	158	7	0.4
boiled	1/2 cup	125	5	0.3
raw	1/2 cup	336	16	0.9
raw	1 oz	94	5	0.2
small, boiled	4 oz	161	2	0.7
small, boiled	1/2 cup	128	2	0.6
small, raw	1/2 cup	363	13	1.3
small, raw	1 oz	95	3	0.3

WHITE BEAN, CANNED

	1/2 cup	153	7	0.4
w/liquid	4 oz	133	515	0.3

WHITE-FLOWERED GOURD. See GOURD, BOTTLE.

WHITE GOURD. See GOURD, WHITE.

WHITEFISH

dry-heat cooked	3 oz	146	55	6.4
dry-heat cooked, approx 7 oz	1 fillet	265	100	11.6
raw	1 lb	610	232	26.6
raw	3 oz	114	43	5.0
raw	1 oz	38	14	1.7
raw, approx 7 oz	1 fillet	265	101	11.6
smoked	4 oz	122	1156	1.1
smoked	3 oz	92	866	0.8
smoked	1 oz	30	285	0.3

WHITING, MIXED SPECIES/silver hake

dry-heat cooked	4 oz	130	150	1.9
dry-heat cooked	3 oz	98	112	1.4
raw	1 lb	408	326	6.0
raw	3 oz	77	61	1.1
raw	1 oz	26	20	0.4

WHITING, MIXED SPECIES, FROZEN

(Booth)	4 oz	100	90	1.0
(Booth) 'Individually Wrapped'	4 oz	80	85	1.0

WILD BERRY DRINK

(Hi-C)	6 oz	92	17	0.1
(Hi-C) aseptic box or chilled	6 oz	90	20	0.0
(Hi-C) boxed	8.45 oz	129	24	0.1

Food Name	Serv. Size	Total Cal.	Sod. MGS	Fat GMS
(Hi-C) chilled	6 oz	90	20	0.0
(Tropicana) 'Juice Sparkler'	8 oz	110	15	0.0
WINE. See ALCOHOLIC BEVERAGES.				
WINE, COOKING. See also ALCOHOLIC BEVERAGES.				
Burgundy *(Regina)*	1/4 cup	2	365	<1.0
Marsala *(Holland House)*	1 oz	9	186	0.0
red *(Holland House)*	1 oz	6	186	0.0
Sauternes *(Regina)*	1/4 cup	2	365	<1.0
sherry *(Holland House)*	1 oz	5	186	0.0
sherry *(Regina)*	1/4 cup	20	70	<1.0
vermouth *(Holland House)*	1 oz	2	186	0.0
white *(Holland House)*	1 oz	2	186	0.0
WINGED BEAN/goa bean				
boiled, drained	4 oz	43	5	0.7
immature seeds, boiled, drained	1/2 cup	12	1	0.2
immature seeds, raw, approx .6 oz	1 pod	8	1	0.1
immature seeds, slices, raw	1 cup	22	2	0.4
mature seeds, boiled, drained	1/2 cup	126	11	5.0
mature seeds, raw	1/2 cup	372	35	14.9
trimmed, raw	1 oz	14	1	0.2
untrimmed, raw	1 lb	218	17	3.9
WINGED BEAN, DRIED				
boiled	4 oz	167	15	6.6
boiled	1/2 cup	126	11	5.0
raw	1/2 cup	372	35	14.9
raw	1 oz	116	11	4.6
WINGED BEAN LEAVES				
trimmed	1 lb	336	na	5.0
trimmed	1 oz	21	na	0.3
WOLF FISH/ocean catfish				
dry-heat cooked	3 oz	105	93	2.6
frozen *(Booth)*	4 oz	115	85	20.0
raw	1 lb	437	386	10.8
raw	3 oz	82	72	2.0
raw	1 oz	27	24	0.7
raw, approx 5.4 oz	1/2 fillet	147	130	3.7
WON TON SKIN				
	1 oz	83	162	0.4
	1 wrapper	23	46	0.1
(Nasoya)	1 wrapper	23	19	0.0
WON TON SOUP. See SOUP.				

Y

Food Name	Serv. Size	Total Cal.	Sod. MGS	Fat GMS
YAM				
boiled and drained, or baked	4 oz	132	9	0.2
boiled and drained, or baked, cubed	1/2 cup	79	5	0.1
raw, cubed	1/2 cup	89	7	0.1
raw, trimmed	1 oz	33	3	<.1
raw, untrimmed	1 lb	460	37	0.7
Mountain/Hawaiian				
raw, approx 8.25 inches long	1 yam	281	55	0.4
raw, cubed	1/2 cup	46	9	0.1
raw, trimmed	1 oz	19	4	<.1
raw, untrimmed	1 lb	253	49	0.4
steamed	4 oz	93	14	0.1
steamed, cubed	1/2 cup	59	9	0.1
YAM, CANNED (Bush's Best)	1/2 cup	120	20	0.0
YAM BEAN TUBER. See JICAMA.				
YARDLONG BEAN/asparagus bean				
boiled, drained	4 oz	53	5	0.1
boiled, drained, approx 13.25 inches long	1 pod	7	1	0.0
boiled, drained, sliced	1 cup	49	4	0.1
boiled, drained, sliced	1/2 cup	25	2	0.1
mature, boiled	1/2 cup	101	4	0.4
mature, raw	1/2 cup	291	14	1.1
raw, approx 13.25 inches long	1 pod	6	0	0.1
raw, sliced	1 cup	43	4	0.4
raw, sliced	1/2 cup	22	2	0.2
raw, trimmed	1 oz	13	1	0.1
raw, untrimmed	1 lb	203	17	1.7
Dried				
boiled	4 oz	134	6	0.5
boiled	1/2 cup	102	4	0.4
raw	1/2 cup	292	14	1.1
raw	1 oz	98	5	0.4
YEAST, BAKER'S				
active dry	1 oz	79	15	0.5
active dry	1 tbsp	35	6	0.6
active dry	.25-oz pkg	21	4	0.3
compressed	100 gm	105	30	1.9
compressed	.6-oz cake	18	5	0.3

Food Name	Serv. Size	Total Cal.	Sod. MGS	Fat GMS
compressed, fortified	1 oz	24	4	0.1
compressed, not fortified	1 oz	24	4	0.1
YEAST, BREWER'S				
debittered	1 oz	79	34	0.3
debittered	1 tbsp	23	10	0.1
(Fleischmann's) 'Active Dry/RapidRise'	1/4 oz	20	10	0.0
(Red Star) 'Active Dry'	1/4 oz	15	5	0.0
YEAST, TORULA	1 oz	78	4	0.3
YELLOW BEAN				
mature, boiled	1/2 cup	127	4	1.0
mature, raw	1/2 cup	338	12	2.5
Dried				
boiled	4 oz	163	6	1.2
boiled	1/2 cup	126	4	1.0
raw	1/2 cup	338	12	2.6
raw	1 oz	98	3	0.7
YELLOW MOMBIN. See JOBO.				
YELLOWEYE BEAN *(B&M)* canned, baked style	8 oz	326	770	7.0
YELLOW-EYED PEAS. See BLACK-EYED PEAS.				
YELLOWTAIL, MIXED SPECIES				
dry-heat cooked	3 oz	159	43	5.7
raw	1 lb	662	177	23.8
raw	3 oz	124	33	4.4
raw	1 oz	41	11	1.5
YOGURT				
(Colombo) 'Fruit on the Bottom' all flavors	8 oz	230	140	6.0
(Colombo) 'Nonfat Fruit on the Bottom' all flavors	8 oz	190	140	<1.0
(Colombo) 'Nonfat Lite Minipack' all flavors	4.4 oz	100	70	0.0
(Crowley) 'Sundae Style' all flavors	8 oz	250	170	2.0
(Crowley) 'Swiss Style' all flavors	8 oz	240	150	2.0
(Dannon) 'Extra Smooth' all flavors	4.4 oz	130	80	2.0
(Dannon) 'Hearty Nuts & Raisins' all flavors except vanilla	8 oz	260	120	3.0
(Knudsen) 'Lowfat' all flavors except strawberry	8 oz	240	135	4.0
(Light n' Lively) 'Free' all flavors except strawberry	4.4 oz	50	60	0.0
(Ripple) '70' fat-free, all flavors	6 oz	70	85	0.0
(Yoplait) 'Fat-free' all flavors	6 oz	150	95	0.0
(Yoplait) 'Light' all flavors	6 oz	90	100	0.0
(Yoplait) 'Light' all flavors	4 oz	60	65	0.0
APPLE CRISP *(New Country)* 'Lowfat'	6 oz	150	85	2.0
BANANA				
(Dannon) 'Sprinkl'ins' lowfat	4.1 oz	140	80	2.0

Food Name	Serv. Size	Total Cal.	Sod. MGS	Fat GMS
(Yoplait) 'Custard Style'	6 oz	180	105	3.0
BANANA BERRY *(Light n' Lively)* lowfat, 1% milkfat, cultured	4.4 oz	130	75	1.0
BERRIES *(Yoplait)* 'Breakfast' w/wheat, raisins, and walnuts	6 oz	200	125	2.0
BLACK CHERRY				
(Alta•Dena) 'Blended European Style'	8 oz	190	140	<1.0
(Alta•Dena) 'Naja' fruit-on-the-bottom	8 oz	240	150	4.0
(Breyers) 'Lowfat'	8 oz	260	120	3.0
(Knudsen) 'Cal 70'	6 oz	70	75	0.0
(Light n' Lively)	8 oz	230	125	2.0
(Light n' Lively) '100'	8 oz	100	100	0.0
(Mountain High) 'Honey Light' natural	8 oz	190	140	1.0
(TCBY) 'Light'	8 oz	100	180	0.0
BLUEBERRY				
(Alta•Dena) 'Maya' fruit-on-the-bottom	8 oz	280	170	9.0
(Breyers) 'Lowfat'	8 oz	250	120	2.0
(Dannon) 'Blended' fat-free	6 oz	160	105	0.0
(Dannon) 'Light' nonfat	8 oz	100	135	0.0
(Knudsen) 'Cal 70'	6 oz	70	80	0.0
(Light n' Lively)	8 oz	240	130	2.0
(Light n' Lively)	4.4 oz	130	79	1.0
(Light n' Lively) 'Free' nonfat	4.4 oz	50	60	0.0
(Light n' Lively) '100'	8 oz	90	110	0.0
(Mountain High) 'Honey Light' natural	8 oz	190	140	<1.0
(Mountain High) w/other natural flavors	8 oz	220	140	6.0
(New Country) 'Supreme'	6 oz	150	90	2.0
(TCBY)	8 oz	220	150	2.0
(TCBY) 'Light' nonfat, w/aspartame	8 oz	100	210	0.0
(Weight Watchers) 'Ultimate 90'	8 oz	90	120	0.0
(Yogi) 'Sundae' cheesecake, w/gelatin	5.6 oz	50	75	<1.0
(Yoplait) 'Fruit-on-the-Bottom'	6 oz	170	105	0,0
(Yoplait) 'Light' fat-free	6 oz	90	70	0.0
(Yoplait) 'Original' 99% fat-free	6 oz	180	130	2.0
(Yoplait) 'Parfait Style' blueberry and vanilla	6 oz	200	120	3.0
BOYSENBERRY *(Yoplait)* 'Original' 99% fat-free	6 oz	180	130	2.0
CAPPUCCINO *(Dannon)* 'Light' nonfat	8 oz	100	135	0.0
CHERRIES JUBILEE *(Weight Watchers)* 'Ultimate 90'	8 oz	90	120	0.0
CHERRY				
(Dannon) 'Sprinkl'ins' lowfat	4.1 oz	140	80	2.0
(Light n' Lively)	4.4 oz	140	70	1.0
(New Country) 'Supreme'	6 oz	150	90	2.0
(Yoplait) 'Breakfast Yogurt' w/almonds	6 oz	200	90	3.0

Food Name	Serv. Size	Total Cal.	Sod. MGS	Fat GMS
(Yoplait) 'Custard Style'	6 oz	180	95	4.0
(Yoplait) 'Light' fat-free	6 oz	90	70	0.0
(Yoplait) 'Original' 99% fat-free	6 oz	180	130	2.0
(Yoplait) 'Parfait Style' cherry and vanilla	6 oz	200	120	3.0
CHERRY-VANILLA				
(Dannon) 'Light' nonfat	8 oz	100	135	0.0
(Dannon) 'Sprinkl'ins' lowfat	4.1 oz	140	95	2.0
(Lite-Line) 'Swiss Style 1%'	8 oz	240	150	2.0
(TCBY)	8 oz	220	150	2.0
(Yogi) w/gelatin 'Sundae'	5.6 oz	50	75	<1.0
(Yoplait) fat-free 'Light Custard Style'	6 oz	90	85	0.0
COFFEE				
(Bison) 'Lowfat'	8 oz	210	160	4.0
(Dannon) 'Fresh Flavors'	8 oz	200	140	3.0
(Friendship) 'Lowfat'	8 oz	210	170	3.0
CRANBERRY-RASPBERRY *(Weight Watchers)* 'Ultimate 90'	8 oz	90	120	0.0
FRUIT CRUNCH *(New Country)* 'Lowfat'	6 oz	150	90	2.0
GRAPE				
(Dannon) lowfat 'Sprinkl'ins'	4.1 oz	140	110	2.0
(Light n' Lively)	4.4 oz	130	70	1.0
HAWAIIAN SALAD *(New Country)* 'Lowfat'	6 oz	150	90	2.0
LEMON				
(Alta•Dena) 'Naja' fruit-on-the-bottom	8 oz	240	150	4.0
(Bison) 'Lowfat'	8 oz	210	160	4.0
(Dannon) 'Fresh Flavors'	8 oz	200	140	3.0
(Knudsen) 'Cal 70'	6 oz	70	125	0.0
(Light n' Lively) '100'	8 oz	100	150	0.0
(Mountain High) 'Natural'	8 oz	220	140	6.0
(New Country) 'Supreme'	6 oz	150	90	2.0
(Weight Watchers) 'Ultimate 90'	1 cup	90	120	0.0
(Yoplait) 'Original' 99% fat-free	6 oz	180	130	2.0
LEMON CHIFFON				
(Dannon) 'Blended' fat-free	6 oz	150	110	0.0
(Dannon) 'Light' non-fat	8 oz	100	135	0.0
(Yogi) 'Sundae' w/gelatin	5.6 oz	50	75	<1.0
MIXED BERRIES				
(Alta•Dena) 'Blended European Style'	8 oz	190	140	<1.0
(Breyers) 'Lowfat'	8 oz	250	120	2.0
(New Country) 'Lowfat'	6 oz	150	85	2.0
(Yoplait) 'Custard Style'	6 oz	180	95	4.0
(Yoplait) 'Original' 99% fat-free	6 oz	180	130	2.0

Food Name	Serv. Size	Total Cal.	Sod. MGS	Fat GMS
ORANGE				
(Dannon) 'Fruit-on-the-Bottom'	8 oz	230	130	3.0
(New Country) 'Supreme'	6 oz	150	90	2.0
ORANGE-PINEAPPLE (Yogi) 'Sundae' w/gelatin	5.6 oz	50	75	<1.0
PEACH				
(Alta•Dena) 'Naja' fruit-on-the-bottom	8 oz	240	150	4.0
(Alta•Dena) nonfat, fruit-on-the-bottom	8 oz	190	128	<1.0
(Breyers) 'Lowfat'	8 oz	250	120	2.0
(Carnation) 'Smooth'n Creamy' fruit on the bottom	8 oz	250	130	3.0
(Dannon) 'Fruit-on-the-Bottom'	8 oz	230	140	3.0
(Dannon) 'Light' nonfat	8 oz	100	135	0.0
(Knudsen) 'Cal 70'	6 oz	70	95	0.0
(Light n' Lively)	8 oz	240	120	2.0
(Light n' Lively)	4.4 oz	130	65	1.0
(Light n' Lively) '100'	8 oz	100	115	0.0
(Lite-Line) 'Swiss Style 1%'	8 oz	230	150	2.0
(Mountain High) 'Natural'	8 oz	220	140	6.0
(New Country) 'Lowfat' 'n cream	6 oz	150	90	2.0
(TCBY)	8 oz	220	150	2.0
(Weight Watchers) 'Ultimate 90'	8 oz	90	120	0.0
(Yogi) 'Sundae' peachy peach, w/gelatin	5.6 oz	50	75	<1.0
(Yoplait) 'Crunch 'N Yogurt' nonfat, w/granola	7 oz	220	125	2.0
(Yoplait) 'Fruit-on-the-Bottom'	6 oz	170	105	0.0
(Yoplait) 'Light' fat-free	6 oz	90	70	0.0
(Yoplait) 'Light Custard Style' fat-free	6 oz	90	85	0.0
(Yoplait) 'Original' 99% fat-free	6 oz	180	130	2.0
(Yoplait) 'Parfait Style' peach and vanilla	6 oz	200	120	3.0
PIÑA COLADA				
(Yoplait)	6 oz	190	110	3.0
(Yoplait) 'Original' 99% fat-free	6 oz	180	130	2.0
PINEAPPLE				
(Breyers) 'Lowfat'	8 oz	250	120	2.0
(Knudsen) 'Cal 70'	6 oz	70	125	0.0
(Light n' Lively)	8 oz	230	120	2.0
(Light n' Lively)	4.4 oz	130	65	1.0
(Yoplait) 'Original' 99% fat-free	6 oz	180	130	2.0
PLAIN				
(Alta•Dena) nonfat	8 oz	100	160	<1.0
(Bison) 'Lowfat'	8 oz	150	180	4.0
(Bison) 'Nonfat'	8 oz	120	170	0.0
(Breyers) 'Lowfat'	8 oz	140	170	3.0

Food Name	Serv. Size	Total Cal.	Sod. MGS	Fat GMS
(Colombo)	8 oz	160	160	8.0
(Colombo) 'Nonfat Lite'	8 oz	110	160	<1.0
(Crowley)	8 oz	160	150	8.0
(Crowley) 'Lowfat'	8 oz	140	180	2.0
(Crowley) 'Nonfat'	8 oz	120	180	<1.0
(Dannon) 'Lowfat'	8 oz	140	160	4.0
(Dannon) 'Nonfat'	8 oz	110	160	0.0
(Friendship) 'Lowfat 1.5%'	8 oz	150	190	3.0
(Knudsen)	8 oz	200	170	9.0
(Knudsen) 'Lowfat'	8 oz	160	180	5.0
(Lite-Line) 'Swiss Style 1.5%'	8 oz	140	150	2.0
(Meadow Gold) lowfat, 2% milkfat	8 oz	160	160	5.0
(Mountain High)	8 oz	200	140	9.0
(Weight Watchers) 'Nonfat'	8 oz	90	135	<1.0
(Yoplait)	6 oz	130	140	3.0
(Yoplait) fat-free	8 oz	120	170	0.0
(Yoplait) 'Nonfat'	8 oz	120	160	0.0
(Yoplait) 'Original' 98% fat-free	6 oz	120	150	2.0
RAINBOW PUNCH (Yoplait) 'Trix'	6 oz	190	120	3.0
RASPBERRY				
(Alta•Dena) 'Blended European Style'	8 oz	180	140	<1.0
(Dannon) 'Blended' fat-free	6 oz	150	110	0.0
(Dannon) 'Fruit-on-the-Bottom'	8 oz	240	140	3.0
(Dannon) 'Light' nonfat	8 oz	100	135	0.0
(Meadow Gold) 'Sundae Style' lowfat, natural	8 oz	250	160	4.0
(Mountain High) 'Honey Light' natural	8 oz	190	140	<1.0
(TCBY)	8 oz	220	150	2.0
(Weight Watchers) 'Ultimate 90'	8 oz	90	120	0.0
(Yoplait) fat-free 'Light'	6 oz	90	70	0.0
(Yoplait) 'Fruit-on-the-Bottom'	6 oz	170	105	0.0
(Yoplait) 'Original' 99% fat-free	6 oz	180	130	2.0
RED RASPBERRY				
(Alta•Dena) 'Naja' fruit-on-the-bottom	8 oz	240	150	4.0
(Breyers) 'Lowfat'	8 oz	250	120	2.0
(Carnation) 'Smooth'n Creamy' fruit on the bottom	8 oz	250	130	3.0
(Knudsen) 'Cal 70'	6 oz	70	80	0.0
(Light n' Lively)	8 oz	230	130	2.0
(Light n' Lively)	4.4 oz	130	70	1.0
(Light n' Lively) 'Free' nonfat	4.4 oz	50	60	0.0
(Light n' Lively) '100'	8 oz	90	105	0.0
(Meadow Gold) lowfat, 1.5% milkfat	8 oz	250	160	4.0

Food Name	Serv. Size	Total Cal.	Sod. MGS	Fat GMS
(New Country) 'Supreme'	6 oz	150	90	2.0
STRAWBERRY				
(Alta•Dena) 'Blended European Style'	8 oz	180	140	<1.0
(Alta•Dena) 'Maya' fruit-on-the-bottom	8 oz	280	170	9.0
(Alta•Dena) 'Naja' fruit-on-the-bottom	8 oz	240	150	4.0
(Breyers) 'Lowfat'	8 oz	250	120	2.0
(Carnation) 'Smooth'n Creamy' fruit on the bottom	8 oz	230	115	3.0
(Colombo)	8 oz	210	140	7.0
(Crowley) 'Nonfat'	8 oz	190	190	<1.0
(Dannon) 'Blended' fat-free	6 oz	150	110	0.0
(Dannon) 'Fruit-on-the-Bottom'	8 oz	230	140	3.0
(Dannon) 'Light' nonfat	8 oz	100	135	0.0
(Dannon) 'Sprinkl'ins' lowfat	4.1 oz	140	95	2.0
(Knudsen) 'Cal 70'	6 oz	70	85	0.0
(Knudsen) 'Lowfat'	8 oz	250	135	4.0
(Light n' Lively)	8 oz	240	130	2.0
(Light n' Lively)	4.4 oz	130	70	1.0
(Light n' Lively) 'Free'	4.4 oz	50	60	0.0
(Light n' Lively) '100'	8 oz	90	105	0.0
(Lite-Line) 'Lowfat 1%'	8 oz	240	150	2.0
(Mountain High) 'Honey Light' natural	8 oz	190	140	<1.0
(New Country) 'Supreme'	6 oz	150	90	2.0
(TCBY)	8 oz	220	150	2.0
(Weight Watchers) 'Ultimate 90'	8 oz	90	120	0.0
(Yoplait) 'Custard Style'	6 oz	180	105	3.0
(Yoplait) 'Fruit-on-the-Bottom'	6 oz	170	105	0.0
(Yoplait) 'Light' fat-free	6 oz	90	70	0.0
(Yoplait) 'Light Custard Style' fat-free	6 oz	90	85	0.0
(Yoplait) 'Original' 99% fat-free	6 oz	180	130	2.0
(Yoplait) 'Parfait Style' strawberry and vanilla	6 oz	200	120	3.0
STRAWBERRY CHEESECAKE *(Yogi)* 'Sundae' w/gelatin	5.6 oz	50	75	<1.0
STRAWBERRY FRUIT BASKET *(Knudsen)* 'Cal 70'	6 oz	70	75	0.0
STRAWBERRY FRUIT CUP				
(Dannon) 'Light' nonfat	8 oz	100	135	0.0
(Light n' Lively)	8 oz	240	120	2.0
(Light n' Lively)	4.4 oz	130	65	1.0
(Light n' Lively) 'Free' nonfat	4.4 oz	50	55	0.0
(Light n' Lively) '100'	8 oz	90	100	0.0
(New Country) 'Lowfat'	6 oz	150	85	2.0
STRAWBERRY-ALMOND *(Yoplait)* 'Breakfast Yogurt'	6 oz	200	90	3.0

Food Name	Serv. Size	Total Cal.	Sod. MGS	Fat GMS
STRAWBERRY-BANANA				
(Alta•Dena) nonfat, fruit-on-the-bottom	8 oz	180	128	<1.0
(Breyers) 'Lowfat'	8 oz	250	120	2.0
(Carnation) 'Smooth'n Creamy' fruit on the bottom	8 oz	240	125	4.0
(Dannon) 'Fruit-on-the-Bottom'	8 oz	230	140	3.0
(Dannon) 'Light' nonfat	8 oz	100	135	0.0
(Dannon) lowfat 'Sprinkl'ins'	4.1 oz	140	95	2.0
(Knudsen) 'Cal 70'	6 oz	70	80	0.0
(Light n' Lively)	8 oz	260	120	2.0
(Light n' Lively)	4.4 oz	140	65	1.0
(Light n' Lively) 'Free' nonfat	4.4 oz	50	60	0.0
(Mountain High) 'Honey Light' natural	8 oz	190	140	<1.0
(New Country)	6 oz	150	85	2.0
(TCBY)	8 oz	220	150	2.0
(Weight Watchers) 'Ultimate 90'	8 oz	90	120	0.0
(Yoplait) 'Breakfast' w/wheat and walnuts	6 oz	200	110	2.0
(Yoplait) 'Fruit-on-the-Bottom'	6 oz	170	105	0.0
(Yoplait) 'Light' fat-free	6 oz	90	70	0.0
(Yoplait) 'Original' 99% fat-free	6 oz	180	130	2.0
(Yoplait) 'Trix' bash	6 oz	190	120	3.0
STRAWBERRY-RHUBARB (Yoplait)	6 oz	190	110	3.0
TRIPLE CHERRY (Yoplait) 'Trix'	6 oz	190	120	3.0
TROPICAL FRUIT				
(Dannon) 'Light' nonfat	8 oz	100	135	0.0
(Ripple) '70'	6 oz	70	85	0.0
(Weight Watchers) 'Ultimate 90'	8 oz	90	120	0.0
(Yoplait) 'Breakfast' w/wheat, raisins, and nuts	6 oz	200	110	3.0
VANILLA				
(Bison) 'Lowfat'	8 oz	210	160	4.0
(Breyers) 'Lowfat' vanilla bean	8 oz	230	150	3.0
(Colombo) French	8 oz	215	140	7.0
(Colombo) 'Nonfat Lite'	8 oz	160	140	<1.0
(Crowley) 'Lowfat'	8 oz	200	170	2.0
(Dannon) 'Blended' French, fat-free	6 oz	150	100	0.0
(Dannon) 'Fresh Flavors'	8 oz	200	140	3.0
(Dannon) 'Fresh Flavors'	4.4 oz	110	90	2.0
(Dannon) 'Hearty Nuts & Raisins' w/wheat	8 oz	270	120	5.0
(Dannon) 'Light' nonfat	8 oz	100	135	0.0
(Friendship) 'Lowfat'	8 oz	210	170	3.0
(Knudsen) 'Cal 70'	6 oz	70	90	0.0
(Knudsen) 'Lowfat'	8 oz	240	135	4.0

Food Name	Serv. Size	Total Cal.	Sod. MGS	Fat GMS
(New Country) 'Lowfat' French	6 oz	150	90	2.0
(Weight Watchers) 'Ultimate 90'	1 cup	90	120	0.0
(Yoplait)	6 oz	180	120	3.0
(Yoplait) 'Crunch 'N Yogurt' w/granola, nonfat	7 oz	220	125	2.0
(Yoplait) 'Custard Style'	6 oz	180	110	4.0
(Yoplait) 'Custard Style'	4 oz	130	70	3.0
(Yoplait) 'Fat-free'	6 oz	150	110	0.0
(Yoplait) 'Light Custard Style' fat-free	6 oz	90	85	0.0
(Yoplait) 'Nonfat'	8 oz	180	140	0.0
WILD BERRY (Light n' Lively) lowfat, 1% milkfat, cultured	4.4 oz	140	70	1.0
YOGURT, FROZEN				
(Alta•Dena) apricot mango, nonfat	4 oz	90	210	0.0
(Baskin Robbins) See Part III.				
(Ben & Jerry's)				
apple pie	1/2 cup	170	90	3.0
banana strawberry	1/2 cup	160	60	2.0
blueberry	1/2 cup	160	60	2.0
cherry Garcia	1/2 cup	170	70	3.0
chocolate fudge brownie	1/2 cup	190	130	4.0
chocolate raspberry swirl	1/2 cup	200	72	2.5
coffee almond fudge	1/2 cup	200	82	7.0
English toffee crunch	1/2 cup	190	110	6.0
(Bison) chocolate	3.5 oz	94	50	2.0
(Breyers)				
black cherry	1/2 cup	120	50	1.0
chocolate	1/2 cup	120	65	1.0
peach	1/2 cup	110	50	1.0
red raspberry	1/2 cup	120	50	1.0
strawberry	1/2 cup	110	45	1.0
strawberry-banana	1/2 cup	110	45	1.0
vanilla	1/2 cup	120	55	1.0
(Colombo)				
banana split, lowfat, 'Sundae Style'	3 oz	100	50	1.0
Bavarian chocolate chunk, 'Gourmet'	3 oz	120	40	4.0
caramel fudge sundae, lowfat, 'Sundae Style'	3 oz	100	60	1.0
caramel-pecan chunk, 'Gourmet'	3 oz	120	150	3.0
chocolate peanut butter twist, 'Sundae Style'	3 oz	110	65	3.0
dream, 'Gourmet'	3 oz	90	45	2.0
Heath bar crunch, 'Gourmet'	3 oz	130	75	5.0
mocha Swiss almond, 'Gourmet'	3 oz	120	45	5.0
nonfat, lite	4 oz	95	70	0.0

Food Name	Serv. Size	Total Cal.	Sod. MGS	Fat GMS
peanut butter cup, 'Gourmet'	3 oz	140	90	7.0
plain, lowfat	4 oz	99	35	2.0
plain, 'Nonfat Lite'	4 oz	95	70	0.0
strawberry passion, 'Gourmet'	3 oz	100	40	2.0
wild raspberry cheesecake, 'Gourmet'	3 oz	100	40	2.0
(Crowley)				
cherry	3 oz	80	40	1.0
chocolate	3 oz	80	40	2.0
peach	3 oz	80	40	1.0
raspberry	3 oz	80	40	1.0
strawberry	3 oz	80	40	1.0
vanilla	3 oz	80	40	2.0
(Dannon)				
cappuccino, nonfat, 'Light'	4 oz	80	70	0.0
caramel pecan, 'Pure Indulgence'	4 oz	180	70	8.0
cherry vanilla swirl, nonfat, 'Light'	4 oz	90	65	0.0
chocolate, nonfat, 'Light'	4 oz	80	70	<1.0
chocolate, 'Pure Indulgence'	3 oz	130	75	3.0
chocolate nut, chunky, 'Pure Indulgence'	4 oz	190	60	9.0
chunky chocolate nut, 'Pure Indulgence'	4 oz	190	60	9.0
cookies and cream, 'Pure Indulgence'	4 oz	180	95	7.0
Heath bar crunch, 'Pure Indulgence'	4 oz	170	100	7.0
peach, nonfat, 'Light'	4 oz	80	70	0.0
red raspberry, nonfat, 'Light'	4 oz	90	65	0.0
strawberry, nonfat, 'Light'	4 oz	80	70	0.0
vanilla, nonfat, 'Light'	4 oz	80	70	0.0
vanilla, 'Pure Indulgence'	3 oz	130	50	3.0
(Dreyer's)				
black cherry vanilla, nonfat, 'Inspirations'	4 oz	90	80	0.0
blueberry, 'Inspirations'	3 oz	80	40	1.0
cherry, 'Inspirations'	3 oz	80	40	1.0
chocolate, 'Inspirations'	3 oz	80	40	1.0
peach, 'Inspirations Perfectly Peach'	3 oz	80	40	1.0
raspberry, 'Inspirations'	3 oz	80	40	1.0
strawberry, 'Inspirations'	3 oz	80	40	1.0
strawberry-banana, 'Inspirations'	3 oz	80	40	1.0
vanilla chocolate swirl, nonfat, 'Inspirations'	4 oz	90	85	0.0
vanilla-raspberry swirl, 'Inspirations'	3 oz	80	45	1.0
(Elan) chocolate almond	1/2 cup	160	65	7.0
(Häagen-Dazs)				
chocolate	3 oz	130	40	3.0

Food Name	Serv. Size	Total Cal.	Sod. MGS	Fat GMS
peach	3 oz	120	30	3.0
praline pandemonium, 'Exträas'	4 oz	240	115	9.0
strawberry	3 oz	120	30	3.0
strawberry cheesecake craze, 'Exträas'	4 oz	210	100	7.0
vanilla almond crunch	3 oz	150	65	5.0
(Natural Nectar) chocolate, 'Fi-Bar Lite'	2.5 oz	190	140	6.0
(Sealtest)				
black cherry, nonfat, 'Free'	1/2 cup	110	50	0.0
chocolate, nonfat, 'Free'	1/2 cup	110	55	0.0
peach, nonfat, 'Free'	1/2 cup	100	35	0.0
red raspberry, nonfat, 'Free'	1/2 cup	100	40	0.0
strawberry, nonfat, 'Free'	1/2 cup	100	35	0.0
(TCBY) See Part III.				

YOGURT, FROZEN, SOFT-SERVE

Food Name	Serv. Size	Total Cal.	Sod. MGS	Fat GMS
(Bresler's)				
'Gourmet' all flavors, 1 oz	1/2 cup	29	15	0.5
'Lite' all flavors, 1 oz	1/2 cup	27	11	0.0
(Crowley)				
banana, 'Peaks of Perfection,' 3.5 oz	1/2 cup	100	50	2.0
chocolate, 'Peaks of Perfection,' 3.5 oz	1/2 cup	100	60	2.0
lemon, 'Peaks of Perfection,' 3.5 oz	1/2 cup	100	50	2.0
plain, 'Peaks of Perfection,' 3.5 oz	1/2 cup	90	40	1.0
raspberry, 'Peaks of Perfection,' 3.5 oz	1/2 cup	100	50	2.0
strawberry, 'Peaks of Perfection,' 3.5 oz	1/2 cup	100	50	2.0
vanilla, 'Peaks of Perfection,' 3.5 oz	1/2 cup	100	50	2.0
(Dannon)				
blueberry	1/2 cup	100	50	2.0
butter pecan	1/2 cup	100	55	2.0
cappuccino	1/2 cup	100	55	2.0
cheesecake	1/2 cup	100	55	2.0
chocolate	1/2 cup	120	65	2.0
lemon meringue	1/2 cup	100	55	2.0
peach	1/2 cup	100	55	2.0
piña colada	1/2 cup	100	55	2.0
raspberry	1/2 cup	100	50	2.0
red raspberry, 'Nonfat'	1/2 cup	90	65	0.0
strawberry	1/2 cup	100	50	2.0
strawberry-banana	1/2 cup	100	50	2.0
(Häagen-Dazs)				
banana, nonfat	1 oz	25	15	0.0
chocolate	1 oz	30	13	1.0

Food Name	Serv. Size	Total Cal.	Sod. MGS	Fat GMS
chocolate, nonfat	1 oz	30	20	0.0
coffee	1 oz	28	13	1.0
raspberry	1 oz	30	15	1.0
strawberry, nonfat	1 oz	25	10	0.0
vanilla	1 oz	28	13	1.0

YOGURT BAR, FROZEN

(Dole)

cherry 'Fruit & Yogurt'	1 bar	80	22	<1.0
raspberry 'Fruit & Yogurt'	1 bar	70	18	<1.0
strawberry 'Fruit & Yogurt'	1 bar	70	16	<1.0

(Häagen-Dazs)

cherry chocolate fudge	1 bar	230	50	12.0
peach	1 bar	100	20	1.0
piña colada	1 bar	100	25	1.0
ràspberry and vanilla	1 bar	100	20	1.0
strawberry daiquiri	1 bar	100	20	1.0
tropical orange passion	1 bar	100	30	1.0

YOGURT DESSERT *(Sara Lee)* 'Free & Light' ... 1/10 pkg ... 120 ... 90 ... 1.0

YOGURT FLAVORED DRINK

(Dannon) all flavors	8 oz	190	110	4.0
(Yogloo) fruit basket	10 oz	170	80	0.0
(Yogloo) original	10 oz	170	80	0.0
(Yogloo) peach	10 oz	170	80	0.0
(Yogloo) strawberry	10 oz	170	80	0.0

YUCA. See CASSAVA.

Z

Food Name	Serv. Size	Total Cal.	Sod. MGS	Fat GMS
ZITI ENTRÉE, FROZEN				
(Budget Gourmet) 'Side Dish' in marinara sauce	6.25 oz	220	380	9.0
ZUCCHINI. See also SQUASH, SUMMER.				
baby, raw	1 large	3	0	0.1
baby, raw	1 med	2	0	0.0
boiled, drained	4 oz	18	3	0.1
raw	1 lb	62	11	0.6
raw, trimmed	1 oz	4	1	<.1
w/skin, boiled, drained, mashed	1/2 cup	19	4	0.1
w/skin, boiled, drained, sliced	1/2 cup	14	3	0.0
w/skin, raw, sliced	1/2 cup	9	2	0.1

Food Name	Serv. Size	Total Cal.	Sod. MGS	Fat GMS
Canned				
in tomato juice	1/2 cup	33	424	0.1
Italian style	1/2 cup	33	426	0.1
(Del Monte) in tomato sauce	1/2 cup	30	485	0.0
(Progresso) Italian style	1/2 cup	50	540	2.0
Frozen				
w/skin, unprepared	10-oz pkg	48	6	0.4
(Seabrook)	3.3 oz	16	2	0.0
(Southern)	3.5 oz	18	20	0.1
(Stilwell) 'Quick Krisp' breaded	3.3 oz	200	410	10.0

FAST FOOD VALUES

Food Name	Serv. Size	Total Cal.	Sod. MGS	Fat GMS
ARBY'S				
AU JUS SAUCE	1 serving	7	750	0.0
BARBECUE SANDWICH, 'Arby Q'	1 serving	389	1268	15.2
BEEF SANDWICH				
'Beef'n Cheddar'	1 serving	508	1166	26.5
'Philly Beef 'n Swiss'	1 serving	467	1144	25.3
BISCUIT, plain	1 serving	280	730	14.9
BREAKFAST				
bacon platter	1 meal	593	880	33.0
'Egg Platter'	1 meal	460	591	24.0
'French Toastix' 3.5 oz	1 serving	420	440	25.0
'Ham Platter'	1 meal	518	1177	26.2
'Sausage Platter'	1 meal	640	861	41.0
BREAKFAST SANDWICH				
'Bacon/Egg Croissant'	1 serving	430	720	30.0
biscuit, w/bacon	1 serving	318	904	17.9
'Ham Biscuit'	1 serving	323	1169	16.6
'Ham/Cheese Croissant'	1 serving	345	939	20.7
'Sausage Biscuit'	1 serving	460	1000	31.9
'Sausage/Egg Croissant'	1 serving	519	632	39.2
BROCCOLI SOUP, cream of	1 serving	166	1050	7.2
CATSUP	1 serving	16	143	0.0
CHEESE SOUP, Wisconsin cheese	1 serving	281	1084	18.0
CHEESEBURGER, 'Bac'n Cheddar Deluxe'	1 serving	512	1094	31.5
CHEESECAKE	1 serving	306	220	22.8
CHICKEN NOODLE SOUP, 'Old Fashioned'	1 serving	99	929	1.8
CHICKEN SANDWICH				
breast, fillet	1 serving	445	958	22.5
cordon bleu	1 serving	518	1463	27.1
grilled, barbecue	1 serving	386	1002	13.1
grilled, 'Deluxe'	1 serving	430	901	19.9
roast, 'Club'	1 serving	503	1143	27.0
roast, 'Deluxe Light'	1 serving	276	777	7.0
CHOWDER, Boston clam	1 serving	193	1032	10.0
COFFEE	8 oz	3	3	0.0
COOKIE, chocolate chip	1 serving	130	95	4.0

Food Name	Serv. Size	Total Cal.	Sod. MGS	Fat GMS
CROISSANT, plain	1 serving	260	300	15.6
CROISSANT SANDWICH, 'Mushroom/Cheese'	1 serving	493	935	37.7
CROUTONS	1 serving	59	155	2.2
DANISH, cinnamon nut	1 serving	360	105	11.0
DESSERT				
'Butterfinger Polar Swirl'	1 serving	457	318	18.1
'Heath Polar Swirl'	1 serving	543	346	21.8
'Oreo Polar Swirl'	1 serving	482	521	19.7
'Peanut Butter Cup Polar Swirl'	1 serving	517	385	24.0
'Snickers Polar Swirl'	1 serving	511	351	18.8
FISH SANDWICH, fillet	1 serving	526	872	27.0
FRENCH DIP SANDWICH				
regular	1 serving	368	1018	15.4
w/Swiss cheese	1 serving	429	1438	19.0
FRENCH FRIES				
cheddar	1 serving	399	443	21.9
curly	1 serving	337	167	17.7
regular, small order, 2.5 oz	1 serving	246	114	13.2
HAM AND CHEESE SANDWICH	1 serving	355	1400	14.2
HORSERADISH SAUCE, 'Horsey Sauce'	1 serving	55	105	5.0
HOT CHOCOLATE	8 oz	110	120	1.2
ICED TEA	16 oz	6	12	0.0
MAYONNAISE	1 serving	90	75	10.0
MILK, 2%	8 oz	121	122	4.4
MILKSHAKE				
chocolate	1 serving	451	341	11.6
jamocha	1 serving	368	262	10.5
vanilla	1 serving	330	281	11.5
MUFFIN, blueberry	1 muffin	240	200	7.0
MUSTARD	1 serving	11	160	0.6
ORANGE JUICE	6 oz	82	2	0.0
POTATO, BAKED				
broccoli and cheddar	1 serving	417	361	17.9
'Deluxe'	1 serving	621	605	36.4
mushroom and cheese	1 serving	515	923	26.7
plain	1 serving	240	58	1.9
w/sour cream and butter	1 serving	463	203	25.2
POTATO CAKES	3 oz	204	397	12.0
POTATO SOUP, w/bacon	1 serving	184	1068	8.8
ROAST BEEF SANDWICH				
'Junior'	1 serving	233	519	10.8

Food Name	Serv. Size	Total Cal.	Sod. MGS	Fat GMS
'Light Deluxe'	1 serving	294	826	10.0
regular, 5.5 oz	1 serving	383	936	18.2
super	1 serving	552	1174	28.3
SALAD				
chef's	1 serving	205	796	9.5
garden	1 serving	117	134	5.2
roast chicken	1 serving	204	508	7.2
side order	1 serving	25	30	0.3
SALAD DRESSING				
blue cheese	1 serving	295	489	31.2
buttermilk ranch	1 serving	349	471	38.5
honey French	1 serving	322	486	26.9
light Italian	1 serving	23	1110	1.1
Thousand Island	1 serving	298	493	29.2
SAUCE, Arby's	1 serving	15	113	0.2
SOFT DRINK				
Coca-Cola Classic	12 oz	141	15	0.0
Diet Coke	12 oz	1	30	0.0
Diet 7Up	12 oz	4	22	0.0
Nehi Orange	12 oz	190	21	0.0
Pepsi Cola	12 oz	159	10	0.0
R.C. Cola	12 oz	173	1	0.0
R.C. Diet Rite	12 oz	1	10	0.0
R.C. Root Beer	12 oz	173	16	0.0
7Up	12 oz	144	34	0.0
Upper Ten	12 oz	169	40	0.0
SUBMARINE SANDWICH				
Italian	1 serving	671	2062	38.8
roast beef	1 serving	623	1847	32.0
tuna	1 serving	663	1342	37.0
turkey	1 serving	486	2033	19.0
SUGAR SUBSTITUTE	1 serving	4	5	0.0
SYRUP, maple, 1.5 oz	1 serving	120	52	0.1
TURKEY SANDWICH, 'Light Roast Turkey Deluxe' 6.8 oz	1 serving	260	1262	6.0
TURNOVER				
apple	1 serving	303	178	18.3
blueberry	1 serving	320	240	19.0
cherry	1 serving	280	200	17.8
VEGETABLE SOUP, mixed vegetable, 'Lumberjack'	1 serving	89	1075	3.6

Food Name	Serv. Size	Total Cal.	Sod. MGS	Fat GMS
BOSTON MARKET				
APPLES, cinnamon, hot	3/4 cup	250	45	4.5
BAKED BEANS, barbecue	3/4 cup	330	630	9.0
BROWNIE	1 brownie	450	190	27.0
CAESAR SALAD				
chicken	13 oz	670	1860	47.0
entree	10 oz	520	1420	43.0
side	4 oz	210	560	17.0
w/o dressing	8 oz	240	780	13.0
CHICKEN				
1/2 chicken, w/skin	10.1 oz	630	960	37.0
1/4 chicken, dark meat, w/skin	4.7 oz	330	460	6.0
1/4 chicken, dark meat, w/o skin	3.7 oz	210	320	10.0
1/4 chicken, white meat, w/skin	5.4 oz	330	530	17.0
1/4 chicken, white meat, w/o skin	3.7 oz	160	350	4.0
CHICKEN ENTRÉE				
1/4 chicken, white meat, corn bread, corn, new potatoes	15.8 oz	690	970	17.0
1/4 chicken, white meat, corn bread, cranberry, new potatoes	18.6 oz	870	850	18.0
1/4 chicken, white meat, corn bread, vegetables, corn	15.0 oz	590	910	15.0
1/4 chicken, white meat, corn bread, vegetables, fruit	15.3 oz	470	790	11.0
CHICKEN GRAVY	1 oz	15	170	1.0
CHICKEN POT PIE, 15 oz	1 pie	750	2380	34.0
CHICKEN SALAD, chunky	3/4 cup	390	790	30.0
CHICKEN SANDWICH				
breast, 9.1 oz	1 sandwich	420	900	5.0
breast, w/fruit salad, 14.6 oz	1 sandwich	490	910	6.0
chunky chicken salad, 10.8 oz	1 sandwich	640	1330	31.0
CHICKEN SOUP	3/4 cup	80	470	3.0
CHICKEN SOUP ENTRÉE				
w/corn bread, steamed vegetables, new potatoes	17.5 oz	470	790	11.0
CHOCOLATE CHIP COOKIE, 2.8 oz	1 cookie	340	240	17.0
COLESLAW	3/4 cup	280	520	16.0
CORN, buttered	3/4 cup	190	130	4.0
CORNBREAD, 2.4 oz	1 loaf	200	390	6.0
CRANBERRY RELISH	3/4 cup	370	5	5.0
CUCUMBER SALAD	4.79 oz	79	182	6.5
FRUIT SALAD	3/4 cup	70	10	0.5
MACARONI AND CHEESE	3/4 cup	280	760	10.0
OATMEAL RAISIN COOKIE, 2.8 oz	1 loaf	320	260	6.0

ood Name	Serv. Size	Total Cal.	Sod. MGS	Fat GMS
PASTA SALAD				
Mediterranean	3/4 cup	170	490	10.0
tortellini	3/4 cup	380	530	24.0
POTATOES				
mashed	2/3 cup	180	390	8.0
mashed, homemade, w/gravy	3/4 cup	200	560	9.0
new	3/4 cup	140	100	3.0
RICE PILAF	2/3 cup	180	600	5.0
SPINACH, creamed	3/4 cup	300	790	24.0
SQUASH, butternut	3/4 cup	160	580	6.0
STUFFING	3/4 cup	310	1140	12.0
TURKEY				
breast, skinless	5.07 oz	170	850	1.0
breast, skinless w/gravy	8.11 oz	200	1370	3.5
sandwich w/o mayo or mustard	9.39 oz	440	1130	8.0
VEGETABLE POT PIE, 17 oz	1 pie	350	1450	12.0
VEGETABLES, steamed	2/3 cup	35	35	0.5
ZUCCHINI, marinara	3/4 cup	80	470	4.0
BURGER KING				
APPLE PIE	1 serving	311	412	14.0
BACON BITS	1 pkt	16	na	1.0
BAGEL				
plain	1 bagel	272	438	6.0
w/cream cheese	1 bagel	370	523	16.0
BARBECUE SAUCE				
	1 oz	36	397	0.0
'Bull's-Eye'	.5 oz	22	47	0.0
BISCUIT, plain	1 serving	332	754	17.0
BREAKFAST				
French toast sticks	1 serving	440	490	27.0
scrambled egg platter, regular	1 serving	549	893	34.0
scrambled egg platter, w/bacon	1 serving	610	1043	39.0
scrambled egg platter, w/sausage	1 serving	768	1271	53.0
BREAKFAST SANDWICH				
bagel, w/bacon, egg, and cheese	1 serving	453	872	20.0
bagel, w/egg and cheese	1 serving	407	759	16.0
bagel, w/ham, egg, and cheese	1 serving	438	1114	17.0
bagel, w/sausage, egg, and cheese	1 serving	626	1137	36.0
biscuit, w/bacon	1 serving	378	867	20.0
biscuit, w/bacon and egg	1 serving	467	1033	27.0

Food Name	Serv. Size	Total Cal.	Sod. MGS	Fc GM
biscuit, w/sausage	1 serving	478	1007	29.
biscuit, w/sausage and egg	1 serving	568	1172	36.
'Breakfast Buddy'	1 serving	255	492	16.
'Croissan'wich' w/bacon, egg, and cheese	1 serving	353	780	23.
'Croissan'wich' w/egg and cheese	1 serving	315	607	20.
'Croissan'wich' w/ham, egg, and cheese	1 serving	351	1373	22.
'Croissan'wich' w/sausage, egg, and cheese	1 serving	534	985	40.
CHEESE				
American	.9 oz	92	312	7.
Swiss	.9 oz	82	352	6.
CHEESEBURGER				
bacon, double	1 serving	515	748	31.
bacon, double, 'Deluxe'	1 serving	592	804	39.
barbecue bacon, double	1 serving	536	795	31.
'Deluxe'	1 serving	390	652	23.
double	1 serving	483	851	27.
'Mushroom Swiss' double	1 serving	473	746	27.
regular	1 serving	318	651	15.0
'Whopper' double, w/cheese	1 serving	935	1245	61.0
'Whopper Jr.'	1 serving	380	660	22.0
'Whopper' w/cheese	1 serving	706	1177	44.0
CHICKEN, 'Chicken Tenders'	6 pieces	236	541	13.0
CHICKEN SANDWICH				
'B.K. Broiler'	1 serving	379	764	18.0
regular	1 serving	685	1417	40.0
CREAM CHEESE	1 oz	98	86	10.0
CROISSANT	1 serving	180	285	10.0
CROUTONS	.25 oz	31	90	1.0
DANISH				
apple cinnamon	1 serving	390	305	13.0
cheese	1 serving	406	454	16.0
cinnamon raisin	1 serving	449	286	18.0
FISH SANDWICH, fillet, 'Ocean Catch'	1 serving	495	879	25.0
FRENCH FRIES, med order	1 serving	372	238	20.0
HAMBURGER				
'Burger Buddies'	1 serving	349	717	17.0
'Deluxe'	1 serving	344	496	19.0
regular	1 serving	272	505	11.0
'Whopper'	1 serving	614	865	36.0
'Whopper' double	1 serving	844	933	53.0
'Whopper Jr.'	1 serving	330	500	19.0

ood Name	Serv. Size	Total Cal.	Sod. MGS	Fat GMS
ONEY SAUCE	1 oz	91	12	0.0
ETTUCE	.75 oz	3	2	0.0
AYONNAISE	1 oz	194	142	21.0
ILKSHAKE				
chocolate	1 serving	326	198	10.0
chocolate, syrup added	1 serving	409	248	11.0
strawberry, syrup added	1 serving	394	230	10.0
vanilla	1 serving	334	213	10.0
MUFFIN				
blueberry, mini	1 serving	292	244	14.0
lemon poppyseed, mini	1 serving	318	253	18.0
MUSTARD	1 pkt	2	34	0.0
ONION	.25 oz	5	0	0.0
ONION RINGS	1 serving	339	628	19.0
PICKLE	.5 oz	1	119	0.0
POTATOES, HASH BROWN, 'Tater Tenders'	1 serving	213	318	12.0
RANCH SAUCE	1 oz	171	208	18.0
SALAD				
chef's, w/o dressing	1 serving	178	568	9.0
chunky chicken, w/o dressing	1 serving	142	443	4.0
garden, w/o dressing	1 serving	95	125	5.0
side salad, w/o dressing	1 serving	25	27	0.0
SALAD DRESSING				
blue cheese, 'Newman's Own'	1 pkt	300	512	32.0
French, 'Newman's Own'	1 pkt	290	400	22.0
Italian, reduced calorie, 'Newman's Own'	1 pkt	170	762	18.0
olive oil and vinegar, 'Newman's Own'	1 pkt	310	214	33.0
ranch, 'Newman's Own'	1 pkt	350	316	37.0
Thousand Island, 'Newman's Own'	1 pkt	290	403	26.0
SANDWICH SAUCE				
'B.K. Broiler'	.5 oz	90	95	10.0
'Burger King A.M. Express'	1 oz	84	18	0.0
SWEET AND SOUR SAUCE	1 oz	45	52	0.0
TARTAR SAUCE	1 oz	134	202	14.0
TOMATO	1 oz	6	3	0.0
JACK-IN-THE-BOX				
APPLE TURNOVER, 3.9 oz	1 serving	354	479	19.0
BARBECUE SAUCE	1-oz pkt	44	300	<1.0
BEEF SANDWICH, gyro	1 serving	620	1310	32.0
BEEF TERIYAKI BOWL	1 serving	640	930	3.0

Food Name	Serv. Size	Total Cal.	Sod. MGS	Fe GM
BREADSTICKS, sesame, .5 oz	1 serving	70	110	2
BREAKFAST				
pancake platter, 8.1 oz	1 serving	612	888	22.
scrambled egg platter, 7.5 oz	1 serving	559	1060	32.
BREAKFAST SANDWICH				
'Breakfast Jack' 4.4 oz	1 serving	307	871	13.
crescent, Canadian bacon, 4.7 oz	1 serving	452	851	31.
crescent, sausage, 5.5 oz	1 serving	584	1012	43.
crescent, supreme, 5.1 oz	1 serving	547	1053	40.
sausage, 5.5 oz	1 serving	584	1012	43.
scrambled egg pocket, 6.5 oz	1 serving	431	1060	21.
sourdough bread, egg, ham, and cheese, 5.2 oz	1 serving	381	1120	20.
CHEESEBURGER				
'Bacon Bacon Cheeseburger' 8.5 oz	1 serving	705	1240	45.
'Jumbo Jack' 8.5 oz	1 serving	677	1090	40.
double, 5.3 oz	1 serving	467	842	27.
patty melt, 'Old Fashioned' 7.6 oz	1 serving	713	1360	46.
regular, 4 oz	1 serving	315	746	14.
Swiss cheese and bacon, 6.6 oz	1 serving	678	1458	47.
'Ultimate' 9.9 oz	1 serving	942	1176	69.
CHEESECAKE, 3.5 oz	1 serving	309	208	18.
CHICKEN SANDWICH				
grilled, fillet, 7.4 oz	1 serving	431	1070	19.0
smoked chicken, cheddar, and bacon	1 serving	540	1520	30.0
spicy crispy chicken	1 serving	560	1020	27.0
supreme, 8.6 oz	1 serving	641	1470	39.0
w/mushrooms, 7.8 oz	1 serving	438	1340	18.0
CHICKEN STRIPS				
4 pieces	4 oz	285	695	13.0
6 pieces	6.2 oz	451	1100	20.0
CHICKEN TERIYAKI BOWL	1 serving	580	1220	1.5
CHICKEN WINGS				
9 pieces	11 oz	1270	2560	66.0
6 pieces	7.3 oz	846	1710	44.0
CHIMICHANGA				
mini, 4 pieces	7.3 oz	571	633	28.0
mini, 6 pieces	11 oz	856	949	42.0
COCKTAIL SAUCE	1 oz	32	206	<1.0
COFFEE, small	8 oz	2	26	0.0
DESSERT, double fudge, 3.0 oz	1 serving	288	259	9.0
EGG ROLL, 5 pieces	10 oz	753	1640	41.0

Food Name	Serv. Size	Total Cal.	Sod. MGS	Fat GMS
FAJITA SANDWICH				
beef fajita pita, 6.2 oz	1 serving	333	635	14.0
chicken fajita pita, 6.7 oz	1 serving	292	703	8.0
FISH SANDWICH, supreme, 7.7 oz	1 serving	510	1040	27.0
FRENCH FRIES				
curly, seasoned, 3.8 oz	1 serving	358	1030	20.0
jumbo order, 4.3 oz	1 serving	396	219	19.0
regular order, 3.8 oz	1 serving	351	194	17.0
small order, 2.4 oz	1 serving	219	121	11.0
GUACAMOLE	1 oz	30	128	3.0
HAMBURGER				
'Jumbo Jack' 7.8 oz	1 serving	584	733	34.0
regular, 3.4 oz	1 serving	267	556	11.0
HOT SAUCE, .5 oz	1 serving	4	112	0.0
ICED TEA, small	16 oz	4	6	0.0
ITALIAN SAUCE	1.5 oz	28	176	<1.0
JELLY, grape	.5 oz	38	3	0.0
MAYO-MUSTARD SAUCE	.7 oz	124	247	13.0
MAYO-ONION SAUCE	.7 oz	143	140	15.0
MILK, 2%	8.6 oz	122	122	5.0
MILKSHAKE				
chocolate	11.4 oz	330	270	7.0
strawberry	11.6 oz	320	240	7.0
vanilla	11.2 oz	320	230	6.0
ONION RINGS, 3.6 oz	1 serving	380	451	23.0
ORANGE JUICE	6.5 oz	80	0	0.0
POTATOES, HASH BROWN, 2.0 oz	1 serving	156	312	11.0
RAVIOLI				
toasted, 7 pieces	5.8 oz	537	639	28.0
toasted, 10 pieces	8.3 oz	768	913	40.0
SALAD				
chef's, 11.7 oz	1 serving	325	900	18.0
Mexican chicken, 14.6 oz	1 serving	442	1500	23.0
side order, 4 oz	1 serving	51	84	3.0
taco, 14.2 oz	1 serving	503	1600	31.0
SALAD DRESSING				
blue cheese	2.5-oz pkt	262	918	22.0
buttermilk, house	2.5-oz pkt	362	694	36.0
French, reduced calorie	2.5-oz pkt	176	600	8.0
Italian, low calorie	2.5-oz pkt	25	810	2.0
Thousand Island	2.5-oz pkt	312	700	30.0

Food Name	Serv. Size	Total Cal.	Sod. MGS	Fat GMS
SALSA	1 oz	8	27	<1.0
SHRIMP				
15 pieces	4.4 oz	404	1003	24.0
10 pieces	3.0 oz	270	669	16.0
SOFT DRINK				
Coca-Cola, small	16 oz	192	19	0.0
Diet Coke, small	16 oz	1	35	0.0
Dr. Pepper, small	16 oz	192	24	0.0
Ramblin' Root Beer, small	16 oz	235	27	0.0
Sprite, small	16 oz	192	61	0.0
STEAK SANDWICH				
country-fried, 5.4 oz	1 serving	450	891	25.0
sirloin, 8.4 oz	1 serving	517	1050	23.0
SWEET AND SOUR SAUCE	1 oz	40	160	<1.0
SYRUP, pancake	1.5 oz	121	6	0.0
TACO				
regular, 3 oz	1 serving	187	414	11.0
super, 4.5 oz	1 serving	281	718	17.0
TAQUITO				
5 pieces	5 oz	363	467	16.0
7 pieces	7 oz	508	654	22.0
TORTILLA CHIPS	1 oz	139	134	6.0
VEGETABLE OIL SPREAD, 'Country Crock'	.2 oz	25	40	2.8
KENTUCKY FRIED CHICKEN				
BARBECUE SAUCE	1 oz	35	450	0.6
BEANS				
barbecue baked	3.9 oz	132	535	2.0
green	3.6 oz	36	563	1.0
BISCUIT				
buttermilk, 2.3 oz	1 biscuit	232	539	11.9
regular, 2.0 oz	1 biscuit	200	564	12.0
BREADSTICKS, 1.2 oz	1 breadstick	110	15	3.0
CHICKEN				
breast, center, 'Extra Tasty Crispy' 4.8 oz	1 serving	342	790	19.7
breast, center, 'Hot & Spicy' 4.3 oz	1 serving	382	905	25.0
breast, center, 'Original Recipe' 3.6 oz	1 serving	260	609	14.0
breast, center, 'Skinfree Crispy'	1 serving	296	435	16.0
breast, side, 'Extra Tasty Crispy' 3.9 oz	1 serving	343	748	22.3
breast, side, 'Hot & Spicy' 4.1 oz	1 serving	398	922	27.0
breast, side, 'Original Recipe'	1 piece	276	654	17.0

Food Name	Serv. Size	Total Cal.	Sod. MGS	Fat GMS
breast, side, 'Skinfree Crispy'	1 serving	293	410	17.0
dark meat quarter, w/skin, 'Rotisserie Gold' 5.1 oz	1 serving	333	980	23.7
dark meat quarter, w/o skin, 'Rotisserie Gold' 4.1 oz	1 serving	217	772	12.2
drumstick, 'Extra Tasty Crispy' 2.4 oz	1 serving	190	260	11.0
drumstick, 'Hot & Spicy' 2.3 oz	1 serving	190	300	11.0
drumstick, 'Original Recipe' 1.8 oz	1 piece	130	210	7.0
drumstick, 'Skinfree Crispy'	1 serving	166	256	9.0
'Hot Wings' 6 pieces, 4.8 oz	1 serving	471	1230	33.0
'Spicy Chicken Bites' small 4.3 oz	1 serving	248	344	12.4
thigh, 'Extra Tasty Crispy' 4.2 oz	1 serving	370	540	25.0
thigh, 'Hot & Spicy' 3.8 oz	1 serving	370	570	27.0
thigh, 'Original Recipe' 3.3 oz	1 piece	260	570	17.0
thigh, 'Skinfree Crispy'	1 serving	256	394	17.0
white meat quarter, w/o skin and wing, 'Rotisserie Gold' 4.1 oz	1 serving	199	667	5.9
white meat quarter, w/skin and wing, 'Rotisserie Gold' 6.2 oz	1 serving	335	1104	18.7
wing, 'Extra Tasty Crispy' 1.9 oz	1 serving	200	290	13.0
wing, 'Hot & Spicy' 1.9 oz	1 serving	210	340	15.0
wing, 'Original Recipe' 1.7 oz	1 piece	150	380	8.0
CHICKEN NUGGETS				
'Kentucky Nuggets' .6 oz	1 nugget	46	140	2.9
'Kentucky Nuggets' 3.4 oz	6 nuggets	284	865	18.0
CHICKEN SANDWICH				
'Chicken Littles'	1.7 oz	169	331	10.1
'Colonel's'	5.9 oz	482	1060	27.3
'Value BBQ Flavored'	5.3 oz	256	782	8.0
COLESLAW	3.2 oz	114	177	6.0
CORN, on the cob	5.3 oz	222	76	12.0
CORNBREAD, 2 oz	1 serving	228	194	13.0
FRENCH FRIES				
'Crispy' 2.5 oz	1 serving	210	493	11.0
'Kentucky Fries'	1 serving	268	81	13.0
regular, 2.7 oz	1 serving	244	139	11.9
GRAVY, chicken	1 serving	59	398	4.0
HONEY SAUCE	.5 oz	49	15	<.1
MACARONI AND CHEESE	4 oz	162	531	8.0
MUSTARD SAUCE	1 oz	36	346	0.9
POTATO WEDGES	3.3 oz	192	428	9.0
POTATOES, MASHED				
plain	1 serving	59	228	tr

Food Name	Serv. Size	Total Cal.	Sod. MGS	Fat GMS
w/gravy	4.2 oz	109	386	5.0
RED BEANS AND RICE	3.9 oz	114	315	3.0
RICE, garden	3.8 oz	75	576	1.0
ROLL, sourdough, 1.7 oz	1 roll	128	236	2.0
SALAD				
garden	3.1 oz	16	10	0.0
macaroni	3.8 oz	248	6	17.0
pasta	3.8 oz	135	663	8.0
potato	4.4 oz	180	423	11.0
vegetable medley	4 oz	126	240	4.0
SALAD DRESSING				
Italian	1 oz	15	420	1.0
ranch	1 oz	170	250	18.0
SWEET AND SOUR SAUCE	1 oz	58	148	0.6
MC DONALD'S				
APPLE JUICE	6 oz	80	30	0.0
APPLE PIE, 3.0 oz	1 serving	260	240	15.0
BACON BITS	1 oz	15	95	1.0
BARBECUE SAUCE	1 serving	50	340	0.5
BISCUIT, w/spread, 2.6 oz	1 serving	260	730	13.0
BREAKFAST				
Cheerios cereal, w/o milk, 3/4 cup	1 serving	80	210	1.0
eggs, scrambled, 3.5 oz	1 serving	140	290	10.0
hotcakes, w/margarine and syrup, 6.2 oz	1 serving	440	685	12.0
sausage, 1.5 oz	1 serving	160	310	15.0
Wheaties cereal, w/o milk, 3/4 cup	1 serving	90	220	1.0
BREAKFAST SANDWICH				
biscuit, bacon, egg, and cheese, 5.4 oz	1 serving	440	1215	26.0
biscuit, sausage and egg, 6.2 oz	1 serving	505	1210	33.0
biscuit, sausage, 4.2 oz	1 serving	420	1040	28.0
egg, ham, and cheese, 'Egg McMuffin' 4.8 oz	1 serving	280	710	11.0
sausage, 'Sausage McMuffin' 4.8 oz	1 serving	345	770	20.0
sausage, 'Sausage Egg McMuffin' 5.6 oz	1 serving	430	920	25.0
CHEESEBURGER				
'McLean Deluxe' 7.7 oz	1 serving	370	890	14.0
'Quarter Pounder' 6.8 oz	1 serving	510	1110	28.0
regular, 4.1 oz	1 serving	305	725	13.0
CHICKEN NUGGET, 'Chicken McNuggets' 6 pieces	1 serving	270	580	15.0
CHICKEN SANDWICH, 'McChicken' 6.6 oz	1 serving	415	830	19.0
CHOW MEIN NOODLES	1 serving	45	60	2.0

Food Name	Serv. Size	Total Cal.	Sod. MGS	Fat GMS
COOKIE				
'Chocolaty Chip' 2 oz	1 serving	330	280	15.0
'McDonaldland' 2 oz	1 serving	290	300	9.0
CROUTONS	.4 oz	50	140	2.0
DANISH				
apple, 4.1 oz	1 serving	390	370	17.0
cinnamon raisin, 3.9 oz	1 serving	440	430	21.0
cheese, iced, 3.9 oz	1 serving	390	420	21.0
raspberry, 4.1 oz	1 serving	410	310	16.0
ENGLISH MUFFIN, w/spread, 2.1 oz	1 muffin	170	285	4.0
FISH SANDWICH, 'Fillet-O-Fish' 5 oz	1 serving	370	730	18.0
FRENCH FRIES				
large order	4.3 oz	400	200	22.0
large order, unsalted	4.3 oz	400	45	22.0
medium order	3.4 oz	320	150	17.0
medium order, unsalted	3.4 oz	320	35	17.0
small order	2.4 oz	220	110	12.0
small order, unsalted	2.4 oz	220	25	12.0
GRAPEFRUIT JUICE	6 oz	80	0	0.0
HAMBURGER				
'Big Mac' 7.6 oz	1 serving	500	890	26.0
'McLean Deluxe' 7.3 oz	1 serving	320	670	10.0
'Quarter Pounder' 5.9 oz	1 serving	410	645	20.0
regular, 3.6 oz	1 serving	255	490	9.0
HAMBURGER PATTY, 'McLean Deluxe' 3 oz	1 serving	130	110	7.0
HONEY SAUCE	1 serving	45	0	0.0
MILK, 1%	8 oz	110	130	2.0
MILKSHAKE				
chocolate, low-fat	10.4 oz	320	240	1.7
strawberry, low-fat	10.4 oz	320	170	1.3
vanilla, low-fat	10.4 oz	290	170	1.3
MUFFIN				
apple bran, fat-free, 2.6 oz	1 muffin	180	200	0.0
blueberry, fat-free, 2.6 oz	1 muffin	170	220	0.0
MUSTARD SAUCE, hot	1 serving	70	250	3.6
ORANGE JUICE	6 oz	80	0	0.0
POTATOES, HASH BROWN 1.9 oz	1 serving	130	330	7.0
SALAD				
chef's, 9.5 oz	1 serving	170	400	9.0
chunky chicken, 9.0 oz	1 serving	150	230	4.0
garden, 6.7 oz	1 serving	50	70	2.0

Food Name	Serv. Size	Total Cal.	Sod. MGS	Fat GMS
side order, 3.7 oz	1 serving	30	35	1.0
SALAD DRESSING				
blue cheese, 1 tbsp	.5 oz	50	150	4.0
French, red, reduced calorie, 1 tbsp	.5 oz	40	115	2.0
Oriental	.5 oz	24	180	tr
ranch, 1 tbsp	.5 oz	55	130	5.0
Thousand Island, 1 tbsp	.5 oz	78	100	8.0
vinaigrette, 1 tbsp	.5 oz	12	60	0.5
SOFT DRINK				
Coca-Cola Classic, extra large	32 oz	380	40	0.0
Coca-Cola Classic, large	22 oz	260	25	0.0
Coca-Cola Classic, medium	16 oz	190	20	0.0
Coca-Cola Classic, small	12 oz	140	15	0.0
Diet Coke, extra large	32 oz	3	80	0.0
Diet Coke, large	22 oz	2	60	0.0
Diet Coke, medium	16 oz	1	40	0.0
Diet Coke, small	12 oz	1	30	0.0
orange, extra large	32 oz	360	25	0.0
orange, large	22 oz	240	20	0.0
orange, medium	16 oz	180	20	0.0
orange, small	12 oz	130	10	0.0
Sprite, extra large	32 oz	380	40	0.0
Sprite, large	22 oz	260	25	0.0
Sprite, medium	16 oz	190	20	0.0
Sprite, small	12 oz	140	15	0.0
SWEET AND SOUR SAUCE	1 serving	60	190	0.2
YOGURT, FROZEN				
cone, vanilla, low-fat	3 oz	105	80	1.0
hot caramel sundae, low-fat	6 oz	270	180	3.0
hot fudge sundae, low-fat	6 oz	240	170	3.0
strawberry sundae, low-fat	6 oz	210	170	1.0

PIZZA HUT
PIZZA
Beef

Food Name	Serv. Size	Total Cal.	Sod. MGS	Fat GMS
hand-tossed	1 slice	261	795	10.0
'Pan Pizza' medium pie	1 slice	288	675	18.0
'Thick 'n Chewy' 10-inch pie	3 slices	620	na	20.0
'Thin 'n Crispy' 10-inch pie	3 slices	490	na	19.0
Cheese				
'Bigfoot'	1 slice	179	959	5.0

Food Name	Serv. Size	Total Cal.	Sod. MGS	Fat GMS
hand-tossed, medium pie	1 slice	253	593	9.0
'Pan Pizza' medium pie	1 slice	279	473	13.0
'Thick 'n Chewy' 10-inch pie	3 slices	560	na	14.0
'Thin 'n Crispy' medium pie	1 slice	223	503	10.0
'Thin 'n Crispy' 10-inch pie	3 slices	450	na	15.0
'Chunky Combo'				
hand-tossed, medium pie	1 slice	280	823	11.6
'Pan Pizza' medium pie	1 slice	306	703	15.5
'Thin 'n Crispy' medium pie	1 slice	250	736	12.7
'Chunky Meat'				
hand-tossed, medium pie	1 slice	325	970	16.0
'Pan Pizza' medium pie	1 slice	352	850	20.0
'Thin 'n Crispy' medium pie	1 slice	295	882	17.0
Italian sausage				
hand-tossed, medium pie	1 slice	313	871	15.0
'Pan Pizza' medium pie	1 slice	399	751	24.0
'Thin 'n Crispy' medium pie	1 slice	282	781	17.0
'Meat Lovers'				
hand-tossed, medium pie	1 slice	321	1106	15.0
'Pan Pizza' medium pie	1 slice	347	986	23.0
'Thin 'n Crispy' medium pie	1 slice	297	1068	16.0
Pepperoni				
'Bigfoot'	1 slice	195	1022	7.0
hand-tossed, medium pie	1 slice	253	738	10.0
'Pan Pizza' medium pie	1 slice	280	618	18.0
'Personal Pan Pizza' 9-oz pie	1 pie	675	1335	29.0
'Thick 'n Chewy' 10-inch pie	3 slices	560	na	18.0
'Thin 'n Crispy' medium pie	1 slice	230	678	11.0
'Thin 'n Crispy' 10-inch pie	3 slices	430	na	17.0
Pepperoni, mushroom, Italian sausage, 'Bigfoot'	1 slice	213	1208	9.0
'Pepperoni Lovers'				
hand-tossed, medium pie	1 slice	335	981	16.0
'Pan Pizza' medium pie	1 slice	362	861	25.0
'Thin 'n Crispy' medium pie	1 slice	320	949	19.0
Pork				
hand-tossed	1 slice	270	803	11.0
'Pan Pizza'	1 slice	296	683	19.0
'Thick 'n Chewy' 10-inch pie	3 slices	640	na	23.0
'Thin 'n Crispy' medium pie	1 slice	240	713	12.0
'Thin 'n Crispy' 10-inch pie	3 slices	520	na	23.0

Food Name	Serv. Size	Total Cal.	Sod. MGS	Fat GMS
'Super Supreme'				
hand-tossed, medium pie	2 slices	463	1336	21.0
hand-tossed, medium pie	1 slice	276	980	10.0
'Pan Pizza' medium pie	1 slice	302	860	19.0
'Thin 'n Crispy' medium pie	1 slice	253	700	12.0
'Supreme'				
hand-tossed, medium pie	1 slice	289	894	12.0
'Pan Pizza' medium pie	1 slice	315	774	16.0
'Personal Pan Pizza' 9.3-oz pie	1 pie	647	1313	28.0
'Thick 'n Chewy' 10-inch pie	3 slices	640	na	22.0
'Thin 'n Crispy' medium pie	1 slice	262	819	14.0
'Thin 'n Crispy' 10-inch pie	3 slices	510	na	21.0
'Veggie Lovers'				
hand-tossed, medium pie	1 slice	222	641	7.0
'Pan Pizza'	1 slice	249	521	15.0
'Thin 'n Crispy' medium pie	1 slice	192	551	8.0
ROY ROGERS				
ALFALFA SPROUTS	2 tbsp	1	<1	tr
BACON BITS	1 tsp	33	189	1.0
BEAN SPROUTS	2 tbsp	4	<1	tr
BEETS, sliced	1/4 cup	18	162	tr
BISCUIT	1 serving	231	575	12.0
BREAKFAST				
egg and biscuit platter	1 serving	557	1020	34.0
egg and biscuit platter, w/bacon	1 serving	607	1236	39.0
egg and biscuit platter, w/ham	1 serving	605	1442	36.0
egg and biscuit platter, w/sausage	1 serving	713	1345	49.0
pancake platter, w/syrup and butter	1 serving	386	547	13.0
pancake platter, w/syrup and butter, w/bacon	1 serving	436	763	17.0
pancake platter, w/syrup and butter, w/ham	1 serving	434	969	15.0
pancake platter, w/syrup and butter, w/sausage	1 serving	542	872	28.0
BREAKFAST SANDWICH				
crescent	1 serving	408	820	27.0
crescent, w/bacon	1 serving	446	982	30.0
crescent, w/ham	1 serving	456	1243	29.0
crescent, w/sausage	1 serving	564	1145	42.0
BROCCOLI, raw	1/4 cup	6	6	tr
CABBAGE, raw	1/4 cup	5	2	tr
CANTALOUPE, cubed	1/4 cup	14	4	tr
CARROT, raw, shredded	1/4 cup	12	2	tr

Food Name	Serv. Size	Total Cal.	Sod. MGS	Fat GMS
CAULIFLOWER, raw	1/4 cup	6	4	tr
CHEESE, cheddar	1/4 cup	100	275	8.0
CHEESEBURGER				
'Express'	1 serving	613	1122	37.0
'Express' w/bacon	1 serving	641	1317	41.0
regular	1 serving	525	830	29.0
small	1 serving	275	558	13.0
w/bacon	1 serving	552	1025	33.0
CHICKEN				
breast, fried	1 serving	412	609	24.0
breast and wing, fried	1 serving	604	894	37.0
breast and wing, w/o skin, 'Roy's Roaster'	1 serving	190	na	6.0
leg, fried	1 serving	140	190	8.0
leg and thigh, fried	1 serving	436	596	28.0
nugget, fried, 6 pieces	1 serving	288	548	18.0
thigh, fried	1 serving	296	406	20.0
wing, fried	1 serving	192	285	13.0
CHICKEN SALAD, grilled	1 serving	120	520	4.0
CHINESE NOODLES	1/4 cup	55	113	3.0
COLESLAW	1 serving	110	261	7.0
COTTAGE CHEESE	2 tbsp	29	114	1.0
CROUTONS	2 tbsp	14	50	tr
CUCUMBER, raw	5-6 slices	4	2	0.0
DANISH				
apple swirl	1 serving	328	279	7.0
cheese swirl	1 serving	383	369	15.0
EGG, boiled, chopped	2 tbsp	55	41	4.0
FISH SANDWICH	1 serving	514	857	24.0
FRENCH FRIES				
large order, 5.5 oz	1 serving	440	225	22.0
regular order, 4 oz	1 serving	320	164	16.0
small order, 3 oz	1 serving	238	122	12.0
FRUIT COCKTAIL	1/4 cup	46	1	tr
GARBANZO BEANS	1/4 cup	55	240	1.0
GELATIN, parfait	1/4 cup	50	23	2.0
GRANOLA	1/4 cup	65	8	3.0
GRAPES	5 grapes	20	<1	tr
GREEK PASTA	1/4 cup	159	328	9.0
HAMBURGER				
'Express'	1 serving	561	899	32.0
regular	1 serving	472	607	25.0

Food Name	Serv. Size	Total Cal.	Sod. MGS	Fat GMS
'Roy Rogers Bar'	1 serving	573	1252	31.0
small	1 serving	222	336	9.0
HONEYDEW MELON, cubed	1/4 cup	15	4	tr
LEMONADE	12 oz	150	na	tr
LETTUCE				
iceberg	1 cup	7	5	tr
romaine	1 cup	9	5	tr
MACARONI SALAD	1/4 cup	93	301	5.0
MILK, 2%	8 oz	120	130	5.0
MILKSHAKE				
chocolate	1 serving	358	290	10.0
strawberry	1 serving	315	261	10.0
vanilla	1 serving	306	282	11.0
ONION, raw, chopped	2 tbsp	7	tr	tr
ORANGE JUICE	8 oz	120	na	tr
PASTA AND NOODLES. See individual listings.				
PASTRY, cinnamon rod	1 serving	376	339	15.0
PEACH, sliced	1/4 cup	48	5	tr
PEAS, green	1/4 cup	28	41	tr
PEPPER, GREEN	2 tbsp	3	tr	tr
PINEAPPLE				
chunks, canned	1/4 cup	48	5	tr
chunks, fresh	1/4 cup	19	<1	tr
POTATO, BAKED, plain 'Hot Topped'	1 serving	211	65	0.0
POTATO SALAD	1/4 cup	54	348	3.0
RADISH, sliced	2 tbsp	2	4	tr
ROAST BEEF SANDWICH				
large	1 serving	373	840	12.0
large, w/cheese	1 serving	427	1062	17.0
regular	1 serving	350	732	11.0
w/cheese	1 serving	403	954	15.0
ROLL, crescent	1 serving	287	547	18.0
SALAD DRESSING				
bacon and tomato	2 tbsp	136	150	12.0
blue cheese	2 tbsp	150	153	16.0
Italian, low-calorie	2 tbsp	70	100	6.0
ranch	2 tbsp	155	100	14.0
Thousand Island	2 tbsp	160	150	16.0
STRAWBERRIES, fresh	1/4 cup	11	<1	tr
SUNDAE				
caramel	1 serving	293	193	9.0

Food Name	Serv. Size	Total Cal.	Sod. MGS	Fat GMS
chocolate	1 serving	358	290	10.0
hot fudge	1 serving	337	186	13.0
strawberry	1 serving	216	99	7.0
vanilla	1 serving	306	282	11.0
TOMATO	3 slices	20	1	tr
WATERMELON, diced	1/4 cup	13	1	tr

TACO BELL
BURRITO

Food Name	Serv. Size	Total Cal.	Sod. MGS	Fat GMS
bean	7.3 oz	447	1148	14.0
beef	7.3 oz	493	1311	21.0
beef, double, 'Supreme'	1 serving	451	928	22.0
beef, 'MexiMelt'	3.7 oz	266	689	15.0
'Cheesarito'	1 serving	312	451	13.0
chicken	6 oz	334	880	12.0
chicken, 'MexiMelt'	3.8 oz	257	779	15.0
combination	7 oz	407	1136	16.0
'Light' bean	7.07 oz	330	na	6.0
'Light' burrito supreme	8.86 oz	350	na	8.0
'Light' 7-layer	9.53 oz	440	na	9.0
'Supreme'	9 oz	503	1181	22.0
CHEESE SAUCE, nacho	2 oz	103	393	8.0
FAJITA, chicken	1 serving	226	619	10.0
FAJITA TACO				
steak	1 serving	235	507	11.0
steak, w/guacamole	1 serving	269	620	13.0
steak, w/sour cream	1 serving	281	507	15.0
GREEN SAUCE	1 oz	4	136	0.0
GUACAMOLE	.75 oz	34	113	2.0
NACHOS				
'Nachos Bellgrande'	10.1 oz	649	997	35.0
'Nachos Supreme'	5.1 oz	367	471	27.0
regular	3.7 oz	346	399	18.0
PASTRY, 'Cinnamon Twists'	1.2 oz	171	234	8.0
PEPPER, JALAPEÑO	3.5 oz	20	1370	0.0
PINTO BEANS, w/cheese and red sauce	4.5 oz	190	642	9.0
PIZZA, Mexican	7.9 oz	575	1031	37.0
RED SAUCE	1 oz	10	261	0.0
RELISH, 'Pico de Gallo'	.7 oz	6	66	0.0
SALAD				
seafood, w/ranch dressing	1 serving	884	1489	66.0

Food Name	Serv. Size	Total Cal.	Sod. MGS	Fat GMS
seafood, w/o dressing	1 serving	648	917	42.0
seafood, w/o dressing, w/o shell	1 serving	217	693	11.0
taco, 21 oz	1 serving	905	910	61.0
taco, w/ranch dressing	1 serving	1167	1959	87.0
taco, w/o beans	1 serving	822	1368	57.0
taco, w/o salsa	1 serving	931	1387	62.0
taco, w/o shell, 18.3 oz	1 serving	484	680	31.0
SALAD DRESSING, ranch	2.6 oz	236	571	25.0
SALSA	.34 oz	18	376	0.0
SOUR CREAM	.75 oz	46	0	4.0
TACO				
'Bellgrande'	5.7 oz	335	472	23.0
chicken	3 oz	171	337	9.0
chicken, soft	3.8 oz	213	615	10.0
'Light' soft taco	5.54 oz	180	na	5.0
'Light' soft taco supreme	4.57 oz	200	na	5.0
'Light' taco	2.79 oz	140	na	5.0
'Light' taco salad w/chips	19.11 oz	680	na	25.0
'Light' taco salad w/o chips	16.57 oz	330	na	9.0
'Light' taco supreme	3.79 oz	160	na	5.0
platter, light	1 serving	1062	2068	58.0
regular	2.75 oz	183	276	11.0
regular, soft	3.25 oz	225	554	12.0
steak, soft	3.5 oz	218	456	11.0
'Supreme'	3.25 oz	230	276	15.0
'Supreme,' soft	4.4 oz	272	554	16.0
TACO SAUCE				
hot	1 pkt	3	82	0.0
regular	1 pkt	2	126	0.0
TOSTADA				
beef	1 serving	322	764	20.0
chicken, w/red sauce	5.8 oz	264	454	15.0
w/red sauce	5.5 oz	243	596	11.0

WENDY'S

Food Name	Serv. Size	Total Cal.	Sod. MGS	Fat GMS
ALFALFA SPROUTS	1 oz	8	na	tr
ALFREDO SAUCE	2 oz	35	300	1.0
APPLE TOPPING	1 serving	130	120	tr
BACON BITS, imitation	1/8 oz	10	100	tr
BARBECUE SAUCE	1 oz	50	100	<1.0
BISCUIT, buttermilk	1 serving	320	860	17.0

Food Name	Serv. Size	Total Cal.	Sod. MGS	Fat GMS
BLUEBERRIES	1 tbsp	6	na	tr
BLUEBERRY TOPPING	1 serving	60	65	tr
BREADSTICKS				
	1 stick	130	250	3.0
salad bar item	2 sticks	35	60	1.0
BREAKFAST				
bacon	1 strip	30	125	2.0
breakfast sandwich	1 serving	370	770	19.0
breakfast sandwich, w/bacon	1 serving	430	1020	23.0
breakfast sandwich, w/sausage	1 serving	570	1175	37.0
eggs, scrambled	2 eggs	190	160	12.0
French toast	2 slices	400	850	19.0
omelet, ham and cheese	1 serving	290	570	21.0
omelet, ham, cheese, and mushroom	1 serving	290	570	21.0
omelet, ham, cheese, onion, and green pepper	1 serving	280	485	19.0
omelet, mushroom, green pepper, and onion	1 serving	210	200	15.0
potatoes	1 serving	360	745	22.0
sausage patty	1 patty	200	405	18.0
BROCCOLI, raw	1/2 cup	12	5	tr
BUN				
Kaiser	1 bun	180	390	2.0
multigrain	1 bun	140	215	3.0
white	1 bun	140	255	2.0
CABBAGE, red, raw	1/4 cup	4	5	tr
CANTALOUPE	2 pieces	18	5	tr
CARROTS, raw	1/4 cup	12	10	0.0
CATSUP	1 tsp	6	50	tr
CAULIFLOWER, raw	1/2 cup	12	10	tr
CELERY, raw	1 tbsp	0	5	tr
CHEESE				
American, salad bar item	1 oz	90	365	7.0
American, sandwich topping	1 slice	60	295	6.0
cheddar, shredded	1 oz	110	175	10.0
imitation, shredded	1 oz	90	125	6.0
mozzarella	1 oz	90	335	7.0
Parmesan, grated	1 oz	130	510	9.0
Parmesan, imitation	1 oz	80	410	3.0
provolone	1 oz	90	335	7.0
Swiss	1 oz	90	365	7.0
CHEESE SAUCE	2 oz	39	305	2.0

Food Name	Serv. Size	Total Cal.	Sod. MGS	Fat GMS
CHEESEBURGER				
bacon, 'Jr.' 5.5 oz	1 serving	430	840	25.0
double	1 serving	620	760	36.0
'Jr.' 4.4 oz	1 serving	310	770	13.0
'Jr. Swiss Deluxe' 5.8 oz	1 serving	360	765	18.0
'Kids Meal' 4.1 oz	1 serving	300	770	13.0
CHICKEN NUGGET				
crispy, 6 pieces	1 serving	310	660	21.0
crispy, 9 pieces	1 serving	465	990	32.0
crispy, 20 pieces	1 serving	1023	2178	69.0
CHICKEN SANDWICH				
breast, on white bun	1 serving	340	565	12.0
club, 7.2 oz	1 serving	506	930	25.0
fried, 6.9 oz	1 serving	440	725	19.0
grilled, 6.2 oz	1 serving	340	815	13.0
CHILI				
8-oz size	1 serving	190	670	6.0
regular, 9 oz	1 serving	220	750	7.0
12-oz size	1 serving	290	1000	9.0
CHIPS				
cheddar	1 oz	160	445	11.0
taco	1.4 oz	260	20	10.0
CHIVES	1/2 tsp	8	na	tr
CHOW MEIN NOODLES	.5 oz	70	105	4.0
COLESLAW				
'California'	2 tbsp	45	60	3.0
salad bar item	1/4 cup	80	165	5.0
COOKIE, chocolate chip	2.25 oz	275	256	13.0
CORN RELISH, 'Old Fashioned'	1/4 cup	35	215	tr
COTTAGE CHEESE	1/2 cup	110	425	4.0
CRACKER, saltines, 2 pieces	1 pkt	25	80	1.0
CROUTONS	.5 oz	70	105	4.0
CUCUMBER	3 slices	2	na	tr
DANISH				
apple	1 serving	360	380	14.0
cheese	1 serving	430	550	21.0
cinnamon raisin	1 serving	430	550	21.0
EGG, hard-cooked, salad topping	1 tbsp	30	25	2.0
FETTUCCINE	2 oz	190	3	3.0
FISH SANDWICH, fillet, 6 oz	1 serving	460	780	25.0

Food Name	Serv. Size	Total Cal.	Sod. MGS	Fat GMS
FRENCH FRIES				
large order	1 serving	390	176	20.0
regular order	1 serving	300	135	15.0
small order, 3.2 oz	1 serving	240	145	12.0
FROZEN DESSERT				
'Frosty Dairy' large	1 serving	680	374	24.0
'Frosty Dairy' small	1 serving	400	220	14.0
GARLIC TOAST	.6-oz piece	70	65	3.0
GRAPEFRUIT	2 oz	10	0	tr
GRAPES	1/4 cup	30	na	tr
HAMBURGER				
'Big Classic' on Kaiser bun	1 serving	470	900	25.0
double, 'Big Classic' on Kaiser bun	1 serving	680	1005	39.0
double, on white bun	1 serving	560	465	30.0
'Kid's Meal' 3.7 oz	1 serving	260	570	9.0
single, 1/4 lb, on white bun	1 serving	350	360	16.0
single, plain, 4.4 oz	1 serving	340	500	15.0
single, w/everything	1 serving	420	890	21.0
HONEY SAUCE	.5 oz	45	tr	0.0
HONEYDEW MELON	2 pieces	20	5	tr
LETTUCE				
iceberg	1 cup	9	5	tr
romaine	1 cup	9	5	tr
sandwich topping	1 leaf	2	tr	0.0
MARGARINE				
liquid	.5 oz	100	100	11.0
whipped	1 tbsp	70	60	8.0
MAYONNAISE	1 tbsp	90	60	10.0
MILK, 2%	8 oz	110	115	4.0
MUSHROOMS, raw	1/4 cup	4	tr	tr
MUSTARD	1 tsp	4	45	tr
MUSTARD SAUCE, sweet	1 oz	50	140	1.0
ONION				
red, raw	3 rings	2	tr	tr
sandwich topping	3 rings	2	tr	tr
ORANGE	2 oz	25	0	tr
ORANGE JUICE	6 oz	80	na	tr
PASTA AND NOODLES. See also individual listings.				
medley	2 oz	60	5	2.0
PEACH	2 pieces	17	0	tr
PEAS, green	1 oz	25	35	tr

Food Name	Serv. Size	Total Cal.	Sod. MGS	Fat GMS
PEPPER, rings	1 tbsp	2	200	tr
PEPPER, CHERRY, mild	1 tbsp	6	180	tr
PEPPER, GREEN	1/4 cup	3	5	tr
PEPPER, JALAPEÑO	1 slice	9	4	tr
PICANTE SAUCE	2 oz	18	5	<1.0
PICKLE, dill	4 slices	2	tr	tr
PINEAPPLE, chunks	1/2 cup	70	0	tr
POTATO, BAKED				
hot stuffed, w/bacon and cheese	12.8 oz	520	1460	18.0
hot stuffed, w/broccoli and cheese	12.3 oz	400	455	16.0
hot stuffed, w/cheese	11.2 oz	420	310	15.0
hot stuffed, w/chili and cheese	14.2 oz	500	630	18.0
hot stuffed, w/sour cream and chives	11.4 oz	500	135	23.0
plain	8.8 oz	270	20	<1.0
PUDDING				
butterscotch	1/4 cup	90	85	4.0
chocolate	1/4 cup	90	70	4.0
RADISH, raw	.5 oz	2	tr	tr
RAVIOLI, cheese, in sauce	2 oz	45	290	1.0
REFRIED BEANS	2 oz	70	215	3.0
RICE, Spanish	2 oz	70	440	1.0
ROTINI	2 oz	90	tr	2.0
SALAD				
Caesar, side order	1 serving	160	700	6.0
chef's	9.1 oz	130	460	5.0
chef's, 'Take Out' approx 11.7 oz	1 serving	180	140	9.0
chicken, grilled	1 serving	200	690	8.0
garden	8.1 oz	70	60	2.0
garden, deluxe	1 serving	110	380	5.0
garden, 'Take Out' approx 9.8 oz	1 serving	102	110	5.0
pasta	1/4 cup	130	190	6.0
pasta, deli	1/4 cup	35	120	tr
'Pick-Up-Window'	1 serving	110	540	6.0
potato, red bliss	1/4 cup	110	265	9.0
side order	1 serving	60	200	3.0
taco	17.3 oz	530	825	23.0
three bean, deluxe	1/4 cup	60	15	tr
SALAD DRESSING				
bacon and tomato, reduced calorie	1 tbsp	45	190	4.0
blue cheese, 1 ladle = 2 tbsp	1 tbsp	60	85	6.0
celery seed, 1 ladle = 2 tbsp	1 tbsp	70	65	6.0

Food Name	Serv. Size	Total Cal.	Sod. MGS	Fat GMS
creamy cucumber, reduced calorie, 1 ladle = 2 tbsp	1 tbsp	50	140	5.0
French, fat-free, 1/2 pkt = 2 tbsp	2 tbsp	35	180	0.0
French, sweet red	1 tbsp	70	125	6.0
French style, 1 ladle = 2 tbsp	1 tbsp	70	130	5.0
Italian, golden, 1 ladle = 2 tbsp	1 tbsp	50	260	4.0
Italian, reduced calorie	1 tbsp	25	185	2.0
Italian caesar	1 tbsp	80	140	8.0
oil, 1 ladle = 2 tbsp	1 tbsp	120	0	14.0
ranch, Hidden Valley	1 tbsp	50	95	5.0
Thousand Island, 1 ladle = 2 tbsp	1 tbsp	70	115	7.0
Thousand Island, reduced calorie, 1 ladle = 2 tbsp	1 tbsp	45	125	4.0
wine vinegar, 1 ladle = 2 tbsp	1 tbsp	2	5	tr
SOUR CREAM				
	1 oz	60	15	6.0
	2 tsp	20	5	2.0
SOUR CREAM, imitation	1 oz	58	30	5.0
SPAGHETTI SAUCE				
regular	1/4 cup	30	340	<1.0
w/meat	2 oz	60	315	2.0
STEAK SANDWICH, country-fried, 5.1 oz	1 serving	440	870	25.0
STRAWBERRIES	2 oz	18	tr	tr
SUNFLOWER SEEDS, w/raisins	1 oz	140	5	10.0
SWEET AND SOUR SAUCE	1 oz	45	55	<1.0
SYRUP	1 pkt	140	5	tr
TACO MEAT	2 oz	110	300	7.0
TACO SAUCE	1 oz	16	140	<1.0
TACO SHELL	.4 oz	45	45	3.0
TARTAR SAUCE	1 tbsp	80	75	9.0
TOMATO, 1-oz slice	1 slice	6	5	tr
TORTELLINI, cheese, in sauce	2 oz	60	280	1.0
TORTILLA, flour 1.3 oz	1 tortilla	110	220	3.0
TURKEY HAM	1/4 cup	50	na	2.0
WATERMELON	3 pieces	18	tr	tr
WHITE CASTLE				
BREAKFAST SANDWICH				
sausage, 1.7 oz	1 serving	196	488	12.0
sausage and egg, 3.4 oz	1 serving	322	698	22.0
BUN, hamburger, .9 oz	1 bun	74	<1	0.9
CHEESE	.3 oz	31	154	1.6
CHEESEBURGER, 2.3 oz	1 serving	200	361	11.0

Food Name	Serv. Size	Total Cal.	Sod. MGS	Fat GMS
CHICKEN SANDWICH, 2.3 oz	1 serving	186	497	7.0
CHIPS, 3.3 oz	1 serving	329	832	17.0
FISH SANDWICH, w/o tartar sauce, 2.1 oz	1 serving	155	201	5.0
FRENCH FRIES, 3.4 oz	1 serving	301	193	15.0
HAMBURGER, 2.0 oz	1 serving	161	266	8.0
ONION RINGS, 2.1 oz	1 serving	245	566	13.0

Free Software Version of this Book!

The NUTRiBASE Guide to Sodium in Your Food

Congratulations! Your purchase of this book entitles you to a free copy of the software edition of the NutriBase Guide to Sodium in Your Food. Get the best of both worlds–the portability and convenience of hard copy, plus the instant analytical capabilities of the NutriBase Series software.

Your free software will provide you with instant access to all of the information in this book including *Food Names, Comments, Brand Names, Serving Sizes, Total Calories, Sodium mgs,* and *Fat Grams.* Harness the power of your DOS or Windows PC and tap into a wide range of capabilities:

 Comprehensive Data - NutriBase software will provide you with information for every food item in this book–a total of 47,547 food items. The software features over 31,000 brand name foods and thousands of generic food entries.

 View - Click on this software icon to instantly display an alphabetized view of food items in a conventional "spreadsheet view." Your NutriBase software also features over 3,100 menu items from more than 70 restaurants.

 Rank - Instantly rank foods based on their values for any nutrient. For instance, rank all of the Frozen Entrees from low-to-high or high-to-low based on *Calorie, Sodium,* or *Fat* content.

Free Software Version of this Book!

Query - *Instantly* locate all foods that meet *all* the criteria you specify. For instance, display all foods from over 70 restaurants that contain no more than 600 *Calories* and contain no more than 500 mgs of *Sodium*–ranked from low-to high based on *Fat Grams!*

Collect Avery Publishing Group's entire NutriBase Series of books and receive the NutriBase software library free.

How to Get Your Free Software
NutriBase Guide to Sodium in Your Food

1. Fill out this order form (photocopy acceptable).

2. Attach the original register receipt for the <u>NutriBase Guide to Sodium in Your Food</u>.

3. Include a $5.00 check or money order (payable to CyberSoft, Inc.) per copy to cover shipping and handling.

4. Send the three items listed above to:

> CyberSoft, Incorporated
> 3646 E. Ray Rd., # B16-8
> Phoenix AZ 85044-7116

Name: _____

Address: _____

Address: _____

City: _____ State: _____ ZIP: _____

Format preference: Windows _____ DOS _____

Software comes on 3.5" HD media only. Windows version requires Windows 3.1 (or greater), 4 Mbytes of hard disk space, 4 Mbytes of RAM. DOS version requires 4 Mbytes of hard disk space, 640K RAM.

Note: *This free software offer is valid only for the book title purchased. Additional free software titles require the purchase of the corresponding NutriBase Series book titles. NutriBase Series software titles are not available for sale–they are available only as free complements to their hard copy book versions. This offer is subject to expiration without notice.*